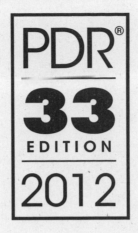

# PDR®

## for Nonprescription Drugs

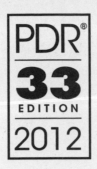

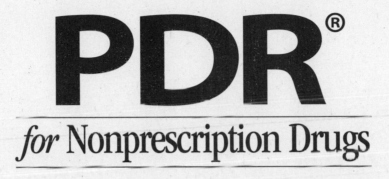

**CEO:** Edward Fotsch, MD

**President:** Richard C. Altus

**Chief Medical Officer:** Steven Merahn, MD

**Chief Technology Officer:** David Cheng

**Chief Financial Officer:** Dawn Carfora

**Senior Vice President, Publishing & Operations:**
Valerie E. Berger

**Senior Vice President, Product Sales, Corporate
Development & General Counsel:** Andrew Gelman

**Senior Vice President, Sales:** John Loucks

**Senior Vice President, Product Management:** Lucian Taylor

**Director of Sales:** Eileen Bruno

**Senior Director, Operations & Client Services:**
Stephanie Struble

**Director, Marketing:** Kim Marich

**Director, Clinical Services:** Sylvia Nashed, PharmD

**Manager, Clinical Services:** Nermin Kerolous, PharmD

**Senior Drug Information Specialist,
Database Management:** Christine Sunwoo, PharmD

**Senior Drug Information Specialist,
Product Development:** Anila Patel, PharmD

**Drug Information Specialists:** Pauline Lee, PharmD;
Peter Leighton, PharmD; Kristine Mecca, PharmD

**Clinical Editor:** Julia Tonelli, MD

**Managing Editor:** J. Harris Fleming, Jr.

**Manager, Art Department:** Livio Udina

**Senior Director, Content Operations:** Jeffrey D. Schaefer

**Associate Director, Manufacturing & Distribution:**
Thomas Westburgh

**Associate Manager, Fulfillment:** Gary Lew

**Web Operations and Customer Service Manager:**
Lee Reynolds

ISBN: 978-1-56363-797-1

# FOREWORD TO THE 33RD EDITION

## PDR Network, LLC

As the nation's leading distributor of drug labeling information, product safety alerts, and pharmaceutical Risk Evaluation and Mitigation Strategy (REMS) programs, PDR Network is committed to ensuring that prescribers have access to the right information at the point of prescribing. PDR Network includes *Physicians' Desk Reference®* ("*PDR®*"), the most highly trusted and commonly used drug information reference available in the U.S.; PDR.net®, the online home of *PDR*; *mobile*PDR®; and PDR Drug Alerts, the only specialty-specific service that provides electronic delivery of FDA-approved Drug Alerts to physicians and other healthcare professionals.

By improving communication of important medication information and FDA-approved Drug Alerts, PDR Network's unique services enhance patient safety and may help to reduce medical liability. For more information or to sign up for electronic PDR® Drug Alerts, visit **PDR.net**.

## About This Book

*PDR® for Nonprescription Drugs* (NPD) is the premier source for drug facts information on the most commonly used over-the-counter medications. These include analgesics, cough and cold preparations, fever reducers, and more. With a new design and name, the 2012 *NPD* offers physicians, residents, and medical students invaluable, easily accessible content.

Formatted similarly to the *PDR*, *NPD* is an invaluable source of information regarding OTC drugs, including manufacturer name, product name, indications and usage, drug warnings, and adverse reactions. In addition, *NPD* also contains comparison tables for quick, at-a-glance dosing, and ingredient information.

*PDR for Nonprescription Drugs* is published annually by PDR Network, LLC. In organizing and presenting the material in *PDR for Nonprescription Drugs*, the Publisher does not warrant or guarantee any of the products described, or perform any independent analysis in connection with any of the product information contained herein. The Publisher does not assume, and expressly disclaims, any obligation to obtain and include any information other than that provided to it by the manufacturers. It should be understood that by making this material available, the Publisher is not advocating the use of any product described herein, nor is the Publisher responsible for the use of any product, or the misuse of any product, due to content or typographical error. Additional information on any product may be obtained from the manufacturer.

## Other Resources from *PDR*

*PDR® for Nonprescription Drugs* enters its 33rd year as part of the products and services of **PDR Network, LLC**, the leading distributor of medical product labeling, FDA-approved Drug Alerts, and REMS program communications. PDR Network includes:

- **Physicians' Desk Reference® (PDR®)**, the most trusted and commonly used drug information reference. To ensure that clinicians have the most current available information at their fingertips, *PDR* also provides:

  - **PDR Update Insert Cards**, a quick reference designed to make prescribers aware of labeling changes, including newly approved labeling, that have occurred since the publication of *PDR*. Mailed every other month, each card lists changes that have occurred in the past 60 days. These updates and the full product information can be viewed at **PDR.net/updates**.

  - **PDR eDrug Updates**, a monthly electronic newsletter that provides specialty-specific drug information including FDA alerts, new drug approvals, and labeling changes that have occurred in the past 30 days. To sign up for this free e-newsletter, send an email to customerservice@pdr.net.

- **PDR.net®**, the online home of *PDR* with weekly updates to FDA-approved full product labeling, manufacturer-supplied product information, and concise drug information based on FDA-approved labeling. Prescribers can earn free Continuing Medical Education (CME) credits for reading product labels and PDR Drug Alerts, as viewed on **PDR.net**.

- **PDR® Drug Alerts** are delivered electronically to physicians and other prescribers who register to receive them at PDR.net, through participating medical societies, or by returning the verification form distributed with complimentary copies of *PDR*. By ensuring that this service is used exclusively for the rapid delivery of PDR Drug Alerts—not advertising or marketing—PDR Network fulfills FDA guidance for electronic delivery of alerts, improves patient safety, and may help reduce liability.

- **RxEvent Adverse Drug Event Reporting System** simplifies previous methods of adverse drug event reporting that have been complicated and inefficient, limiting the number of adverse drug event reports submitted each year. Using RxEvent—a new, web- and EHR based reporting service by PDR Network—reporting adverse drug events is quick and convenient. RxEvent empowers healthcare professionals to contribute significantly toward increasing drug safety by making the reporting process more efficient. For more information, visit **RxEvent.org**.

- **mobilePDR®** provides the only single source for FDA-approved full product labeling and concise point-of-care information from *PDR* directly on your mobile device. Information on over 2,400 drugs, full-color product images, and weekly updates provide up-to-date drug information. *mobile*PDR is free for U.S.-based MDs, DOs, NPs, and PAs in full-time patient practice and can be downloaded at **PDR.net**.

- A wide range of prescribing references and clinical decision publications including the 2012 *PDR® for Ophthalmic Medicines* and 2012 *PDR® Nurse's Drug Handbook*. For more information, a complete list of titles, or to order, visit **PDRBooks.com**.

- For more information on these or any other members of the growing family of *PDR* products, please call, toll-free, 800-232-7379; fax 201-722-2680; or visit **PDRBooks.com**.

For more information about licensing PDR Network content, please contact Andrew Gelman at 201-358-7540 or andrew.gelman@pdr.net.

# CONTENTS

# HOW TO USE THIS BOOK

The 2012 edition of *PDR® for Nonprescription Drugs* features a format designed to help you find the information you need as quickly and easily as possible. In addition to consulting the index, you can go directly to a specific product comparison table to find the relevant over-the-counter (OTC) products for a particular condition.

The **Product Name Index** provides the page number of each product description in the Nonprescription Drug Information section. Listings appear alphabetically by brand name.

### NONPRESCRIPTION DRUG INFORMATION
**Organized alphabetically by product name.** The product labeling in this section includes brand-name OTC products marketed for home use. **Please keep in mind that the product information included herein is valid as of press time (October 2011).** Additional information, as well as updates to the product labeling, can be obtained from the manufacturer.

### PRODUCT COMPARISON TABLES
**Organized alphabetically by therapeutic category or condition and brand name.** These tables provide a quick and easy way to compare the active ingredients and dosages of common brand-name OTC drugs.

# NONPRESCRIPTION DRUG INFORMATION

This section presents information on nonprescription products marketed for home use by consumers.

The descriptions of over-the-counter products in this section reflect the manufacturers' Drug Facts, as included in the product labeling provided to consumers. Those descriptions are designed to provide the information necessary for informed use by consumers, including, when applicable, active ingredients, uses (indications), specific warnings (including when a product should not be used under any circumstances, when it is appropriate to consult a doctor or pharmacist, side effects that could occur, and substances or activities to avoid), dosage instructions, and inactive ingredients.

The function of the Publisher is solely the compilation, organization, and distribution of this information. The descriptions seen here include all information made available by the manufacturer. The Publisher does not warrant or guarantee any product described herein, and does not perform any independent analysis of the information provided. Inclusion of a product in this book does not represent an endorsement, and the Publisher does not advocate the use of any product listed.

## 4 WAY FAST ACTING (phenylephrine hydrochloride) spray

Novartis Consumer Health, Inc.

### DRUG FACTS

| Active ingredient | Purpose |
|---|---|
| Phenylephrine hydrochloride | Nasal decongestant |

### USES
- temporarily relieves nasal congestion due to:
  - common cold
  - hay fever
  - upper respiratory allergies

### WARNINGS

#### ASK DOCTOR BEFORE USE IF YOU HAVE
- heart disease
- high blood pressure
- thyroid disease
- diabetes
- trouble urinating due to an enlarged prostate gland

#### WHEN USING THIS PRODUCT
- do not use more than directed
- do not use more than 3 days
- use only as directed
- frequent or prolonged use may cause nasal congestion to recur or worsen
- temporary discomfort such as burning, stinging, sneezing, or an increase in nasal discharge may occur
- infection may spread if this container is used by more than one person

#### STOP USE AND ASK A DOCTOR IF
- symptoms persist

**Pregnancy or breastfeeding,** ask a health professional before use.

**Keep out of reach of children.** If swallowed, get medical help or contact a Poison Control Center right away.

### DIRECTIONS

| adults and children 12 years of age and over | 2 or 3 sprays in each nostril not more often than every 4 hours |
|---|---|
| children under 12 years of age | ask a doctor |

### OTHER INFORMATION
- store at controlled room temperature 20-25°C (68-77°F)
- container is filled to proper level for best spray action

### INACTIVE INGREDIENTS
benzalkonium chloride, boric acid, sodium borate, water

### QUESTIONS OR COMMENTS
Call **1-800-452-0051**

---

## 4 WAY MOISTURIZING RELIEF (xylometazoline hydrochloride) nasal spray

Novartis Consumer Health, Inc.

### DRUG FACTS

| Active ingredient | Purpose |
|---|---|
| Xylometazoline hydrochloride | Nasal decongestant |

### USES
- temporarily relieves nasal congestion due to:
  - a cold
  - hay fever
  - upper respiratory allergies
- soothes nasal discomfort caused by dryness

### WARNINGS

#### ASK DOCTOR BEFORE USE IF YOU HAVE
- heart disease
- high blood pressure
- thyroid disease
- diabetes
- trouble urinating due to an enlarged prostate gland

#### WHEN USING THIS PRODUCT
- do not use more than directed
- do not use more than 3 days
- use only as directed
- frequent or prolonged use may cause nasal congestion to recur or worsen
- temporary discomfort such as burning, stinging, sneezing, or an increase in nasal discharge may occur
- infection may spread if this container is used by more than one person

#### STOP USE AND ASK A DOCTOR IF
- symptoms persist

**Pregnancy or breast feeding,** ask a health professional before use.

**Keep out of reach of children.** If swallowed, get medical help or contact a Poison Control Center right away.

### DIRECTIONS

| adults and children 12 years of age and over | 2 or 3 sprays in each nostril not more often than every 8 to 10 hours do not use more than 3 doses in 24 hours |
|---|---|
| children under 12 years of age | ask a doctor |

### OTHER INFORMATION
- store at controlled room temperature 20-25°C (68-77°F)
- container is filled to proper level for best spray action
- non-USP for assay

### INACTIVE INGREDIENTS
benzalkonium chloride, dibasic sodium phosphate, edetate disodium, hypromellose, monobasic sodium phosphate, purified water, sodium chloride, sorbitol solution

### QUESTIONS OR COMMENTS
Call **1-800-452-0051**

---

## A AND D ORIGINAL (lanolin and petrolatum) ointment

MSD Consumer Care, Inc.

### DRUG FACTS

| Active ingredients | Purpose |
|---|---|
| Lanolin 15.5% | Diaper rash ointment |
| Petrolatum 53.4% | Skin protectant |

## USES
- helps treat and prevent diaper rash
- temporarily protects minor:
  - cuts
  - scrapes
  - burns
- temporarily protects and helps relieve chapped, chafed or cracked skin and lips
- protect chafed skin due to diaper rash and helps seal out wetness

## WARNINGS
**For external use only.**

## DO NOT USE ON
- deep or puncture wounds
- animal bites
- serious burns

## WHEN USING THIS PRODUCT
- do not get into eyes

## STOP USE AND ASK A DOCTOR IF
- condition worsens
- symptoms last more than 7 days or clear up and occur again within a few days

**Keep out of reach of children.** If swallowed, get medical help or contact a Poison Control Center right away.

## DIRECTIONS
- for skin protectant use apply as needed
- for diaper rash use:
  - change wet and soiled diapers promptly
  - cleanse the diaper area, and allow to dry
  - apply ointment liberally as often as necessary, with each diaper change, especially at bedtime or anytime when exposure to wet diapers may be prolonged

## OTHER INFORMATION
- store between 20°-25°C ( 68°-77°F)
- store upright when not in use

## INACTIVE INGREDIENTS
cod liver oil (contains vitamin A & vitamin D), fragrance, light mineral oil, microcrystalline wax, paraffin

## ABREVA (docosanol) cream
GlaxoSmithKline Consumer Healthcare LP

## DRUG FACTS

| Active ingredient | Purpose |
|---|---|
| Docosanol 10% | Cold sore/fever blister treatment |

## USES
- treats cold sores/fever blisters on the face or lips
- shortens healing time and duration of symptoms:
  - tingling, pain, burning, and/or itching

## WARNINGS
**For external use only.**

## DO NOT USE
- if you are allergic to any ingredient in this product

## WHEN USING THIS PRODUCT
- apply only to affected areas

- do not use in or near the eyes
- avoid applying directly inside your mouth
- do not share this product with anyone. This may spread infection

## STOP USE AND ASK A DOCTOR IF
- your cold sore gets worse or the cold sore is not healed within 10 days

**Keep out of reach of children.** If swallowed, get medical help or contact a Poison Control Center right away.

## DIRECTIONS

| adults and children 12 years or over | wash hands before and after applying cream |
| | apply to affected area on face or lips at the first sign of cold sore/ fever blister |
| | early treatment ensures the best results |
| | rub in gently but completely |
| | use 5 times a day until healed |
| children under 12 years | ask a doctor |

## OTHER INFORMATION
- store at 20-25°C (68-77°F)
- do not freeze

## INACTIVE INGREDIENTS
benzyl alcohol, light mineral oil, propylene glycol, purified water, sucrose distearate, sucrose stearate

## QUESTIONS OR COMMENTS
Call toll-free **1-877-709-3539** (English/Spanish) weekdays visit us at www.abreva.com

## ACTIFED COLD & ALLERGY TABLETS
(chlorpheniramine maleate and phenylephrine hydrochloride)
Pfizer Consumer Healthcare

## DRUG FACTS

| Active ingredients (in each tablet) | Purpose |
|---|---|
| Chlorpheniramine maleate 4 mg | Antihistamine |
| Phenylephrine hydrochloride 10 mg | Nasal decongestant |

## USES
- temporarily relieves these symptoms due to hay fever (allergic rhinitis) or other upper respiratory allergies:
  - runny nose
  - sneezing
  - itchy, watery eyes
  - nasal congestion
  - itching of the nose or throat
- temporarily relieves these symptoms due to the common cold:
  - runny nose
  - sneezing
  - nasal congestion

## WARNINGS

## DO NOT USE
- if you are now taking a prescription monoamine oxidase inhibitor (MAOI) (certain drugs for depression, psychiatric, or

emotional conditions, or Parkinson's disease), or for 2 weeks after stopping the MAOI drug
- if you do not know if your prescription drug contains an MAOI, ask a doctor or pharmacist before taking this product

**ASK A DOCTOR BEFORE USE IF YOU HAVE**
- heart disease
- high blood pressure
- thyroid disease
- diabetes
- trouble urinating due to an enlarged prostate gland
- a breathing problem such as emphysema or chronic bronchitis
- glaucoma

**ASK A DOCTOR OR PHARMACIST BEFORE USE IF YOU ARE**
- taking sedatives or tranquilizers

**WHEN USING THIS PRODUCT**
- do not exceed recommended dose
- excitability may occur, especially in children
- drowsiness may occur
- alcohol, sedatives, and tranquilizers may increase drowsiness
- avoid alcoholic drinks
- be careful when driving a motor vehicle or operating machinery

**STOP USE AND ASK A DOCTOR IF**
- nervousness, dizziness, or sleeplessness occur
- symptoms do not improve within 7 days or occur with fever

**If pregnant or breastfeeding,** ask a health professional before use.

**Keep out of reach of children.** In case of overdose, get medical help or contact a Poison Control Center right away. (1-800-222-1222)

**DIRECTIONS**

| adults and children 12 years and over | take 1 tablet every 4 hours |
| | do not take more than 6 tablets in 24 hours |
| children under 12 years | do not use this product |

**OTHER INFORMATION**
- store between 20-25°C (68-77°F)

**INACTIVE INGREDIENTS**
carnauba wax, corn starch, magnesium stearate, microcrystalline cellulose, polyethylene glycol, polyvinyl alcohol, powdered cellulose, pregelatinized starch, sodium starch glycolate, talc, titanium dioxide

**QUESTIONS OR COMMENTS**
Call 1-800-524-2624

---

# ACTIVON ULTRA STRENGTH JOINT AND MUSCLE (menthol) stick

Family First Pharmaceuticals, Inc.

## DRUG FACTS

| Active ingredient | Purpose |
|---|---|
| Menthol 5.138% | Topical analgesic |

**USES**
- For the temporary relief of minor aches and pains of muscles and joints associated with:
  - simple backache
  - arthritis
  - strains
  - bruises
  - sprains

**WARNINGS**
**For external use only.**

**DO NOT USE**
- otherwise than as directed
- if you are allergic to any ingredient in this product
- on a child under 12 years of age with arthritis-like conditions
- with a heating pad

**WHEN USING THIS PRODUCT**
- avoid contact with eyes, wounds, mucous membranes, broken or irritated skin
- do not share this product with anyone
- do not bandage tightly

**STOP USE AND ASK A DOCTOR IF**
- condition worsens, or if symptoms persist for more than 7 days or clear up and occur again within a few days
- skin redness or excessive irritation of the skin develops

**If pregnant or breastfeeding,** ask a health professional before use.

**Keep out of the reach of children.** If swallowed, get medical help or contact a Poison Control Center right away.

**DIRECTIONS**

| adults and children 12 years of age and older | apply to affected area not more than 3 to 4 times daily |
| children under 12 years of age | ask a doctor |

**OTHER INFORMATION**
- keep away from heat
- store between 15°C-30°C (59°F-86°F)

**INACTIVE INGREDIENTS**
diazolidinyl urea, ethyl alcohol, iodopropynyl butylcarbamate, menthyl lactate, propylene glycol, sodium stearate, steareth-21, tetrasodium EDTA, triethanolamine, water

**QUESTIONS OR COMMENTS**
Call **1-800-379-8870**, Weekdays 9 AM to 5PM EST or visit us online at activ-on.com

---

# ADVANCED EYE RELIEF/DRY EYE/ ENVIRONMENTAL LUBRICANT (glycerin)
solution/ drops

Bausch & Lomb Incorporated

## DRUG FACTS

| Active ingredient | Purpose |
|---|---|
| Glycerin (1.0%) | Lubricant |

**USES**
- relieves dryness of the eye
- prevents further irritation

## WARNINGS

**DO NOT USE**
- if solution changes color or becomes cloudy

**WHEN USING THIS PRODUCT**
- do not touch tip of container to any surface to avoid contamination
- remove contact lenses before using
- replace cap after use

**STOP USE AND ASK A DOCTOR IF**
- you experience eye pain, changes in vision, continued redness or irritation of the eye
- condition worsens or persists for more than 72 hours

**Keep out of reach of children.** If swallowed, get medical help or contact a Poison Control Center right away.

**DIRECTIONS**
- instill 1 or 2 drops in the affected eye(s) as needed

**OTHER INFORMATION**
- store at 15-30°C (59-86°F)
- keep tightly closed
- use before expiration date marked on the carton and bottle

**INACTIVE INGREDIENTS**
benzalkonium chloride (0.01%) boric acid, edetate disodium, potassium chloride, purified water, sodium borate, sodium chloride. Hydrochloric acid and/or sodium hydroxide may be used to adjust pH

**QUESTIONS OR COMMENTS**
Toll-free product information or to report a serious side effect associated with use of this product
Call: **1-800-553-5340**

## ADVANCED EYE RELIEF/DRY EYE/ REJUVENATION LUBRICANT (propylene glycol) solution/drops

Bausch & Lomb Incorporated

### DRUG FACTS

| Active ingredient | Purpose |
|---|---|
| Propylene glycol (0.95%) | Lubricant |

**USES**
- temporary relief of burning and irritation due to dryness of the eye
- prevents further irritation

**WARNINGS**

**DO NOT USE**
- if solution changes color or becomes cloudy
- if single-use dispenser is not intact

**WHEN USING THIS PRODUCT**
- do not touch tip of container to any surface to avoid contamination
- do not reuse
- once applied, discard

**STOP USE AND ASK A DOCTOR IF**
- you experience eye pain, changes in vision, continued redness or irritation of the eye
- condition worsens or persists for more than 72 hours

**Keep out of reach of children.** If swallowed, get medical help or contact a Poison Control Center right away.

**DIRECTIONS**
- to open, completely twist off tab
- squeeze 1 to 2 drops in the affected eye(s) as needed
- throw away dispenser immediately after use
- do not reuse

**OTHER INFORMATION**
- store at 15-30°C (59-86°F)
- keep tightly closed
- use before expiration date on dispenser

**INACTIVE INGREDIENTS**
boric acid, edetate disodium, potassium chloride, purified water, sodium borate, sodium chloride, hydrochloric acid and/or sodium hydroxide may be used to adjust pH

**QUESTIONS OR COMMENTS**
Toll-free product information or to report a serious side effect associated with use of this product call: **1-800-553-5340**

## ADVANCED EYE RELIEF/REDNESS INSTANT RELIEF (naphazoline hydrochloride and polyethylene glycol 300) solution/drops

Bausch & Lomb Incorporated

### DRUG FACTS

| Active ingredients | Purpose |
|---|---|
| Naphazoline hydrochloride (0.012%) | Redness reliever |
| Polyethylene glycol 300 (0.2%) | Lubricant |

**USES**
- relieves redness of the eye due to minor eye irritations
- temporary relief of burning and irritation due to dryness of the eye
- protects against further irritation

**WARNINGS**

**DO NOT USE**
- if solution changes color or becomes cloudy

**ASK A DOCTOR BEFORE USE IF YOU HAVE**
- narrow angle glaucoma

**WHEN USING THIS PRODUCT**
- do not touch tip of container to any surface to avoid contamination
- do not overuse as it may produce increased redness of the eye
- pupils may become enlarged temporarily
- remove contact lenses before using
- replace cap after use

**STOP USE AND ASK A DOCTOR IF**
- you experience eye pain, changes in vision, continued redness or irritation of the eye
- condition worsens or persists for more than 72 hours

**Keep out of reach of children.** If swallowed, get medical help or contact a Poison Control Center right away.

**DIRECTIONS**
- instill 1 to 2 drops in the affected eye(s) up to four times daily

## OTHER INFORMATION
- store at 15-25°C (59-77°F)
- keep tightly closed
- use before expiration date marked on the carton and bottle

## INACTIVE INGREDIENTS
benzalkonium chloride (0.01%), boric acid, edetate disodium, sodium borate, sodium chloride

## QUESTIONS OR COMMENTS
Toll-free product information or to report a serious side effect associated with use of this product call: **1-800-553-5340**

---

# ADVANCED EYE RELIEF/REDNESS MAXIMUM RELIEF (naphazoline hydrochloride and hypromellose) solution/drops
Bausch & Lomb Incorporated

## DRUG FACTS

| Active ingredients | Purpose |
|---|---|
| Hypromellose (0.5%) | Lubricant |
| Naphazoline hydrochloride (0.03%) | Redness reliever |

## USES
- temporary relief of redness and discomfort due to:
  - minor eye irritations
  - exposure to wind or sun
  - dryness of the eye
- prevents further irritation

## WARNINGS

### DO NOT USE
- if solution changes color or becomes cloudy

### ASK A DOCTOR BEFORE USE IF YOU HAVE
- narrow angle glaucoma

### WHEN USING THIS PRODUCT
- do not touch tip of container to any surface to avoid contamination
- do not overuse as it may produce increased redness of the eye
- pupils may become enlarged temporarily
- remove contact lenses before using
- replace cap after use

### STOP USE AND ASK A DOCTOR IF
- you experience eye pain, changes in vision, continued redness or irritation of the eye
- condition worsens or persists for more than 72 hours

**Keep out of reach of children.** If swallowed, get medical help or contact a Poison Control Center right away.

## DIRECTIONS
- instill 1 to 2 drops in the affected eye(s) up to four times daily

## OTHER INFORMATION
- store at 15-25°C (59-77°F)
- keep tightly closed
- use before expiration date marked on the carton and bottle

## INACTIVE INGREDIENTS
benzalkonium chloride (0.01%), boric acid, edetate disodium, purified water, sodium borate, sodium chloride, hydrochloric acid and/or sodium hydroxide may be used to adjust pH

## QUESTIONS OR COMMENTS
Toll-free product information or to report a serious side effect associated with use of this product call: **1-800-553-5340**

---

# ADVIL (ibuprofen) capsule, liquid filled
Pfizer Consumer Healthcare

## DRUG FACTS

| Active ingredient (in each capsule) | Purpose |
|---|---|
| Solubilized ibuprofen equal to 200 mg ibuprofen (NSAID)* (present as the free acid and potassium salt) | Pain reliever/fever reducer |

*nonsteroidal anti-inflammatory drug

## USES
- temporarily relieves minor aches and pains due to:
  - headache
  - toothache
  - backache
  - menstrual cramps
  - the common cold
  - muscular aches
  - minor pain of arthritis
- temporarily reduces fever

## WARNINGS
### Allergy alert
Ibuprofen may cause a severe allergic reaction, especially in people allergic to aspirin. Symptoms may include:

- hives
- facial swelling
- asthma (wheezing)
- shock
- skin reddening
- rash
- blisters

If an allergic reaction occurs, stop use and seek medical help right away.

### Stomach bleeding warning
This product contains an NSAID, which may cause severe stomach bleeding. The chance is higher if you:
- are age 60 or older
- have had stomach ulcers or bleeding problems
- take a blood thinning (anticoagulant) or steroid drug
- take other drugs containing prescription or nonprescription NSAIDs [aspirin, ibuprofen, naproxen, or others]
- have 3 or more alcoholic drinks every day while using this product
- take more or for a longer time than directed

### DO NOT USE
- if you have ever had an allergic reaction to any other pain reliever/fever reducer
- right before or after heart surgery

### ASK A DOCTOR BEFORE USE IF
- stomach bleeding warning applies to you
- you have problems or serious side effects from taking pain relievers or fever reducers
- you have a history of stomach problems, such as heartburn
- you have high blood pressure, heart disease, liver cirrhosis, kidney disease, or asthma
- you are taking a diuretic

## ASK A DOCTOR OR PHARMACIST BEFORE USE IF YOU ARE
- under a doctor's care for any serious condition
- taking aspirin for heart attack or stroke, because ibuprofen may decrease this benefit of aspirin
- taking any other drug

## WHEN USING THIS PRODUCT
- take with food or milk if stomach upset occurs
- the risk of heart attack or stroke may increase if you use more than directed or for longer than directed

## STOP USE AND ASK A DOCTOR IF
- you experience any of the following signs of stomach bleeding
  - feel faint
  - vomit blood
  - have bloody or black stools
  - have stomach pain that does not get better
- pain gets worse or lasts more than 10 days
- fever gets worse or lasts more than 3 days
- redness or swelling is present in the painful area
- any new symptoms appear

**If pregnant or breastfeeding,** ask a health professional before use.

**It is especially important not to use ibuprofen during the last 3 months of pregnancy unless definitely directed to do so by a doctor because it may cause problems in the unborn child or complications during delivery.**

**Keep out of reach of children.** In case of overdose, get medical help or contact a Poison Control Center right away.

## DIRECTIONS
- do not take more than directed
- the smallest effective dose should be used

| adults and children 12 years and over | take 1 capsule every 4 to 6 hours while symptoms persist |
| --- | --- |
| | if pain or fever does not respond to 1 capsule, 2 capsules may be used |
| | do not exceed 6 capsules in 24 hours, unless directed by a doctor |
| children under 12 years | ask a doctor |

## OTHER INFORMATION
- each capsule contains: potassium 20 mg
- read all warnings and directions before use. Keep carton
- store at 20-25°C (68-77°F)
- avoid excessive heat above 40°C (104°F)

## INACTIVE INGREDIENTS
FD&C green no. 3, gelatin, light mineral oil, pharmaceutical ink, polyethylene glycol, potassium hydroxide, purified water, sorbitan, sorbitol

## QUESTIONS OR COMMENTS
Call toll-free **1-800-88-ADVIL**

# CHILDREN'S ADVIL (ibuprofen) suspension
Pfizer Consumer Healthcare

## DRUG FACTS

| Active ingredient (in each 5 ml) | Purpose |
| --- | --- |
| Ibuprofen 100 mg (NSAID)* | Fever reducer/pain reliever |

*nonsteroidal anti-inflammatory drug

## USES
- temporarily:
  - reduces fever
  - relieves minor aches and pains due to the common cold, flu, sore throat, headaches and toothaches

## WARNINGS
**Allergy alert**
Ibuprofen may cause a severe allergic reaction, especially in people allergic to aspirin. Symptoms may include:

- hives
- facial swelling
- asthma (wheezing)
- shock
- skin reddening
- rash
- blisters

If an allergic reaction occurs, stop use and seek medical help right away.

**Stomach bleeding warning**
This product contains an NSAID, which may cause severe stomach bleeding. The chance is higher if the child

- has had stomach ulcers or bleeding problems
- takes a blood thinning (anticoagulant) or steroid drug
- takes other drugs containing prescription or nonprescription NSAIDs [aspirin, ibuprofen, naproxen, or others]
- takes more or for a longer time than directed

**Sore throat warning**
Severe or persistent sore throat or sore throat accompanied by high fever, headache, nausea, and vomiting may be serious. Consult doctor promptly. Do not use more than 2 days or administer to children under 3 years of age unless directed by doctor.

## DO NOT USE
- if the child has ever had an allergic reaction to any other pain reliever/fever reducer
- right before or after heart surgery

## ASK A DOCTOR BEFORE USE IF
- stomach bleeding warning applies to the child
- child has problems or serious side effects from taking pain relievers or fever reducers
- child has a history of stomach problems, such as heartburn
- child has high blood pressure, heart disease, liver cirrhosis, kidney disease, or asthma
- child has not been drinking fluids
- child has lost a lot of fluid due to vomiting or diarrhea
- child is taking a diuretic

## ASK A DOCTOR OR PHARMACIST BEFORE USE IF THE CHILD IS
- under a doctor's care for any serious condition
- taking any other drug

**WHEN USING THIS PRODUCT**
- take with food or milk if stomach upset occurs
- the risk of heart attack or stroke may increase if you use more than directed or for longer than directed

**STOP USE AND ASK A DOCTOR IF**
- child experiences any of the following signs of stomach bleeding:
  - feels faint
  - vomits blood
  - has bloody or black stools
  - has stomach pain that does not get better
- the child does not get any relief within first day (24 hours) of treatment
- fever or pain gets worse or lasts more than 3 days
- redness or swelling is present in the painful area
- any new symptoms appear

**Keep out of reach of children.** In case of overdose, get medical help or contact a Poison Control Center right away.

**DIRECTIONS**
- this product does not contain directions or complete warnings for adult use
- do not give more than directed
- shake well before using
- find right dose on chart below. If possible, use weight to dose; otherwise use age
- repeat dose every 6-8 hours, if needed
- do not use more than 4 times a day
- measure only with the dosing cup provided. Dosing cup to be used with Children's Advil Suspension only. Do not use with other products. Dose lines account for product remaining in cup due to thickness of suspension

### Dosing Chart

| Weight (lb) | Age (yr) | Dose (tsp) |
|---|---|---|
| under 24 lb | under 2 yr | ask a doctor |
| 24-35 lb | 2-3 yr | 1 tsp |
| 36-47 lb | 4-5 yr | 1½ tsp |
| 48-59 lb | 6-8 yr | 2 tsp |
| 60-71 lb | 9-10 yr | 2½ tsp |
| 72-95 lb | 11 yr | 3 tsp |

**OTHER INFORMATION**
- Children's Advil Suspension Fruit Flavor; Children's Advil Suspension Grape Flavor
  - each teaspoon contains: sodium 3 mg
  - one dose lasts 6-8 hours
  - store at 20-25°C (68-77°F)
  - see bottom of box for lot number and expiration date
- Children's Advil Suspension Blue Raspberry Flavor
  - each teaspoon contains: sodium 10 mg
  - one dose lasts 6-8 hours
  - store at 20-25°C (68-77°F)
  - see bottom of box for lot number and expiration date

**INACTIVE INGREDIENTS**
**Children's Advil Suspension Fruit Flavor**
artificial flavors, carboxymethylcellulose sodium, citric acid monohydrate, edetate disodium, FD&C red no. 40, glycerin, microcrystalline cellulose, polysorbate 80, purified water, sodium benzoate, sorbitol solution, sucrose, xanthan gum

**Children's Advil Suspension Grape Flavor**
acetic acid, artificial flavor, butylated hydroxytoluene, carboxymethylcellulose sodium, citric acid monohydrate, edetate disodium, FD&C blue no.1, FD&C red no. 40, glycerin, microcrystalline cellulose, polysorbate 80, propylene glycol, purified water, sodium benzoate, sorbitol solution, sucrose, xanthan gum

**Children's Advil Suspension Blue Raspberry Flavor**
artificial and natural flavors, carboxymethylcellulose sodium, citric acid monohydrate, edetate disodium, FD&C blue no. 1, glycerin, microcrystalline cellulose, polysorbate 80, propylene glycol, purified water, sodium benzoate, sodium citrate, sorbitol solution, sucrose, xanthan gum

**QUESTIONS OR COMMENTS**
Call toll-free **1-800-88-ADVIL** or ask your pharmacist, doctor or health care professional

# JUNIOR STRENGTH ADVIL (ibuprofen) tablet, chewable
## Pfizer Consumer Healthcare

### DRUG FACTS

| Active ingredient (in each tablet) | Purpose |
|---|---|
| Ibuprofen 100 mg (NSAID)* | Fever reducer/pain reliever |

*nonsteroidal anti-inflammatory drug

**USES**
- temporarily.
  - reduces fever
  - relieves minor aches and pains due to the common cold, flu, sore throat, headaches and toothaches

**WARNINGS**
**Allergy alert**
Ibuprofen may cause a severe allergic reaction, especially in people allergic to aspirin. Symptoms may include:

- hives
- facial swelling
- asthma (wheezing)
- shock
- skin reddening
- rash
- blisters

If an allergic reaction occurs, stop use and seek medical help right away.

**Stomach bleeding warning**
This product contains an NSAID, which may cause severe stomach bleeding. The chance is higher if the child:

- has had stomach ulcers or bleeding problems
- takes a blood thinning (anticoagulant) or steroid drug
- takes other drugs containing prescription or nonprescription NSAIDs [aspirin, ibuprofen, naproxen, or others]
- takes more or for a longer time than directed

**Sore throat warning**
Severe or persistent sore throat or sore throat accompanied by high fever, headache, nausea, and vomiting may be serious. Consult doctor promptly. Do not use more than 2 days or administer to children under 3 years of age unless directed by doctor.

**DO NOT USE**
- if the child has ever had an allergic reaction to any other pain reliever/fever reducer
- right before or after heart surgery

## ASK A DOCTOR BEFORE USE IF

- stomach bleeding warning applies to the child
- child has problems or serious side effects from taking pain relievers or fever reducers
- child has a history of stomach problems, such as heartburn
- child has high blood pressure, heart disease, liver cirrhosis, kidney disease, or asthma
- child has not been drinking fluids
- child has lost a lot of fluid due to vomiting or diarrhea
- child is taking a diuretic

## ASK A DOCTOR OR PHARMACIST BEFORE USE IF THE CHILD IS

- under a doctor's care for any serious condition
- taking any other drug

## WHEN USING THIS PRODUCT

- take with food or milk if stomach upset occurs
- the risk of heart attack or stroke may increase if you use more than directed or for longer than directed

## STOP USE AND ASK A DOCTOR IF

- child experiences any of the following signs of stomach bleeding:
  - feels faint
  - vomits blood
  - has bloody or black stools
  - has stomach pain that does not get better
- child does not get any relief within first day (24 hours) of treatment
- fever or pain gets worse or lasts more than 3 days
- redness or swelling is present in the painful area
- any new symptoms appear

**Keep out of reach of children.** In case of overdose, get medical help or contact a Poison Control Center right away.

## DIRECTIONS

- this product does not contain directions or complete warnings for adult use
- do not give more than directed
- find right dose on chart below. If possible, use weight to dose; otherwise use age
- repeat dose every 6-8 hours, if needed
- do not use more than 4 times a day

### Dosing Chart

| Weight (lb) | Age (yr) | Dose (tablets) |
|---|---|---|
| under 48 lb | under 6 yr | ask a doctor |
| 48-59 lb | 6-8 yr | 2 tablets |
| 60-71 lb | 9-10 yr | 2 ½ tablets |
| 72-95 lb | 11 yr | 3 tablets |

## OTHER INFORMATION

- **Phenylketonurics:** contains phenylalanine 4.2 mg per tablet
- one dose lasts 6-8 hours store
- store at 20-25°C (68-77°F)
- see side of box for lot number and expiration date

## INACTIVE INGREDIENTS

aspartame, cellacefate, colloidal silicon dioxide, D&C red no. 30 aluminum lake, FD&C blue no. 2 aluminum lake, gelatin, magnesium stearate, mannitol, microcrystalline cellulose, natural and artificial flavors, sodium starch glycolate

## QUESTIONS OR COMMENTS

Call toll-free **1-800-88-ADVIL** or ask your pharmacist, doctor or health care professional

## ADVIL ALLERGY SINUS (chlorpheniramine maleate, ibuprofen, and pseudoephedrine hydrochloride) caplets

Wyeth

### DRUG FACTS

| Active ingredients (in each caplet) | Purpose |
|---|---|
| Chlorpheniramine maleate 2 mg | Antihistamine |
| Ibuprofen 200 mg (NSAID)* | Pain reliever/fever reducer |
| Pseudoephedrine hydrochloride 30 mg | Nasal decongestant |

*nonsteroidal anti-inflammatory drug

### USES

- temporarily relieves these symptoms associated with hay fever or other upper respiratory allergies, and the common cold:
  - runny nose
  - itchy, watery eyes
  - itching of the nose or throat
  - sneezing
  - nasal congestion
  - sinus pressure
  - headache
  - minor aches and pains
  - fever

### WARNINGS
#### Allergy alert
Ibuprofen may cause a severe allergic reaction, especially in people allergic to aspirin. Symptoms may include:

- hives
- facial swelling
- asthma (wheezing)
- shock
- skin reddening
- rash
- blisters

If an allergic reaction occurs, stop use and seek medical help right away.

#### Stomach bleeding warning
This product contains an NSAID, which may cause severe stomach bleeding. The chance is higher if you:
- are age 60 or older
- have had stomach ulcers or bleeding problems
- take a blood thinning (anticoagulant) or steroid drug
- take other drugs containing prescription or nonprescription NSAIDs [aspirin, ibuprofen, naproxen, or others]
- have 3 or more alcoholic drinks every day while using this product
- take more or for a longer time than directed

### DO NOT USE
- in children under 12 years of age
- if you have ever had an allergic reaction to any other pain reliever/fever reducer
- right before or after heart surgery
- if you are now taking a prescription monoamine oxidase inhibitor (MAOI) (certain drugs for depression, psychiatric, or emotional conditions, or Parkinson's disease), or for 2 weeks after stopping the MAOI drug. If you do not know if your prescription drug contains an MAOI, ask a doctor or pharmacist before taking this product

## ASK A DOCTOR BEFORE USE IF
- you have a breathing problem such as emphysema or chronic bronchitis
- stomach bleeding warning applies to you
- you have problems or serious side effects from taking pain relievers or fever reducers
- you have a history of stomach problems, such as heartburn
- you have high blood pressure, heart disease, liver cirrhosis, kidney disease, asthma, thyroid disease, diabetes, glaucoma, or trouble urinating due to an enlarged prostate gland
- you are taking a diuretic

## ASK A DOCTOR OR PHARMACIST BEFORE USE IF YOU ARE
- under a doctor's care for any serious condition
- taking sedatives or tranquilizers
- taking any other product that contains pseudoephedrine, chlorpheniramine or any other nasal decongestant or antihistamine
- taking aspirin for heart attack or stroke, because ibuprofen may decrease this benefit of aspirin
- taking any other drug

## WHEN USING THIS PRODUCT
- take with food or milk if stomach upset occurs
- the risk of heart attack or stroke may increase if you use more than directed or for longer than directed
- avoid alcoholic drinks
- be careful when driving a motor vehicle or operating machinery
- drowsiness may occur
- alcohol, sedatives, and tranquilizers may increase drowsiness

## STOP USE AND ASK A DOCTOR IF
- you experience any of the following signs of stomach bleeding:
  - feel faint
  - vomit blood
  - have bloody or black stools
  - have stomach pain that does not get better
- fever gets worse or lasts more than 3 days
- nasal congestion lasts for more than 7 days
- redness or swelling is present in the painful area
- you get nervous, dizzy, or sleepless
- symptoms continue or get worse
- any new symptoms appear

**If pregnant or breastfeeding,** ask a health professional before use.

**It is especially important not to use ibuprofen during the last 3 months of pregnancy unless definitely directed to do so by a doctor because it may cause problems in the unborn child or complications during delivery.**

**Keep out of reach of children.** In case of overdose, get medical help or contact a Poison Control Center right away.

## DIRECTIONS
- do not take more than directed
- the smallest effective dose should be used

| adults | take 1 caplet every 4-6 hours while symptoms persist |
| | do not take more than 6 caplets in any 24-hour period, unless directed by a doctor |
| children under 12 years of age | do not use |

## OTHER INFORMATION
- read all warnings and directions before use. Keep carton
- store at 20-25°C (68-77°F)
- avoid excessive heat above 40°C (104°F)

## INACTIVE INGREDIENTS:
carnauba wax, colloidal silicon dioxide, corn starch, croscarmellose sodium, FD&C red no. 40 aluminum lake, FD&C yellow no. 6 aluminum lake, glyceryl behenate, hypromellose microcrystalline cellulose, pharmaceutical ink, polydextrose, polyethylene glycol, pregelatinized starch, propylene glycol, silicon dioxide, titanium dioxide

## QUESTIONS OR COMMENTS
Call weekdays from 9 AM to 5 PM EST at **1-800-88-ADVIL**

---

## ADVIL ALLERGY SINUS (chlorpheniramine maleate, ibuprofen, pseudoephedrine hydrochloride) tablet, coated
Pfizer Consumer Healthcare

## DRUG FACTS

| Active ingredients (in each caplet) | Purpose |
| --- | --- |
| Chlorpheniramine maleate 2 mg | Antihistamine |
| Ibuprofen 200 mg (NSAID)* | Pain reliever/fever reducer |
| Pseudoephedrine hydrochloride 30 mg | Nasal decongestant |

*nonsteroidal anti-inflammatory drug

## USES
- temporarily relieves these symptoms associated with hay fever or other upper respiratory allergies, and the common cold:
  - runny nose
  - itchy, watery eyes
  - itching of the nose or throat
  - sneezing
  - nasal congestion
  - sinus pressure
  - headache
  - minor aches and pains
  - fever

## WARNINGS
**Allergy alert**
Ibuprofen may cause a severe allergic reaction, especially in people allergic to aspirin. Symptoms may include:

- hives
- facial swelling
- asthma (wheezing)
- shock
- skin reddening
- rash
- blisters

If an allergic reaction occurs, stop use and seek medical help right away.

**Stomach bleeding warning**
This product contains an NSAID, which may cause severe stomach bleeding. The chance is higher if you:
- are age 60 or older
- have had stomach ulcers or bleeding problems
- take a blood thinning (anticoagulant) or steroid drug

- take other drugs containing prescription or nonprescription NSAIDs [aspirin, ibuprofen, naproxen, or others]
- have 3 or more alcoholic drinks every day while using this product
- take more or for a longer time than directed

## DO NOT USE
- in children under 12 years of age
- if you have ever had an allergic reaction to any other pain reliever/fever reducer
- right before or after heart surgery
- if you are now taking a prescription monoamine oxidase inhibitor (MAOI) (certain drugs for depression, psychiatric, or emotional conditions, or Parkinson's disease), or for 2 weeks after stopping the MAOI drug. If you do not know if your prescription drug contains an MAOI, ask a doctor or pharmacist before taking this product

## ASK A DOCTOR BEFORE USE IF
- you have a breathing problem such as emphysema or chronic bronchitis
- stomach bleeding warning applies to you
- you have problems or serious side effects from taking pain relievers or fever reducers
- you have a history of stomach problems, such as heartburn
- you have high blood pressure, heart disease, liver cirrhosis, kidney disease, asthma, thyroid disease, diabetes, glaucoma, or trouble urinating due to an enlarged prostate gland
- you are taking a diuretic

## ASK A DOCTOR OR PHARMACIST BEFORE USE IF YOU ARE
- under a doctor's care for any serious condition
- taking sedatives or tranquilizers
- taking any other product that contains pseudoephedrine, chlorpheniramine or any other nasal decongestant or antihistamine
- taking aspirin for heart attack or stroke, because ibuprofen may decrease this benefit of aspirin
- taking any other drug

## WHEN USING THIS PRODUCT
- take with food or milk if stomach upset occurs
- the risk of heart attack or stroke may increase if you use more than directed or for longer than directed
- avoid alcoholic drinks
- be careful when driving a motor vehicle or operating machinery
- drowsiness may occur
- alcohol, sedatives, and tranquilizers may increase drowsiness

## STOP USE AND ASK A DOCTOR IF
- you experience any of the following signs of stomach bleeding:
  - feel faint
  - vomit blood
  - have bloody or black stools
  - have stomach pain that does not get better
- fever gets worse or lasts more than 3 days
- nasal congestion lasts for more than 7 days
- redness or swelling is present in the painful area
- you get nervous, dizzy, or sleepless
- symptoms continue or get worse
- any new symptoms appear

**If pregnant or breastfeeding,** ask a health professional before use.

**It is especially important not to use ibuprofen during the last 3 months of pregnancy unless definitely directed to do so by a doctor because it may cause problems in the unborn child or complications during delivery.**

**Keep out of reach of children.** In case of overdose, get medical help or contact a Poison Control Center right away.

## DIRECTIONS
- do not take more than directed
- the smallest effective dose should be used

| adults | take 1 caplet every 4-6 hours while symptoms persist. do not take more than 6 caplets in any 24-hour period, unless directed by a doctor |
| --- | --- |
| children under 12 years of age | do not use |

## OTHER INFORMATION
- read all warnings and directions before use. Keep carton
- store at 20-25°C (68-77°F)
- avoid excessive heat above 40°C (104°F)

## INACTIVE INGREDIENTS
carnauba wax, colloidal silicon dioxide, corn starch, croscarmellose sodium, FD&C red no. 40 aluminum lake, FD&C yellow no. 6 aluminum lake, glyceryl behenate, hypromellose, microcrystalline cellulose, pharmaceutical ink, polydextrose, polyethylene glycol, pregelatinized starch, propylene glycol, silicon dioxide, titanium dioxide

## QUESTIONS OR COMMENTS
Call weekdays from 9 AM to 5 PM EST at **1-800-88-ADVIL**

---

# ADVIL COLD AND SINUS (ibuprofen, pseudoephedrine hydrochloride) capsule, liquid filled
Pfizer Consumer Healthcare

## DRUG FACTS

| Active ingredients (in each liquid-filled capsule) | Purpose |
| --- | --- |
| Solubilized ibuprofen equal to 200 mg ibuprofen (NSAID)* (present as the free acid and potassium salt) | Pain reliever/fever reducer |
| Pseudoephedrine hydrochloride 30 mg | Nasal decongestant |

*nonsteroidal anti-inflammatory drug

## USES
- temporarily relieves these symptoms associated with the common cold or flu:
  - headache
  - fever
  - sinus pressure
  - nasal congestion
  - minor body aches and pains

## WARNINGS
**Allergy alert**
Ibuprofen may cause a severe allergic reaction, especially in people allergic to aspirin. Symptoms may include:

- hives
- facial swelling
- asthma (wheezing)
- shock
- skin reddening
- rash
- blisters

If an allergic reaction occurs, stop use and seek medical help right away.

## Stomach bleeding warning

This product contains an NSAID, which may cause severe stomach bleeding. The chance is higher if you:

- are age 60 or older
- have had stomach ulcers or bleeding problems
- take a blood thinning (anticoagulant) or steroid drug
- take other drugs containing prescription or nonprescription NSAIDs [aspirin, ibuprofen, naproxen, or others]
- have 3 or more alcoholic drinks every day while using this product
- take more or for a longer time than directed

## DO NOT USE

- in children under 12 years of age
- if you have ever had an allergic reaction to any other pain reliever/fever reducer
- right before or after heart surgery
- if you are now taking a prescription monoamine oxidase inhibitor (MAOI) (certain drugs for depression, psychiatric, or emotional conditions, or Parkinson's disease), or for 2 weeks after stopping the MAOI drug. If you do not know if your prescription drug contains an MAOI, ask a doctor or pharmacist before taking this product

## ASK A DOCTOR BEFORE USE IF

- stomach bleeding warning applies to you
- you have problems or serious side effects from taking pain relievers or fever reducers
- you have a history of stomach problems, such as heartburn
- you have high blood pressure, heart disease, liver cirrhosis, kidney disease, asthma, thyroid disease, diabetes or trouble urinating due to an enlarged prostate gland
- you are taking a diuretic

## ASK A DOCTOR OR PHARMACIST BEFORE USE IF YOU ARE

- under a doctor's care for any serious condition
- taking any other product that contains pseudoephedrine or any other nasal decongestant
- taking aspirin for heart attack or stroke, because ibuprofen may decrease this benefit of aspirin
- taking any other drug

## WHEN USING THIS PRODUCT

- take with food or milk if stomach upset occurs
- the risk of heart attack or stroke may increase if you use more than directed or for longer than directed

## STOP USE AND ASK A DOCTOR IF

- you experience any of the following signs of stomach bleeding:
  - feel faint
  - vomit blood
  - have bloody or black stools
  - have stomach pain that does not get better
- fever gets worse or lasts more than 3 days
- nasal congestion lasts for more than 7 days
- symptoms continue or get worse
- redness or swelling is present in the painful area
- you get nervous, dizzy, or sleepless
- any new symptoms appear

**If pregnant or breastfeeding,** ask a health professional before use.

**It is especially important not to use ibuprofen during the last 3 months of pregnancy unless definitely directed to do so by a doctor because it may cause problems in the unborn child or complications during delivery.**

**Keep out of reach of children.** In case of overdose, get medical help or contact a Poison Control Center right away.

## DIRECTIONS

- do not take more than directed
- the smallest effective dose should be used

| adults and children 12 years of age and over | take 1 capsule every 4 to 6 hours while symptoms persist. If symptoms do not respond to 1 capsule, 2 capsules may be used. |
| --- | --- |
| | do not use more than 6 capsules in any 24-hour period unless directed by a doctor |
| children under 12 years of age | do not use |

## OTHER INFORMATION

- each capsule contains: potassium 20 mg
- store at 20-25°C (68-77°F). Avoid excessive heat above 40°C (104°F)
- read all warnings and directions before use. Keep carton

## INACTIVE INGREDIENTS

D&C yellow no. 10, FD&C red no. 40, fractionated coconut oil, gelatin, pharmaceutical ink, polyethylene glycol, potassium hydroxide, purified water, sorbitan, sorbitol

## QUESTIONS OR COMMENTS

Call toll-free **1-800-88-ADVIL**

---

# ADVIL COLD AND SINUS (ibuprofen, pseudoephedrine hydrochloride) tablet, coated

Pfizer Consumer Healthcare

## DRUG FACTS

| Active ingredients (in each caplet) | Purpose |
| --- | --- |
| Ibuprofen 200 mg (NSAID)* | Pain reliever/fever reducer |
| Pseudoephedrine hydrochloride 30 mg | Nasal decongestant |

*nonsteroidal anti-inflammatory drug

## USES

- temporarily relieves these symptoms associated with the common cold or flu:
  - headache
  - fever
  - sinus pressure
  - nasal congestion
  - minor body aches and pains

## WARNINGS

**Allergy alert**

Ibuprofen may cause a severe allergic reaction, especially in people allergic to aspirin. Symptoms may include:

- hives
- facial swelling
- asthma (wheezing)
- shock
- skin reddening
- rash
- blisters

If an allergic reaction occurs, stop use and seek medical help right away.

**Stomach bleeding warning**
This product contains an NSAID, which may cause severe stomach bleeding. The chance is higher if you:
- are age 60 or older
- have had stomach ulcers or bleeding problems
- take a blood thinning (anticoagulant) or steroid drug
- take other drugs containing prescription or nonprescription NSAIDs [aspirin, ibuprofen, naproxen, or others]
- have 3 or more alcoholic drinks every day while using this product
- take more or for a longer time than directed

## DO NOT USE
- in children under 12 years of age
- if you have ever had an allergic reaction to any other pain reliever/fever reducer
- right before or after heart surgery
- if you are now taking a prescription monoamine oxidase inhibitor (MAOI) (certain drugs for depression, psychiatric, or emotional conditions, or Parkinson's disease), or for 2 weeks after stopping the MAOI drug. If you do not know if your prescription drug contains an MAOI, ask a doctor or pharmacist before taking this product

## ASK A DOCTOR BEFORE USE IF
- stomach bleeding warning applies to you
- you have problems or serious side effects from taking pain relievers or fever reducers
- you have a history of stomach problems, such as heartburn
- you have high blood pressure, heart disease, liver cirrhosis, kidney disease, asthma, thyroid disease, diabetes or have trouble urinating due to an enlarged prostate gland
- you are taking a diuretic

## ASK A DOCTOR OR PHARMACIST BEFORE USE IF YOU ARE
- under a doctor's care for any serious condition
- taking any other product that contains pseudoephedrine or any other nasal decongestant
- taking aspirin for heart attack or stroke, because ibuprofen may decrease this benefit of aspirin
- taking any other drug

## WHEN USING THIS PRODUCT
- take with food or milk if stomach upset occurs
- the risk of heart attack or stroke may increase if you use more than directed or for longer than directed

## STOP USE AND ASK A DOCTOR IF
- you experience any of the following signs of stomach bleeding:
  - feel faint
  - vomit blood
  - have bloody or black stools
  - have stomach pain that does not get better
- fever gets worse or lasts more than 3 days
- nasal congestion lasts for more than 7 days
- symptoms continue or get worse
- redness or swelling is present in the painful area
- you get nervous, dizzy, or sleepless
- any new symptoms appear

**If pregnant or breastfeeding,** ask a health professional before use.

**It is especially important not to use ibuprofen during the last 3 months of pregnancy unless definitely directed to do so by a doctor because it may cause problems in the unborn child or complications during delivery.**

**Keep out of reach of children.** In case of overdose, get medical help or contact a Poison Control Center right away.

## DIRECTIONS
- do not take more than directed
- the smallest effective dose should be used

| adults and children 12 years of age and over | take 1 caplet every 4 to 6 hours while symptoms persist. If symptoms do not respond to 1 caplet, 2 caplets may be used. do not use more than 6 caplets in any 24-hour period unless directed by a doctor |
| --- | --- |
| children under 12 years of age | do not use |

## OTHER INFORMATION
- store at 20-25°C (68-77°F). Avoid excessive heat above 40°C (104°F)
- read all warnings and directions before use. Keep carton

## INACTIVE INGREDIENTS
acetylated monoglycerides, carnauba wax, colloidal silicon dioxide, corn starch, croscarmellose sodium, methylparaben, microcrystalline cellulose, pharmaceutical glaze, pharmaceutical ink, povidone, pregelatinized starch, propylparaben, sodium benzoate, sodium lauryl sulfate, stearic acid, sucrose, synthetic iron oxides, titanium dioxide

## QUESTIONS OR COMMENTS
Call toll-free **1-800-88-ADVIL**

# CHILDREN'S ADVIL COLD (ibuprofen, pseudoephedrine hydrochloride) suspension
Pfizer Consumer Healthcare

## DRUG FACTS

| Active ingredients (in each 5 mL teaspoon) | Purpose |
| --- | --- |
| Ibuprofen 100 mg (NSAID)* | Fever reducer/pain reliever |
| Pseudoephedrine hydrochloride 15 mg | Nasal decongestant |

*nonsteroidal anti-inflammatory drug

## USES
- temporarily relieves these cold, sinus and flu symptoms:
  - nasal and sinus congestion
  - headache
  - stuffy nose
  - sore throat
  - minor aches and pains
  - fever

## WARNINGS
**Allergy alert**
Ibuprofen may cause a severe allergic reaction, especially in people allergic to aspirin. Symptoms may include:
- hives
- facial swelling
- asthma (wheezing)
- shock
- skin reddening
- rash
- blisters

If an allergic reaction occurs, stop use and seek medical help right away.

### Stomach bleeding warning
This product contains an NSAID, which may cause severe stomach bleeding. The chance is higher if your child:
- has had stomach ulcers or bleeding problems
- takes a blood thinning (anticoagulant) or steroid drug
- takes other drugs containing prescription or nonprescription NSAIDs [aspirin, ibuprofen, naproxen, or others]
- takes more or for a longer time than directed

### Sore throat warning
Severe or persistent sore throat or sore throat accompanied by high fever, headache, nausea, and vomiting may be serious. Consult doctor promptly. Do not use more than 2 days or administer to children under 3 years of age unless directed by a doctor.

### DO NOT USE
- in a child under 2 years of age
- if the child has ever had an allergic reaction to any other pain reliever/fever reducer
- right before or after heart surgery
- in a child who is taking a prescription monoamine oxidase inhibitor (MAOI) (certain drugs for depression, psychiatric, or emotional conditions, or Parkinson's disease), or for 2 weeks after stopping the MAOI drug. If you do not know if the child's prescription drug contains an MAOI, ask a doctor or pharmacist before giving this product

### ASK A DOCTOR BEFORE USE IF
- stomach bleeding warning applies to your child
- child has problems or serious side effects from taking pain relievers or fever reducers
- child has a history of stomach problems, such as heartburn
- child has not been drinking fluids
- child has lost a lot of fluid due to vomiting or diarrhea
- child has high blood pressure, heart disease, liver cirrhosis, kidney disease, thyroid disease, diabetes or asthma
- child is taking a diuretic

### ASK A DOCTOR OR PHARMACIST BEFORE USE IF THE CHILD IS
- under a doctor's care for any serious condition
- taking any other product that contains pseudoephedrine or any other nasal decongestant
- taking any other drug

### WHEN USING THIS PRODUCT
- take with food or milk if stomach upset occurs
- the risk of heart attack or stroke may increase if you use more than directed or for longer than directed

### STOP USE AND ASK A DOCTOR IF
- the child experiences any of the following signs of stomach bleeding:
  - feels faint
  - vomits blood
  - has bloody or black stools
  - has stomach pain that does not get better
- the child does not get any relief within first day (24 hours) of treatment
- symptoms continue or get worse
- fever or pain or nasal congestion gets worse or lasts more than 3 days
- redness or swelling is present in the painful area
- the child gets nervous, dizzy, or sleepless or sleepy
- any new symptoms appear

**Keep out of reach of children.** In case of overdose, get medical help or contact a Poison Control Center right away.

### DIRECTIONS
- this product does not contain directions or complete warnings for adult use
- do not give more than directed
- shake well before using
- find right dose on chart. If possible, use weight to dose; otherwise use age
- if needed, repeat dose every 6 hours
- do not use more than 4 times a day
- replace original bottle cap to maintain child resistance
- measure only with dosing cup provided. Dosing cup to be used with Children's Advil Cold Suspension only. Do not use with other products. Dose lines account for product remaining in cup due to thickness of suspension

| Dosing Chart | | |
|---|---|---|
| **Weight (lb)** | **Age (yr)** | **Dose (teaspoons)** |
| under 24 | under 2 yr | do not use |
| 24-47 | 2-5 yr | 1 teaspoon |
| 48-95 | 6-11 yr | 2 teaspoons |

### OTHER INFORMATION
- each teaspoon contains: sodium 3 mg
- store at room temperature 20-25°C (68-77°F)
- alcohol free
- read all warnings and directions before use. Keep carton

### INACTIVE INGREDIENTS
artificial flavor, carboxymethylcellulose sodium, citric acid monohydrate, edetate disodium, FD&C blue no. 1, FD&C red no. 40, glycerin, microcrystalline cellulose, polysorbate 80, purified water, sodium benzoate, sorbitol solution, sucrose, xanthan gum

### QUESTIONS OR COMMENTS
Call weekdays from 9 AM to 5 PM EST at **1-800-88-ADVIL** or ask your pharmacist, doctor or health care professional.

---

## ADVIL CONGESTION RELIEF (ibuprofen, phenylephrine hydrochloride) tablet, film coated
Pfizer Consumer Healthcare

### DRUG FACTS

| Active ingredients (in each tablet) | Purpose |
|---|---|
| Ibuprofen 200 mg (NSAID)* | Pain reliever/fever reducer |
| Phenylephrine hydrochloride 10 mg | Nasal decongestant |

\* nonsteroidal anti-inflammatory drug

### USES
- temporarily relieves these symptoms associated with the common cold or flu:
  - headache
  - fever
  - sinus pressure
  - nasal congestion
  - minor body aches and pains
- reduces swelling of the nasal passages
- temporarily restores freer breathing through the nose

## WARNINGS

### Allergy alert

Ibuprofen may cause a severe allergic reaction, especially in people allergic to aspirin. Symptoms may include:

- hives
- facial swelling
- asthma (wheezing)
- shock
- skin reddening
- rash
- blisters

If an allergic reaction occurs, stop use and seek medical help right away.

### Stomach bleeding warning

This product contains an NSAID, which may cause severe stomach bleeding. The chance is higher if you:

- are age 60 or older
- have had stomach ulcers or bleeding problems
- take a blood thinning (anticoagulant) or steroid drug
- take other drugs containing prescription or nonprescription NSAIDs [aspirin, ibuprofen, naproxen, or others]
- have 3 or more alcoholic drinks every day while using this product
- take more or for a longer time than directed

### DO NOT USE

- in children under 12 years of age because this product contains too much medication for children under this age
- if you have ever had an allergic reaction to any other pain reliever/fever reducer
- right before or after heart surgery
- if you are now taking a prescription monoamine oxidase inhibitor (MAOI) (certain drugs for depression, psychiatric, or emotional conditions, or Parkinson's disease), or for 2 weeks after stopping the MAOI drug. If you do not know if your prescription drug contains an MAOI, ask a doctor or pharmacist before taking this product

### ASK A DOCTOR BEFORE USE IF

- stomach bleeding warning applies to you
- you have problems or serious side effects from taking pain relievers or fever reducers
- you have a history of stomach problems, such as heartburn
- you have high blood pressure, heart disease, liver cirrhosis, kidney disease, asthma, thyroid disease, diabetes, or have trouble urinating due to an enlarged prostate gland
- you are taking a diuretic

### ASK A DOCTOR OR PHARMACIST BEFORE USE IF YOU ARE

- under a doctor's care for any serious condition
- taking any other product that contains phenylephrine or any other nasal decongestant
- taking aspirin for heart attack or stroke, because ibuprofen may decrease this benefit of aspirin
- taking any other drug

### WHEN USING THIS PRODUCT

- take with food or milk if stomach upset occurs
- the risk of heart attack or stroke may increase if you use more than directed or for longer than directed

### STOP USE AND ASK A DOCTOR IF

- you experience any of the following signs of stomach bleeding:
  - feel faint
  - vomit blood
  - have bloody or black stools
  - have stomach pain that does not get better
- pain gets worse or lasts more than 7 days
- fever gets worse or lasts more than 3 days

- nasal congestion lasts for more than 7 days
- symptoms continue or get worse
- redness or swelling is present in the painful area
- you get nervous, dizzy, or sleepless
- any new symptoms appear

**If pregnant or breastfeeding,** ask a health professional before use.

**It is especially important not to use ibuprofen during the last 3 months of pregnancy unless definitely directed to do so by a doctor because it may cause problems in the unborn child or complications during delivery.**

**Keep out of reach of children.** In case of overdose, get medical help or contact a Poison Control Center right away.

## DIRECTIONS

- do not take more than directed

| adults and children 12 years of age and over | take 1 tablet every 4 hours while symptoms persist.<br><br>do not use more than 6 tablets in any 24-hour period unless directed by a doctor |
| --- | --- |
| children under 12 years of age | do not use because this product contains too much medication for children under this age |

## OTHER INFORMATION

- store at 20-25°C (68-77°F)
- avoid excessive heat above 40°C (104°F)
- read all warnings and directions before use. Keep carton

## INACTIVE INGREDIENTS

acesulfame potassium, artificial flavor, carnauba wax, colloidal silicon dioxide, corn starch, croscarmellose sodium, glycerin, hypromellose, lactic acid, lecithin, maltodextrin, medium-chain triglycerides, microcrystalline cellulose, pharmaceutical ink, polydextrose, polyvinyl alcohol, pregelatinized starch, propyl gallate, sodium lauryl sulfate, stearic acid, sucralose, synthetic iron oxide, talc, titanium dioxide, triacetin, xanthan gum

## QUESTIONS OR COMMENTS

Call weekdays from 9 AM to 5 PM toll-free at **1-800-88-ADVIL**

---

## ADVIL MIGRAINE (ibuprofen) capsule, liquid filled
### Pfizer Consumer Healthcare

### DRUG FACTS

| Active ingredient (in each brown oval capsule) | Purpose |
| --- | --- |
| Solubilized ibuprofen equal to 200 mg ibuprofen (NSAID)* (present as the free acid and potassium salt) | Pain reliever |

*nonsteroidal anti-inflammatory drug

### USE

- treats migraine

### WARNINGS

#### Allergy alert

Ibuprofen may cause a severe allergic reaction, especially in people allergic to aspirin. Symptoms may include:

- hives
- facial swelling
- asthma (wheezing)
- shock
- skin reddening
- rash
- blisters

If an allergic reaction occurs, stop use and seek medical help right away.

**Stomach bleeding warning**
This product contains an NSAID, which may cause severe stomach bleeding. The chance is higher if you:
- are age 60 or older
- have had stomach ulcers or bleeding problems
- take a blood thinning (anticoagulant) or steroid drug
- take other drugs containing prescription or nonprescription NSAIDs [aspirin, ibuprofen, naproxen, or others]
- have 3 or more alcoholic drinks every day while using this product
- take more or for a longer time than directed

**DO NOT USE**
- if you have ever had an allergic reaction to any other pain reliever/fever reducer
- right before or after heart surgery

**ASK A DOCTOR BEFORE USE IF**
- you have never had migraines diagnosed by a health professional
- you have a headache that is different from your usual migraines
- you have the worst headache of your life
- you have fever and stiff neck
- you have headaches beginning after or caused by head injury, exertion, coughing or bending
- you have experienced your first headache after the age of 50
- you have daily headaches
- you have a migraine so severe as to require bed rest
- stomach bleeding warning applies to you
- you have problems or serious side effects from taking pain relievers or fever reducers
- you have a history of stomach problems, such as heartburn
- you have high blood pressure, heart disease, liver cirrhosis, kidney disease, or asthma
- you are taking a diuretic

**ASK A DOCTOR OR PHARMACIST BEFORE USE IF YOU ARE**
- under a doctor's care for any serious condition
- taking aspirin for heart attack or stroke, because ibuprofen may decrease this benefit of aspirin
- taking any other drug

**WHEN USING THIS PRODUCT**
- take with food or milk if stomach upset occurs
- the risk of heart attack or stroke may increase if you use more than directed or for longer than directed

**STOP USE AND ASK A DOCTOR IF**
- you experience any of the following signs of stomach bleeding:
  - feel faint
  - vomit blood
  - have bloody or black stools
  - have stomach pain that does not get better
- migraine headache pain is not relieved or gets worse after the first dose
- any new symptoms appear

**If pregnant or breastfeeding,** ask a health professional before use.

**It is especially important not to use ibuprofen during the last 3 months of pregnancy unless definitely directed to** do so by a doctor because it may cause problems in the unborn child or complications during delivery.

**Keep out of reach of children.** In case of overdose, get medical help or contact a Poison Control Center right away.

**DIRECTIONS**
- do not take more than directed
- the smallest effective dose should be used

| adults | take 2 capsules with a glass of water |
| | if symptoms persist of worsen, ask your doctor |
| | do not take more than 2 capsules in 24 hours, unless directed by a doctor |
| under 18 years of age | ask a doctor |

**OTHER INFORMATION**
- each capsule contains: potassium 20 mg
- read all directions and warnings before use. Keep carton
- store at 20-25°C (68-77°F)
- avoid excessive heat above 40°C (104°F)

**INACTIVE INGREDIENTS**
D&C yellow no. 10, FD&C green no. 3, FD&C red no. 40, gelatin, light mineral oil, pharmaceutical ink, polyethylene glycol, potassium hydroxide, purified water, sorbitan, sorbitol

**QUESTIONS OR COMMENTS**
Call toll-free **1-800-88-ADVIL**

---

## ADVIL PM (ibuprofen and diphenhydramine citrate) tablet, coated

Pfizer Consumer Healthcare

### DRUG FACTS

| Active ingredient (in each tablet) | Purpose |
|---|---|
| Diphenhydramine citrate 38 mg | Nighttime sleep-aid |
| Ibuprofen 200 mg (NSAID) | Pain reliever |
| *nonsteroidal anti-inflammatory drug | |

**USES**
- for relief of occasional sleeplessness when associated with minor aches and pains
- helps you fall asleep and stay asleep

**WARNINGS**
**Allergy alert**
Ibuprofen may cause a severe allergic reaction, especially in people allergic to aspirin. Symptoms may include:

- hives
- facial swelling
- asthma (wheezing)
- shock
- skin reddening
- rash
- blisters

If an allergic reaction occurs, stop use and seek medical help right away.

**Stomach bleeding warning**
This product contains an NSAID, which may cause severe stomach bleeding. The chance is higher if you:
- are age 60 or older
- have had stomach ulcers or bleeding problems
- take a blood thinning (anticoagulant) or steroid drug
- take other drugs containing prescription or nonprescription NSAIDs [aspirin, ibuprofen, naproxen, or others]
- have 3 or more alcoholic drinks every day while using this product
- take more or for a longer time than directed

**DO NOT USE**
- if you have ever had an allergic reaction to any other pain reliever/fever reducer
- unless you have time for a full night's sleep
- in children under 12 years of age
- right before or after heart surgery
- with any other product containing diphenhydramine, even one used on skin
- if you have sleeplessness without pain

**ASK A DOCTOR BEFORE USE IF**
- stomach bleeding warning applies to you
- you have problems or serious side effects from taking pain relievers or fever reducers
- you have a history of stomach problems, such as heartburn
- you have high blood pressure, heart disease, liver cirrhosis, kidney disease, or asthma
- you are taking a diuretic
- you have a breathing problem such as emphysema or chronic bronchitis
- you have glaucoma
- you have trouble urinating due to an enlarged prostate gland

**ASK A DOCTOR OR PHARMACIST BEFORE USE IF YOU ARE**
- taking sedatives or tranquilizers, or any other sleep-aid
- under a doctor's care for any continuing medical illness
- taking any other antihistamines
- taking aspirin for heart attack or stroke, because ibuprofen may decrease this benefit of aspirin
- taking any other drug

**WHEN USING THIS PRODUCT**
- drowsiness will occur
- avoid alcoholic drinks
- do not drive a motor vehicle or operate machinery
- take with food or milk if stomach upset occurs
- the risk of heart attack or stroke may increase if you use more than directed or for longer than directed

**STOP USE AND ASK A DOCTOR IF**
- you experience any of the following signs of stomach bleeding:
  - feel faint
  - vomit blood
  - have bloody or black stools
  - have stomach pain that does not get better
- pain gets worse or lasts more than 10 days
- sleeplessness persists continuously for more than 2 weeks. Insomnia may be a symptom of a serious underlying medical illness
- redness or swelling is present in the painful area
- any new symptoms appear

**If pregnant or breastfeeding,** ask a health professional before use.

**It is especially important not to use ibuprofen during the last 3 months of pregnancy unless definitely directed to do so by a doctor because it may cause problems in the unborn child or complications during delivery.**

**Keep out of reach of children.** In case of overdose, get medical help or contact a Poison Control Center right away.

**DIRECTIONS**
- do not take more than directed

| adults and children 12 years and over | take 2 tablets at bedtime<br>do not take more than 2 tablets in 24 hours |
|---|---|

**OTHER INFORMATION**
- read all warnings and directions before use. Keep carton
- store at 20-25°C (68-77°F)
- avoid excessive heat above 40°C (104°F)

**INACTIVE INGREDIENTS**
calcium stearate, carnauba wax, colloidal silicon dioxide, corn starch, croscarmellose sodium, FD&C blue no. 2 aluminum lake, glyceryl behenate, hypromellose, lactose monohydrate, microcrystalline cellulose, pharmaceutical ink, polydextrose, polyethylene glycol, pregelatinized starch, sodium lauryl sulfate, sodium starch glycolate, stearic acid, titanium dioxide

**QUESTIONS OR COMMENTS**
Call weekdays 9 AM to 5 PM EST at **1-800-88-ADVIL** or www.lildrugstore.com

# AFRIN NODRIP ORIGINAL PUMP MIST
(oxymetazoline hydrochloride) nasal spray, solution
MSD Consumer Care, Inc

## DRUG FACTS

| Active ingredient | Purpose |
|---|---|
| Oxymetazoline hydrochloride 0.05% | Nasal decongestant |

**USES**
- temporarily relieves nasal congestion due to:
  - common cold
  - hay fever
  - upper respiratory allergies
- temporarily relieves sinus congestion and pressure
- shrinks swollen nasal membranes so you can breathe more freely

**WARNINGS**

**ASK A DOCTOR BEFORE USE IF YOU HAVE**
- heart disease
- high blood pressure
- thyroid disease
- diabetes
- trouble urinating due to an enlarged prostate gland

**WHEN USING THIS PRODUCT**
- do not use more than directed
- do not use for more than 3 days. Use only as directed. Frequent or prolonged use may cause nasal congestion to recur or worsen
- temporary discomfort such as burning, stinging, sneezing or an increase in nasal discharge may occur
- use of this container by more than one person may spread infection

**STOP USE AND ASK A DOCTOR IF**
- symptoms persist

**If pregnant or breastfeeding,** ask a health professional before use.

**Keep out of reach of children.** If swallowed, get medical help or contact a Poison Control Center right away.

## DIRECTIONS

| adults and children 6 to under 12 years of age (with adult supervision) | 2 or 3 sprays in each nostril not more often than every 10 to 12 hours<br><br>do not exceed 2 doses in any 24-hour period |
|---|---|
| children under 6 years of age | ask a doctor |

- Shake well before use. Before using the first time, remove the protective cap from the tip and prime metered pump by depressing pump firmly several times. To spray, hold bottle with thumb at base and nozzle between first and second fingers. Without tilting head, insert nozzle into nostril. Fully depress rim with a firm, even stroke and sniff deeply. Wipe nozzle clean after use

## OTHER INFORMATION
- store between 20°C-25°C (68°F-77°F)
- retain carton for future reference on full labeling

## INACTIVE INGREDIENTS
benzalkonium chloride solution, benzyl alcohol, edetate disodium, flavor, microcrystalline cellulose and carboxymethylcellulose sodium, polyethylene glycol, povidone, purified water, sodium phosphate dibasic, sodium phosphate monobasic

---

## AFTERBITE (ammonia)
Tender Corporation

## DRUG FACTS

| Active ingredient | Purpose |
|---|---|
| Ammonia 3.5% | Counterirritant |

## USES
- for the temporary relief of pain and itching associated with
  - insect bites & stings
  - minor skin irritations & rashes

## WARNINGS
**For external use only.**

## WHEN USING THIS PRODUCT
- do not get in eyes
- do not bandage of cover tightly until dry

## STOP USE AND ASK A DOCTOR IF
- rash, redness, swelling occurs or pain increases

**Keep out of reach of children.** If swallowed, get medical help or contact a Poison Control Center right away

If in eyes flush with water 10 to 15 minutes and consult a doctor.

## DIRECTIONS
- dab directly on bite or sting and rub gently
- if itching persists re-apply as necessary
- for a bee sting, remove stinger before treatment

| adults and children 2 years and older | apply to affected area |
|---|---|
| children under 2 years | consult a doctor |

## INACTIVE INGREDIENTS
alcohol ethoxylate, dimethicone, natural oil and purified water

---

## AKWA TEARS (polyvinyl alcohol) solution
Preferred Pharmaceuticals, Inc

## DRUG FACTS

| Active ingredients | Purpose |
|---|---|
| Polyvinyl alcohol 1.4% | Relief of burning and irritation and protectant of further irritation |
| Benzalkonium chloride 0.005% | |

## USES
- for the temporary relief of burning and irritation of the eye and for use as a protectant against further irritation
- for the temporary relief of discomfort due to minor irritations of the eye or to exposure to wind or sun

## WARNINGS

## DO NOT USE
- if imprinted seal on the bottle neck is broken or missing
- if solution changes color or becomes cloudy
- to avoid contamination, do not touch tip of container to any surface
- replace cap after using

## WHEN USING THIS PRODUCT
- remove contact lenses before using
- to avoid contamination, do not touch tip
- replace cap after each use

## STOP USE AND ASK A DOCTOR IF
- you feel eye pain
- changes in vision occur
- redness or irritation of the eye gets worse or lasts more than 72 hours

**If pregnant or breastfeeding,** ask a health professional before use.

**Keep out of the reach of children.** If swallowed, get medical help or contact a Poison Control Center right away.

## DIRECTIONS
- instill 1 or 2 drops in the affected eye(s) as needed
- store at room temperature

## OTHER INFORMATION
- store at 20°C-25°C (68°F-77°F)
- store away from heat
- protect from freezing
- keep tightly closed

## INACTIVE INGREDIENT
- Benzalkonium Chloride 0.005% (preservative), Edetate Disodium, Sodium Chloride, Sodium Phosphate Dibasic, Sodium Phosphate Monobasic, Purified Water, USP, Sodium Hydroxide and/or Hydrochloric Acid to adjust pH

## ALAVERT ALLERGY (loratadine) tablet, orally disintegrating

Pfizer Consumer Healthcare

### DRUG FACTS

| Active ingredient (in each tablet) | Purpose |
|---|---|
| Loratadine 10 mg | Antihistamine |

### USES
- temporarily relieves these symptoms due to hay fever or other upper respiratory allergies:
  - runny nose
  - sneezing
  - itchy, watery eyes
  - itching of the nose or throat

### WARNINGS

### DO NOT USE
- if you have ever had an allergic reaction to this product or any of its ingredients

### ASK A DOCTOR BEFORE USE IF YOU HAVE
- liver or kidney disease. Your doctor should determine if you need a different dose

### WHEN USING THIS PRODUCT
- do not use more than directed. Taking more than recommended may cause drowsiness

### STOP USE AND ASK A DOCTOR IF
- an allergic reaction to this product occurs. Seek medical help right away

**If pregnant or breastfeeding,** ask a health professional before use.

**Keep out of reach of children.** In case of overdose, get medical help or contact a Poison Control Center right away

### DIRECTIONS
- tablet melts in mouth. Can be taken with or without water

| Age | Dose |
|---|---|
| adults and children 6 years and over | 1 tablet daily; do not use more than 1 tablet daily |
| children under 6 | ask a doctor |
| consumers who have liver or kidney disease | ask a doctor |

### OTHER INFORMATION
- **Phenylketonurics:** Contains phenylalanine 8.4 mg per tablet
- store at 20-25°C (68-77°F)
- keep in a dry place

### INACTIVE INGREDIENTS
**Alavert Allergy Fresh Mint**
anhydrous citric acid, aspartame, colloidal silicon dioxide, corn syrup solids, crospovidone, magnesium stearate, mannitol, microcrystalline cellulose, modified starch, natural and artificial flavors, sodium bicarbonate

**Alavert Allergy Citrus Burst**
anhydrous citric acid, aspartame, butylated hydroxyanisole, colloidal silicon dioxide, corn syrup solids, crospovidone, dextrin, ferric oxides, magnesium stearate, maltodextrin, mannitol, microcrystalline cellulose, modified starch, natural and artificial flavors, sodium bicarbonate

### QUESTIONS OR COMMENTS
Call weekdays from 9 AM to 5 PM EST at **1-800-ALAVERT (1-800-252-8378)**

## ALAVERT ALLERGY SINUS D-12 (loratadine, pseudoephedrine sulfate) tablet, film coated, extended release

Wyeth Consumer Healthcare

### DRUG FACTS

| Active ingredients (in each tablet) | Purpose |
|---|---|
| Loratadine 5 mg | Antihistamine |
| Pseudoephedrine sulfate 120 mg | Nasal decongestant |

### USES
- temporarily relieves these symptoms due to hay fever or other upper respiratory allergies:
  - runny nose
  - sneezing
  - itchy, watery eyes
  - itching of the nose or throat
- temporarily relieves nasal congestion due to the common cold, hay fever or other respiratory allergies
- reduces swelling of nasal passages
- temporarily relieves sinus congestion and pressure
- temporarily restores freer breathing through the nose

### WARNINGS

### DO NOT USE
- if you have ever had an allergic reaction to this product or any of its ingredients
- if you are now taking a prescription monoamine oxidase inhibitor (MAOI) (certain drugs for depression, psychiatric, or emotional conditions, or Parkinson's disease), or for 2 weeks after stopping the MAOI drug. If you do not know if your prescription drug contains an MAOI, ask a doctor or pharmacist before taking this product

### ASK A DOCTOR BEFORE USE IF YOU HAVE
- heart disease
- high blood pressure
- thyroid disease
- diabetes
- trouble urinating due to an enlarged prostate gland
- liver or kidney disease. Your doctor should determine if you need a different dose

### WHEN USING THIS PRODUCT
- Do not take more than directed. Taking more than directed may cause drowsiness

### STOP USE AND ASK A DOCTOR IF
- an allergic reaction to this product occurs. Seek medical help right away
- symptoms do not improve within 7 days or are accompanied by a fever
- nervousness, dizziness or sleeplessness occurs

**If pregnant or breastfeeding,** ask a health professional before use.

**Keep out of reach of children.** In case of overdose, get medical help or contact a Poison Control Center right away.

**DIRECTIONS**
• do not divide, crush, chew or dissolve the tablet

| adults and children 12 years and over | 1 tablet every 12 hours; not more than 2 tablets in 24 hours |
| --- | --- |
| children under 12 years of age | ask a doctor |
| consumers with liver or kidney disease | ask a doctor |

**OTHER INFORMATION**
• each tablet contains: calcium 30 mg
• store between 15°C-25°C (59°F-77°F)
• keep in a dry place

**INACTIVE INGREDIENTS**
croscarmellose sodium, dibasic calcium phosphate, hypromellose, lactose monohydrate, magnesium stearate, pharmaceutical ink, povidone, titanium dioxide

**QUESTIONS OR COMMENTS**
Call weekdays from 9 AM to 5 PM EST at **1-800-ALAVERT (1-800-252-8378)**

---

# ALAVERT BUBBLE GUM FLAVOR (loratadine) tablet
Pfizer Consumer Healthcare

## DRUG FACTS

| Active ingredient (in each tablet) | Purpose |
| --- | --- |
| Loratadine 10 mg | Antihistamine |

**USES**
• temporarily relieves these symptoms due to hay fever or other upper respiratory allergies:
  • runny nose
  • sneezing
  • itchy, watery eyes
  • itching of the nose or throat

**WARNINGS**

**DO NOT USE**
• if you have ever had an allergic reaction to this product or any of its ingredients

**ASK A DOCTOR BEFORE USE IF YOU HAVE**
• liver or kidney disease. Your doctor should determine if you need a different dose

**WHEN USING THIS PRODUCT**
• do not use more than directed. Taking more than recommended may cause drowsiness

**STOP USE AND ASK A DOCTOR IF**
• an allergic reaction to this product occurs. Seek medical help right away

**If pregnant or breastfeeding,** ask a health professional before use.

**Keep out of reach of children.** In case of overdose, get medical help or contact a Poison Control Center right away.

**DIRECTIONS**
• tablet melts in mouth. Can be taken with or without water

| Age | Dose |
| --- | --- |
| adults and children 6 years and over | 1 tablet daily; do not use more than 1 tablet daily |
| children under 6 | ask a doctor |
| consumers who have liver or kidney disease | ask a doctor |

**OTHER INFORMATION**
• **Phenylketonurics:** Contains phenylalanine 8.4 mg per tablet
• store at 20-25°C (68-77°F)
• keep in a dry place

**INACTIVE INGREDIENTS**
anhydrous citric acid, artificial and natural flavor, ascorbic acid, aspartame, colloidal silicon dioxide, crospovidone, ferric oxide, magnesium stearate, maltodextrin, mannitol, microcrystalline cellulose, modified starch, sodium bicarbonate

**QUESTIONS OR COMMENTS**
Call weekdays from 9 AM to 5 PM EST at **1-800- ALAVERT (1-800-252-8378)**

---

# ALAVERT CITRUS BURST (loratadine) tablet
Pfizer Consumer Healthcare

## DRUG FACTS

| Active ingredient (in each tablet) | Purpose |
| --- | --- |
| Loratadine 10 mg | Antihistamine |

**USES**
• temporarily relieves these symptoms due to hay fever or other upper respiratory allergies:
  • runny nose
  • sneezing
  • itchy, watery eyes
  • itching of the nose or throat

**WARNINGS**

**DO NOT USE**
• if you have ever had an allergic reaction to this product or any of its ingredients

**ASK A DOCTOR BEFORE USE IF YOU HAVE**
• liver or kidney disease. Your doctor should determine if you need a different dose

**WHEN USING THIS PRODUCT**
• do not use more than directed. Taking more than recommended may cause drowsiness

**STOP USE AND ASK A DOCTOR IF**
• an allergic reaction to this product occurs. Seek medical help right away

**If pregnant or breastfeeding,** ask a health professional before use.

**Keep out of reach of children.** In case of overdose, get medical help or contact a Poison Control Center right away.

**DIRECTIONS**
• tablet melts in mouth. Can be taken with or without water

| adults and children 6 years and over | 1 tablet daily; do not use more than 1 tablet daily |
|---|---|
| children under 6 | ask a doctor |
| consumers who have liver or kidney disease | ask a doctor |

## OTHER INFORMATION
- **Phenylketonurics:** contains phenylalanine 8.4 mg per tablet
- store at 20-25°C (68-77°F)
- keep in a dry place

## INACTIVE INGREDIENTS
anhydrous citric acid, aspartame, butylated hydroxyanisole, colloidal silicon dioxide, corn syrup solids, crospovidone, dextrin, ferric oxides, magnesium stearate, maltodextrin, mannitol, microcrystalline cellulose, modified starch, natural and artificial flavors, sodium bicarbonate

## QUESTIONS OR COMMENTS
Call weekdays from 9 AM to 5 PM EST at **1-800- ALAVERT (1-800-252-8378)**

---

# ALAWAY (ketotifen fumarate) solution/drops
Bausch & Lomb Incorporated

SIFAVITOR SRL

## DRUG FACTS

| Active ingredient | Purpose |
|---|---|
| Ketotifen 0.025% (equivalent to ketotifen fumarate 0.035%) | Antihistamine |

## USES
- for the temporary relief of itchy eyes due to ragweed, pollen, grass, animal hair and dander

## WARNINGS
### DO NOT USE
- if you are sensitive to any ingredient in this product
- if solution changes color or becomes cloudy
- to treat contact lens related irritation

### WHEN USING THIS PRODUCT
- remove contact lenses before use
- wait at least 10 minutes before re-inserting contact lenses after use
- do not touch tip of container to any surface to avoid contamination
- replace cap after each use

### STOP USE AND ASK DOCTOR IF YOU EXPERIENCE ANY OF THE FOLLOWING
- eye pain
- changes in vision
- redness of the eyes
- itching that worsens or lasts more than 72 hours

**Keep out of reach of children.** If swallowed, get medical help or contact a Poison Control Center right away.

## DIRECTIONS

| adults and children 3 years and older | put 1 drop in the affected eye(s) twice daily, every 8-12 hours, no more than twice per day |
|---|---|
| children under 3 years of age | consult a doctor |

## OTHER INFORMATION
- Store at 4-25°C (39-77°F)

## INACTIVE INGREDIENTS
benzalkonium chloride, 0.01%, glycerin, sodium hydroxide and/or hydrochloric acid and water for injection

## QUESTIONS OR COMMENTS
Toll-free Product Information Call: **1-800-553-5340**

---

# ALEVE GELCAPS (naproxen sodium)
Bayer HealthCare

## DRUG FACTS

| Active ingredient (in each gelcap) | Purpose |
|---|---|
| Naproxen sodium 220 mg (naproxen 200 mg) (NSAID)* | Pain reliever/fever reducer |

*nonsteroidal anti-inflammatory drug

## USES
- temporarily relieves minor aches and pains due to:
  - minor pain of arthritis
  - muscular aches
  - backache
  - menstrual cramps
  - headache
  - toothache
  - the common cold
- temporarily reduces fever

## WARNINGS
### Allergy alert
Naproxen sodium may cause a severe allergic reaction, especially in people allergic to aspirin. Symptoms may include:

- hives
- facial swelling
- asthma (wheezing)
- shock
- skin reddening
- rash
- blisters

If an allergic reaction occurs, stop use and seek medical help right away.

### Stomach Bleeding Warning
This product contains an NSAID, which may cause severe stomach bleeding. The chance is higher if you:
- are age 60 or older
- have had stomach ulcers or bleeding problems
- take a blood thinning (anticoagulant) or steroid drug
- take other drugs containing prescription or nonprescription NSAIDs (aspirin, ibuprofen, naproxen, or others)
- have 3 or more alcoholic drinks every day while using this product
- take more or for a longer time than directed

## DO NOT USE
- if you have ever had an allergic reaction to any other pain reliever/fever reducer
- right before or after heart surgery

## ASK A DOCTOR BEFORE USE IF
- the stomach bleeding warning applies to you
- you have a history of stomach problems, such as heartburn
- you have high blood pressure, heart disease, liver cirrhosis, or kidney disease
- you are taking a diuretic
- you have problems or serious side effects from taking pain relievers or fever reducers
- you have asthma

## ASK A DOCTOR OR PHARMACIST BEFORE USE IF YOU ARE
- under a doctor's care for any serious condition
- taking any other drug

## WHEN USING THIS PRODUCT
- take with food or milk if stomach upset occurs
- the risk of heart attack or stroke may increase if you use more than directed or for longer than directed

## STOP USE AND ASK A DOCTOR IF
- you experience any of the following signs of stomach bleeding:
  - feel faint
  - vomit blood
  - have bloody or black stools
  - have stomach pain that does not get better
- pain gets worse or lasts more than 10 days
- fever gets worse or lasts more than 3 days
- you have difficulty swallowing
- it feels like the pill is stuck in your throat
- redness or swelling is present in the painful area
- any new symptoms appear

**If pregnant or breastfeeding,** ask a health professional before use.

**It is especially important not to use naproxen sodium during the last 3 months of pregnancy unless definitely directed to do so by a doctor because it may cause problems in the unborn child or complications during delivery.**

**Keep out of reach of children.** In case of overdose, get medical help or contact a Poison Control Center right away.

## DIRECTIONS
- do not take more than directed
- the smallest effective dose should be used
- drink a full glass of water with each dose

| adults and children 12 years and older | take 1 gelcap every 8 to 12 hours while symptoms last |
| --- | --- |
| | for the first dose you may take 2 gelcaps within the first hour |
| | do not exceed 2 gelcaps in any 8- to 12-hour period |
| | do not exceed 3 gelcaps in a 24-hour period |
| children under 12 years | ask a doctor |

## OTHER INFORMATION
- each tablet contains: sodium 20 mg
- store at 20-25°C (68-77°F). Avoid high humidity and excessive heat above 40°C(104°F)

## INACTIVE INGREDIENTS
D&C yellow no. 10 aluminum lake, edetate disodium, edible ink, FD&C blue no. 1, FD&C yellow no. 6 aluminum lake, gelatin, glycerin, hypromellose, magnesium stearate, microcrystalline cellulose, polyethylene glycol, povidone, stearic acid, talc, titanium dioxide

## QUESTIONS OR COMMENTS
Call **1-800-395-0689** (Mon-Fri 9 AM-5 PM EST) or www.aleve.com

## ALEVE LIQUID GELS (Naproxen sodium) capsule
Bayer HealthCare

## DRUG FACTS

| Active ingredient (in each capsule) | Purpose |
| --- | --- |
| Naproxen sodium 220 mg (naproxen 200 mg) (NSAID)* | Pain reliever/fever reducer |

*nonsteroidal anti-inflammatory drug

## USES
- temporarily relieves minor aches and pains due to:
  - minor pain of arthritis
  - muscular aches
  - backache
  - menstrual cramps
  - headache
  - toothache
  - the common cold
- temporarily reduces fever

## WARNINGS
**Allergy alert**
Naproxen sodium may cause a severe allergic reaction, especially in people allergic to aspirin. Symptoms may include:

- hives
- facial swelling
- asthma (wheezing)
- shock
- skin reddening
- rash
- blisters

If an allergic reaction occurs, stop use and seek medical help right away.

**Stomach Bleeding Warning**
This product contains an NSAID, which may cause severe stomach bleeding. The chance is higher if you:
- are age 60 or older
- have had stomach ulcers or bleeding problems
- take a blood thinning (anticoagulant) or steroid drug
- take other drugs containing prescription or nonprescription NSAIDs (aspirin, ibuprofen, naproxen, or others)
- have 3 or more alcoholic drinks every day while using this product
- take more or for a longer time than directed

## DO NOT USE
- if you have ever had an allergic reaction to any other pain reliever/fever reducer
- right before or after heart surgery

## ASK A DOCTOR BEFORE USE IF

- the stomach bleeding warning applies to you
- you have a history of stomach problems, such as heartburn
- you have high blood pressure, heart disease, liver cirrhosis, or kidney disease
- you are taking a diuretic
- you have problems or serious side effects from taking pain relievers or fever reducers
- you have asthma

## ASK A DOCTOR OR PHARMACIST BEFORE USE IF YOU ARE

- under a doctor's care for any serious condition
- taking any other drug

## WHEN USING THIS PRODUCT

- take with food or milk if stomach upset occurs
- the risk of heart attack or stroke may increase if you use more than directed or for longer than directed

## STOP USE AND ASK A DOCTOR IF

- you experience any of the following signs of stomach bleeding:
  - feel faint
  - vomit blood
  - have bloody or black stools
  - have stomach pain that does not get better
- pain gets worse or lasts more than 10 days
- fever gets worse or lasts more than 3 days
- redness or swelling is present in the painful area
- any new symptoms appear
- you have difficulty swallowing
- it feels like the capsule is stuck in your throat

**If pregnant or breastfeeding,** ask a health professional before use.

**It is especially important not to use naproxen sodium during the last 3 months of pregnancy unless definitely directed to do so by a doctor because it may cause problems in the unborn child or complications during delivery.**

**Keep out of reach of children.** In case of overdose, get medical help or contact a Poison Control Center right away.

## DIRECTIONS

- do not take more than directed
- the smallest effective dose should be used
- drink a full glass of water with each dose
- if taken with food, this product may take longer to work

| adults and children 12 years and older | take 1 capsule every 8 to 12 hours while symptoms last |
| --- | --- |
| | for the first dose you may take 2 capsules within the first hour |
| | do not exceed 2 capsules in any 8- to 12-hour period |
| | do not exceed 3 capsules in a 24-hour period |
| children under 12 years | ask a doctor |

## OTHER INFORMATION

- each capsule contains: sodium 20 mg
- store at 20-25°C (68-77°F) avoid high humidity and excessive heat above 40°C (104°F)
- read all directions and warnings before use. Keep carton

## INACTIVE INGREDIENTS

FD&C blue no. 1, gelatin, glycerin, lactic acid, mannitol, pharmaceutical ink, polyethylene glycol, povidone, propylene glycol, purified water, sorbitan, sorbitol

## QUESTIONS OR COMMENTS

Call **1-800-395-0689** (Mon-Fri 9 AM-5 PM EST) or www.aleve.com

---

# ALEVE-D SINUS & COLD (naproxen sodium and pseudoephedrine hydrochloride)

## Bayer HealthCare

## DRUG FACTS

| Active ingredient (in each caplet) | Purpose |
| --- | --- |
| Naproxen sodium 220 mg (naproxen 200 mg) (NSAID)* | Pain reliever/fever reducer |
| Pseudoephedrine hydrochloride 120 mg, extended-release. | Nasal decongestant |

*nonsteroidal anti-inflammatory drug

## USES

- temporarily relieves these cold, sinus, and flu symptoms:
  - sinus pressure
  - minor body aches and pains
  - headache
  - nasal and sinus congestion (promotes sinus drainage and restores freer breathing through the nose)
  - fever

## WARNINGS

**Allergy alert**
Naproxen sodium may cause a severe allergic reaction, especially in people allergic to aspirin. Symptoms may include:

- hives
- facial swelling
- asthma (wheezing)
- shock
- skin reddening
- rash
- blisters

If an allergic reaction occurs, stop use and seek medical help right away.

**Stomach Bleeding Warning**
This product contains an NSAID, which may cause stomach bleeding. The chance is higher if you:

- are age 60 or older
- have had stomach ulcers or bleeding problems
- take a blood thinning (anticoagulant) or steroid drug
- take other drugs containing an NSAID (aspirin, ibuprofen, naproxen, or others)
- have 3 or more alcoholic drinks every day while using this product
- take more or for a longer time than directed

## DO NOT USE

- if you have ever had an allergic reaction to any other pain reliever/fever reducer
- right before or after heart surgery
- if you are now taking a prescription monoamine oxidase inhibitor (MAOI) (certain drugs for depression, psychiatric, or emotional conditions, or Parkinson's disease), or for 2 weeks after stopping the MAOI drug. If you do not know if your prescription drug contains an MAOI, ask a doctor or pharmacist before taking this product

## ASK A DOCTOR BEFORE USE IF YOU HAVE
- problems or serious side effects from taking pain relievers or fever reducers
- stomach problems that last or come back, such as heartburn, upset stomach, or stomach pain
- ulcers
- bleeding problems
- high blood pressure
- heart or kidney disease
- taken a diuretic
- reached age 60 or older
- thyroid disease
- diabetes
- trouble urinating due to an enlarged prostate gland

## ASK A DOCTOR OR PHARMACIST BEFORE USE IF YOU ARE
- taking any other drug containing an NSAID (prescription or nonprescription)
- taking a blood thinning (anticoagulant) or steroid drug
- under a doctor's care for any serious condition
- using any other product that contains naproxen or pseudoephedrine
- taking any other pain reliever/fever reducer or nasal decongestant
- taking any other drug

## WHEN USING THIS PRODUCT
- take with food or milk if stomach upset occurs
- long term continuous use may increase the risk of heart attack or stroke

## STOP USE AND ASK A DOCTOR IF
- you feel faint, vomit blood, or have bloody or black stools. These are signs of stomach bleeding
- fever gets worse or lasts more than 3 days
- stomach pain or upset gets worse or lasts
- redness or swelling is present in the painful area
- any new symptoms appear
- you have difficulty swallowing or the caplet feels stuck in your throat
- you develop heartburn
- you get nervous, dizzy, or sleepless
- nasal congestion lasts more than 7 days

**If pregnant or breastfeeding,** ask a health professional before use.

**It is especially important not to use naproxen sodium during the last 3 months of pregnancy unless definitely directed to do so by a doctor because it may cause problems in the unborn child or complications during delivery.**

**Keep out of reach of children.** In case of overdose, get medical help or contact a Poison Control Center right away.

## DIRECTIONS
- do not take more than directed
- the smallest effective dose should be used
- do not take longer than 7 days, unless directed by a doctor (see Warnings)
- swallow whole; do not crush or chew
- drink a full glass of water with each dose

| adults and children 12 years and older | 1 caplet every 12 hours; do not take more than 2 caplets in 24 hours |
|---|---|
| children under 12 years | ask a doctor |

## OTHER INFORMATION
- each caplet contains: sodium 20 mg
- store at 20-25°C (68-77°F)
- store in a dry place

## INACTIVE INGREDIENTS
colloidal silicon dioxide, hypromellose, lactose monohydrate, magnesium stearate, microcrystalline cellulose, polyethylene glycol, polysorbate 80, povidone, talc, titanium dioxide

## QUESTIONS OR COMMENTS
Call **1-800-986-0369** (Mon-Fri 9 AM-5 PM EST) or www.aleved.com

## ALEVE (naproxen sodium) tablets
Bayer HealthCare

## DRUG FACTS

| Active ingredient (in each tablet) | Purpose |
|---|---|
| Naproxen sodium 220 mg (naproxen 200 mg) (NSAID)* | Pain reliever/fever reducer |

*nonsteroidal anti-inflammatory drug

## USES
- temporarily relieves minor aches and pains due to:
  - minor pain of arthritis
  - muscular aches
  - backache
  - menstrual cramps
  - headache
  - toothache
  - the common cold
- temporarily reduces fever

## WARNINGS
**Allergy alert**
Naproxen sodium may cause a severe allergic reaction, especially in people allergic to aspirin. Symptoms may include:
- hives
- facial swelling
- asthma (wheezing)
- shock
- skin reddening
- rash
- blisters

If an allergic reaction occurs, stop use and seek medical help right away.

**Stomach Bleeding Warning**
This product contains an NSAID, which may cause severe stomach bleeding. The chance is higher if you:
- are age 60 or older
- have had stomach ulcers or bleeding problems
- take a blood thinning (anticoagulant) or steroid drug
- take other drugs containing prescription or nonprescription NSAIDs (aspirin, ibuprofen, naproxen, or others)
- have 3 or more alcoholic drinks every day while using this product
- take more or for a longer time than directed

## DO NOT USE
- if you have ever had an allergic reaction to any other pain reliever/fever reducer
- right before or after heart surgery

## ASK A DOCTOR BEFORE USE IF

- the stomach bleeding warning applies to you
- you have a history of stomach problems, such as heartburn
- you have high blood pressure, heart disease, liver cirrhosis, or kidney disease
- you are taking a diuretic
- you have problems or serious side effects from taking pain relievers or fever reducers
- you have asthma

## ASK A DOCTOR OR PHARMACIST BEFORE USE IF YOU ARE

- under a doctor's care for any serious condition
- taking any other drug

## WHEN USING THIS PRODUCT

- take with food or milk if stomach upset occurs
- the risk of heart attack or stroke may increase if you use more than directed or for longer than directed

## STOP USE AND ASK A DOCTOR IF

- you experience any of the following signs of stomach bleeding:
  - feel faint
  - vomit blood
  - have bloody or black stools
  - have stomach pain that does not get better
- pain gets worse or lasts more than 10 days
- fever gets worse or lasts more than 3 days
- you have difficulty swallowing
- it feels like the tablet is stuck in your throat
- redness or swelling is present in the painful area
- any new symptoms appear

**If pregnant or breastfeeding,** ask a health professional before use.

**It is especially important not to use naproxen sodium during the last 3 months of pregnancy unless definitely directed to do so by a doctor because it may cause problems in the unborn child or complications during delivery.**

**Keep out of reach of children.** In case of overdose, get medical help or contact a Poison Control Center right away.

## DIRECTIONS

- do not take more than directed
- the smallest effective dose should be used
- drink a full glass of water with each dose

| adults and children 12 years and older | take 1 tablet every 8 to 12 hours while symptoms last |
| | for the first dose you may take 2 tablets within the first hour |
| | do not exceed 2 tablets in any 8- to 12-hour period |
| | do not exceed 3 tablets in a 24-hour period |
| children under 12 years | ask a doctor |

## OTHER INFORMATION

- each tablet contains: sodium 20 mg
- store at 20-25°C (68-77°F). Avoid high humidity and excessive heat above 40°C(104°F)

## INACTIVE INGREDIENTS

FD&C blue no. 2 lake, hypromellose, magnesium stearate, microcrystalline cellulose, polyethylene glycol, povidone, talc, titanium dioxide

## QUESTIONS OR COMMENTS

Call **1-800-395-0689** (Mon-Fri 9 AM-5 PM EST) or www.aleve.com

---

# ALKA-SELTZER HEARTBURN (anhydrous citric acid and sodium bicarbonate) granule, effervescent

BAYER HealthCare

## DRUG FACTS

| Active ingredients (in each tablet) | Purpose |
|---|---|
| Anhydrous citric acid 1000 mg | Antacid |
| Sodium bicarbonate (heat-treated) 1940 mg | Antacid |

## USES

- for the relief of:
  - heartburn
  - acid indigestion
  - upset stomach associated with these symptoms

## WARNINGS

### ASK A DOCTOR BEFORE USE IF YOU HAVE

- a sodium-restricted diet

### ASK A DOCTOR OR PHARMACIST BEFORE USE IF YOU ARE

- presently taking a prescription drug. Antacids may interact with certain prescription drugs

### WHEN USING THIS PRODUCT

- do not exceed recommended dosage

### STOP USE AND ASK A DOCTOR IF

- you have taken the maximum dose for 2 weeks

**If pregnant or breastfeeding,** ask a health professional before use.

**Keep out of reach of children.**

## DIRECTIONS

- fully dissolve 2 tablets in 4 ounces of water before taking

| adults and children 12 years and over | 2 tablets every 4 hours as needed, or as directed by a doctor |
| | do not exceed 8 tablets in 24 hours |
| adults 60 years and over | 2 tablets every 4 hours as needed, or as directed by a doctor |
| | do not exceed 4 tablets in 24 hours |
| children under 12 years | consult a doctor |

## OTHER INFORMATION

- each tablet contains: sodium 575 mg
- **Phenylketonurics:** contains phenylalanine 5.6 mg per tablet
- store at room temperature. Avoid excessive heat
- Alka-Seltzer Heartburn in water contains the antacid sodium citrate as the principal active ingredient

## INACTIVE INGREDIENTS

acesulfame potassium, aspartame, flavors, magnesium stearate, mannitol

## QUESTIONS OR COMMENTS

**1-800-986-0369** (Mon-Fri 9 AM-5 PM EST) or www.alkaseltzer.com

## ALKA-SELTZER XTRA STRENGTH (anhydrous citric acid, sodium bicarbonate, and aspirin) granule, effervescent

Bayer HealthCare

### DRUG FACTS

| Active ingredients (in each tablet) | Purpose |
|---|---|
| Anhydrous citric acid 1000 mg | Antacid |
| Aspirin 500 mg | Analgesic |
| Sodium bicarbonate (heat-treated) 1985 mg | Antacid |

### USES
- for the relief of:
  - heartburn, acid indigestion, and sour stomach when accompanied with headache or body aches and pains
  - upset stomach with headache from overindulgence in food or drink
  - headache, body aches, and pain alone

### WARNINGS
**Reye's syndrome**
Children and teenagers should not use this medicine for chicken pox or flu symptoms before a doctor is consulted about Reye's syndrome, a rare but serious illness reported to be associated with aspirin.

**Allergy alert**
Aspirin may cause a severe allergic reaction which may include:
- hives
- facial swelling
- asthma (wheezing)
- shock

**Alcohol warning**
- If you consume 3 or more alcoholic drinks every day, ask your doctor whether you should take aspirin or other pain relievers/fever reducers
- Aspirin may cause stomach bleeding

### DO NOT USE
- if you are allergic to aspirin or any other pain reliever/fever reducer

### ASK A DOCTOR BEFORE USE IF YOU HAVE
- asthma
- ulcers
- bleeding problems
- stomach problems that last or come back frequently, such as heartburn, upset stomach, or pain
- a sodium-restricted diet

### ASK A DOCTOR OR PHARMACIST BEFORE USE IF YOU ARE
- presently taking a prescription drug. Antacids may interact with certain prescription drugs
- taking a prescription drug for anticoagulation (blood thinning), diabetes, gout, or arthritis

### WHEN USING THIS PRODUCT
- do not exceed recommended dosage

### STOP USE AND ASK A DOCTOR IF
- an allergic reaction occurs. Seek medical help right away
- symptoms get worse or last more than 10 days
- redness or swelling is present
- ringing in the ears or loss of hearing occurs
- new symptoms occur

**If pregnant or breastfeeding,** ask a health professional before use.

**It is especially important not to use aspirin during the last 3 months of pregnancy unless definitely directed to do so by a doctor because it may cause problems in the unborn child or complications during delivery.**

**Keep out of reach of children.** In case of overdose, get medical help or contact a Poison Control Center right away.

### DIRECTIONS
- fully dissolve 2 tablets in 4 ounces of water before taking

| adults and children 12 years and over | 2 tablets every 6 hours, or as directed by a doctor |
|---|---|
| | do not exceed 7 tablets in 24 hours |
| adults 60 years and over | 2 tablets every 6 hours, or as directed by a doctor |
| | do not exceed 3 tablets in 24 hours |
| children under 12 years | consult a doctor |

### OTHER INFORMATION
- each tablet contains: sodium 588 mg
- store at room temperature. Avoid excessive heat
- Alka-Seltzer Xtra Strength in water contains principally the antacid sodium citrate and the analgesic sodium acetylsalicylate

### INACTIVE INGREDIENT
flavor

### QUESTIONS OR COMMENTS
**1-800-986-0369** (Mon - Fri 9 AM-5 PM EST) or www.alkaseltzer.com

## ALKA-SELTZER PLUS CHERRY BURST COLD FORMULA (aspirin, chlorpheniramine maleate, and phenylephrine bitartrate) effervescent tablets

Bayer HealthCare

### DRUG FACTS

| Active ingredients (in each tablet) | Purpose |
|---|---|
| Aspirin 325 mg (NSAID)* | Pain reliever/fever reducer |
| Chlorpheniramine maleate 2 mg | Antihistamine |
| Phenylephrine bitartrate 7.8 mg | Nasal decongestant |

*nonsteroidal anti-inflammatory drug

### USES
- temporarily relieves these symptoms due to a cold:
  - minor aches and pains
  - headache
  - runny nose
  - nasal and sinus congestion
  - sneezing
  - sore throat
- temporarily reduces fever

### WARNINGS
**Reye's syndrome**
Children and teenagers who have or are recovering from chicken pox or flu-like symptoms should not use this product. When

using this product, if changes in behavior with nausea and vomiting occur, consult a doctor because these symptoms could be an early sign of Reye's syndrome, a rare but serious illness.

### Allergy alert
Aspirin may cause a severe allergic reaction which may include:
- hives
- facial swelling
- asthma (wheezing)
- shock

### Stomach bleeding warning
This product contains an NSAID, which may cause severe stomach bleeding. The chance is higher if you:
- are age 60 or older
- have had stomach ulcers or bleeding problems
- take a blood thinning (anticoagulant) or steroid drug
- take other drugs containing prescription or nonprescription NSAIDs (aspirin, ibuprofen, naproxen, or others)
- have 3 or more alcoholic drinks every day while using this product
- take more or for a longer time than directed

### Sore throat warning
If sore throat is severe, persists for more than 2 days, is accompanied or followed by fever, headache, rash, nausea, or vomiting, consult a doctor promptly.

### Do not use to sedate children.

### DO NOT USE
- if you are allergic to aspirin or any other pain reliever/fever reducer
- if you are now taking a prescription monoamine oxidase inhibitor (MAOI) (certain drugs for depression, psychiatric, or emotional conditions, or Parkinson's disease), or for 2 weeks after stopping the MAOI drug. If you do not know if your prescription drug contains an MAOI, ask a doctor or pharmacist before taking this product
- in children under 12 years of age

### ASK A DOCTOR BEFORE USE IF
- stomach bleeding warning applies to you
- you have a history of stomach problems, such as heartburn
- you have high blood pressure, heart disease, liver cirrhosis, or kidney disease
- you are taking a diuretic
- you have:
  - asthma
  - diabetes
  - thyroid disease
  - glaucoma
  - difficulty in urination due to enlargement of the prostate gland
  - a breathing problem such as emphysema or chronic bronchitis
  - a sodium-restricted diet

### ASK A DOCTOR OR PHARMACIST BEFORE USE IF YOU ARE
- taking a prescription drug for
  - gout
  - diabetes
  - arthritis
- taking sedatives or tranquilizers

### WHEN USING THIS PRODUCT
- do not exceed recommended dosage
- excitability may occur, especially in children
- you may get drowsy
- avoid alcoholic drinks
- alcohol, sedatives, and tranquilizers may increase drowsiness
- be careful when driving a motor vehicle or operating machinery

### STOP USE AND ASK A DOCTOR IF
- an allergic reaction occurs. Seek medical help right away
- you experience any of the following signs of stomach bleeding:
  - feel faint
  - vomit blood
  - have bloody or black stools
  - have stomach pain that does not get better
- pain or nasal congestion gets worse or lasts more than 7 days
- fever gets worse or lasts more than 3 days
- redness or swelling is present
- new symptoms occur
- ringing in the ears or a loss of hearing occurs
- nervousness, dizziness, or sleeplessness occurs

**If pregnant or breastfeeding,** ask a health professional before use.

**It is especially important not to use aspirin during the last 3 months of pregnancy unless definitely directed to do so by a doctor because it may cause problems in the unborn child or complications during delivery.**

**Keep out of reach of children.** In case of overdose, get medical help or contact a Poison Control Center right away.

### DIRECTIONS

| adults and children 12 years and over | take 2 tablets fully dissolved in 4 ounces of water every 4 hours |
| | do not exceed 8 tablets in 24 hours or as directed by a doctor |
| children under 12 years | do not use |

### OTHER INFORMATION
- each tablet contains: sodium 476 mg
- **Phenylketonurics:** contains phenylalanine 10 mg per tablet
- store at room temperature. Avoid excessive heat

### INACTIVE INGREDIENTS
acesulfame potassium, anhydrous citric acid, aspartame, calcium silicate, dimethylpolysiloxane, docusate sodium, FD&C red no. 40, flavors, mannitol, povidone, sodium benzoate, sodium bicarbonate

### QUESTIONS OR COMMENTS
Call 1 -800-986-0369 (Mon-Fri 9 AM-5 PM EST) or www.alkaseltzerplus.com

---

## ALKA-SELTZER PLUS COLD AND COUGH
(acetaminophen, dextromethorphan hydrobromide, chlorpheniramine maleate, and phenylephrine hydrochloride) capsule, liquid filled effervescent
Bayer HealthCare

### DRUG FACTS

| Active ingredients (in each capsule) | Purpose |
| --- | --- |
| Acetaminophen 325 mg | Pain reliever/fever reducer |
| Chlorpheniramine maleate 2 mg | Antihistamine |
| Dextromethorphan hydrobromide 10 mg | Cough suppressant |
| Phenylephrine hydrochloride 5 mg | Nasal decongestant |

## USES

- temporarily relieves these symptoms due to a cold or flu:
  - minor aches and pains
  - headache
  - nasal and sinus congestion
  - cough
  - runny nose
  - sneezing
  - sore throat
- temporarily reduces fever

## WARNINGS
### Liver warning
This product contains acetaminophen. Severe liver damage may occur if you take:
- more than 12 capsules in 24 hours, which is the maximum daily amount
- with other drugs containing acetaminophen
- 3 or more alcoholic drinks every day while using this product

### Sore throat warning
If sore throat is severe, persists for more than 2 days, is accompanied or followed by fever, headache, rash, nausea, or vomiting, consult a doctor promptly.

**Do not use to sedate children.**

## DO NOT USE
- with any other drug containing acetaminophen (prescription or nonprescription). If you are not sure whether a drug contains acetaminophen, ask a doctor or pharmacist
- if you are now taking a prescription monoamine oxidase inhibitor (MAOI) (certain drugs for depression, psychiatric, or emotional conditions, or Parkinson's disease), or for 2 weeks after stopping the MAOI drug. If you do not know if your prescription drug contains an MAOI, ask a doctor or pharmacist before taking this product
- in children under 12 years of age

## ASK A DOCTOR BEFORE USE IF YOU HAVE
- liver disease
- heart disease
- high blood pressure
- thyroid disease
- diabetes
- glaucoma
- cough with excessive phlegm (mucus)
- a breathing problem such as emphysema or chronic bronchitis
- difficulty in urination due to enlargement of the prostate gland
- persistent or chronic cough such as occurs with smoking, asthma, or emphysema

## ASK A DOCTOR OR PHARMACIST BEFORE USE IF YOU ARE
- taking the blood thinning drug warfarin
- taking sedatives or tranquilizers

## WHEN USING THIS PRODUCT
- do not exceed recommended dosage
- may cause marked drowsiness
- avoid alcoholic drinks
- alcohol, sedatives, and tranquilizers may increase drowsiness
- be careful when driving a motor vehicle or operating machinery
- excitability may occur, especially in children

## STOP USE AND ASK A DOCTOR IF
- pain, cough, or nasal congestion gets worse or lasts more than 7 days
- fever gets worse or lasts more than 3 days
- redness or swelling is present
- new symptoms occur
- cough comes back or occurs with rash or headache that lasts. These could be signs of a serious condition
- nervousness, dizziness, or sleeplessness occurs

**If pregnant or breastfeeding,** ask a health professional before use.

**Keep out of reach of children.** In case of overdose, get medical help or contact a Poison Control Center right away. Quick medical attention is critical for adults as well as for children even if you do not notice any signs or symptoms.

## DIRECTIONS
- do not take more than the recommended dose

| adults and children 12 years and over | take 2 capsules with water every 4 hours<br><br>do not exceed 12 capsules in 24 hours or as directed by a doctor |
|---|---|
| children under 12 years | do not use |

## OTHER INFORMATION
- store at room temperature
- avoid excessive heat

## INACTIVE INGREDIENTS
butylated hydroxyanisole, butylated hydroxytoluene, D&C red no. 33, FD&C blue no. 1, gelatin, glycerin, hypromellose, mannitol, polyethylene glycol 400, polyethylene glycol 600, povidone, propylene glycol, purified water, sorbitan, sorbitol, titanium dioxide

## QUESTIONS OR COMMENTS
Call **1-800-986-0369** (Mon-Fri 9 AM-5 PM EST) or visit www.alkaseltzerplus.com

---

# ALKA-SELTZER PLUS DAY & NIGHT COLD FORMULA (aspirin, dextromethorphan hydrobromide, and phenylephrine bitartrate)
Bayer HealthCare

# DAY FORMULA
## DRUG FACTS

| Active ingredients (in each tablet) | Purpose |
|---|---|
| Aspirin 325 mg (NSAID)* | Pain reliever/fever reducer |
| Dextromethorphan hydrobromide 10 mg | Cough suppressant |
| Phenylephrine bitartrate 7.8 mg | Nasal decongestant |

*nonsteroidal anti-inflammatory drug

## USES
- temporarily relieves these symptoms due to a cold with cough:
  - minor aches and pains
  - headache
  - cough
  - nasal and sinus congestion
  - sore throat
- temporarily reduces fever

## WARNINGS

### Reye's syndrome

Children and teenagers who have or are recovering from chicken pox or flu-like symptoms should not use this product. When using this product, if changes in behavior with nausea and vomiting occur, consult a doctor because these symptoms could be an early sign of Reye's syndrome, a rare but serious illness.

### Allergy alert

Aspirin may cause a severe allergic reaction which may include:
- hives
- facial swelling
- asthma (wheezing)
- shock

### Stomach bleeding warning

This product contains an NSAID, which may cause severe stomach bleeding. The chance is higher if you:
- are age 60 or older
- have had stomach ulcers or bleeding problems
- take a blood thinning (anticoagulant) or steroid drug
- take other drugs containing prescription or nonprescription NSAIDs (aspirin, ibuprofen, naproxen, or others)
- have 3 or more alcoholic drinks every day while using this product
- take more or for a longer time than directed

### Sore throat warning

If sore throat is severe, persists for more than 2 days, is accompanied or followed by fever, headache, rash, nausea, or vomiting, consult a doctor promptly.

## DO NOT USE

- if you are allergic to aspirin or any other pain reliever/fever reducer
- if you are now taking a prescription monoamine oxidase inhibitor (MAOI) (certain drugs for depression, psychiatric, or emotional conditions, or Parkinson's disease), or for 2 weeks after stopping the MAOI drug. If you do not know if your prescription drug contains an MAOI, ask a doctor or pharmacist before taking this product
- in children under 12 years of age

## ASK A DOCTOR BEFORE USE IF

- stomach bleeding warning applies to you
- you have a history of stomach problems, such as heartburn
- you have high blood pressure, heart disease, liver cirrhosis, or kidney disease
- you are taking a diuretic
- you have:
  - asthma
  - thyroid disease
  - diabetes
  - cough with excessive phlegm (mucus)
  - difficulty in urination due to enlargement of the prostate gland
  - persistent or chronic cough such as occurs with smoking, asthma, or emphysema
  - a sodium-restricted diet

## ASK A DOCTOR OR PHARMACIST BEFORE USE IF YOU ARE

- taking a prescription drug for:
  - gout
  - diabetes
  - arthritis

## WHEN USING THIS PRODUCT

- do not exceed recommended dosage

## STOP USE AND ASK A DOCTOR IF

- an allergic reaction occurs. Seek medical help right away
- you experience any of the following signs of stomach bleeding
  - feel faint
  - vomit blood
  - have bloody or black stools
  - have stomach pain that does not get better
- pain, cough, or nasal congestion gets worse or lasts more than 7 days
- fever gets worse or lasts more than 3 days
- redness or swelling is present
- new symptoms occur
- ringing in the ears or loss of hearing occurs
- cough comes back or occurs with rash or headache that lasts. These could be signs of a serious condition
- nervousness, dizziness, or sleeplessness occurs

**If pregnant or breastfeeding,** ask a health professional before use.

**It is especially important not to use aspirin during the last 3 months of pregnancy unless definitely directed to do so by a doctor because it may cause problems in the unborn child or complications during delivery.**

**Keep out of reach of children.** In case of overdose, get medical help or contact a Poison Control Center right away.

## DIRECTIONS

| adults and children 12 years and over | take 2 tablets fully dissolved in 4 ounces of water every 4 hours |
| | do not exceed 8 tablets in 24 hours or as directed by a doctor |
| children under 12 years | do not use |

## OTHER INFORMATION

- each tablet contains: sodium 416 mg
- **Phenylketonurics:** contains phenylalanine 9 mg per tablet
- store at room temperature. Avoid excessive heat

## INACTIVE INGREDIENTS

acesulfame potassium, anhydrous citric acid, aspartame, calcium silicate, dimethylpolysiloxane, docusate sodium, flavors, mannitol, povidone, sodium benzoate, sodium bicarbonate

## QUESTIONS OR COMMENTS

Call **1-800-986-0369** (Mon-Fri 9 AM-5 PM EST) or www.alkaseltzerplus.com

# NIGHT FORMULA

## DRUG FACTS

| Active ingredients (in each tablet) | Purpose |
| --- | --- |
| Aspirin 500 mg (NSAID)* | Pain reliever/fever reducer |
| Dextromethorphan hydrobromide 10 mg | Cough suppressant |
| Doxylamine succinate 6.25 mg | Antihistamine |
| Phenylephrine bitartrate 7.8 mg | Nasal decongestant |

*nonsteroidal anti-inflammatory drug

## USES

- temporarily relieves these symptoms due to a cold:
  - minor aches and pains
  - headache
  - runny nose
  - sinus congestion and pressure

- cough
- sneezing
- sore throat
- nasal congestion
- temporarily reduces fever

## WARNINGS
### Reye's syndrome
Children and teenagers who have or are recovering from chicken pox or flu-like symptoms should not use this product. When using this product, if changes in behavior with nausea and vomiting occur, consult a doctor because these symptoms could be an early sign of Reye's syndrome, a rare but serious illness.

### Allergy alert
Aspirin may cause a severe allergic reaction which may include:
- hives
- facial swelling
- asthma (wheezing)
- shock

### Stomach bleeding warning
This product contains an NSAID, which may cause severe stomach bleeding. The chance is higher if you:
- are age 60 or older
- have had stomach ulcers or bleeding problems
- take a blood thinning (anticoagulant) or steroid drug
- take other drugs containing prescription or nonprescription NSAIDs (aspirin, ibuprofen, naproxen, or others)
- have 3 or more alcoholic drinks every day while using this product
- take more or for a longer time than directed

### Sore throat warning
- If sore throat is severe, persists for more than 2 days, is accompanied or followed by fever, headache, rash, nausea, or vomiting, consult a doctor promptly
- Do not use to sedate children

## DO NOT USE
- if you are allergic to aspirin or any other pain reliever/fever reducer
- if you are now taking a prescription monoamine oxidase inhibitor (MAOI) (certain drugs for depression, psychiatric, or emotional conditions, or Parkinson's disease), or for 2 weeks after stopping the MAOI drug. If you do not know if your prescription drug contains an MAOI, ask a doctor or pharmacist before taking this product.
- in children under 12 years of age

## ASK A DOCTOR BEFORE USE IF
- stomach bleeding warning applies to you
- you have a history of stomach problems, such as heartburn
- you have high blood pressure, heart disease, liver cirrhosis, or kidney disease
- you are taking a diuretic
- you have
  - asthma
  - diabetes
  - thyroid disease
  - glaucoma
  - cough with excessive phlegm (mucus)
  - a breathing problem such as emphysema or chronic bronchitis
  - difficulty in urination due to enlargement of the prostate gland
  - persistent or chronic cough such as occurs with smoking, asthma, or emphysema
  - a sodium-restricted diet

## ASK A DOCTOR OR PHARMACIST BEFORE USE IF YOU ARE
- taking a prescription drug for
  - gout
  - diabetes
  - arthritis
- taking sedatives or tranquilizers

## WHEN USING THIS PRODUCT
- do not exceed recommended dosage
- may cause marked drowsiness
- avoid alcoholic drinks
- alcohol, sedatives, and tranquilizers may increase drowsiness
- be careful when driving a motor vehicle or operating machinery
- excitability may occur, especially in children

## STOP USE AND ASK A DOCTOR IF
- an allergic reaction occurs. Seek medical help right away.
- you experience any of the following signs of stomach bleeding
  - feel faint
  - vomit blood
  - have bloody or black stools
  - have stomach pain that does not get better
- pain, cough, or nasal congestion gets worse or lasts more than 7 days
- fever gets worse or lasts more than 3 days
- redness or swelling is present
- new symptoms occur
- ringing in the ears or loss of hearing occurs
- cough comes back or occurs with rash or headache that lasts. These could be signs of a serious condition. nervousness, dizziness, or sleeplessness occurs

**If pregnant or breastfeeding,** ask a health professional before use.

**It is especially important not to use aspirin during the last 3 months of pregnancy unless definitely directed to do so by a doctor because it may cause problems in the unborn child or complications during delivery.**

**Keep out of reach of children.** In case of overdose, get medical help or contact a Poison Control Center right away.

## DIRECTIONS

| adults and children 12 years and over | take 2 tablets fully dissolved in 4 ounces of water at bedtime (may be taken every 4 to 6 hours) |
| --- | --- |
| | do not exceed 8 tablets in 24 hours or as directed by a doctor |
| children under 12 years | do not use |

## OTHER INFORMATION
- each tablet contains: sodium 474 mg
- **Phenylketonurics:** Contains phenylalanine 5.6 mg per tablet
- store at room temperature. Avoid excessive heat

## INACTIVE INGREDIENTS
acesulfame potassium, anhydrous citric acid, aspartame, calcium silicate, dimethylpolysiloxane, docusate sodium, flavors, mannitol, povidone, sodium benzoate, sodium bicarbonate

## QUESTIONS OR COMMENTS
Call **1-800-986-0369** (Mon-Fri 9 AM-5 PM EST) or www.alkaseltzerplus.com

# ALKA-SELTZER PLUS DAY NON-DROWSY COLD MEDICINE CITRUS (aspirin, dextromethorphan hydrobromide, and phenylephrine bitartrate) tablet, effervescent

Bayer HealthCare

## DRUG FACTS

| Active ingredients (in each tablet) | Purpose |
|---|---|
| Aspirin 325 mg | Pain reliever/fever reducer |
| Dextromethorphan hydrobromide 10 mg | Cough suppressant |
| Phenylephrine bitartrate 7.8 mg | Nasal decongestant |

## USES
- temporarily relieves these symptoms due to a cold or flu with cough:
  - minor aches and pains
  - nasal and sinus congestion
  - headache
  - sore throat
  - cough
- temporarily reduces fever

## WARNINGS
**Reye's syndrome**
Children and teenagers should not use this medicine for chicken pox or flu symptoms before a doctor is consulted about Reye's syndrome, a rare but serious illness reported to be associated with aspirin.

**Allergy alert**
Aspirin may cause a severe allergic reaction which may include:
- hives
- facial swelling
- asthma (wheezing)
- shock

**Alcohol warning**
If you consume 3 or more alcoholic drinks every day, ask your doctor whether you should take aspirin or other pain relievers/fever reducers. Aspirin may cause stomach bleeding.

**Sore throat warning**
If sore throat is severe, persists for more than 2 days, is accompanied or followed by fever, headache, rash, nausea, or vomiting, consult a doctor promptly.

## DO NOT USE
- if you are allergic to aspirin or any other pain reliever/fever reducer
- if you are now taking a prescription monoamine oxidase inhibitor (MAOI) (certain drugs for depression, psychiatric, or emotional conditions, or Parkinson's disease), or for 2 weeks after stopping the MAOI drug. If you do not know if your prescription drug contains an MAOI, ask a doctor or pharmacist before taking this product
- in children under 12 years of age

## ASK A DOCTOR BEFORE USE IF YOU HAVE
- stomach problems (such as heartburn, upset stomach, or stomach pain) that last or come back
- bleeding problems
- heart disease
- diabetes
- ulcers
- high blood pressure
- glaucoma
- asthma
- thyroid disease
- cough with excessive phlegm (mucus)
- difficulty in urination due to enlargement of the prostate gland
- persistent or chronic cough such as occurs with smoking, asthma, or emphysema
- a sodium-restricted diet

## ASK A DOCTOR OR PHARMACIST BEFORE USE IF YOU ARE
- taking a prescription drug for:
  - anticoagulation (blood thinning)
  - diabetes
  - gout
  - arthritis

## WHEN USING THIS PRODUCT
- do not exceed recommended dosage

## STOP USE AND ASK A DOCTOR IF
- an allergic reaction occurs. Seek medical help right away
- pain, cough, or nasal congestion gets worse or lasts more than 7 days
- fever gets worse or lasts more than 3 days
- redness or swelling is present
- new symptoms occur
- ringing in the ears or loss of hearing occurs
- cough comes back or occurs with rash or headache that lasts. These could be signs of a serious condition
- nervousness, dizziness, or sleeplessness occurs

**If pregnant or breastfeeding,** ask a health professional before use.

**It is especially important not to use aspirin during the last 3 months of pregnancy unless definitely directed to do so by a doctor because it may cause problems in the unborn child or complications during delivery.**

**Keep out of reach of children.** In case of overdose, get medical help or contact a Poison Control Center right away.

## DIRECTIONS

| adults and children 12 years and over | take 2 tablets fully dissolved in 4 ounces of water every 4 hours<br><br>do not exceed 8 tablets in 24 hours or as directed by a doctor |
|---|---|
| children under 12 years | do not use |

## OTHER INFORMATION
- each tablet contains: sodium 416 mg
- **Phenylketonurics:** contains phenylalanine 9 mg per tablet
- store at room temperature. Avoid excessive heat

## INACTIVE INGREDIENTS
acesulfame potassium, anhydrous citric acid, aspartame, calcium silicate, dimethylpolysiloxane, docusate sodium, flavors, mannitol, povidone, sodium benzoate, sodium bicarbonate

## QUESTIONS OR COMMENTS
Call **1-800-986-0369** (Mon-Fri 9 AM-5 PM EST) or visit www.alkaseltzerplus.com

## ALKA-SELTZER PLUS FAST CRYSTALS PACKS COLD FORMULA (acetaminophen, chlorpheniramine maleate, and phenylephrine hydrochloride) granule, effervescent

Bayer HealthCare

### DRUG FACTS

| Active ingredients (in each powder packet) | Purpose |
|---|---|
| Acetaminophen 650 mg | Pain reliever/fever reducer |
| Chlorpheniramine maleate 4 mg | Antihistamine |
| Phenylephrine hydrochloride 10 mg | Nasal decongestant |

### USES
- temporarily relieves these symptoms due to a cold:
  - minor aches and pains
  - headache
  - nasal and sinus congestion
  - runny nose
  - sneezing
  - sore throat
- temporarily reduces fever

### WARNINGS
**Alcohol warning**
If you consume 3 or more alcoholic drinks every day, ask your doctor whether you should take acetaminophen or other pain relievers/fever reducers. Acetaminophen may cause liver damage.

**Sore throat warning**
If sore throat is severe, persists for more than 2 days, is accompanied or followed by fever, headache, rash, nausea, or vomiting, consult a doctor promptly.

**Do not use to sedate children.**

### DO NOT USE
- with any other products containing acetaminophen
- if you are now taking a prescription monoamine oxidase inhibitor (MAOI) (certain drugs for depression, psychiatric, or emotional conditions, or Parkinson's disease), or for 2 weeks after stopping the MAOI drug. If you do not know if your prescription drug contains an MAOI, ask a doctor or pharmacist before taking this product
- in children under 12 years of age

### ASK A DOCTOR BEFORE USE IF YOU HAVE
- heart disease
- high blood pressure
- diabetes
- thyroid disease
- glaucoma
- difficulty in urination due to enlargement of the prostate gland
- a breathing problem such as emphysema or chronic bronchitis

### ASK A DOCTOR OR PHARMACIST BEFORE USE IF YOU ARE
- taking sedatives or tranquilizers

### WHEN USING THIS PRODUCT
- do not exceed recommended dosage
- excitability may occur, especially in children
- you may get drowsy
- avoid alcoholic drinks
- alcohol, sedatives, and tranquilizers may increase drowsiness
- be careful when driving a motor vehicle or operating machinery

### STOP USE AND ASK A DOCTOR IF
- pain or nasal congestion gets worse or lasts more than 7 days
- fever gets worse or lasts more than 3 days
- redness or swelling is present
- new symptoms occur
- nervousness, dizziness, or sleeplessness occurs

**If pregnant or breastfeeding,** ask a health professional before use.

**Keep out of reach of children.**

### OVERDOSE WARNING
Taking more than the recommended dose can cause serious health problems. In case of overdose, get medical help or contact a Poison Control Center right away. Quick medical attention is critical for adults as well as for children even if you do not notice any signs or symptoms.

### DIRECTIONS
- do not take more than the recommended dose (see Overdose Warning)

| adults and children 12 years and over | dissolve contents of 1 powder packet in 6-8 ounces of hot or cold beverage: juice, soda, tea, coffee, or water<br><br>consume entire beverage within 15 minutes<br><br>take every 4 hours as needed<br><br>do not exceed 6 powder packets in 24 hours |
|---|---|
| children under 12 years | do not use |

### OTHER INFORMATION
- **Phenylketonurics:** contains phenylalanine 6 mg per powder packet
- store at room temperature

### INACTIVE INGREDIENTS
acesulfame potassium, aspartame, calcium silicate, citric acid, dimethicone, docusate sodium, flavor, povidone, sucralose, sucrose

### QUESTIONS OR COMMENTS
Call **1-800-986-0369** (Mon-Fri 9 AM-5 PM EST) or visit www.alkaseltzerplus.com

---

## ALKA-SELTZER PLUS FAST PACKS COLD AND FLU FORMULA (acetaminophen, chlorpheniramine maleate, and phenylephrine hydrochloride) granule, effervescent

Bayer HealthCare

### DRUG FACTS

| Active ingredients (in each powder packet) | Purpose |
|---|---|
| Acetaminophen 650 mg | Pain reliever/fever reducer |
| Chlorpheniramine maleate 4 mg | Antihistamine |
| Phenylephrine hydrochloride 10 mg | Nasal decongestant |

## USES
- temporarily relieves these symptoms due to a cold or flu:
  - minor aches and pains
  - headache
  - nasal and sinus congestion
  - runny nose
  - sneezing
  - sore throat
- temporarily reduces fever

## WARNINGS
### Liver warning
This product contains acetaminophen. Severe liver damage may occur if you take:
- more than 5 powder packets in 24 hours, which is the maximum daily amount for this product
- with other drugs containing acetaminophen
- 3 or more alcoholic drinks every day while using this product

### Sore throat warning
If sore throat is severe, persists for more than 2 days, is accompanied or followed by fever, headache, rash, nausea, or vomiting, consult a doctor promptly.

### Do not use to sedate children.

## DO NOT USE
- with any other drug containing acetaminophen (prescription or nonprescription). If you are not sure whether a drug contains acetaminophen, ask a doctor or pharmacist
- if you are now taking a prescription monoamine oxidase inhibitor (MAOI) (certain drugs for depression, psychiatric, or emotional conditions, or Parkinson's disease), or for 2 weeks after stopping the MAOI drug. If you do not know if your prescription drug contains an MAOI, ask a doctor or pharmacist before taking this product
- in children under 12 years of age

## ASK A DOCTOR BEFORE USE IF YOU HAVE
- liver disease
- heart disease
- high blood pressure
- diabetes
- thyroid disease
- glaucoma
- difficulty in urination due to enlargement of the prostate gland
- a breathing problem such as emphysema or chronic bronchitis

## ASK A DOCTOR OR PHARMACIST BEFORE USE IF YOU ARE
- taking the blood thinning drug warfarin
- taking sedatives or tranquilizers

## WHEN USING THIS PRODUCT
- do not exceed recommended dosage
- excitability may occur, especially in children
- you may get drowsy
- avoid alcoholic drinks
- alcohol, sedatives, and tranquilizers may increase drowsiness
- be careful when driving a motor vehicle or operating machinery

## STOP USE AND ASK A DOCTOR IF
- pain or nasal congestion gets worse or lasts more than 7 days
- fever gets worse or lasts more than 3 days
- redness or swelling is present
- new symptoms occur
- nervousness, dizziness, or sleeplessness occurs

**If pregnant or breastfeeding,** ask a health professional before use.

**Keep out of reach of children.** In case of overdose, get medical help or contact a Poison Control Center right away. Quick medical attention is critical for adults as well as for children even if you do not notice any signs or symptoms.

## DIRECTIONS

| adults and children 12 years and over | dissolve contents of 1 powder packet in 6-8 ounces of hot or cold beverage: juice, tea, black coffee, or water |
|---|---|
|  | consume entire beverage within 15 minutes |
|  | take every 4 hours as needed |
|  | do not exceed 5 powder packets in 24 hours |
| children under 12 years | do not use |

## OTHER INFORMATION
- **Phenylketonurics:** contains phenylalanine 6 mg per powder packet
- store at room temperature

## INACTIVE INGREDIENTS
acesulfame potassium, anhydrous citric acid, aspartame, calcium silicate, dimethicone, docusate sodium, flavor, povidone, sucralose, sucrose

## QUESTIONS OR COMMENTS
Call **1-800-986-0369** (Mon-Fri 9 AM-5 PM EST) or visit www.alkaseltzerplus.com

---

# ALKA-SELTZER PLUS FLU FORMULA
(acetaminophen, chlorpheniramine maleate, phenylephrine hydrochloride, and dextromethorphan hydrobromide) tablet, effervescent

Bayer HealthCare

## DRUG FACTS

| Active ingredients (in each tablet) | Purpose |
|---|---|
| Acetaminophen 250 mg | Pain reliever/fever reducer |
| Chlorpheniramine maleate 2 mg | Antihistamine |
| Dextromethorphan hydrobromide 10 mg | Cough suppressant |
| Phenylephrine hydrochloride 5 mg | Nasal decongestant |

## USES
- temporarily relieves these symptoms due to a cold or flu:
  - minor aches and pains
  - headache
  - cough
  - sore throat
  - runny nose
  - sneezing
  - nasal and sinus congestion
- temporarily reduces fever

## WARNINGS
### Liver warning
This product contains acetaminophen. Severe liver damage may occur if you take:
- more than 8 tablets in 24 hours, which is the maximum daily amount for this product

- with other drugs containing acetaminophen
- 3 or more alcoholic drinks every day while using this product

**Sore throat warning**
If sore throat is severe, persists for more than 2 days, is accompanied or followed by fever, headache, rash, nausea, or vomiting, consult a doctor promptly.

**Do not use to sedate children**

**DO NOT USE**
- with any other drug containing acetaminophen (prescription or nonprescription). If you are not sure whether a drug contains acetaminophen, ask a doctor or pharmacist
- if you are now taking a prescription monoamine oxidase inhibitor (MAOI) (certain drugs for depression, psychiatric, or emotional conditions, or Parkinson's disease), or for 2 weeks after stopping the MAOI drug. If you do not know if your prescription drug contains an MAOI, ask a doctor or pharmacist before taking this product
- in children under 12 years of age

**ASK A DOCTOR BEFORE USE IF YOU HAVE**
- liver disease
- heart disease
- high blood pressure
- thyroid disease
- diabetes
- glaucoma
- cough with excessive phlegm (mucus)
- a breathing problem such as emphysema or chronic bronchitis
- difficulty in urination due to enlargement of the prostate gland
- persistent or chronic cough such as occurs with smoking, asthma, or emphysema
- a sodium restricted diet

**ASK A DOCTOR OR PHARMACIST BEFORE USE IF YOU ARE**
- taking the blood thinning drug warfarin
- taking sedatives or tranquilizers

**WHEN USING THIS PRODUCT**
- do not exceed recommended dosage
- may cause marked drowsiness
- avoid alcoholic drinks
- alcohol, sedatives, and tranquilizers may increase drowsiness
- be careful when driving a motor vehicle or operating machinery
- excitability may occur, especially in children

**STOP USE AND ASK A DOCTOR IF**
- pain, cough, or nasal congestion gets worse or lasts more than 7 days
- fever gets worse or lasts more than 3 days
- redness or swelling is present
- new symptoms occur
- cough comes back or occurs with rash or headache that lasts. These could be signs of a serious condition
- nervousness, dizziness, or sleeplessness occurs

**If pregnant or breastfeeding,** ask a health professional before use.

**Keep out of reach of children.** In case of overdose, get medical help or contact a Poison Control Center right away. Quick medical attention is critical for adults as well as for children even if you do not notice any signs or symptoms.

**DIRECTIONS**
- do not take more than the recommended dose

| | |
|---|---|
| adults and children 12 years and over | take 2 tablets fully dissolved in 4 ounces of water every 4 hours |
| | do not exceed 8 tablets in 24 hours or as directed by a doctor |
| children under 12 years | do not use |

**OTHER INFORMATION**
- each tablet contains: sodium 416 mg
- **Phenylketonurics:** Contain phenylalanine 5.6 mg per tablet
- store at room temperature. Avoid excessive heat

**INACTIVE INGREDIENTS**
acesulfame potassium, anhydrous citric acid, aspartame, FD&C red no. 40, flavors, magnesium stearate, maltodextrin, mannitol, saccharin sodium, sodium bicarbonate

**QUESTIONS OR COMMENTS**
Call **1-800-986-0369** (Mon-Fri 9 AM-5 PM EST) or visit www.alkaseltzerplus.com

# ALKA-SELTZER PLUS MUCUS & CONGESTION (dextromethorphan hydrobromide and guaifenesin) liquid filled capsules
Bayer HealthCare

## DRUG FACTS

| Active ingredients (in each capsule) | Purpose |
|---|---|
| Dextromethorphan hydrobromide 10 mg | Cough suppressant |
| Guaifenesin 200 mg | Expectorant |

**USES**
- helps loosen phlegm (mucus) and thin bronchial secretions to rid the bronchial passageways of bothersome mucus and make coughs more productive
- temporarily relieves:
  - cough due to minor throat and bronchial irritation as may occur with a cold
  - the intensity of coughing
  - the impulse to cough to help you get to sleep

**WARNINGS**

**DO NOT USE**
- if you are now taking a prescription monoamine oxidase inhibitor (MAOI) (certain drugs for depression, psychiatric, or emotional conditions, or Parkinson's disease), or for 2 weeks after stopping the MAOI drug. If you do not know if your prescription drug contains an MAOI, ask a doctor or pharmacist before taking this product
- in children under 12 years of age

**ASK A DOCTOR BEFORE USE IF YOU HAVE**
- cough with excessive phlegm (mucus)
- persistent or chronic cough such as occurs with smoking, asthma, chronic bronchitis, or emphysema

**STOP USE AND ASK A DOCTOR IF**
- cough lasts more than 7 days, comes back, or is accompanied by a fever, rash, or persistent headache. These could be signs of a serious condition

**If pregnant or breastfeeding,** ask a health professional before use.

**Keep out of reach of children.** In case of overdose, get medical help or contact a Poison Control Center right away.

## DIRECTIONS
• do not take more than the recommended dose

| adults and children 12 years and over | take 2 capsules every 4 to 6 hours |
|---|---|
| | do not exceed 12 capsules in 24 hours |
| children under 12 years | do not use |

## OTHER INFORMATION
• store at room temperature
• avoid excessive heat

## INACTIVE INGREDIENTS
FD&C blue no. 1, FD&C red no. 40, gelatin, glycerin, hypromellose, mannitol, polyethlene glycol 400, polyethylene glycol 600, providone, propylene glycol, purified water, sorbitol, titanium dioxide

## QUESTIONS OR COMMENTS
Call **1-800-986-0369** (Mon-Fri 9 AM-5 PM EST) or www.alkaseltzerplus.com

---

# ALKA-SELTZER PLUS NIGHT COLD FORMULA (aspirin, doxylamine succinate, phenylephrine bitartrate, and dextromethorphan hydrobromide) tablet, effervescent

Bayer HealthCare

## DRUG FACTS

| Active ingredients (in each tablet) | Purpose |
|---|---|
| Aspirin 500 mg | Pain reliever/fever reducer |
| Dextromethorphan hydrobromide 10 mg | Cough suppressant |
| Doxylamine succinate 6.25 mg | Antihistamine |
| Phenylephrine bitartrate 7.8 mg | Nasal decongestant |

## USES
• temporarily relieves these symptoms due to a cold:
  • minor aches and pains
  • sinus congestion and pressure
  • sore throat
  • headache
  • cough
  • nasal congestion
  • runny nose
  • sneezing
• temporarily reduces fever

## WARNINGS
### Reye's syndrome
Children and teenagers should not use this medicine for chicken pox or flu symptoms before a doctor is consulted about Reye's syndrome, a rare but serious illness reported to be associated with aspirin.

### Allergy alert
Aspirin may cause a severe allergic reaction which may include:
• hives
• facial swelling
• asthma (wheezing)
• shock

### Alcohol warning
If you consume 3 or more alcoholic drinks every day, ask your doctor whether you should take aspirin or other pain relievers/fever reducers. Aspirin may cause stomach bleeding.

### Sore throat warning
If sore throat is severe, persists for more than 2 days, is accompanied or followed by fever, headache, rash, nausea, or vomiting, consult a doctor promptly.

**Do not use to sedate children.**

## DO NOT USE
• if you are allergic to aspirin or any other pain reliever/fever reducer
• if you are now taking a prescription monoamine oxidase inhibitor (MAOI) (certain drugs for depression, psychiatric, or emotional conditions, or Parkinson's disease), or for 2 weeks after stopping the MAOI drug. If you do not know if your prescription drug contains an MAOI, ask a doctor or pharmacist before taking this product
• in children under 12 years of age

## ASK A DOCTOR BEFORE USE IF YOU HAVE
• stomach problems (such as heartburn, upset stomach, or stomach pain) that last or come back
• bleeding problems
• ulcers
• asthma
• heart disease
• high blood pressure
• diabetes
• thyroid disease
• glaucoma
• cough with excessive phlegm (mucus)
• a breathing problem such as emphysema or chronic bronchitis
• difficulty in urination due to enlargement of the prostate gland
• persistent or chronic cough such as occurs with smoking, asthma, or emphysema
• a sodium-restricted diet

## ASK A DOCTOR OR PHARMACIST BEFORE USE IF YOU ARE
• taking a prescription drug for
  • anticoagulation (blood thinning)
  • diabetes
  • gout
  • arthritis
• taking sedatives or tranquilizers

## WHEN USING THIS PRODUCT
• **do not exceed recommended dosage**
• may cause marked drowsiness
• avoid alcoholic drinks
• alcohol, sedatives, and tranquilizers may increase drowsiness
• be careful when driving a motor vehicle or operating machinery
• excitability may occur, especially in children

## STOP USE AND ASK A DOCTOR IF
• an allergic reaction occurs. Seek medical help right away
• pain, cough, or nasal congestion gets worse or lasts more than 7 days
• fever gets worse or lasts more than 3 days
• redness or swelling is present
• new symptoms occur
• ringing in the ears or loss of hearing occurs
• cough comes back or occurs with rash or headache that lasts. These could be signs of a serious condition
• nervousness, dizziness, or sleeplessness occurs

**If pregnant or breastfeeding,** ask a health professional before use.

**It is especially important not to use aspirin during the last 3 months of pregnancy unless definitely directed to do so by a doctor because it may cause problems in the unborn child or complications during delivery.**

**Keep out of reach of children.** In case of overdose, get medical help or contact a Poison Control Center right away.

## DIRECTIONS

| adults and children 12 years and over | take 2 tablets fully dissolved in 4 ounces of water at bedtime (may be taken every 4 to 6 hours) |
| | do not exceed 8 tablets in 24 hours or as directed by a doctor |
| children under 12 years | do not use |

## OTHER INFORMATION
- each tablet contains: sodium 474 mg
- **Phenylketonurics:** contains phenylalanine 5.6 mg per tablet
- store at room temperature. Avoid excessive heat

## INACTIVE INGREDIENTS
acesulfame potassium, anhydrous citric acid, aspartame, calcium silicate, dimethylpolysiloxane, docusate sodium, flavors, mannitol, povidone, sodium benzoate, sodium bicarbonate

## QUESTIONS OR COMMENTS
Call **1-800-986-0369** (Mon-Fri 9 AM-5 PM EST) or visit www.alkaseltzerplus.com

## ALKA-SELTZER PLUS ORANGE ZEST COLD FORMULA (aspirin, chlorpheniramine maleate, and phenylephrine bitartrate) tablet, effervescent
Bayer HealthCare LLC

## DRUG FACTS

| Active ingredients (in each tablet) | Purpose |
| --- | --- |
| Aspirin 325 mg (NSAID)* | Pain reliever/fever reducer |
| Chlorpheniramine maleate 2 mg | Antihistamine |
| Phenylephrine bitartrate 7.8 mg | Nasal decongestant |

*nonsteroidal anti-inflammatory drug

## USES
- temporarily relieves these symptoms due to a cold:
  - minor aches and pains
  - headache
  - runny nose
  - nasal and sinus congestion
  - sneezing
  - sore throat
- temporarily reduces fever

## WARNINGS
### Reye's syndrome
Children and teenagers who have or are recovering from chicken pox or flu-like symptoms should not use this product. When using this product, if changes in behavior with nausea and vomiting occur, consult a doctor because these symptoms could be an early sign of Reye's syndrome, a rare but serious illness.

### Allergy alert
Aspirin may cause a severe allergic reaction which may include:
- hives
- facial swelling
- asthma (wheezing)
- shock

### Stomach bleeding warning
This product contains an NSAID, which may cause severe stomach bleeding. The chance is higher if you:
- are age 60 or older
- have had stomach ulcers or bleeding problems
- take a blood thinning (anticoagulant) or steroid drug
- take other drugs containing prescription or nonprescription NSAIDs (aspirin, ibuprofen, naproxen, or others)
- have 3 or more alcoholic drinks every day while using this product
- take more or for a longer time than directed

### Sore throat warning
If sore throat is severe, persists for more than 2 days, is accompanied or followed by fever, headache, rash, nausea, or vomiting, consult a doctor promptly.

**Do not use to sedate children.**

### DO NOT USE
- if you are allergic to aspirin or any other pain reliever/fever reducer
- if you are now taking a prescription monoamine oxidase inhibitor (MAOI) (certain drugs for depression, psychiatric, or emotional conditions, or Parkinson's disease), or for 2 weeks after stopping the MAOI drug. If you do not know if your prescription drug contains an MAOI, ask a doctor or pharmacist before taking this product
- in children under 12 years of age

### ASK A DOCTOR BEFORE USE IF
- stomach bleeding warning applies to you
- you have a history of stomach problems, such as heartburn
- you have high blood pressure, heart disease, liver cirrhosis, or kidney disease
- you are taking a diuretic
- you have:
  - asthma
  - diabetes
  - thyroid disease
  - glaucoma
  - difficulty in urination due to enlargement of the prostate gland
  - a breathing problem such as emphysema or chronic bronchitis
  - a sodium-restricted diet

### ASK A DOCTOR OR PHARMACIST BEFORE USE IF YOU ARE
- taking a prescription drug for:
  - gout
  - diabetes
  - arthritis
- taking sedatives or tranquilizers

### WHEN USING THIS PRODUCT
- do not exceed recommended dosage
- excitability may occur, especially in children
- you may get drowsy
- avoid alcoholic drinks
- alcohol, sedatives, and tranquilizers may increase drowsiness
- be careful when driving a motor vehicle or operating machinery

### STOP USE AND ASK A DOCTOR IF
- an allergic reaction occurs. Seek medical help right away
- you experience any of the following signs of stomach bleeding:
  - feel faint
  - vomit blood
  - have bloody or black stools

- have stomach pain that does not get better
- pain or nasal congestion gets worse or lasts more than 7 days
- fever gets worse or lasts more than 3 days
- redness or swelling is present
- new symptoms occur
- ringing in the ears or a loss of hearing occurs
- nervousness, dizziness, or sleeplessness occurs

**If pregnant or breastfeeding,** ask a health professional before use.

**It is especially important not to use aspirin during the last 3 months of pregnancy unless definitely directed to do so by a doctor because it may cause problems in the unborn child or complications during delivery.**

**Keep out of reach of children.** In case of overdose, get medical help or contact a Poison Control Center right away.

## DIRECTIONS

| adults and children 12 years and over | take 2 tablets fully dissolved in 4 ounces of water every 4 hours |
| | do not exceed 8 tablets in 24 hours or as directed by a doctor |
| children under 12 years | do not use |

## OTHER INFORMATION
- each tablet contains: sodium 476 mg
- **Phenylketonurics:** contains phenylalanine 9 mg per tablet
- store at room temperature. Avoid excessive heat

## INACTIVE INGREDIENTS
acesulfame potassium, anhydrous citric acid, aspartame, calcium silicate, dimethylpolysiloxane, docusate sodium, FD&C red no. 40, FD&C yellow no. 6, flavors, mannitol, povidone, sodium benzoate, sodium bicarbonate

## QUESTIONS OR COMMENTS
Call **1-800-986-0369** (Mon-Fri 9 AM-5 PM EST) or www.alkaseltzerplus.com

---

# ALKA-SELTZER PLUS SEVERE SINUS CONGESTION AND COUGH (acetaminophen, dextromethorphan hydrobromide, and phenylephrine hydrochloride) capsule, liquid filled
Bayer HealthCare

## DRUG FACTS

| Active ingredients (in each capsule) | Purpose |
| --- | --- |
| Acetaminophen 325 mg | Pain reliever/fever reducer |
| Dextromethorphan hydrobromide 10 mg | Cough suppressant |
| Phenylephrine hydrochloride 5 mg | Nasal decongestant |

## USES
- temporarily relieves these symptoms due to a cold or flu:
  - minor aches and pains
  - headache
  - cough
  - sore throat
  - nasal congestion
- temporarily relieves sinus congestion and pressure
- helps clear nasal passages and shrinks swollen membranes

- temporarily reduces fever

## WARNINGS
**Liver warning**
This product contains acetaminophen. Severe liver damage may occur if you take:
- more than 12 capsules in 24 hours, which is the maximum daily amount
- with other drugs containing acetaminophen
- 3 or more alcoholic drinks every day while using this product

**Sore throat warning**
If sore throat is severe, persists for more than 2 days, is accompanied or followed by fever, headache, rash, nausea, or vomiting, consult a doctor promptly.

## DO NOT USE
- with any other drug containing acetaminophen (prescription or nonprescription). If you are not sure whether a drug contains acetaminophen, ask a doctor or pharmacist
- if you are now taking a prescription monoamine oxidase inhibitor (MAOI) (certain drugs for depression, psychiatric, or emotional conditions, or Parkinson's disease), or for 2 weeks after stopping the MAOI drug. If you do not know if your prescription drug contains an MAOI, ask a doctor or pharmacist before taking this product
- in children under 12 years of age

## ASK A DOCTOR BEFORE USE IF YOU HAVE
- liver disease
- heart disease
- high blood pressure
- thyroid disease
- diabetes
- cough with excessive phlegm (mucus)
- difficulty in urination due to enlargement of the prostate gland
- persistent or chronic cough such as occurs with smoking, asthma, or emphysema

## ASK A DOCTOR OR PHARMACIST BEFORE USE IF YOU ARE
- taking the blood thinning drug warfarin

## WHEN USING THIS PRODUCT
- do not exceed recommended dosage

## STOP USE AND ASK A DOCTOR IF
- pain, cough, or nasal congestion gets worse or lasts more than 7 days
- fever gets worse or lasts more than 3 days
- redness or swelling is present
- new symptoms occur
- cough comes back or occurs with rash or headache that lasts. These could be signs of a serious condition
- nervousness, dizziness, or sleeplessness occurs

**If pregnant or breastfeeding,** ask a health professional before use.

**Keep out of reach of children.** In case of overdose, get medical help or contact a Poison Control Center right away. Quick medical attention is critical for adults as well as for children even if you do not notice any signs or symptoms.

## DIRECTIONS
- do not take more than the recommended dose

| adults and children 12 years and over | take 2 capsules with water every 4 hours |
| | do not exceed 12 capsules in 24 hours or as directed by a doctor |
| children under 12 years | do not use |

## OTHER INFORMATION
- store at room temperature
- avoid excessive heat

## INACTIVE INGREDIENTS
FD&C blue no. 1, FD&C red no. 40, gelatin, glycerin, lecithin, mannitol, polyethylene glycol 400, povidone, propylene glycol, purified water, shellac, simethicone, sorbitan, sorbitol, titanium dioxide

## QUESTIONS OR COMMENTS
Call **1-800-986-0369** (Mon-Fri 9 AM-5 PM EST) or www.alkaseltzerplus.com

---

# ALKA-SELTZER PLUS SINUS FORMULA
(aspirin and phenylephrine bitartrate) tablet, effervescent

Bayer HealthCare

## DRUG FACTS

| Active ingredients (in each tablet) | Purpose |
|---|---|
| Aspirin 325 mg (NSAID)* | Pain reliever/fever reducer |
| Phenylephrine bitartrate 7.8 mg | Nasal decongestant |

*nonsteroidal anti-inflammatory drug

## USES
- temporarily relieves these symptoms due to a cold:
  - minor aches and pains
  - headache
  - nasal congestion
  - sinus congestion and pressure
- temporarily reduces fever

## WARNINGS
**Reye's syndrome**
Children and teenagers who have or are recovering from chicken pox or flu-like symptoms should not use this product. When using this product, if changes in behavior with nausea and vomiting occur, consult a doctor because these symptoms could be an early sign of Reye's syndrome, a rare but serious illness.

**Allergy alert**
Aspirin may cause a severe allergic reaction which may include:
- hives
- facial swelling
- asthma (wheezing)
- shock

**Stomach bleeding warning**
This product contains an NSAID, which may cause severe stomach bleeding. The chance is higher if you:
- are age 60 or older
- have had stomach ulcers or bleeding problems
- take a blood thinning (anticoagulant) or steroid drug
- take other drugs containing prescription or nonprescription NSAIDs (aspirin, ibuprofen, naproxen, or others)
- have 3 or more alcoholic drinks every day while using this product
- take more or for a longer time than directed

## DO NOT USE
- if you are allergic to aspirin or any other pain reliever/fever reducer
- if you are now taking a prescription monoamine oxidase inhibitor (MAOI) (certain drugs for depression, psychiatric, or emotional conditions, or Parkinson's disease), or for 2 weeks after stopping the MAOI drug. If you do not know if your prescription drug contains an MAOI, ask a doctor or pharmacist before taking this product

## ASK A DOCTOR BEFORE USE IF
- stomach bleeding warning applies to you
- you have a history of stomach problems, such as heartburn
- you have high blood pressure, heart disease, liver cirrhosis, or kidney disease
- you are taking a diuretic
- you have:
  - asthma
  - thyroid disease
  - diabetes
  - difficulty in urination due to enlargement of the prostate gland
  - a sodium-restricted diet

## ASK A DOCTOR OR PHARMACIST BEFORE USE IF YOU ARE
- taking a prescription drug for:
  - gout
  - diabetes
  - arthritis

## WHEN USING THIS PRODUCT
- do not exceed recommended dosage

## STOP USE AND ASK A DOCTOR IF
- an allergic reaction occurs. Seek medical help right away
- you experience any of the following signs of stomach bleeding:
  - feel faint
  - vomit blood
  - have bloody or black stools
  - have stomach pain that does not get better
- pain or nasal congestion gets worse or lasts more than 7 days
- fever gets worse or lasts more than 3 days
- redness or swelling is present
- new symptoms occur
- ringing in the ears or a loss of hearing occurs
- nervousness, dizziness, or sleeplessness occurs

**If pregnant or breastfeeding,** ask a health professional before use.

**It is especially important not to use aspirin during the last 3 months of pregnancy unless definitely directed to do so by a doctor because it may cause problems in the unborn child or complications during delivery.**

**Keep out of reach of children.** In case of overdose, get medical help or contact a Poison Control Center right away.

## DIRECTIONS

| adults and children 12 years and over | take 2 tablets fully dissolved in 4 ounces of water every 4 hours |
| | do not exceed 8 tablets in 24 hours or as directed by a doctor |
| children under 12 years | consult a doctor |

## OTHER INFORMATION
- each tablet contains: sodium 476 mg
- **Phenylketonurics:** contains phenylalanine 9 mg per tablet
- protect from excessive heat

## INACTIVE INGREDIENTS
acesulfame potassium, anhydrous citric acid, aspartame, calcium silicate, dimethylpolysiloxane, docusate sodium, flavors, mannitol, povidone, sodium benzoate, sodium bicarbonate

## QUESTIONS OR COMMENTS
Call **1-800-986-0369** (Mon-Fri 9 AM-5 PM EST) or www.alkaseltzerplus.com

# ALKA-SELTZER PLUS SPARKLING ORIGINAL COLD FORMULA (aspirin, chlorpheniramine maleate, and phenylephrine bitartrate) tablet, effervescent

Bayer HealthCare

## DRUG FACTS

| Active ingredients (in each tablet) | Purpose |
|---|---|
| Aspirin 325 mg (NSAID)* | Pain reliever/fever reducer |
| Chlorpheniramine maleate 2 mg | Antihistamine |
| Phenylephrine bitartrate 7.8 mg | Nasal decongestant |

*nonsteroidal anti-inflammatory drug

## USES
- temporarily relieves these symptoms due to a cold:
  - minor aches and pains
  - headache
  - runny nose
  - nasal and sinus congestion
  - sneezing
  - sore throat
- temporarily reduces fever

## WARNINGS
**Reye's syndrome**
Children and teenagers who have or are recovering from chicken pox or flu-like symptoms should not use this product. When using this product, if changes in behavior with nausea and vomiting occur, consult a doctor because these symptoms could be an early sign of Reye's syndrome, a rare but serious illness.

**Allergy alert**
Aspirin may cause a severe allergic reaction which may include:
- hives
- facial swelling
- asthma (wheezing)
- shock

**Stomach bleeding warning**
This product contains an NSAID, which may cause severe stomach bleeding. The chance is higher if you:
- are age 60 or older
- have had stomach ulcers or bleeding problems
- take a blood thinning (anticoagulant) or steroid drug
- take other drugs containing prescription or nonprescription NSAIDs (aspirin, ibuprofen, naproxen, or others)
- have 3 or more alcoholic drinks every day while using this product
- take more or for a longer time than directed

**Sore throat warning**
If sore throat is severe, persists for more than 2 days, is accompanied or followed by fever, headache, rash, nausea, or vomiting, consult a doctor promptly.

**Do not use to sedate children.**

## DO NOT USE
- if you are allergic to aspirin or any other pain reliever/fever reducer
- if you are now taking a prescription monoamine oxidase inhibitor (MAOI) (certain drugs for depression, psychiatric, or emotional conditions, or Parkinson's disease), or for 2 weeks after stopping the MAOI drug. if you do not know if your prescription drug contains an MAOI, ask a doctor or pharmacist before taking this product
- in children under 12 years of age

## ASK A DOCTOR BEFORE USE IF
- stomach bleeding warning applies to you
- you have a history of stomach problems, such as heartburn
- you have high blood pressure, heart disease, liver cirrhosis, or kidney disease
- you are taking a diuretic
- you have:
  - asthma
  - diabetes
  - thyroid disease
  - glaucoma
  - difficulty in urination due to enlargement of the prostate gland
  - a breathing problem such as emphysema or chronic bronchitis
  - a sodium-restricted diet

## ASK A DOCTOR OR PHARMACIST BEFORE USE IF YOU ARE
- taking a prescription drug for:
  - gout
  - diabetes
  - arthritis
- taking sedatives or tranquilizers

## WHEN USING THIS PRODUCT
- do not exceed recommended dosage
- excitability may occur, especially in children
- you may get drowsy
- avoid alcoholic drinks
- alcohol, sedatives, and tranquilizers may increase drowsiness
- be careful when driving a motor vehicle or operating machinery

## STOP USE AND ASK A DOCTOR IF
- an allergic reaction occurs. Seek medical help right away
- you experience any of the following signs of stomach bleeding
  - feel faint
  - vomit blood
  - have bloody or black stools
  - have stomach pain that does not get better
- pain or nasal congestion gets worse or lasts more than 7 days
- fever gets worse or lasts more than 3 days
- redness or swelling is present
- new symptoms occur
- ringing in the ears or a loss of hearing occurs
- nervousness, dizziness, or sleeplessness occurs

**If pregnant or breastfeeding,** ask a health professional before use.

**It is especially important not to use aspirin during the last 3 months of pregnancy unless definitely directed to do so by a doctor because it may cause problems in the unborn child or complications during delivery.**

**Keep out of reach of children.** In case of overdose, get medical help or contact a Poison Control Center right away.

## DIRECTIONS

| adults and children 12 years and over | take 2 tablets fully dissolved in 4 ounces of water every 4 hours |
|---|---|
| | do not exceed 8 tablets in 24 hours or as directed by a doctor |
| children under 12 years | do not use |

## OTHER INFORMATION
- each tablet contains: sodium 474 mg
- **Phenylketonurics:** contains phenylalanine 8.4 mg per tablet
- store at room temperature. Avoid excessive heat

## INACTIVE INGREDIENTS

acesulfame potassium, anhydrous citric acid, aspartame, calcium silicate, dimethylpolysiloxane, docusate sodium, flavors, mannitol, povidone, sodium benzoate, sodium bicarbonate

## QUESTIONS OR COMMENTS

Call **1-800-986-0369** (Mon-Fri 9 AM-5 PM EST) or www.alkaseltzerplus.com

---

# ALLI (orlistat) capsule

## GlaxoSmithKline Consumer Healthcare

## DRUG FACTS

| Active ingredient (in each sealed capsule) | Purpose |
|---|---|
| Orlistat 60 mg | Weight loss aid |

## USE

- for weight loss in overweight adults, 18 years and older, when used along with a reduced-calorie and low-fat diet

## WARNINGS

**Organ transplant alert**
- do not use if you have had an organ transplant
- Orlistat interferes with the medicines used to prevent transplant rejection

**Allergy alert**
- Do not use if you are allergic to any of the ingredients in orlistat capsules

## DO NOT USE

- if you are taking cyclosporine
- if you have been diagnosed with problems absorbing food
- if you are not overweight

## ASK A DOCTOR BEFORE USE IF YOU HAVE EVER HAD

- gallbladder problems
- kidney stones
- pancreatitis

## ASK A DOCTOR OR PHARMACIST BEFORE USE IF YOU ARE

- taking warfarin (blood thinning medicine), or taking medicine for diabetes or thyroid disease. Your medication dose may need to be adjusted
- taking other weight loss products

## WHEN USING THIS PRODUCT

- take a multivitamin once a day, at bedtime. Orlistat can reduce the absorption of some vitamins
- follow a well-balanced, reduced-calorie, low-fat diet. Try starting this diet before taking orlistat
- orlistat works by preventing the absorption of some of the fat you eat. The fat passes out of your body, so you may have bowel changes. You may get:
  - gas with oily spotting
  - loose stools
  - more frequent stools that may be hard to control
- eating a low-fat diet lowers the chances of having these bowel changes
- for every 5 pounds you lose from diet alone, orlistat can help you lose 2-3 pounds more. In studies, most people lost 5-10 pounds over 6 months

## STOP USE AND ASK A DOCTOR IF

- you develop itching, yellow eyes or skin, dark urine or loss of appetite. There have been rare reports of liver injury in people taking orlistat

- severe or continuous abdominal pain occurs. This may be a sign of a serious medical condition

**If pregnant or breastfeeding,** do not use.

**Keep out of reach of children.** In case of overdose, get medical help or contact a Poison Control Center right away.

## DIRECTIONS

- read the enclosed brochure for other important information
- diet and exercise are the starting points for any weight loss program. Try these first before adding orlistat. Check with your doctor before starting any exercise program
- to see if orlistat capsules are right for you, find your height on the chart below. You may consider starting a weight loss program with orlistat if your weight is the same or more than the weight shown for your height
- for overweight adults 18 years and older:
  - take 1 capsule with each meal containing fat
  - do not take more than 3 capsules daily
- use with a reduced-calorie, low-fat diet and exercise program until you reach your weight loss goal. Most weight loss occurs in the first 6 months
- if you stop taking orlistat, continue with your diet and exercise program
- if you start to regain weight after you stop taking orlistat, you may need to start taking orlistat again along with your diet and exercise program
- take a multivitamin once a day, at bedtime, when using orlistat

| Ht./Wt | | Ht./Wt | |
|---|---|---|---|
| 4'10" | 129 lbs. | 5'8" | 177 lbs. |
| 4'11" | 133 lbs. | 5'9" | 182 lbs. |
| 5'0" | 138 lbs. | 5'10" | 188 lbs. |
| 5'1" | 143 lbs. | 5'11" | 193 lbs. |
| 5'2" | 147 lbs. | 6'0" | 199 lbs. |
| 5'3" | 152 lbs. | 6'1" | 204 lbs. |
| 5'4" | 157 lbs. | 6'2" | 210 lbs. |
| 5'5" | 162 lbs. | 6'3" | 216 lbs. |
| 5'6" | 167 lbs. | 6'4" | 221 lbs. |
| 5'7" | 172 lbs. | 6'5" | 227 lbs. |

## OTHER INFORMATION

- store at 20-25°C (68-77°F)
- protect drug from excessive light, humidity and temperatures over 30°C (86°F)

## INACTIVE INGREDIENTS

FD&C Blue no. 2, edible ink, gelatin, iron oxide, microcrystalline cellulose, povidone, sodium lauryl sulfate, sodium starch glycolate, talc, titanium dioxide

## QUESTIONS OR COMMENTS

Call toll-free **1-800-671-2554** (English/Spanish) weekdays (10:00 AM-4:30 PM EST)

## AMERICAINE (benzocaine) aerosol, spray
Insight Pharmaceuticals Corp.

### DRUG FACTS

| Active ingredient | Purpose |
|---|---|
| Benzocaine 20% | Topical Anesthetic |

### USES
- temporarily relieves pain and itching associated with:
  - minor cuts
  - scrapes
  - minor burns
  - insect bites

### WARNINGS
**For external use only.**

**Flammability Warning**
Contents under pressure. Do not puncture or incinerate. Flammable mixture; do not use near fire or flame, or expose to heat or temperatures above 49°C (120°F). Use only as directed. Intentional misuse by deliberately concentrating and inhaling contents can be harmful or fatal.

### WHEN USING THIS PRODUCT
- avoid contact with the eyes

### STOP USE AND ASK A DOCTOR IF
- condition worsens, or symptoms persists for more than 7 days
- symptoms do not get better, or if redness, irritation, swelling, pain or other symptoms occur or increase

**Keep out of reach of children.** If swallowed, get medical help or contact a Poison Control Center right away.

### DIRECTIONS
- shake can well, hold 6" to 12" from affected area; spray liberally

| adults and children 2 years of age and older | apply to affected area not more than 3 to 4 times daily |
|---|---|
| children under 2 years of age | consult a physician |

### INACTIVE INGREDIENTS
Polyethylene glycol 300, Propellant: Isobutane, normal butane, propane

### OTHER INFORMATION
- store at room temperature 15-25°C (59-77°F)

### QUESTIONS OR COMMENTS
Call **1-800-344-7239** or visit our website at www.insightpharma.com

## AMERICAINE (benzocaine) ointment
Insight Pharmaceuticals Corp.

### DRUG FACTS

| Active ingredient | Purpose |
|---|---|
| Benzocaine 20% | Hemorrhoidal ointment |

### USES
- temporarily relieves these symptoms associated with hemorrhoids:
  - inflammation
  - itching
  - local pain
  - soreness

### WARNINGS
**For external use only.**

### WHEN USING THIS PRODUCT
- certain persons can develop allergic reactions to ingredients in this product
- do not put this product into the rectum by using fingers or any mechanical device or applicator
- do not exceed dosage unless directed by a doctor

### STOP USE AND ASK A DOCTOR IF
- condition worsens or does not improve in 7 days
- bleeding occurs
- symptoms do not get better, or if redness, irritation, swelling, pain or other symptoms occur or increase

**Keep out of reach of children.** If swallowed, get medical help or contact a Poison Control Center right away.

### DIRECTIONS
- when practical, cleanse affected area with mild soap and warm water and rinse thoroughly. Gently dry by patting or blotting with toilet tissue or soft cloth before application of this product
- apply externally to the affected area up to 6 times daily
- children under 12 years: ask a doctor

### OTHER INFORMATION
- if ointment contacts clothing or other fabrics, wash in warm water only; do not use bleach
- store at room temperature 15-25°C (59-77°F)
- tube is sealed for your protection
- do not use if foil seal is broken or missing

### INACTIVE INGREDIENTS
benzethonium chloride, polyethylene glycol 300, polyethylene glycol 3350

### QUESTIONS OR COMMENTS
Call **1-800-344-7239** or visit our website at www.insightpharma.com

## ANACIN AF (acetaminophen, aspirin and caffeine) tablet, coated
Insight Pharmaceuticals Corp.

### DRUG FACTS

| Active ingredient (in each tablet) | Purpose |
|---|---|
| Acetaminophen 250 mg | Pain reliever |
| Aspirin 250 mg | Pain reliever |
| Caffeine 65 mg | Pain reliever aid |

### USES
- temporarily relieves minor aches and pains due to:
  - headache
  - a cold
  - toothache
  - muscular aches
  - arthritis
  - menstrual cramps

# WARNINGS

**Reye's syndrome**
Children and teenagers who have or are recovering from chicken pox or flu-like symptoms should not use this product. When using this product, if changes in behavior with nausea and vomiting occur, consult a doctor because these symptoms could be an early sign of Reye's syndrome, a rare but serious illness.

**Allergy alert**
Aspirin may cause a severe allergic reaction which may include:
* hives
* facial swelling
* asthma (wheezing)
* shock

**Alcohol warning**
If you consume 3 or more alcoholic drinks every day, ask your doctor whether you should take acetaminophen and aspirin or other pain relievers/fever reducers. Acetaminophen and aspirin may cause liver damage and stomach bleeding.

## DO NOT USE
* if you have ever had an allergic reaction to any other pain reliever/fever reducer
* with any other products containing acetaminophen. Taking more than directed may cause liver damage

## ASK A DOCTOR BEFORE USE IF YOU HAVE
* asthma
* ulcers
* bleeding problems
* stomach problems such as heartburn, upset stomach, or stomach pain that do not go away or return

## ASK A DOCTOR OR PHARMACIST BEFORE USE IF YOU ARE
* taking a prescription drug for:
  * anticoagulation (thinning of the blood)
  * diabetes
  * gout
  * arthritis

## STOP USE AND ASK A DOCTOR IF
* an allergic reaction occurs. Seek medical help right away
* new symptoms occur
* symptoms do not get better or worsen
* ringing in the ears or loss of hearing occurs
* painful area is red or swollen
* pain gets worse or lasts more than 10 days
* fever gets worse or lasts more than 3 days

**Caffeine warning**
The recommended dose of this product contains about as much caffeine as a cup of coffee. Limit the use of caffeine-containing medications, foods, or beverages while taking this product because too much caffeine may cause nervousness, irritability, sleeplessness, and occasionally, rapid heart beat.

**If pregnant or breastfeeding,** ask a health professional before use.

**It is especially important not to use aspirin during the last 3 months of pregnancy unless definitely directed to do so by a doctor because it may cause problems in the unborn child or complications during delivery.**

**Keep out of reach of children.**

## OVERDOSE WARNING
Taking more than the recommended dose can cause serious health problems. In the case of overdose, get medical help or contact a Poison Control Center right away. Quick medical attention is critical for adults as well as for children even if you do not notice any signs or symptoms.

# DIRECTIONS
* do not use more than directed (see OVERDOSE WARNING)
* drink a full glass of water with each dose

| adults and children 12 years of age and over | take 2 tablets every 6 hours; not more than 8 tablets in 24 hours, or as directed by a doctor |
|---|---|
| children under 12 years | ask a doctor |

## OTHER INFORMATION
* read all product information before using
* store at 20-25°C (68-77°F). Protect from moisture

## INACTIVE INGREDIENTS
colloidal silicon dioxide, crospovidone, lecithin, microcrystalline cellulose, polyvinyl alcohol, povidone, pregelatinized starch, sodium starch glycolate, starch, stearic acid, talc, titanium dioxide

## QUESTIONS OR COMMENTS
Call **1-800-344-7239** or visit us at www.anacin.com

---

# ANBESOL BABY (benzocaine) gel
Wyeth Consumer Healthcare

## DRUG FACTS

| Active ingredient | Purpose |
|---|---|
| Benzocaine 7.5% | Oral anesthetic |

## USE
* temporarily relieves sore gums due to teething in infants and children 4 months of age and older

## WARNINGS
**Allergy alert**
Do not use this product if you have a history of allergy to local anesthetics such as procaine, butacaine, benzocaine, or other "caine" anesthetics.

## DO NOT USE
* to treat fever and nasal congestion. These are not symptoms of teething and may indicate the presence of infection. If these symptoms persist, consult your doctor

## WHEN USING THIS PRODUCT
* avoid contact with the eyes
* do not exceed recommended dosage
* do not use for more than 7 days unless directed by a doctor/dentist

## STOP USE AND ASK A DOCTOR IF
* sore mouth symptoms do not improve in 7 days
* irritation, pain, or redness persists or worsens
* swelling, rash, or fever develops

**Keep out of reach of children.** If more than used for pain is accidentally swallowed, get medical help or contact a Poison Control Center right away.

## DIRECTIONS
- to open tube, cut tip of the tube on score mark with scissors

| children 4 months of age and older | apply to the affected area not more than 4 times daily or as directed by a doctor/dentist |
|---|---|
| infants under 4 months of age | no recommended dosage or treatment except under the advice and supervision of a doctor/dentist |

## OTHER INFORMATION
- store at 20-25°C (68-77°F)

## INACTIVE INGREDIENTS
artificial flavor, benzoic acid, carbomer 934P, D&C red no. 33, edetate disodium, FD&C blue no. 1, glycerin, methylparaben, polyethylene glycol, propylparaben, purified water, saccharin

## QUESTIONS OR COMMENTS
Call weekdays 9 AM to 5 PM EST at **1-888-797-5638** or visit www.anbesol.com

---

# ANBESOL COLD SORE THERAPY (allantoin, benzocaine, camphor, petrolatum) ointment
Pfizer Consumer Healthcare

## DRUG FACTS

| Active ingredients | Purpose |
|---|---|
| Allantoin 1% | Skin protectant |
| Benzocaine 20% | Fever blister/cold sore treatment |
| Camphor 3% | Fever blister/cold sore treatment |
| White petrolatum 64.9% | Skin protectant |

## USES
- temporarily relieves pain associated with fever blisters and cold sores
- relieves dryness and softens fever blisters and cold sores

## WARNINGS
**For external use only.**

**Allergy alert**
Do not use this product if you have a history of allergy to local anesthetics such as procaine, butacaine, benzocaine, or other "caine" anesthetics.

## DO NOT USE
- over deep or puncture wounds, infections, or lacerations consult a doctor

## WHEN USING THIS PRODUCT
- avoid contact with the eyes
- do not exceed recommended dosage

## STOP USE AND ASK A DOCTOR IF
- condition worsens
- symptoms persist for more than 7 days
- symptoms clear up and occur again within a few days

**Keep out of reach of children.** If swallowed, get medical help or contact a Poison Control Center right away.

## DIRECTIONS
- to open tube, cut tip of the tube on score mark with scissors

| adults and children 2 years of age and older | apply to the affected area not more than 3 to 4 times daily |
|---|---|
| children under 12 years of age | adult supervision should be given in the use of this product |
| children under 2 years of age | consult a doctor |

## OTHER INFORMATION
- store at 20-25°C (68-77°F)

## INACTIVE INGREDIENTS
aloe barbadenis leaf extract, benzyl alcohol, butylparaben, glyceryl monostearate, isocetyl stearate, menthol, methylparaben, mineral oil, propylparaben, sodium lauryl sulfate, vitamin E, white wax

## QUESTIONS OR COMMENTS
Call weekdays 9 AM to 5 PM EST at **1-888-797-5638**

---

# ANBESOL REGULAR STRENGTH LIQUID
(benzocaine) liquid
Wyeth Consumer Healthcare

## DRUG FACTS

| Active ingredient | Purpose |
|---|---|
| Benzocaine 10% | Oral anesthetic |

## USES
- temporarily relieves pain associated with the following mouth and gum irritations:
  - toothache
  - sore gums
  - canker sores
  - braces
  - minor dental procedures
  - dentures

## WARNINGS
**Allergy alert**
Do not use this product if you have a history of allergy to local anesthetics such as procaine, butacaine, benzocaine, or other "caine" anesthetics

## WHEN USING THIS PRODUCT
- avoid contact with the eyes
- do not exceed recommended dosage
- do not use for more than 7 days unless directed by a doctor/dentist
- do not use if plastic blister or backing material is separated from the plastic

## STOP USE AND ASK A DOCTOR IF
- sore mouth symptoms do not improve in 7 days
- irritation, pain, or redness persists or worsens
- swelling, rash, or fever develops

**Keep out of reach of children.** If more than used for pain is accidentally swallowed, get medical help or contact a Poison Control Center right away.

## DIRECTIONS

| adults and children 2 years of age and older | wipe liquid on with cotton, or cotton swab, or fingertip |
|---|---|
| | apply to the affected area up to 4 times daily or as directed by a doctor/dentist |
| children under 12 years of age | adult supervision should be given in the use of this product |
| children under 2 years of age | consult a doctor/dentist |

## OTHER INFORMATION
• store at 20-25°C (68-77°F)

## INACTIVE INGREDIENTS
benzyl alcohol, D&C red no. 33, D&C yellow no. 10, FD&C blue no. 1, FD&C yellow no. 6, flavor, methylparaben, polyethylene glycol, propylene glycol, saccharin

## QUESTIONS OR COMMENTS
Call weekdays 9 AM to 5 PM EST at **1-888-797-5638** or visit www.anbesol.com

## ANBESOL JR (benzocaine) gel
Wyeth Consumer Healthcare

### DRUG FACTS

| Active ingredient | Purpose |
|---|---|
| Benzocaine 10% | Oral anesthetic |

## USES
• temporarily relieves pain associated with the following mouth and gum irritations:
  • toothache
  • sore gums
  • canker sores
  • braces
  • minor dental procedures
  • dentures

## WARNINGS
**Allergy alert**
Do not use this product if you have a history of allergy to local anesthetics such as procaine, butacaine, benzocaine, or other "caine" anesthetics

## WHEN USING THIS PRODUCT
• avoid contact with the eyes
• do not exceed recommended dosage
• do not use for more than 7 days unless directed by a doctor/dentist

## STOP USE AND ASK A DOCTOR IF
• sore mouth symptoms do not improve in 7 days
• irritation, pain, or redness persists or worsens
• swelling, rash, or fever develops

**Keep out of reach of children.** If more than used for pain is accidentally swallowed, get medical help or contact a Poison Control Center right away.

## DIRECTIONS
• to open tube, cut tip of the tube on score mark with scissors

| adults and children 2 years of age and older | apply to the affected area up to 4 times daily or as directed by a doctor/dentist |
|---|---|
| children under 12 years of age | adult supervision should be given in the use of this product |
| children under 2 years of age | consult a doctor/dentist |

## OTHER INFORMATION
• store at 20-25°C (68-77°F)

## INACTIVE INGREDIENTS
artificial flavor, benzyl alcohol, carbomer 934P, D&C red no. 33, glycerin, methylparaben, polyethylene glycol, potassium acesulfame

## QUESTIONS OR COMMENTS
Call weekdays 9 AM to 5 PM EST at **1-888-797-5638** or visit www.anbesol.com

## AQUAPHOR ORIGINAL (petrolatum) ointment
Beiersdorf Inc

### DRUG FACTS

| Active ingredient | Purpose |
|---|---|
| Petrolatum 41% | Skin protectant ointment |

## USES
• temporarily protects minor:
  • cuts
  • scrapes
  • burns
• temporarily protects and helps relieve chapped or cracked skin and lips
• helps protect from the drying effects of wind and cold weather

## WARNING
**For external use only.**

## WHEN USING THIS PRODUCT
• do not get into eyes

## DO NOT USE ON
• deep or puncture wounds
• animal bites
• serious burns

## STOP USE AND ASK A DOCTOR IF
• condition worsens
• symptoms last more than 7 days or clear up and occur again within a few days

**Keep out of reach of children.** If swallowed, get medical help or contact a Poison Control Center right away.

## DIRECTIONS
• apply as needed

## INACTIVE INGREDIENTS
mineral oil, ceresin, lanolin alcohol

## QUESTIONS OR COMMENTS
Call **1-800-227-4703**

# ASPERCREME MAX NO MESS ROLL ON
(menthol) liquid
Chattem, Inc.

## DRUG FACTS

| Active ingredient | Purpose |
|---|---|
| Menthol 16% | Topical analgesic |

### USES
- temporarily relieves minor pain associated with:
  - arthritis
  - simple backache
  - muscle strains
  - sprains
  - bruises
  - cramps

### WARNINGS
**For external use only.**

**Flammable**
- Keep away from fire or flame

### WHEN USING THIS PRODUCT
- use only as directed
- do not bandage tightly or use with a heating pad
- avoid contact with eyes and mucous membranes
- do not apply to wounds or damaged, broken or irritated skin
- a transient burning sensation or redness may occur upon application but generally disappears in several days
- if severe burning sensation occurs, discontinue use immediately
- do not expose the area treated with product to heat or direct sunlight

### STOP USE AND ASK A DOCTOR IF
- condition worsens
- redness is present
- irritation develops
- symptoms persist for more than 7 days or clear up and occur again within a few days

**If pregnant or breastfeeding,** ask a health professional before use.

**Keep out of reach of children.** If swallowed, get medical help or contact a Poison Control Center right away.

### DIRECTIONS

| adults and children over 12 years | apply generously to affected area |
|---|---|
| | massage into painful area until thoroughly absorbed into skin |
| | repeat as necessary, but no more than 3 to 4 times daily |
| | if medicine comes in contact with hands, wash with soap and water |
| children 12 years or younger | ask a doctor |

### INACTIVE INGREDIENTS
acrylates/C10-30 alkyl acrylate crosspolymer, capsaicin, glycerin, isopropyl myristate, propylene glycol, SD alcohol 40 (30%), triethanolamine, water (245-256)

### OTHER INFORMATION
- Close cap tightly after use
- Keep carton as it contains important information

# AXID AR (nizatidine) tablet, film coated
Wyeth Consumer Healthcare

## DRUG FACTS

| Active ingredient (in each tablet) | Purpose |
|---|---|
| Nizatidine 75 mg | Acid reducer |

### USES
- relieves heartburn associated with acid indigestion and sour stomach
- prevents heartburn associated with acid indigestion and sour stomach brought on by eating or drinking certain food and beverages

### WARNINGS
**Allergy alert**
Do not use if you are allergic to nizatidine or other acid reducers

### DO NOT USE
- if you have trouble or pain swallowing food, vomiting with blood, or bloody or black stools. These may be signs of a serious condition. See your doctor
- with other acid reducers

### ASK A DOCTOR BEFORE USE IF YOU HAVE
- had heartburn over 3 months. This may be a sign of a more serious condition
- heartburn with lightheadedness, sweating or dizziness
- chest pain or shoulder pain with shortness of breath; sweating; pain spreading to arms, neck or shoulders; or lightheadedness
- frequent chest pain
- frequent wheezing, particularly with heartburn
- unexplained weight loss
- nausea or vomiting
- stomach pain

### STOP USE AND ASK A DOCTOR IF
- your heartburn continues or worsens
- you need to take this product for more than 14 days

**If pregnant or breastfeeding,** ask a health professional before use.

**Keep out of reach of children.** In case of overdose, get medical help or contact a Poison Control Center right away

### DIRECTIONS

| adults and children 12 years and over | to relieve symptoms, swallow 1 tablet with a full glass of water |
|---|---|
| | to prevent symptoms, swallow 1 tablet with a full glass of water right before eating or up to 60 minutes before consuming food and beverages that cause you heartburn |
| | do not use more than 2 tablets in 24 hours |
| children under 12 years | ask a doctor |

## OTHER INFORMATION
- store at 20-25°C (68-77°F)
- protect from light
- replace cap tightly after opening bottle
- keep the carton and package insert. They contain important information

## INACTIVE INGREDIENTS
colloidal silicon dioxide, corn starch, hypromellose, magnesium stearate, microcrystalline cellulose, pharmaceutical ink, polyethylene glycol, pregelatinized starch, propylene glycol, synthetic iron oxides, titanium dioxide

## QUESTIONS OR COMMENTS
Call **1-800-555-2943** Monday through Friday 9 AM to 5 PM EST

---

# AYR SALINE NASAL MIST (sodium chloride [0.65%]) nasal spray
B.F. Ascher & Company Inc.

## DRUG FACTS

| Active ingredient | Purpose |
|---|---|
| Sodium chloride (0.65%) | Nasal moisturizer |

## USES
- relieves dry, crusty, and inflamed nasal membranes due to:
  - central heating
  - low-humidity environments
  - colds
  - overuse of nasal decongestant drops or sprays

## WARNINGS
- use of bottle by more than one person may spread infection
- take care not to aspirate nasal contents back into bottle
- if spray tip touches nose, rinse with hot water before replacing cap

## DIRECTIONS
- to spray, hold bottle upright and give short, firm squeezes in each nostril as often as needed
- for drops, hold bottle upside down

## INACTIVE INGREDIENTS
- deionized water, potassium phosphate, sodium hydroxide buffer, disodium EDTA, benzalkonium chloride

---

# AZO STANDARD & AZO STANDARD MAXIMUM STRENGTH (phenazopyridine hydrochloride)
I-Health, Inc.

## DRUG FACTS

| Active ingredients (each tablet) | Purpose |
|---|---|
| Phenazopyridine hydrochloride (standard): 95 mg. (Maximum Strength): 97.5 mg | Urinary analgesic |

## USE
- provides fast relief from urinary pain, burning, urgency and frequency associated with urinary tract infections

## WARNINGS

### ASK A DOCTOR BEFORE USE IF YOU HAVE
- kidney disease
- allergies to foods, preservatives or dyes
- had a hypersensitive reaction to phenazopyridine

### WHEN USING THIS PRODUCT
- stomach upset may occur, taking this product with or after meals may reduce stomach upset
- your urine will become reddish-orange in color. This is not harmful, but care should be taken to avoid staining clothing or other items

### STOP USE AND ASK A DOCTOR IF
- your symptoms last for more than 2 days
- you suspect you are having an adverse reaction to the medication

**If you are pregnant or breastfeeding,** ask a health professional before use.

**Keep out of reach of children.** In case of an overdose, get medical help or contact a Poison Control Center right away.

## DIRECTIONS

| adults and children over 12 years | take 2 tablets 3 times daily with or after meals as needed |
|---|---|
| | take with a full glass of water |
| | do not use for more than 2 days (12 tablets) without consulting a doctor |
| children under 12 years | do not use without consulting a doctor |

## OTHER INFORMATION
- this product can interfere with laboratory tests including urine, glucose (sugar), and ketones tests
- this product may stain soft contact lenses and other items if handled after touching tablets
- store at room temperature (59-86°F) in a dry place and protect from light
- Tamper evident: tablets sealed in cellophane or blister foil. Do not use if cellophane or blister foil is open or damaged

## INACTIVE INGREDIENTS
microcrystalline cellulose, pregelatinized corn starch, hypromellose, PVP, croscarmellose sodium, polyethylene glycol, carnauba wax and vegetable magnesium stearate, may also contain corn starch

## QUESTIONS OR COMMENTS
Visit www.azoproducts.com

---

# BACITRACIN (bacitracin zinc) ointment
Qualitest Pharmaceuticals

## DRUG FACTS

| Active ingredient (in each gram) | Purpose |
|---|---|
| Bacitracin zinc, USP 500 units | First aid antibiotic |

## USES
- First aid to help reduce the risk of infection in minor:
  - cuts
  - scrapes
  - burns

## WARNINGS
**For external use only.**

### DO NOT USE
- if you are allergic to any of the ingredients

### ASK A DOCTOR BEFORE USE IF YOU HAVE
- deep or puncture wounds
- animal bites
- serious burns

### WHEN USING THIS PRODUCT
- do not use in the eyes
- do not apply over large areas of the body

### STOP USE AND ASK A DOCTOR IF
- you need to use more than 1 week
- condition persists or gets worse
- rash or other allergic reaction develops

**Keep out of reach of children.** If swallowed, get medical help or contact a Poison Control Center right away.

### DIRECTIONS
- clean the affected area
- apply a small amount of this product (an amount equal to the surface area of the tip of a finger) on the area 1 to 3 times daily
- may be covered with a sterile bandage

### OTHER INFORMATION
- store at 15-30°C (59-86°F)
- lot number and expiration date: See crimp of tube or box

### INACTIVE INGREDIENTS
mineral oil, white petrolatum

### QUESTIONS OR COMMENTS
You may report serious side effects to: 130 Vintage Drive, Huntsville, AL 35811.

---

## BACITRACIN ZINC (bacitracin zinc) ointment
E. Fougera & Co., a division of Nycomed US Inc.

### DRUG FACTS

| Active ingredient (in each gram) | Purpose |
|---|---|
| Bacitracin zinc (equal to 500 bacitracin units) | Antibiotic |

### USE
- first aid to help prevent infection in minor cuts, scrapes, and burns

### WARNINGS
**For external use only.**

### DO NOT USE
- in the eyes
- over large areas of the body if you are allergic to any of the ingredients

### ASK A DOCTOR BEFORE USE
- in case of deep or puncture wounds, animal bites or serious burns

### WHEN USING THIS PRODUCT
- do not use longer than 1 week unless directed by a doctor

### STOP USE AND ASK A DOCTOR IF
- the condition persists or gets worse if a rash or other allergic reaction develops

**Keep out of reach of children.** If swallowed, get medical help or contact a Poison Control Center right away.

### DIRECTIONS
Clean the affected area, apply a small amount of this product (an amount equal to the surface area of the tip of a finger) on the area 1 to 3 times daily. May be covered with a sterile bandage.

### OTHER INFORMATION
- store at room temperature

### INACTIVE INGREDIENT
white petrolatum

### QUESTIONS OR COMMENTS
Call toll-free **1-800-645-9833**

---

## BACTINE (benzalkonium chloride and lidocaine hydrochloride) liquid
Bayer HealthCare

### DRUG FACTS

| Active ingredients | Purpose |
|---|---|
| Benzalkonium Cl 0.13% w/w | First aid antiseptic |
| Lidocaine hydrochloride 2.5% w/w | Pain relieving liquid |

### USES
- first aid to help prevent skin infection, and for temporary relief of pain and itching associated with minor:
  - cuts
  - scrapes
  - burns
  - sunburn
  - skin irritations

### WARNINGS
**For external use only.**

### ASK A DOCTOR BEFORE USE IF YOU HAVE
- deep or puncture wounds
- animal bites
- serious burns

### WHEN USING THIS PRODUCT
- do not use in or near the eyes
- do not apply over large areas of the body or in large quantities
- do not apply over raw surfaces or blistered areas

### STOP USE AND ASK A DOCTOR IF
- condition worsens
- symptoms persist for more than 7 days, or clear up and occur again within a few days

**Keep out of reach of children.** If swallowed, get medical help or contact a Poison Control Center right away.

## DIRECTIONS

| adults and children 2 years and older | clean the affected area |
|---|---|
| | apply a small amount on the area 1 to 3 times daily |
| | may be covered with a sterile bandage |
| | if bandaged, let dry first |
| children under 2 years | ask a doctor |

## OTHER INFORMATION
• avoid excessive heat

## INACTIVE INGREDIENTS
edetate disodium, fragrances, nonoxynol 9, propylene glycol, purified water

## QUESTIONS OR COMMENTS
Call **1-800-986-0369** (Mon-Fri 9 AM-5 PM EST) or www.bactine.com

# BACTINE PAIN RELIEVING CLEANSING SPRAY (benzalkonium chloride and lidocaine hydrochloride)
Bayer

## DRUG FACTS

| Active ingredients | Purpose |
|---|---|
| Benzalkonium Cl 0.13% w/w | First aid antiseptic |
| Lidocaine hydrochloride 2.5% w/w | Pain relieving spray |

## USES
• first aid to help prevent bacterial contamination or skin infection, and temporary relief of pain and itching associated with minor:
  • cuts
  • scrapes
  • burns
  • sunburn
  • skin irritations

## WARNINGS
**For external use only.**

## ASK A DOCTOR BEFORE USE IF YOU HAVE
• deep or puncture wounds
• animal bites
• serious burns

## WHEN USING THIS PRODUCT
• do not use in or near the eyes
• do not apply over large areas of the body or in large quantities
• do not apply over raw surfaces or blistered areas

## STOP USE AND ASK A DOCTOR IF
• condition worsens
• symptoms persist for more than 7 days, or clear up and occur again within a few days

**Keep out of reach of children.** If swallowed, get medical help or contact a Poison Control Center right away

## DIRECTIONS

| adults and children 2 years and older | clean the affected area |
|---|---|
| | apply a small amount on the area 1 to 3 times daily |
| | may be covered with a sterile bandage |
| | if bandaged (let dry first) |
| children under 2 years | ask a doctor |

## OTHER INFORMATION
• avoid excessive heat

## INACTIVE INGREDIENTS
edetate disodium, fragrances, nonoxynol 9, propylene glycol, purified water

## QUESTIONS OR COMMENTS
Call **1-800-986-0369** (Mon-Fri 9 AM-5 PM EST) or www.bactine.com

# BALMEX DIAPER RASH STICK (zinc oxide)
cream

Chattem, Inc.

## DRUG FACTS

| Active ingredient | Purpose |
|---|---|
| Zinc oxide 11.3% | Skin protectant |

## USES
• helps treat and prevent diaper rash
• protects chafed skin due to diaper rash and helps seal out wetness

## WARNINGS
**For external use only.**

## WHEN USING THIS PRODUCT
• avoid contact with eyes

## STOP USE AND ASK A DOCTOR IF
• condition worsens or lasts more than 7 days

**Keep out of reach of children.** If swallowed, get medical help or contact a Poison Control Center immediately.

## DIRECTIONS
• change wet or soiled diapers promptly
• cleanse the diaper area and allow to dry
• apply cream liberally as often as necessary, with each diaper change, especially at bedtime or anytime when exposure to wet diapers may be prolonged

## OTHER INFORMATION
• do not use if quality seal is broken
• see bottom of carton for expiration date

## INACTIVE INGREDIENTS
beeswax, benzoic acid, dimethicone, fragrance, glycine soja (soybean) oil, magnesium aspartate, methylparaben, microcrystalline wax, mineral oil, oenothera biennis (evening primrose) seed extract, olea europaea (olive) leaf extract, panthenol potassium aspartate, potassium hydroxide, propylene glycol, propylparaben, sarcosine, sodium cocoyl amino acids, sorbitan sesquioleate, synthetic beeswax, tocopherol, water (245-230)

# BAYER ADVANCED ASPIRIN EXTRA STRENGTH (aspirin) tablet, coated

Bayer Corporation Consumer Care Division

## DRUG FACTS

| Active ingredient (in each tablet) | Purpose |
|---|---|
| Aspirin 500 mg (NSAID) | Pain reliever/fever reducer |
| *nonsteroidal anti-inflammatory drug | |

## USES

- temporarily relieves:
  - headache
  - menstrual pain
  - minor pain of arthritis
  - muscle pain
  - pain and fever of colds
  - toothache

## WARNINGS

### Reye's syndrome

Children and teenagers who have or are recovering from chicken pox or flu-like symptoms should not use this product. When using this product, if changes in behavior with nausea and vomiting occur, consult a doctor because these symptoms could be an early sign of Reye's syndrome, a rare but serious illness.

### Allergy alert

Aspirin may cause a severe allergic reaction which may include:
- hives
- facial swelling
- asthma (wheezing)
- shock

### Stomach bleeding warning

This product contains an NSAID, which may cause severe stomach bleeding. The chance is higher if you:
- are age 60 or older
- have had stomach ulcers or bleeding problems
- take a blood thinning (anticoagulant) or steroid drug
- take other drugs containing prescription or nonprescription NSAIDs (aspirin, ibuprofen, naproxen, or others)
- have 3 or more alcoholic drinks every day while using this product
- take more or for a longer time than directed

## DO NOT USE

- if you are allergic to aspirin or any other pain reliever/fever reducer

## ASK A DOCTOR BEFORE USE IF

- stomach bleeding warning applies to you
- you have a history of stomach problems, such as heartburn
- you have high blood pressure, heart disease, liver cirrhosis, or kidney disease
- you are taking a diuretic
- you have asthma
- you have a sodium-restricted diet

## ASK A DOCTOR OR PHARMACIST BEFORE USE IF YOU ARE

- taking a prescription drug for:
  - gout
  - diabetes
  - arthritis

## STOP USE AND ASK A DOCTOR IF

- an allergic reaction occurs. Seek medical help right away
- you experience any of the following signs of stomach bleeding:
  - feel faint
  - vomit blood
  - have bloody or black stools
  - have stomach pain that does not get better
- pain gets worse or lasts more than 10 days
- redness or swelling is present
- fever lasts more than 3 days
- new symptoms occur
- ringing in the ears or a loss of hearing occurs

**If pregnant or breastfeeding,** ask a health professional before use.

**It is especially important not to use aspirin during the last 3 months of pregnancy unless definitely directed to do so by a doctor because it may cause problems in the unborn child or complications during delivery.**

**Keep out of reach of children.** In case of overdose, get medical help or contact a Poison Control Center right away.

## DIRECTIONS

- drink a full glass of water with each dose

| adults and children 12 years and over | take 1 or 2 tablets every 4 to 6 hours, not to exceed 8 tablets in 24 hours |
|---|---|
| children under 12 years | consult a doctor |

## OTHER INFORMATION

- each tablet contains: sodium 72 mg
- store at room temperature. Avoid excessive heat and moisture. Keep desiccant and product in original bottle. Immediately close cap tightly after use
- save carton for full directions and warnings

## INACTIVE INGREDIENTS

carnauba wax, colloidal silicon dioxide, hypromellose, sodium carbonate, zinc stearate

## QUESTIONS OR COMMENTS

Call **1-800-331-4536** (Mon - Fri 9 AM-5 PM EST) or visit www.bayeraspirin.com

# BAYER ADVANCED ASPIRIN REGULAR STRENGTH (aspirin) tablet

Bayer Corporation Consumer Care Division

## DRUG FACTS

| Active ingredient (in each tablet) | Purpose |
|---|---|
| Aspirin 325 mg (NSAID) | Pain reliever/fever reducer |
| *nonsteroidal anti-inflammatory drug | |

## USES

- temporarily relieves:
  - headache
  - menstrual pain
  - minor pain of arthritis
  - muscle pain
  - pain and fever of colds
  - toothache

## WARNINGS

### Reye's syndrome

Children and teenagers who have or are recovering from chicken pox or flu-like symptoms should not use this product. When using this product, if changes in behavior with nausea and vomiting occur, consult a doctor because these symptoms could be an early sign of Reye's syndrome, a rare but serious illness.

### Allergy alert

Aspirin may cause a severe allergic reaction which may include:
- hives
- facial swelling
- asthma (wheezing)
- shock

### Stomach bleeding warning

This product contains an NSAID, which may cause severe stomach bleeding. The chance is higher if you:
- are age 60 or older
- have had stomach ulcers or bleeding problems
- take a blood thinning (anticoagulant) or steroid drug
- take other drugs containing prescription or nonprescription NSAIDs (aspirin, ibuprofen, naproxen, or others)
- have 3 or more alcoholic drinks every day while using this product
- take more or for a longer time than directed

## DO NOT USE
- if you are allergic to aspirin or any other pain reliever/fever reducer

## ASK A DOCTOR BEFORE USE IF
- stomach bleeding warning applies to you
- you have a history of stomach problems, such as heartburn
- you have high blood pressure, heart disease, liver cirrhosis, or kidney disease
- you are taking a diuretic
- you have asthma
- you have a sodium-restricted diet

## ASK A DOCTOR OR PHARMACIST BEFORE USE IF YOU ARE
- taking a prescription drug for:
  - gout
  - diabetes
  - arthritis

## STOP USE AND ASK A DOCTOR IF
- an allergic reaction occurs. Seek medical help right away
- you experience any of the following signs of stomach bleeding:
  - feel faint
  - vomit blood
  - have bloody or black stools
  - have stomach pain that does not get better
- pain gets worse or lasts more than 10 days
- redness or swelling is present
- fever lasts more than 3 days
- new symptoms occur
- ringing in the ears or a loss of hearing occurs

**If pregnant or breastfeeding,** ask a health professional before use.

**It is especially important not to use aspirin during the last 3 months of pregnancy unless definitely directed to do so by a doctor because it may cause problems in the unborn child or complications during delivery.**

**Keep out of reach of children.** In case of overdose, get medical help or contact a Poison Control Center right away.

## DIRECTIONS
- drink a full glass of water with each dose

| adults and children 12 years and over | take 1 or 2 tablets every 4 hours or 3 tablets every 6 hours, not to exceed 12 tablets in 24 hours |
| --- | --- |
| children under 12 years | consult a doctor |

## OTHER INFORMATION
- each tablet contains: sodium 47 mg
- store at room temperature. Avoid excessive heat and moisture. Keep desiccant and product in original bottle. Immediately close cap tightly after use
- save carton for full directions and warnings

## INACTIVE INGREDIENTS
carnauba wax, colloidal silicon dioxide, hypromellose, sodium carbonate, zinc stearate

## QUESTIONS OR COMMENTS
Call **1-800-331-4536** (Mon-Fri 9 AM-5 PM EST) or visit www.bayeraspirin.com

# BAYER AM EXTRA STENGTH (aspirin and caffeine) tablet
Bayer HealthCare

## DRUG FACTS

| Active ingredients (in each tablet) | Purpose |
| --- | --- |
| Aspirin 500 mg (NSAID) | Pain reliever |
| Caffeine 65 mg | Alertness aid |
| *nonsteroidal anti-inflammatory drug | |

## USES
- for the temporary relief of minor aches and pains associated with a hangover
- helps restore mental alertness or wakefulness when experiencing fatigue or drowsiness associated with a hangover
- also effective for headache, body aches and pains alone

## WARNINGS

### Reye's syndrome

Children and teenagers who have or are recovering from chicken pox or flu-like symptoms should not use this product. When using this product, if changes in behavior with nausea and vomiting occur, consult a doctor because these symptoms could be an early sign of Reye's syndrome, a rare but serious illness.

### Allergy alert

Aspirin may cause a severe allergic reaction which may include:
- hives
- facial swelling
- asthma (wheezing)
- shock

### Stomach bleeding warning

This product contains an NSAID, which may cause severe stomach bleeding. The chance is higher if you:
- are age 60 or older
- have had stomach ulcers or bleeding problems
- take a blood thinning (anticoagulant) or steroid drug
- take other drugs containing prescription or nonprescription NSAIDs (aspirin, ibuprofen, naproxen, or others)
- have 3 or more alcoholic drinks every day while using this product

- take more or for a longer time than directed

**DO NOT USE**
- if you are allergic to aspirin or any other pain reliever/fever reducer
- in children under 12 years of age

**ASK A DOCTOR BEFORE USE IF**
- stomach bleeding warning applies to you
- you have a history of stomach problems, such as heartburn
- you have high blood pressure, heart disease, liver cirrhosis, or kidney disease
- you are taking a diuretic
- you have asthma

**ASK A DOCTOR OR PHARMACIST BEFORE USE IF YOU ARE**
- taking a prescription drug for:
  - gout
  - diabetes
  - arthritis

**WHEN USING THIS PRODUCT**
- the recommended dose of this product contains about as much caffeine as a cup of coffee. Limit the use of caffeine-containing medications, foods, or beverages while taking this product because too much caffeine may cause nervousness, irritability, sleeplessness, and, occasionally, rapid heartbeat
- take for occasional use only. Do not use for more than 2 days for a hangover unless directed by a doctor. Not intended for use as a substitute for sleep. If fatigue or drowsiness persists or continues to recur, consult a doctor

**STOP USE AND ASK A DOCTOR IF**
- an allergic reaction occurs. Seek medical help right away
- you experience any of the following signs of stomach bleeding:
  - feel faint
  - vomit blood
  - have bloody or black stools
  - have stomach pain that does not get better
- pain gets worse or lasts more than 10 days
- redness or swelling is present
- new symptoms occur
- ringing in the ears or a loss of hearing occurs

**If pregnant or breastfeeding,** ask a health professional before use.

**It is especially important not to use aspirin during the last 3 months of pregnancy unless definitely directed to do so by a doctor because it may cause problems in the unborn child or complications during delivery.**

**Keep out of reach of children.** In case of overdose, get medical help or contact a Poison Control Center right away.

**DIRECTIONS**
- drink a full glass of water with each dose

| adults and children 12 years and over | take 2 tablets every 6 hours not to exceed 8 tablets in 24 hours |
| --- | --- |
| children under 12 years | consult a doctor |

**OTHER INFORMATION**
- store at room temperature

**INACTIVE INGREDIENTS**
carnauba wax, corn starch, hypromellose, powdered cellulose, triacetin

**QUESTIONS OR COMMENTS**
Call **1-800-331-4536** (Mon-Fri 9-5 EST) or visit www.bayeraspirin.com

## BAYER FAST RELEASE (aspirin) powder
Bayer Corporation Consumer Care Division

### DRUG FACTS

| Active ingredient (in each powder pouch) | Purpose |
| --- | --- |
| Aspirin 500 mg (NSAID) | Pain reliever/fever reducer |
| *nonsterodial anti-inflammatory drug | |

**USES**
- temporarily relieves
  - headache
  - toothache
  - pain and fever of colds
  - minor pain of arthritis
  - muscle pain
  - menstrual pain

**WARNINGS**
**Reye's syndrome**
Children and teenagers who have or are recovering from chicken pox or flu-like symptoms should not use this product.

**Allergy alert**
Aspirin may cause a severe allergic reaction which may include:
- hives
- asthma (wheezing)
- facial swelling
- shock

**Stomach bleeding warning**
This product contains an NSAID, which may cause severe stomach bleeding. The chance is higher if you:

- are age 60 or older
- have had stomach ulcers or bleeding problems
- take a blood thinning (anticoagulant) or steroid drug
- take other drugs containing prescription or nonprescription NSAIDs (aspirin, ibuprofen, naproxen, or others)
- have 3 or more alcoholic drinks every day while using this product
- take more or for a longer time than directed

**DO NOT USE**
- if you are allergic to aspirin or any other pain reliever/fever reducer
- this product for at least 7 days after tonsillectomy or oral surgery unless directed by a doctor

**ASK A DOCTOR BEFORE USE IF**
- stomach bleeding warning applies to you
- you have a history of stomach problems, such as heartburn
- you have high blood pressure, heart disease, liver cirrhosis, or kidney disease
- you are taking a diuretic
- you have asthma

**ASK A DOCTOR OR PHARMACIST BEFORE USE IF YOU ARE**
- taking a prescription drug for:
  - gout
  - diabetes
  - arthritis

**WHEN USING THIS PRODUCT**
- if changes in behavior with nausea and vomiting occur, consult a doctor because these symptoms could be an early sign of Reye's syndrome, a rare but serious illness

**STOP USE AND ASK A DOCTOR IF**
- an allergic reaction occurs. Seek medical help right away
- you experience any of the following signs of stomach bleeding:
  - feel faint
  - vomit blood
  - have bloody or black stools
  - have stomach pain that does not get better
- pain gets worse or lasts more than 10 days
- redness or swelling is present
- fever lasts more than 3 days
- new symptoms occur
- ringing in the ears or a loss of hearing occurs

**If pregnant or breastfeeding,** ask a health professional before use.

**It is especially important not to use aspirin during the last 3 months of pregnancy unless definitely directed to do so by a doctor because it may cause problems in the unborn child or complications during delivery.**

**Keep out of reach of children.** In case of overdose, get medical help or contact a Poison Control Center right away.

**DIRECTIONS**

| adults and children 12 years and over | take contents of 1 powder pouch every 4 hours; dissolve powder on tongue, followed by a full glass of water; do not exceed 8 powder pouches in 24 hours |
|---|---|
| children under 12 years | consult a doctor |

**OTHER INFORMATION**
- **Phenylketonurics:** contains phenylalanine 5.6 mg per powder pouch
- save carton for full directions and warnings
- store at room temperature

**INACTIVE INGREDIENTS**
acesulfame potassium, anhydrous citric acid, aspartame, flavor, isomalt

**QUESTIONS OR COMMENTS**
Call **1-800-331-4536** (Mon-Fri 9 AM-5 PM EST) or visit www.bayeraspirin.com

## BC (aspirin and caffeine) powder
GlaxoSmithKline Consumer Healthcare LP

**DRUG FACTS**

| Active ingredient (in each powder) | Purpose |
|---|---|
| FAST PAIN RELIEF<br>• Aspirin (NSAID*) 845 mg<br>• Caffeine 65 mg | Pain reliever aid |

*nonsteroidal anti-inflammatory drug

**USES**
- temporarily relieves minor aches and pains due to:
  - headache
  - muscular aches
  - minor arthritis pain
  - colds
- temporarily reduces fever

**WARNINGS**
**Reye's syndrome**
Children and teenagers who have or are recovering from chicken pox or flu-like symptoms should not use this product. When using this product, if changes in behavior with nausea and vomiting occur, consult a doctor because these symptoms could be an early sign of Reye's syndrome, a rare but serious illness.

**Allergy alert**
Aspirin may cause a severe allergic reaction which may include:
- hives
- facial swelling
- shock
- asthma (wheezing)

**Stomach bleeding warning**
This product contains an NSAID, which may cause severe stomach bleeding. The chance is higher if you:
- are age 60 or older
- have had stomach ulcers or bleeding problems
- take a blood thinning (anticoagulant) or steroid drug
- take other drugs containing prescription or nonprescription NSAIDs (aspirin, ibuprofen, naproxen, or others)
- have 3 or more alcoholic drinks every day while using this product
- take more or for a longer time than directed

**DO NOT USE**
- if you have ever had an allergic reaction to aspirin or any other pain reliever/fever reducer

**ASK A DOCTOR BEFORE USE IF**
- stomach bleeding warning applies to you
- you have a history of stomach problems, such as heartburn
- you have high blood pressure, heart disease, liver cirrhosis, or kidney disease
- you are taking a diuretic
- you have asthma

**ASK A DOCTOR OR PHARMACIST BEFORE USE IF YOU ARE** taking a prescription drug for:
- diabetes
- gout
- arthritis

**WHEN USING THIS PRODUCT**
- limit the use of caffeine-containing drugs, foods, or drinks because too much caffeine may cause nervousness, irritability, sleeplessness, and, occasionally, rapid heart beat
- The recommended dose of this product contains about as much caffeine as a cup of coffee

**STOP USE AND ASK A DOCTOR IF**
- an allergic reaction occurs. Seek medical help right away
- you experience any of the following signs of stomach bleeding:
  - feel faint
  - have stomach pain that does not get better
  - vomit blood
  - have bloody or black stools
- pain gets worse or lasts more than 10 days
- fever gets worse or lasts more than 3 days
- redness or swelling is present
- any new symptoms appear
- ringing in the ears or a loss of hearing occurs

These could be signs of a serious condition.

**If pregnant or breastfeeding,** ask a health professional before use.

**It is especially important not to use aspirin during the last 3 months of pregnancy unless definitely directed to do so by a doctor because it may cause problems in the unborn child or complications during delivery.**

**Keep out of reach of children.** In case of overdose, get medical help or contact a Poison Control Center right away.

## DIRECTIONS

| adults and children 12 years of age and over | place 1 powder on tongue every 6 hours, while symptoms persist |
| | drink a full glass of water with each dose, or may stir powder into a glass of water or other liquid |
| | do not take more than 4 powders in 24 hours unless directed by a doctor |
| children under 12 years of age | ask a doctor |

## OTHER INFORMATION

**Fast Pain Relief**
- each powder contains: potassium 55 mg
- store below 25°C (77°F)

## INACTIVE INGREDIENTS

docusate sodium, fumaric acid, lactose monohydrate, potassium chloride

## QUESTIONS OR COMMENTS

Call **1-866-255-5197** (English/Spanish) weekdays or www.bcpowder.com

---

# BC ARTHRITIS
(aspirin and caffeine) powder

GlaxoSmithKline Consumer Healthcare LP

## DRUG FACTS

| Active ingredient (in each powder) | Purpose |
|---|---|
| **Arthritis Formula**<br>• Aspirin (NSAID*) 1000 mg<br>• Caffeine 65 mg | Pain reliever/fever reducer |

*nonsteroidal anti-inflammatory drug

## USES
- temporarily relieves minor aches and pains due to:
  - headache
  - muscular aches
  - minor arthritis pain
  - colds
- temporarily reduces fever

## WARNINGS
**Reye's syndrome**
Children and teenagers who have or are recovering from chicken pox or flu-like symptoms should not use this product. When using this product, if changes in behavior with nausea and vomiting occur, consult a doctor because these symptoms could be an early sign of Reye's syndrome, a rare but serious illness.

**Allergy alert**
Aspirin may cause a severe allergic reaction which may include:
- hives
- facial swelling
- shock
- asthma (wheezing)

**Stomach bleeding warning**
This product contains an NSAID, which may cause severe stomach bleeding. The chance is higher if you:
- are age 60 or older
- have had stomach ulcers or bleeding problems
- take a blood thinning (anticoagulant) or steroid drug
- take other drugs containing prescription or nonprescription NSAIDs (aspirin, ibuprofen, naproxen, or others)
- have 3 or more alcoholic drinks every day while using this product
- take more or for a longer time than directed

## DO NOT USE
- if you have ever had an allergic reaction to aspirin or any other pain reliever/fever reducer

## ASK A DOCTOR BEFORE USE IF
- stomach bleeding warning applies to you
- you have a history of stomach problems, such as heartburn
- you have high blood pressure, heart disease, liver cirrhosis, or kidney disease
- you are taking a diuretic
- you have asthma

## ASK A DOCTOR OR PHARMACIST BEFORE USE IF YOU ARE
taking a prescription drug for:
- diabetes
- gout
- arthritis

## WHEN USING THIS PRODUCT
- limit the use of caffeine-containing drugs, foods, or drinks because too much caffeine may cause nervousness, irritability, sleeplessness, and, occasionally, rapid heart beat
- The recommended dose of this product contains about as much caffeine as a cup of coffee

## STOP USE AND ASK A DOCTOR IF
- an allergic reaction occurs. Seek medical help right away
- you experience any of the following signs of stomach bleeding:
  - feel faint
  - have stomach pain that does not get better
  - vomit blood
  - have bloody or black stools
- pain gets worse or lasts more than 10 days
- fever gets worse or lasts more than 3 days
- redness or swelling is present
- any new symptoms appear
- ringing in the ears or a loss of hearing occurs

These could be signs of a serious condition.

**If pregnant or breastfeeding,** ask a health professional before use.

**It is especially important not to use aspirin during the last 3 months of pregnancy unless definitely directed to do so by a doctor because it may cause problems in the unborn child or complications during delivery.**

**Keep out of reach of children.** In case of overdose, get medical help or contact a Poison Control Center right away.

## DIRECTIONS

| adults and children 12 years of age and over | place 1 powder on tongue every 6 hours, while symptoms persist |
| | drink a full glass of water with each dose, or may stir powder into a glass of water or other liquid |
| | do not take more than 4 powders in 24 hours unless directed by a doctor |
| children under 12 years of age | ask a doctor |

## OTHER INFORMATION
**Arthritis Formula**
• each powder contains: potassium 65 mg
• store below 25°C (77°F)

## INACTIVE INGREDIENTS
docusate sodium, fumaric acid, lactose monohydrate, potassium chloride

## QUESTIONS OR COMMENTS
Call **1-866-255-5197** (English/Spanish) weekdays or www.bcpowder.com

# BENADRYL ALLERGY (diphenhydramine hydrochloride) gelcap, coated
McNeil Consumer Healthcare, Division of McNeil-PPC, Inc

## DRUG FACTS

| Active ingredient (in each gelcap) | Purpose |
| --- | --- |
| Diphenhydramine hydrochloride 25 mg | Antihistamine |

## USES
• temporarily relieves these symptoms due to hay fever or other upper respiratory allergies:
  • runny nose
  • sneezing
  • itchy, watery eyes
  • itching of the nose or throat
• temporarily relieves these symptoms due to the common cold:
  • runny nose
  • sneezing

## WARNINGS

### DO NOT USE
• to make a child sleepy
• with any other product containing diphenhydramine, even one used on skin

### ASK A DOCTOR BEFORE USE IF YOU HAVE
• glaucoma
• trouble urinating due to an enlarged prostate gland
• a breathing problem such as emphysema or chronic bronchitis

### ASK A DOCTOR OR PHARMACIST BEFORE USE IF YOU ARE
taking sedatives or tranquilizers

### WHEN USING THIS PRODUCT
• marked drowsiness may occur
• avoid alcoholic drinks
• alcohol, sedatives, and tranquilizers may increase drowsiness
• be careful when driving a motor vehicle or operating machinery
• excitability may occur, especially in children

**If pregnant or breastfeeding,** ask a health professional before use.

**Keep out of reach of children.** In case of overdose, get medical help or contact a Poison Control Center right away. (1-800-222-1222)

### DIRECTIONS
• if needed, repeat dose every 4 to 6 hours
• do not take more than 6 times in 24 hours

| adults and children 12 years of age and over | 1 to 2 gelcaps |
| --- | --- |
| children 6 to under 12 years of age | 1 gelcap |
| children under 6 years of age | do not use this product in children under 6 years of age |

### OTHER INFORMATION
• each gelcap contains: calcium 35 mg
• store between 20-25°C (68-77°F). Avoid high humidity
• do not use if carton is open or if blister unit is broken
• see side panel for lot number and expiration date

### INACTIVE INGREDIENTS
benzyl alcohol, black iron oxide, butylparaben, carboxymethylcellulose sodium, crospovidone, D&C red no. 28, dibasic calcium phosphate dihydrate, edetate calcium disodium, FD&C red no. 40, gelatin, hypromellose, magnesium stearate, methylparaben, microcrystalline cellulose, polyethylene glycol, polysorbate 80, propylparaben, red iron oxide, sodium lauryl sulfate, sodium propionate, titanium dioxide, yellow iron oxide

### QUESTIONS OR COMMENTS
Call **1-877-717-2824**

# BENADRYL ALLERGY (diphenhydramine hydrochloride) tablet, film coated
McNeil Consumer Healthcare, Division of McNeil-PPC, Inc

## DRUG FACTS

| Active ingredient (in each tablet) | Purpose |
| --- | --- |
| Diphenhydramine hydrochloride 25 mg | Antihistamine |

## USES
• temporarily relieves these symptoms due to hay fever or other upper respiratory allergies:
  • runny nose
  • sneezing
  • itchy, watery eyes
  • itching of the nose or throat
• temporarily relieves these symptoms due to the common cold:
  • runny nose
  • sneezing

## WARNINGS

**DO NOT USE**
- with any other product containing diphenhydramine, even one used on skin

**ASK A DOCTOR BEFORE USE IF YOU HAVE**
- a breathing problem such as emphysema or chronic bronchitis
- glaucoma
- trouble urinating due to an enlarged prostate gland

**ASK A DOCTOR OR PHARMACIST BEFORE USE IF YOU ARE**
- taking sedatives or tranquilizers

**WHEN USING THIS PRODUCT**
- marked drowsiness may occur
- avoid alcoholic drinks
- alcohol, sedatives, and tranquilizers may increase drowsiness
- be careful when driving a motor vehicle or operating machinery
- excitability may occur, especially in children

**If pregnant or breastfeeding,** ask a health professional before use.

**Keep out of reach of children.** In case of overdose, get medical help or contact a Poison Control Center right away. (1-800-222-1222)

## DIRECTIONS
- take every 4 to 6 hours
- do not take more than 6 times in 24 hours

| adults and children 12 years and over | 1 to 2 tablets |
|---|---|
| children 6 to under 12 years | 1 tablet |
| children under 6 years | do not use this product in children under 6 years of age |

## OTHER INFORMATION
- each tablet contains: calcium 15 mg
- store between 20-25°C (68-77°F). Avoid high humidity. Protect from light
- do not use if carton is opened or if blister unit is broken
- see side panel for lot number and expiration date

## INACTIVE INGREDIENTS
carnauba wax, crospovidone, D&C red no. 27 aluminum lake, dibasic calcium phosphate dihydrate, hypromellose, magnesium stearate, microcrystalline cellulose, polyethylene glycol, polysorbate 80, pregelatinized starch, stearic acid, titanium dioxide

## QUESTIONS OR COMMENTS
Call **1-877-717-2824**

# BENADRYL ALLERGY DYE-FREE LIQUI-GELS
(diphenhydramine hydrochloride)

McNeil Consumer Healthcare, Division of McNeil-PPC, Inc.

## DRUG FACTS

| Active ingredient (in each capsule) | Purpose |
|---|---|
| Diphenhydramine hydrochloride 25 mg | Antihistamine |

## USES
- temporarily relieves these symptoms due to hay fever or other upper respiratory allergies:
  - runny nose
  - sneezing
  - itchy, watery eyes
  - itching of the nose or throat
- temporarily relieves these symptoms due to the common cold:
  - runny nose
  - sneezing

## WARNINGS

**DO NOT USE**
- to make a child sleepy
- with any other product containing diphenhydramine, even one used on skin

**ASK A DOCTOR BEFORE USE IF YOU HAVE**
- a breathing problem such as emphysema or chronic bronchitis
- glaucoma
- trouble urinating due to an enlarged prostate gland

**ASK A DOCTOR OR PHARMACIST BEFORE USE IF YOU ARE**
- taking sedatives or tranquilizers

**WHEN USING THIS PRODUCT**
- marked drowsiness may occur
- avoid alcoholic drinks
- alcohol, sedatives, and tranquilizers may increase drowsiness
- be careful when driving a motor vehicle or operating machinery
- excitability may occur, especially in children

**If pregnant or breastfeeding,** ask a health professional before use.

**Keep out of reach of children.** In case of overdose, get medical help or contact a Poison Control Center right away. (1-800-222-1222)

## DIRECTIONS
- take every 4 to 6 hours
- do not take more than 6 doses in 24 hours

| adults and children 12 years and over | 1 to 2 capsules |
|---|---|
| children 6 to under 12 years | 1 capsule |
| children under 6 years | do not use this product |

## OTHER INFORMATION
- store at 59°F-77°F in a dry place
- protect from heat, humidity, and light

## INACTIVE INGREDIENTS
gelatin, glycerin, polyethylene glycol, purified water, and sorbitol. Capsules are imprinted with edible dye-free ink

## QUESTIONS OR COMMENTS
Call **1-877-717-2824**

# BENADRYL ALLERGY QUICK DISSOLVE
(diphenhydramine hydrochloride) strip

McNeil Consumer Healthcare, Division of McNeil-PPC, Inc.

## DRUG FACTS

| Active ingredient (in each film strip) | Purpose |
|---|---|
| Diphenhydramine hydrochloride 25 mg | Antihistamine |

## USES
- temporarily relieves these symptoms due to hay fever or other upper respiratory allergies:
  - runny nose
  - sneezing
  - itchy, watery eyes
  - itching of the nose or throat
- temporarily relieves these symptoms due to the common cold:
  - runny nose
  - sneezing

## WARNINGS

### DO NOT USE
- to make a child sleepy
- with any other product containing diphenhydramine, even one used on skin

### ASK A DOCTOR BEFORE USE IF YOU HAVE
- a breathing problem such as emphysema or chronic bronchitis
- glaucoma
- trouble urinating due to an enlarged prostate gland

### ASK A DOCTOR OR PHARMACIST BEFORE USE IF YOU ARE
- taking sedatives or tranquilizers

### WHEN USING THIS PRODUCT
- marked drowsiness may occur
- avoid alcoholic drinks
- alcohol, sedatives, and tranquilizers may increase drowsiness
- be careful when driving a motor vehicle or operating machinery
- excitability may occur, especially in children

**If pregnant or breastfeeding,** ask a health professional before use.

**Keep out of reach of children.** In case of overdose, get medical help or contact a Poison Control Center right away. (1-800-222-1222)

## DIRECTIONS
- if needed, repeat dose every 4 to 6 hours
- do not take more than 6 times in 24 hours

| adults and children 12 years and over | place one film strip on tongue and allow it to dissolve |
|---|---|
| | A second film strip may be taken after the first strip has dissolved |
| children 6 to 11 years | place one film strip on tongue and allow it to dissolve |
| children under 6 years | do not use this product in children under 6 years of age |

## OTHER INFORMATION
- each film strip contains: sodium 4 mg
- store at 59-77°F in a dry place. Protect from light
- do not use if individual carton or pouch is open or torn
- see bottom panel for lot number and expiration date

## INACTIVE INGREDIENTS
acesulfame potassium, carrageenan, FD&C blue no. 2 aluminum lake, flavors, glycerin, glyceryl oleate, locust bean gum, medium chain triglycerides, polysorbate 80, povidone, propylene glycol, pullulan, sodium polystyrene sulfonate, sucralose and xanthan gum

## QUESTIONS OR COMMENTS
Call **1-877-717-2824**

# CHILDREN'S BENADRYL ALLERGY
(diphenhydramine hydrochloride) liquid

McNeil Consumer Healthcare, Division of McNeil-PPC, Inc.

## DRUG FACTS

| Active ingredient (in each 5 mL)* | Purpose |
|---|---|
| Diphenhydramine hydrochloride 12.5 mg | Antihistamine |

*5 mL = one pre-filled spoon also 5mL = 1 teaspoon (tsp)

## USES
- temporarily relieves these symptoms due to hay fever or other upper respiratory allergies:
  - runny nose
  - sneezing
  - itchy, watery eyes
  - itching of the nose or throat

## WARNINGS

### DO NOT USE
- to make a child sleepy
- with any other product containing diphenhydramine, even one used on skin

### ASK A DOCTOR BEFORE USE IF THE CHILD HAS
- a breathing problem such as emphysema or chronic bronchitis
- glaucoma
- trouble urinating due to an enlarged prostate gland
- a sodium-restricted diet

### ASK A DOCTOR OR PHARMACIST BEFORE USE IF YOU ARE
- taking sedatives or tranquilizers

### WHEN USING THIS PRODUCT
- marked drowsiness may occur
- avoid alcoholic drinks
- sedatives and tranquilizers may increase drowsiness
- excitability may occur, especially in children
- be careful when driving a motor vehicle or operating machinery

**If pregnant or breastfeeding,** ask a health professional before use.

**Keep out of reach of children.** In case of overdose, get medical help or contact a Poison Control Center right away. (1-800-222-1222)

## DIRECTIONS
- use only enclosed cup designed for use with this product
- do not use any other dosing device
- find right dose on chart below
- take every 4 to 6 hours
- do not take more than 6 doses in 24 hours

| | |
|---|---|
| children under 2 years | do not use |
| children 2 to 5 years | do not use unless directed by a doctor |
| children 6 to 11 years | 1 to 2 pre-filled spoons |
| adults and children 12 years and over | 2 to 4 pre-filled spoons |

## OTHER INFORMATION
- each tsp contains: sodium 14 mg
- store between 20-25°C (68-77°F). Protect from light. Store in outer carton until contents used

## INACTIVE INGREDIENTS
anhydrous citric acid, D&C red no. 33, FD&C red no. 40, flavors, glycerin, monoammonium glycyrrhizinate, poloxamer 407, purified water, sodium benzoate, sodium chloride, sodium citrate, sucrose

## QUESTIONS OR COMMENTS
Call **1-877-717-2824**

# BENADRYL EXTRA STRENGTH SPRAY
(diphenhydramine hydrochloride and zinc acetate)
McNeil Consumer Healthcare, Division of McNeil-PPC, Inc.

## DRUG FACTS

| Active ingredients | Purpose |
|---|---|
| Diphenhydramine hydrochloride 2% | Topical analgesic |
| Zinc acetate 0.1% | Skin protectant |

## USES
- temporarily relieves pain and itching associated with:
  - insect bites
  - minor bums
  - sunburn
  - minor skin irritations
  - minor cuts
  - scrapes
  - rashes due to poison ivy, poison oak, and poison sumac
- dries the oozing and weeping of poison ivy, poison oak, and poison sumac

## WARNINGS
**For external use only.**

**Flammable. Keep away from fire or flame.**

## DO NOT USE
- on large areas of your body
- with any other product containing diphenhydramine, even one taken by mouth

## ASK A DOCTOR BEFORE USE
- on chicken pox
- on measles

## WHEN USING THIS PRODUCT
- avoid contact with eyes

## STOP USE AND ASK A DOCTOR IF
- condition worsens or does not improve within 7 days
- symptoms persist for more than 7 days or clear up and occur again within a few days

**Keep out of reach of children.** If swallowed, get medical help or contact a Poison Control Center right away. (1-800-222-1222)

## DIRECTIONS
- Do not use more than directed

| | |
|---|---|
| adults and children 2 years of age and older | spray on affected area not more than 3 to 4 times daily |
| children under 2 years of age | ask a doctor |

## OTHER INFORMATION
- store at 20°C-25°C (68°F-77°F)

## INACTIVE INGREDIENTS
alcohol, glycerin, povidone, purified water, and tromethamine

## QUESTIONS OR COMMENTS
Call **1-800-524-2624**

# BENADRYL ORIGINAL STRENGTH ITCH STOPPING CREAM (diphenhydramine hydrochloride and zinc acetate) cream
McNeil Consumer Healthcare, Division of McNeil-PPC, Inc.

## DRUG FACTS

| Active ingredient | Purpose |
|---|---|
| Diphenhydramine hydrochloride 1% | Topical analgesic |
| Zinc acetate 0.1% | Skin protectant |

## USES
- temporarily relieves pain and itching associated with:
  - insect bites
  - minor burns
  - sunburn
  - minor skin irritations
  - minor cuts
  - scrapes
  - rashes due to poison ivy, poison oak, and poison sumac
- dries the oozing and weeping of poison ivy, poison oak, and poison sumac

## WARNINGS
**For external use only.**

## DO NOT USE
- on large areas of the body
- with any other product containing diphenhydramine, even one taken by mouth

## ASK A DOCTOR BEFORE USE
- on chicken pox
- on measles

## WHEN USING THIS PRODUCT
- avoid contact with eyes

**STOP USE AND ASK A DOCTOR IF**
- condition worsens or does not improve within 7 days
- symptoms persist for more than 7 days or clear up and occur again within a few days

**Keep out of reach of children.** If swallowed, get medical help or contact a Poison Control Center right away. (1-800-222-1222)

**DIRECTIONS**
- do not use more than directed

| adults and children 2 years of age and older | apply to affected area not more than 3 to 4 times daily |
|---|---|
| children under 2 years of age | ask a doctor |

**OTHER INFORMATION**
- store at 20°C-25°C (68°F-77°F)

**INACTIVE INGREDIENTS**
cetyl alcohol, diazolidinyl urea, methylparaben, polyethylene glycol monostearate 1000, propylene glycol, propylparaben, and purified water

**QUESTIONS OR COMMENTS**
Call 1-800-524-2624

---

# BENADRYL-D ALLERGY PLUS SINUS
(diphenhydramine hydrochloride and phenylephrine hydrochloride) tablet
McNeil Consumer Healthcare, Division of McNeil-PPC, Inc.

## DRUG FACTS

| Active ingredients (in each tablet) | Purpose |
|---|---|
| Diphenhydramine hydrochloride 25 mg | Antihistamine |
| Phenylephrine hydrochloride 10 mg | Nasal decongestant |

**USES**
- temporarily relieves these symptoms due to hay fever (allergic rhinitis) or other upper respiratory allergies:
  - runny nose
  - sneezing
  - itchy, watery eyes
  - nasal congestion
  - sinus congestion and pressure
  - itching of the nose or throat
- temporarily relieves these symptoms due to the common cold:
  - runny nose
  - sneezing
  - nasal congestion
  - sinus congestion and pressure

**WARNINGS**

**DO NOT USE**
- with any other product containing diphenhydramine, even one used on skin
- if you are now taking a prescription monoamine oxidase inhibitor (MAOI) (certain drugs for depression, psychiatric or emotional conditions, or Parkinson's disease), or for 2 weeks after stopping the MAOI drug. If you do not know if your prescription drug contains an MAOI, ask a doctor or pharmacist before taking this product

**ASK A DOCTOR BEFORE USE IF YOU HAVE**
- heart disease
- high blood pressure
- thyroid disease
- diabetes
- trouble urinating due to an enlarged prostate gland
- a breathing problem such as emphysema or chronic bronchitis
- glaucoma

**ASK A DOCTOR OR PHARMACIST BEFORE USE IF YOU ARE**
- taking sedatives or tranquilizers

**WHEN USING THIS PRODUCT**
- do not exceed recommended dose
- excitability may occur, especially in children
- marked drowsiness may occur
- alcohol, sedatives, and tranquilizers may increase drowsiness
- avoid alcoholic drinks
- be careful when driving a motor vehicle or operating machinery

**STOP USE AND ASK A DOCTOR IF**
- nervousness, dizziness, or sleeplessness occur
- symptoms do not improve within 7 days or occur with a fever

**If pregnant or breastfeeding,** ask a health professional before use.

**Keep out of reach of children.** In case of overdose, get medical help or contact a Poison Control Center right away. (1-800-222-1222)

**DIRECTIONS**

| adults and children 12 years and over | take 1 tablet every 4 hours |
| | do not take more than 6 tablets in 24 hours |
| children under 12 years | do not use this product in children under 12 years of age |

**OTHER INFORMATION**
- store between 20-25°C (68-77°F)

**INACTIVE INGREDIENTS**
carnauba wax, corn starch, FD&C blue no. 1 aluminum lake, magnesium stearate, microcrystalline cellulose, polyethylene glycol, polyvinyl alcohol, powdered cellulose, pregelatinized starch, sodium starch glycolate, talc, titanium dioxide

**QUESTIONS OR COMMENTS**
Call 1-877-717-2824

---

# BENGAY COLD THERAPY WITH PRO-COOL TECHNOLOGY (menthol) gel
Johnson & Johnson Consumer Companies, Inc.

## DRUG FACTS

| Active ingredient | Purpose |
|---|---|
| Menthol 5% | Topical analgesic |

**USES**
- temporarily relieves the minor aches and pains of muscles and joints associated with:
  - simple backache
  - bruises
  - arthritis
  - sprains
  - strains

**WARNINGS**
For external use only.

**Flammable: Keep away from fire or flame.**

**DO NOT USE**
- on wounds or damaged skin
- with a heating pad
- on a child under 12 years of age with arthritis-like conditions

**ASK A DOCTOR BEFORE USE IF YOU HAVE**
- redness over the affected area

**WHEN USING THIS PRODUCT**
- avoid contact with eyes or mucous membranes
- do not bandage tightly

**STOP USE AND ASK A DOCTOR IF**
- condition worsens or symptoms persist for more than 7 days
- symptoms clear up and occur again within a few days
- excessive skin irritation occurs

**Keep out of reach of children.** If swallowed, get medical help or contact a Poison Control Center immediately.

**DIRECTIONS**

| adults and children 12 years of age and older | apply to affected area not more than 3 to 4 times daily |
| --- | --- |
| children under 12 years of age | ask a doctor |

**OTHER INFORMATION**
- store at 20°C-25°C (68°F-77°F)

**INACTIVE INGREDIENTS**
alcohol, aminomethyl propanol, camphor, carbomer, disteareth-75 IPDI, ethylhexyl isononanoate, FD&C blue no. 1, glycerin, isopropyl alcohol, PEG-7 caprylic/capric glycerides, polysorbate 60, water

**QUESTIONS OR COMMENTS**
Call **1-800-223-0182**

## BENGAY GREASELESS PAIN RELIEVING CREAM (menthol and methyl salicylate)

Johnson & Johnson Consumer Companies, Inc.

### DRUG FACTS

| Active ingredients | Purpose |
| --- | --- |
| Menthol 10% | Topical analgesic |
| Methyl salicylate 15% | Topical analgesic |

**USES**
- temporarily relieves the minor aches and pains of muscles and joints associated with:
  - simple backache
  - arthritis
  - strains
  - bruises
  - sprains

**WARNINGS**
For external use only.

**DO NOT USE**
- on wounds or damaged skin
- with a heating pad
- on a child under 12 years of age with arthritis-like conditions

**ASK A DOCTOR BEFORE USE IF**
- you have redness over the affected area

**WHEN USING THIS PRODUCT**
- avoid contact with eyes or mucous membranes
- do not bandage tightly

**STOP USE AND ASK A DOCTOR IF**
- condition worsens or symptoms persist for more than 7 days
- symptoms clear up and occur again within a few days
- excessive skin irritation occurs

**Keep out of reach of children to avoid accidental ingestion.** If swallowed, get medical help or contact a Poison Control Center immediately.

**DIRECTIONS**
- use only as directed

| adults and children 12 years of age and older | apply to affected area not more than 3 to 4 times daily |
| --- | --- |
| children under 12 years of age | ask a doctor |

**OTHER INFORMATION**
- store between 20°C-25°C (68°F-77°F)

**INACTIVE INGREDIENTS**
carbomer, cetyl alcohol, glycerin, glyceryl stearate se, isopropyl palmitate, methylparaben, potassium cetyl phosphate, propylparaben, stearic acid, stearyl alcohol, trolamine, water.

**QUESTIONS OR COMMENTS**
Call **1-800-223-0182**

## BENGAY PAIN RELIEF AND MASSAGE (menthol) gel

Johnson & Johnson Consumer Companies, Inc.

### DRUG FACTS

| Active ingredient | Purpose |
| --- | --- |
| Menthol 2.5% | Topical analgesic |

**USES**
- temporarily relieves the minor aches and pains of muscles and joints associated with:
  - simple backache
  - bruises
  - arthritis
  - sprains
  - strains

**WARNINGS**
For external use only.

**DO NOT USE**
- on wounds or damaged skin
- with a heating pad
- on a child under 12 years of age with arthritis-like conditions

**ASK A DOCTOR BEFORE USE IF YOU HAVE**
- redness over the affected area

**WHEN USING THIS PRODUCT**
- avoid contact with eyes or mucous membranes
- do not bandage tightly

**STOP USE AND ASK A DOCTOR IF**
- condition worsens or symptoms persist for more than 7 days
- symptoms clear up and occur again within a few days
- excessive skin irritation occurs

**Keep out of reach of children.** If swallowed, get medical help or contact a Poison Control Center immediately.

### DIRECTIONS

| adults and children 12 years of age and older | apply to affected area not more than 3 to 4 times daily |
|---|---|
| | remove protective cap |
| | to open: twist applicator counter-clockwise until it stops |
| | squeeze tube to dispense gel |
| | to close: twist applicator clockwise until it stops |
| | after closing, use applicator to massage in gel |
| | after use, clean applicator with damp cloth or paper towel – do not rinse under or immerse in water |
| | replace protective cap |
| children under 12 years of age | ask a doctor |

### OTHER INFORMATION
- store at 20°C-25°C (68°F-77°F)

### INACTIVE INGREDIENTS
camphor, carbomer, DMDM hydantoin, isoceteth-20, isopropyl alcohol, PEG-40 hydrogenated castor oil, sodium hydroxide, water

### QUESTIONS OR COMMENTS
Call **1-800-223-0182**

---

## BENGAY VANISHING SCENT (menthol) gel
Johnson & Johnson Consumer Companies, Inc.

### DRUG FACTS

| Active ingredient | Purpose |
|---|---|
| Menthol 2.5% | Topical analgesic |

### USES
- temporarily relieves the minor aches and pains of muscles and joints associated with:
  - simple backache
  - arthritis
  - strains
  - bruises
  - sprains

### WARNINGS
**For external use only.**

### DO NOT USE
- on wounds or damaged skin
- with a heating pad
- on a child under 12 years of age with arthritis-like conditions

### ASK A DOCTOR BEFORE USE IF YOU HAVE
- redness over the affected area

**WHEN USING THIS PRODUCT**
- avoid contact with eyes or mucous membranes
- do not bandage tightly

**STOP USE AND ASK A DOCTOR IF**
- condition worsens or symptoms persist for more than 7 days
- symptoms clear up and occur again within a few days
- excessive skin irritation occurs

**Keep out of reach of children.** If swallowed, get medical help or contact a Poison Control Center immediately.

### DIRECTIONS

| adults and children 12 years of age and older | apply to affected area not more than 3 to 4 times daily |
|---|---|
| children under 12 years of age | ask a doctor |

### OTHER INFORMATION
- store at 20°C-25°C (68°F-77°F)

### INACTIVE INGREDIENTS
camphor, carbomer, DMDM hydantoin, isoceteth-20, isopropyl alcohol, PEG-40 hydrogenated castor oil, sodium hydroxide, water

### QUESTIONS OR COMMENTS
Call **1-800-223-0182**

---

## BETADINE (povidone-iodine) solution
Purdue Products LP

### DRUG FACTS

| Active ingredient | Purpose |
|---|---|
| Povidone-iodine, 10% (1% available iodine) | Antiseptic |

### USES
- for preparation of the skin prior to surgery
- helps reduce bacteria that potentially can cause skin infection

### WARNINGS
**For external use only.**

### DO NOT USE
- in the eyes
- if you are allergic to povidone-iodine or any other ingredients in this preparation

### WHEN USING THIS PRODUCT
- prolonged exposure to wet solution may cause irritation or, rarely, severe skin reactions
- in pre-operative prepping, avoid "pooling" beneath the patient

### STOP USE AND ASK A DOCTOR IF
- irritation, sensitization, or allergic reaction occurs and lasts for 72 hours. These may be signs of a serious condition

**Keep out of reach of children.** If swallowed, get medical help or contact a Poison Control Center right away.

### DIRECTIONS
- clean the operative site prior to surgery
- apply product and allow to dry
- may be covered with a bandage

**OTHER INFORMATION**
- store at 25°C (77°F); excursions permitted between 15-30°C (59-86°F)
- store in original container

**INACTIVE INGREDIENTS**
purified water, sodium hydroxide

---

## BETADINE SKIN CLEANSER (povidone-iodine)
solution
Purdue Products LP

### DRUG FACTS

| Active ingredient | Purpose |
|---|---|
| Povidone-iodine, 7.5% (equal to 0.75% available iodine) | Antiseptic |

**USES**
- disinfectant hand wash and skin cleanser
- significantly reduces bacteria on the skin

**WARNINGS**
**For external use only.**

**DO NOT USE THIS PRODUCT**
- if you are sensitive to iodine or other product ingredients
- in the eyes
- over large areas of the body
- longer than 1 week unless directed by a doctor

**ASK A DOCTOR BEFORE USE IF YOU HAVE**
- deep or puncture wounds
- serious burns
- animal bites

**STOP USING THIS PRODUCT AND ASK A DOCTOR IF**
- redness, irritation, swelling, or pain continues or increases
- infection occurs

**Keep out of reach of children.** If swallowed, get medical help or contact a Poison Control Center right away.

**DIRECTIONS**
- wet skin and apply a sufficient amount for lather to cover all surfaces
- wash vigorously for at least 15 seconds
- rinse and dry thoroughly

**OTHER INFORMATION**
- store at 25°C (77°F); excursions permitted between 15-30°C (59-86°F)

**INACTIVE INGREDIENTS**
ammonium nonoxynol-4 sulfate, nonoxynol-9, purified water, sodium hydroxide

---

## BIOFREEZE (menthol) spray
Performance Health Inc.

### DRUG FACTS

| Active ingredients | Purpose |
|---|---|
| Menthol USP 10% | Cooling pain reliever |

**USES**
- soothing on-the-go temporary relief from minor aches and pains of sore muscles and joints associated with:
  - arthritis
  - backache
  - strains
  - sprains

**WARNINGS**
**For external use only.**

**Flammable: Keep away from excessive heat or open flame**

**ASK A DOCTOR BEFORE USE IF YOU HAVE**
- sensitive skin, are pregnant or are breastfeeding

**WHEN USING THIS PRODUCT**
- avoid contact with the eyes or mucous membranes
- do not apply to wounds or damaged skin
- do not use with other ointments, creams, sprays or liniments
- do not apply to irritated skin or if excessive irritation develops
- do not bandage
- wash hands after use with cool water
- do not use with heating pad or device

**STOP USE AND ASK A DOCTOR IF**
- condition worsens, or if
- symptoms persist for more than 7 days, or clear up and reoccur

**If pregnant or breastfeeding,** ask a health professional before use.

**Keep out of reach of children.** If accidentally ingested, get medical help or contact a Poison Control Center immediately.

**DIRECTIONS**

| adults and children 12 years of age and older | apply on to the affected areas not more than 4 times daily |
|---|---|
| children under 12 years of age | consult physician |

**OTHER INFORMATION**
- store in a cool dry place with lid closed tightly

**INACTIVE INGREDIENTS**
arnica montana, calendula, chamomile, dimethyl sulfone, echinacea, ethanol, ILEX paraguariensis, isopropyl myristate, juniper berry, water, white tea

**QUESTIONS OR COMMENTS**
Call **1-800-246-3733**

---

## BIOFREEZE PAIN RELIEVING (menthol) gel
Performance Health Inc.

### DRUG FACTS

| Active ingredient | Purpose |
|---|---|
| Natural menthol USP 3.5% | Cooling pain reliever |

**USES**
- temporary relief from minor aches and pains of sore muscles and joints associated with:
  - arthritis
  - backache
  - strains
  - sprains

## WARNINGS
For external use only.

Flammable: Keep away from excessive heat or open flame

### ASK A DOCTOR BEFORE USE IF YOU HAVE
- sensitive skin

### WHEN USING THIS PRODUCT
- avoid contact with the eyes or mucous membranes
- do not apply to wounds or damaged skin
- do not use with other ointments, creams, sprays or liniments
- do not apply to irritated skin or if excessive irritation develops
- do not bandage
- wash hands after use with cool water
- do not uses with heating pad or device

### STOP USE AND ASK A DOCTOR IF
- condition worsens, or symptoms persist for more than 7 days, or clear up and reoccur

If pregnant or breastfeeding, ask a health professional before use.

Keep out of the reach of children. If accidentally ingested, get medical help or contact a Poison Control Center immediately.

### DIRECTIONS

| adults and children 2 years of age and older | rub a thin film over affected areas not more than 4 times daily; massage not necessary |
|---|---|
| children under 2 years of age | consult physician |

### OTHER INFORMATION
- store in a cool dry place with lid closed tightly

### INACTIVE INGREDIENTS
carbomer, FD&C blue no. 1, FD&C yellow no. 5, glycerine, herbal extract Ilex paraguariensis, isopropyl alcohol USP, methylparaben, natural camphor USP for scent, propylene glycol, silicon dioxide, triethanolamine, purified water USP

### QUESTIONS OR COMMENTS
Call 1-800-246-3733

---

## BIOFREEZE PAIN RELIEVING WIPES (menthol)
gel

Performance Health Inc.

### DRUG FACTS

| Active ingredient | Purpose |
|---|---|
| Natural menthol USP 10.5% | Cooling pain reliever |

### USES
- temporary relief from minor aches and pains of sore muscles and joints associated with:
  - arthritis
  - backache
  - strains
  - sprains

### WARNINGS
For external use only.

Flammable: Keep away from excessive heat or open flame.

### ASK A DOCTOR BEFORE USE IF YOU HAVE
- sensitive skin

### WHEN USING THIS PRODUCT
- avoid contact with the eyes or mucous membranes
- do not apply to wounds or damaged skin
- do not use with other ointments, creams, sprays or liniments
- do not apply to irritated skin or if excessive irritation develops
- do not bandage
- wash hands after use with cool water
- do not use with heating pad or device

### STOP USE AND ASK A DOCTOR IF
- condition worsens, symptoms persist more than 7 days, or clear up and reoccur

Keep out of reach of children. If accidentally ingested, get medical help or contact a Poison Control Center immediately.

### DIRECTIONS

| adults and Children 12 years and older | wipe onto affected area |
|---|---|
| | discard wipe and clean hands following use |
| | do not use more than 4 times daily |
| children under 12 years of age | consult physician |

### OTHER INFORMATION
- Store in a cool dry place

### OTHER INFORMATION
arnica montana, calendula, chamomile, dimethyl sulfone msm, echinacea, ethanol, ilex paraguariensis, isopropyl myristate, juniper berry, purified water USP, white tea

### QUESTIONS OR COMMENTS
Call 1-800-246-3733

---

## BLINK (polyethylene glycol)
Abbott

### DRUG FACTS

| Active ingredient | Purpose |
|---|---|
| Polyethylene glycol 400 0.25% | Eye lubricant |

### USES
- for the temporary relief of burning, irritation, and discomfort due to dryness of the eye or exposure to wind or sun
- May be used as a protectant against further irritation

### WARNINGS
For external use only.
- to avoid contamination, do not touch tip of container to any surface. Replace cap after using
- do not use if solution changes color or becomes cloudy
- do not use if carton or unit dose vial is broken or damaged
- do not reuse. Once vial is opened, discard

### CONTRAINDICATIONS (REASONS NOT TO USE)
- if you are allergic to any ingredient in Blink Tears Lubricating Eye Drops, do not use this product

## STOP USE AND ASK A DOCTOR IF

- you experience eye pain, changes in vision, continued redness or irritation of the eye, or if the condition worsens or persists for more than 72 hours

**Keep out of the reach of children.** If swallowed, get medical help or contact a Poison Control Center right away.

## DIRECTIONS

- to open, twist and pull tab to remove
- instill 1 or 2 drops in the affected eye(s) as needed or as directed by your eye care practitioner

## OTHER INFORMATION

- store at room temperature

## INACTIVE INGREDIENTS

boric acid, calcium chloride, magnesium chloride, potassium chloride, purified water, sodium borate, sodium chloride, sodium hyaluronate

---

# BLISTEX FIVE STAR (petrolatum, hemosalate, octinoxate, oxybenzone, octisalate) stick

Blistex Inc.

## DRUG FACTS

| Active ingredients | Purpose |
|---|---|
| Petrolatum 30.1 grams | Skin protectant/sunscreen |
| Hemosalate 9.6 grams | |
| Octinoxate 5.0 grams | |
| Oxybenzone 7.5 grams | |
| Octisalate 5.0 grams | |

## USES

- temporarily protects and helps relieve chapped or cracked lips
- helps protect lips from the drying effects of wind, cold weather
- helps prevent sunburn

## WARNINGS
**For external use only.**

## DO NOT USE ON

- deep puncture wounds
- animal bites
- serious burns

## STOP USE IF

- skin rash occurs

## DIRECTIONS

| adults and children 2 years of age and older | apply liberally to affected area not more than 3 to 4 times daily |
|---|---|
| children under 2 years of age | consult a doctor |

# BLISTEX KANK-A SOOTHING BEADS
(benzocaine) bead

Blistex Inc.

## DRUG FACTS

| Active ingredient | Purpose |
|---|---|
| Benzocaine 3 mg per bead | Oral anesthetic |

## USES

- for the temporary relief of pain due to canker sores, minor dental procedures, dentures or orthodontic appliances, or minor irritation or injury of the mouth or gums

## WARNINGS
**For oral use only**

**Allergy alert**
This product if you have a history of allergy to local anesthetics such as procaine butacaine, benzocaine, or other caine anesthetics.

## WHEN USING THIS PRODUCT

- do not use for more than 7 days unless directed by a dentist or doctor
- if sore mouth symptoms do not improve in 7 days
- if irritation, pain or redness persists or worsens or if swelling, rash or fever develops, see your doctor or dentist promptly
- Do not exceed recommended dosage

**Keep out of reach of children.** In cases of overdose, get medical help or contact a Poison Control Center right away.

## DIRECTIONS

| adults and children 2 years of age and older | for all over discomfort, including multiple mouth sores brace or denture pain, oral abrasions or minor burns inside the mouth: |
|---|---|
| | place 1 dose 5 beads, in mouth and circulate the mini beads until they dissolve |
| | for targeted pain relief from individual canker sores, accidental bites, etc.: |
| | place 1 dose 5 beads over the affected area and hold in place until dissolved |
| | may be repeated every 2 hours as needed or as directed by a dentist or a doctor |
| children under 12 years of age | should be supervised in the use of this product |
| children under 2 years of age | consult a dentist or doctor |

## OTHER INFORMATION

- do not purchase if package has been opened
- store in a cool, dry place, protect from moisture and humidity

## INACTIVE INGREDIENTS
caprylic capric triglyceride, eugenol, flavor, gelatin, glycerin, hydrogenated coco glycerides, PEG 90, polysorbate 80, sorbitol sucralose, sucrose acetate isobutyrate

QUESTIONS OR COMMENTS
Call toll-free **1-800-837-1800**

# BLISTEX LIP MASSAGE (pertolatum, octinoxate, avobenzone, octocrylene, oxybenzone) gel

Blistex Inc

## DRUG FACTS

| Active ingredients | Purpose |
|---|---|
| Petrolatum 42.33<br>Octinoxate 7.5%<br>Avobenzone 3.0%<br>Octocrylene 2.7%<br>Oxybenzone 2.5% | Skin protectant/sunscreen |

### USES
- temporarily protects and helps relieve chapped or cracked lips
  - helps protect lips from the drying effects of wind and cold weather
  - helps prevent sunburn
  - apply liberally before sun exposure and as needed
  - first use may take up to 10 turns to dispense, subsequent uses should require only 1 turn

### DO NOT USE
- on deep or puncture wounds
- animal bites
- serious burns

### STOP USE IF
- skin rash occurs

### DIRECTIONS
- children under six months of age ask a doctor

# BLISTEX REVIVE AND RESTORE (dimethicone, octinoxate, oxybenzone, and lanolin) kit

Blistex Inc.

## DRUG FACTS - REVIVE

| Active ingredients | Purpose |
|---|---|
| Dimethicone 1.0% (w/w) | Skin protectant |
| Octinoxate 7.5% (w/w) | Sunscreen |
| Oxybenzone 2.5% (w/w) | Sunscreen |

### USES
- temporarily protects and helps relieve chapped or cracked lips
- helps protect lips from the drying effects of wind and cold weather
- helps prevent sunburn

### WARNINGS
- stop use if skin rash occurs

### DIRECTIONS
- apply liberally before sun exposure and as needed
- children under six months of age: ask a doctor

### INACTIVE INGREDIENTS
acer saccharum (sugar maple) extract, aloe barbadensis leaf extract, beeswax, bis-diglyceryl polyacyladipate-2, butyrospermum parkii (shea butter), C10-30 cholesterol/lanosterol esters, caprylic/capric triglyceride, cholesteryl/behenyl/octyldodecyl lauroyl glutamate, citrus aurantium dulcis (orange) fruit extract, citrus medica limonum (lemon) extract, flavors, menthol, microcrystalline wax, myristyl myristate, octyldodecanol, phenoxyethanol, polybutene, purified water, ricinus communis (castor) seed oil, saccharin, saccharum officinarum (sugar cane) extract, vaccinium myrtillus (bilberry) extract

## DRUG FACTS - RESTORE

| Active ingredients | Purpose |
|---|---|
| Lanolin 15.0% (w/w) | Skin protectant |

### USES
- temporarily protects and helps relieve chapped or cracked lips
- helps protect lips from the drying effects of wind and cold weather

### DIRECTIONS
- apply as needed

### INACTIVE INGREDIENTS
beeswax, bis-diglyceryl polyacyladipate-2, brassica campestris/aleurites fordi oil copolymer, C10-30 cholesterol/lanosterol esters, flavors, hydrogenated polyisobutene, jojoba esters, microcrystalline wax, myristyl myristate, octyldodecanol, phenoxyethanol, polybutene, saccharin, simmondsia chinensis (jojoba) seed oil, squalane, theobroma cacao (cocoa) seed butter, tocopheryl acetate

# BONINE (meclizine hydrochloride) tablet, chewable

Insight Pharmaceuticals Corp.

## DRUG FACTS

| Active ingredient<br>(in each tablet) | Purpose |
|---|---|
| Meclizine hydrochloride 25 mg | Antiemetic |

### USES
- prevents and treats nausea, vomiting or dizziness associated with motion sickness

### WARNINGS

**DO NOT USE**
- for children under 12 years of age unless directed by a doctor

**DO NOT TAKE UNLESS DIRECTED BY A DOCTOR IF YOU HAVE**
- glaucoma
- trouble urinating due to an enlarged prostate gland
- a breathing problem such as emphysema or chronic bronchitis

**DO NOT TAKE IF YOU ARE**
- taking sedatives or tranquilizers, without first consulting your doctor

**WHEN USING THIS PRODUCT**
- do not exceed recommended dosage
- drowsiness may occur
- alcohol, sedatives, and tranquilizers may increase drowsiness
- avoid alcoholic drinks
- be careful when driving a motor vehicle or operating machinery

**If pregnant or breastfeeding,** ask a health professional before use.

**Keep out of reach of children.** In case of overdose, get medical help or contact a Poison Control Center right away.

## DIRECTIONS
- dosage should be taken one hour before travel starts

| adults and children 12 years of age and over: | take 1 to 2 tablets once daily or as directed by a doctor |
|---|---|

## OTHER INFORMATION
- store at room temperature 20-25°C (68-77°F)

## INACTIVE INGREDIENTS
croscarmellose sodium, crospovidone, FD&C red no. 40 lake, lactose, magnesium stearate, raspberry flavor, silica, sodium saccharin, stearic acid, vanilla flavor

## QUESTIONS OR COMMENTS
Call **1-800-344-7239** or visit us on the web at www.insightpharma.com

---

## BONINE KIDS (chlorcyclizine hydrochloride) tablet, chewable
Insight Pharmaceuticals Corp.

### DRUG FACTS

| Active ingredient (in each tablet) | Purpose |
|---|---|
| Cyclizine hydrochloride 25 mg | Antiemetic |

## USES
- prevents and treats nausea, vomiting or dizziness associated with motion sickness

## WARNINGS

**DO NOT USE**
- in children under 6 years of age unless directed by a doctor

**DO NOT TAKE OR GIVE TO CHILDREN IF THEY HAVE**
- a breathing problem such as chronic bronchitis or glaucoma without first consulting a doctor

**DO NOT TAKE OR GIVE TO CHILDREN IF THEY ARE**
- taking sedatives or tranquilizers without first consulting a doctor

**WHEN USING THIS PRODUCT**
- do not exceed recommended dosage
- drowsiness may occur
- alcohol, sedatives, and tranquilizers may increase drowsiness
- be careful when driving a motor vehicle or operating machinery

**Keep out of reach of children.** In case of overdose, get medical help or contact a Poison Control Center right away.

## DIRECTIONS
- children 6 years of age and older: chew 1 tablet thoroughly every 6 to 8 hours
- do not exceed 3 tablets in 24 hours or as directed by a doctor
- dosage should be taken up to one hour before travel starts or at onset of symptoms

## OTHER INFORMATION
- store at room temperature 20-25°C (86-77°F)

---

## INACTIVE INGREDIENTS
croscarmellose sodium, ethylcellulose, D&C red no. 27 lake, FD&C blue no. 2 lake, hydroxypropylcellulose, hypromellose, magnesium stearate, mannitol, N&A flavors, sorbitol, sucralose

## QUESTIONS OR COMMENTS
Call **1-800-344-7239**
www.insightpharma.com

---

## BOUDREAUX'S BUTT PASTE (zinc oxide) paste
Blairex

### DRUG FACTS

| Active Ingredient | Purpose |
|---|---|
| Zinc oxide, 16% | prevent diaper rash |

## USES
- helps treat and prevent diaper rash
- protects chafed skin due to diaper rash and helps seal out wetness

## WARNINGS
**For external use only.**
- Avoid contact with the eyes

**STOP USE AND ASK A DOCTOR IF**
- condition worsens or does not improve after 7 days

**Keep out of the reach of children.** If swallowed seek medical help or call Poison Control Center immediately.

## DIRECTIONS FOR USE
- change wet and soiled diaper immediately
- cleanse the diaper area and allow to dry
- apply ointment liberally and often as necessary with each diaper change and especially when exposed to wet diapers for a prolonged period of time, such as bedtime

## OTHER INFORMATION
- store at room temperature, 20-27°C (68-80°F)
- use with infants, children and adults
- will stain clothing and fabric

## INACTIVE INGREDIENTS
castor oil, mineral oil, paraffin, peruvian balsam, petrolatum

---

## BRIOSCHI EFFERVESCENT ANTACID (sodium bicarbonate, tartaric acid) granule, effervescent
Brioschi Pharmaceuticals International, LLC

### DRUG FACTS

| Active ingredients (in each dose) | Purpose |
|---|---|
| Sodium bicarbonate 1.80 grams | Antacid |
| Tartaric acid 1.62 grams | Antacid |

## USES
- provides relief of:
  - heartburn
  - acid indigestion
  - upset stomach associated with above conditions.

## WARNINGS
- do not exceed recommended dosage

### DO NOT USE
- this product if you are on a sodium restricted diet, unless directed by a physician

### DO NOT TAKE
- more than the recommended daily dosage (see Directions) in a 24 hour period, or use the maximum dosage of this product for more than 2 weeks, except under the advice & supervision of a physician

### ASK A DOCTOR OR PHARMACIST BEFORE USE
- if you are presently taking a prescription drug. Antacids may interact with certain prescription drugs

### STOP USE AND ASK A DOCTOR
- if symptoms last for more than 2 weeks

**If pregnant or breastfeeding,** ask a health professional before use.

**Keep out of reach of children.**

### DIRECTIONS
- fully dissolve one capful (approx. 6 grams) in 4-6 ounces of water before drinking

| adults and children 12 years and older | one dose each hour<br>do not exceed 6 doses in 24 hours |
|---|---|
| adults 60 years and older | one dose each hour<br>do not exceed 3 doses in 24 hours |
| children under 12 | ask a doctor |

### OTHER INFORMATION
- each 6 gram dose contains 500 mg of sodium
- BRIOSCHI Effervescent antacid in water contains the antacid sodium tartrate as the principal active ingredient
- store in a cool dry place
- reseal cap tightly

### INACTIVE INGREDIENTS
sugar, corn syrup, natural lemon flavor

### QUESTIONS OR COMMENTS
Call **1-800**-BRIOSCHI or visit www.brioschi.com

---

# BRONKAID HERBAL ADVANTAGE (ephedrine sulfate and guaifenesin) caplet
Bayer HealthCare

## DRUG FACTS

| Active ingredients (in each caplet) | Purpose |
|---|---|
| Ephedrine sulfate 25 mg | Bronchodilator |
| Guaifenesin 400 mg | Expectorant |

### USES
- temporarily relieves shortness of breath, tightness of chest, and wheezing due to bronchial asthma
- helps loosen phlegm (mucus) and thin bronchial secretions to rid the bronchial passageways of bothersome mucus, drain bronchial tubes and make coughs more productive

## WARNINGS

### DO NOT USE
- unless a diagnosis of asthma has been made by a doctor
- if you are now taking a prescription monoamine oxidase inhibitor (MAOI) (certain drugs for depression, psychiatric, or emotional conditions, or Parkinson's disease), or for 2 weeks after stopping the MAOI drug. If you do not know if your prescription drug contains an MAOI, ask a doctor or pharmacist before taking this product
- in children under 12 years of age

### ASK A DOCTOR BEFORE USE IF YOU HAVE
- heart disease
- high blood pressure
- thyroid disease
- diabetes
- difficulty in urination due to enlargement of the prostate gland
- ever been hospitalized for asthma or if you are taking a prescription drug for asthma
- persistent or chronic cough such as occurs with smoking, asthma, chronic bronchitis, or emphysema
- a cough which is accompanied by excessive phlegm (mucus)

### WHEN USING THIS PRODUCT
- you may experience nervousness, tremor, sleeplessness, nausea, and loss of appetite. If these symptoms persist or become worse, consult your doctor

### STOP USE AND ASK A DOCTOR IF
- symptoms are not relieved within 1 hour or become worse
- cough persists for more than 1 week, tends to recur, or is accompanied by a fever, rash, or persistent headache. These could be signs of a serious condition

**If pregnant or breastfeeding,** ask a health professional before use.

**Keep out of reach of children.** In case of overdose, get medical help or contact a Poison Control Center right away.

### DIRECTIONS

| adults and children 12 years and over | take one caplet every 4 hours as needed<br>do not exceed 6 caplets in 24 hours or as directed by a doctor |
|---|---|
| children under 12 years | do not use |

### INACTIVE INGREDIENTS
carnauba wax, corn starch, croscarmellose sodium, hypromellose, magnesium stearate, magnesium trisilicate, microcrystalline cellulose, polyethylene glycol, povidone, pregelatinized starch

### OTHER INFORMATION
- each caplet contains: 15 mg magnesium

---

# BUFFERIN LOW DOSE (aspirin) tablet
Novartis Consumer Health, Inc.

## DRUG FACTS

| Active ingredient (in each tablet) | Purpose |
|---|---|
| Buffered aspirin equal to 81 mg aspirin (NSAID)* (buffered with calcium carbonate, magnesium carbonate and magnesium oxide) | Pain reliever |

*nonsteroidal anti-inflammatory drug

## USES
- temporarily relieves minor aches and pains or as recommended by your doctor
- ask your doctor about other uses of buffered aspirin 81 mg

## WARNINGS
**Reye's syndrome**
Children and teenagers who have or are recovering from chicken pox or flu-like symptoms should not use this product. When using this product if changes in behavior with nausea and vomiting occur, consult a doctor because these symptoms could be an early sign of Reye's syndrome, a rare but serious illness.

**Allergy alert**
Aspirin may cause a severe allergic reaction which may include:
- hives
- facial swelling
- asthma (wheezing)
- shock

**Stomach bleeding warning**
This product contains an NSAID, which may cause severe stomach bleeding. The chance is higher if you:
- are age 60 or older
- have had stomach ulcers or bleeding problems
- take a blood thinning (anticoagulant) or steroid drug
- take other drugs containing prescription or nonprescription NSAIDs (aspirin, ibuprofen, naproxen, or others)
- have 3 or more alcoholic drinks every day while using this product
- take more or for a longer time than directed

## DO NOT USE
- if you have ever had an allergic reaction to aspirin or any other pain reliever/fever reducer

## ASK A DOCTOR BEFORE USE IF
- stomach bleeding warning applies to you
- you have a history of stomach problems, such as heartburn
- you have high blood pressure, heart disease, liver cirrhosis, or kidney disease
- you are taking a diuretic
- you are on a magnesium-restricted diet
- you have asthma

## ASK DOCTOR OR PHARMACIST BEFORE USE IF YOU ARE TAKING
- any other drug containing an NSAID (prescription or nonprescription)
- a blood thinning (anticoagulant) or steroid drug
- a prescription drug for diabetes, gout, or arthritis
- any other drug, or are under a doctor's care for any serious condition

## STOP USE AND ASK A DOCTOR IF
- an allergic reaction occurs. Seek medical help right away
- you experience any of the following signs of stomach bleeding:
  - feel faint
  - vomit blood
  - have bloody or black stools
  - have stomach pain that does not get better
- ringing in the ears or loss of hearing occurs
- painful area is red or swollen
- pain gets worse or lasts for more than 10 days
- fever gets worse or lasts for more than 3 days
- any new symptoms appear

**If pregnant or breastfeeding,** ask a health professional before use.

**It is especially important not to use aspirin during the last 3 months of pregnancy unless definitely directed to** do so by a doctor because it may cause problems in the unborn child or complications during delivery.

**Keep out of reach of children.** In case of overdose, get medical help or contact a Poison Control Center right away.

## DIRECTIONS
- do not use more than directed
- drink a full glass of water with each dose

| adults and children 12 years and over | take 4 to 8 tablets every 4 hours; not more than 48 tablets in 24 hours or as directed by a doctor |
| children under 12 years | ask a doctor |

## OTHER INFORMATION
- each tablet contains: calcium 18 mg and magnesium 15 mg
- store at controlled room temperature 20-25° C (68-77° F)
- protect from freezing
- read all product information before using. Keep box for important information

## INACTIVE INGREDIENTS
benzoic acid, carnauba wax, corn starch, FD&C blue no. 1, hypromellose, light mineral oil, magnesium stearate, microcrystalline cellulose, polysorbate 20, polysorbate 80, povidone, pregelatinized starch, propylene glycol, simethicone emulsion, sorbitan monolaurate, talc, titanium dioxide

## QUESTIONS OR COMMENTS
Call **1-800-468-7746**

---

# CALADRYL ANTI-ITCH LOTION (calamine and pramoxine hydrochloride) lotion
Johnson & Johnson

## DRUG FACTS

| Active ingredients | Purpose |
| --- | --- |
| Calamine 8% | Skin protectant |
| Pramoxine hydrochloride 1% | Topical analgesic |

## USES
- temporarily relieves pain and itching associated with:
  - rashes due to poison ivy, poison oak, or poison sumac
  - insect bites
  - minor skin irritation
  - minor cuts
- dries the oozing and weeping of poison ivy, poison oak and poison sumac

## WARNINGS
**For external use only**

## WHEN USING THIS PRODUCT
- avoid contact with eyes

## STOP USE AND ASK A DOCTOR IF
- condition worsens or does not improve within 7 days
- symptoms persist for more than 7 days or clear up and occur again within a few days

**Keep out of reach of children.** If swallowed, get medical help or contact a Poison Control Center right away.

## DIRECTIONS
- shake well before use

| adults and children 2 years of age and older | apply to affected area not more than 3 to 4 times daily |
|---|---|
| children under 2 years of age | ask a doctor |

### OTHER INFORMATION
- store at 20°C-25°C (68°F-77°F)

### INACTIVE INGREDIENTS
SD alcohol 38-B, camphor, diazolidinyl urea, fragrance, hypromellose, methylparaben, polysorbate 80, propylene glycol, propylparaben, purified water, xanthan gum

### QUESTIONS OR COMMENTS
Call **1-800-223-0182**

## CALAGEL MEDICATED ANTI-ITCH GEL
(diphenhydramine hydrochloride, zinc acetate, and benzethonium chloride) gel

Iec Labs

### DRUG FACTS

| Active ingredients | Purpose |
|---|---|
| Diphenhydramine Hydrochloride 1.8% | First aid antiseptic |
| Zinc acetate 0.21% | Skin protectant |
| Benzethonium chloride 0.1% | Topical analgesic |

### USES
- For temporary relief of pain and itching associated with minor burns, sunburn, minor cuts, scrapes, insect bites, and minor skin irritations.
- Dries the oozing and weeping of poison ivy, oak, and sumac.

### WARNINGS
- In case of accidental ingestion, seek professional assistance or contact a Poison Control Center immediately
- Keep this and all drugs out of the reach of children

**For external use only.**
- avoid contact with eyes. If condition worsens or if symptoms persist for more than 7 days or clear up and occur again within a few days, discontinue use of this product and consult a physician
- do not apply over large areas of the body. In case of deep or puncture wounds, animal bites or serious burns, consult a physician
- do not use on children under 2 without consulting a physician
- do not use on chicken pox or measles unless supervised by a physician

### DIRECTIONS
- before each application cleanse skin with Techu (for poison oak, ivy & sumac) or soap and warm water, and dry affected area
- may be covered with a sterile bandage
- if bandage let dry first

| adults and children 2 years of age and older | apply to affected area not more than three times daily |
|---|---|
| children under 2 years of age | consult a physician |

### OTHER INFORMATION
- preventative measures should be taken to prevent reintroduction of poison ivy, poison oak and sumac from personal belongings
- unfortunately, urushiol, the skin irritant oil produced from those plants can last up to one year
- store at room temperature (59-86°F)

### INACTIVE INGREDIENTS
purified water, polysorbate 20, hydroxypropl, methylcellulose, disodium EDTA, sodium metabisulfite, menthol and other fragrance

## CALMOSEPTINE (menthol and zinc oxide) ointment
Calmoseptine, Inc.

### DRUG FACTS

| Active ingredients | Purpose |
|---|---|
| Menthol 0.44% | External analgesic/anti-itch |
| Zinc oxide 20.6% | Skin protectant/anorectal astringent |

### USES
- a moisture barrier that prevents & helps heal skin irritations from:
  - urine
  - diarrhea
  - perspiration
  - fistula drainage
  - feeding tube site leakage
  - wound drainage (peri-wound skin)
  - minor burns
  - cuts
  - scrapes
  - itching

### WARNINGS
**For external use only.**

- not for deep or puncture wounds
- avoid contact with eyes
- if condition worsens or does not improve within 7 days, consult a doctor

**Keep out of reach of children.** In case of accidental ingestion contact a physician or Poison Control Center immediately

### DIRECTIONS
- cleanse skin gently with mild skin cleanser
- pat dry or allow to air dry
- apply a thin layer of Calmoseptine Ointment to reddened or irritated skin 2-4 times daily, or after each incontinent episode or diaper change to promote comfort and long lasting protection

### INACTIVE INGREDIENTS
calamine, chlorothymol, glycerin, lanolin, phenol, sodium bicarbonate, and thymol

# CAPZASIN ARTHRITIS PAIN RELIEF
(capsaicin) cream
Chattem, Inc.

## DRUG FACTS

| Active ingredient | Purpose |
|---|---|
| Capsaicin 0.035% | Topical analgesic |

### USES
- temporarily relieves minor pain associated with:
  - arthritis
  - simple backache
  - strains
  - sprains
  - bruises

### WARNINGS
**For external use only.**

### WHEN USING THIS PRODUCT
- use only as directed
- do not bandage
- do not use with a heating pad
- avoid contact with eyes and mucous membranes
- do not apply to wounds or damaged skin

### STOP USE AND ASK A DOCTOR IF
- condition worsens
- symptoms persist for more than 7 days or clear up and occur again within a few days
- redness is present
- irritation develops

**If pregnant or breastfeeding,** ask a health professional before use.

**Keep out of reach of children.** In case of accidental ingestion, get medical help or contact a Poison Control Center right away.

### DIRECTIONS

| adults and children over 18 years | apply to affected area |
|---|---|
| | massage into painful area until thoroughly absorbed |
| | repeat as necessary, but no more than 4 times daily |
| | wash hands with soap and water after applying |
| children 18 years or younger | ask a doctor |

### OTHER INFORMATION
- read package insert before using
- keep carton and insert as it contains important information

### INACTIVE INGREDIENTS
benzyl alcohol, cetyl alcohol, glyceryl stearate, isopropyl myristate, PEG-40 stearate, petrolatum, sorbitol, water (238-9)

### QUESTIONS OR COMMENTS
www.chattem.com

# CAPZASIN HP ARTHRITIS PAIN RELIEF
(capsaicin) cream
Chattem, Inc.

## DRUG FACTS

| Active ingredient | Purpose |
|---|---|
| Capsaicin 0.1% | Topical analgesic |

### USES
- temporarily relieves minor pain of muscles and joints associated with:
  - arthritis
  - simple backache
  - strains
  - sprains
  - bruises

### WARNINGS
**For external use only.**

### WHEN USING THIS PRODUCT
- use only as directed
- do not bandage tightly or use with a heating pad
- avoid contact with eyes and mucous membranes
- do not apply to wounds, damaged, broken or irritated skin
- a transient burning sensation may occur upon application but generally disappears in several days
- if severe burning sensation occurs, discontinue use immediately and read important information printed inside carton
- do not expose the area treated with product to heat or direct sunlight

### STOP USE AND ASK A DOCTOR IF
- condition worsens
- symptoms persist for more than 7 days or clear up and occur again within a few days
- redness is present
- irritation develops

**If pregnant or breastfeeding,** ask a health professional before use.

**Keep out of reach of children.** If swallowed, get medical help or contact a Poison Control Center right away.

### DIRECTIONS

| adults and children over 18 years | apply to affected area |
|---|---|
| | massage into painful area until thoroughly absorbed |
| | repeat as necessary, but no more than 3 to 4 times daily |
| | wash hands with soap and water after applying |
| children 18 years or younger | ask a doctor |

### INACTIVE INGREDIENTS
benzyl alcohol, cetyl alcohol, glyceryl stearate, isopropyl myristate, PEG-40 stearate, petrolatum, sorbitol, water (238-10)

### QUESTIONS OR COMMENTS
www.chattem.com

## CAPZASIN NO MESS APPLICATOR (capsaicin)
liquid

Chattem, Inc.

### DRUG FACTS

| Active ingredient | Purpose |
|---|---|
| Capsaicin 0.15% | Topical analgesic |

### USES
- temporarily relieves minor pain associated with:
  - arthritis
  - simple backache
  - muscle strains
  - sprains
  - bruises
  - cramps

### WARNINGS
**For external use only.**

### WHEN USING THIS PRODUCT
- read inside of carton before using
- use only as directed
- do not bandage
- do not use with a heating pad
- avoid contact with eyes and mucous membranes
- do not apply to wounds, damaged, broken or irritated skin
- a transient burning sensation may occur upon application but generally disappears in several days
- if severe burning sensation occurs, discontinue use immediately and read information printed inside carton
- do not expose the area treated with product to heat or direct sunlight

### STOP USE AND ASK A DOCTOR IF
- condition worsens
- redness is present
- irritation develops
- symptoms persist for more than 7 days or clear up and occur again within a few days

**Flammable.** Keep away from fire or flame.

**If pregnant or breastfeeding,** ask a health professional before use.

**Keep out of reach of children.** If swallowed, get medical help or contact a Poison Control Center right away.

### DIRECTIONS

| adults and children over 18 years | apply to affected area |
|---|---|
| | place applicator on skin, press firmly and hold to activate the dispensing of liquid |
| | massage into painful area until thoroughly absorbed |
| | repeat as necessary, but no more than 3 to 4 times daily |
| | if medicine comes in contact with hands, wash with soap and water |
| children 18 years or younger | ask a doctor |

### OTHER INFORMATION
- keep carton as it contains important information

### INACTIVE INGREDIENTS
carbomer, glycerin, propylene glycol, SD alcohol 40-2 (35%), triethanolamine, water (245-130)

### QUESTIONS OR COMMENTS
www.chattem.com

## CAPZASIN QUICK RELIEF (capsaicin and menthol)
gel

Chattem, Inc.

### DRUG FACTS

| Active ingredient | Purpose |
|---|---|
| Capsaicin 0.025% | Topical analgesic |
| Menthol 10% | Topical analgesic |

### USES
- temporarily relieves minor pain associated with:
  - arthritis
  - simple backache
  - muscle strains
  - sprains
  - bruises
  - cramps

### WARNINGS
**For external use only.**

### WHEN USING THIS PRODUCT
- read inside of carton before using
- use only as directed
- do not bandage tightly or use with a heating pad
- avoid contact with eyes and mucous membranes
- do not apply to wounds or damaged, broken or irritated skin
- a transient burning sensation may occur upon application but generally disappears in several days
- if severe burning sensation occurs, discontinue use immediately and read inside carton for important information
- do not expose the area treated with product to heat or direct sunlight

### STOP USE AND ASK A DOCTOR IF
- condition worsens
- redness is present
- irritation develops
- symptoms persist for more than 7 days or clear up and occur again within a few days

**If pregnant or breastfeeding,** ask a health professional before use.

**Keep out of reach of children.** If swallowed, get medical help or contact a Poison Control Center right away.

## DIRECTIONS

| adults and children over 18 years | squeeze desired amount of Capzasin Quick Relief Gel onto affected area |
| --- | --- |
| | using the sponge-top applicator, massage dispensed gel into painful area until thoroughly absorbed |
| | repeat as necessary, but no more than 3 to 4 times daily |
| | if medicine comes in contact with hands, wash with soap and water |
| children 18 years or younger | ask a doctor |

## OTHER INFORMATION
• keep carton and insert as it contains important information

## INACTIVE INGREDIENTS
acrylates/C10-30 alkyl acrylate crosspolymer, allantoin, aloe barbadensis leaf juice, DMDM hydantoin, fragrance, glycerin, methylparaben, phenoxyethanol, propylene glycol, propylparaben, SD alcohol 40-2 (15%), steareth-2, steareth-21, triethanolamine, water (245-285)

## QUESTIONS OR COMMENTS
www.chattem.com

## CEPACOL ANTIBACTERIAL (cetylpyridinium chloride) liquid
Reckitt Benckiser LLC

### DRUG FACTS

| Active ingredient | Purpose |
| --- | --- |
| Cetylpyridinium chloride 0.05% | Antigingivitis/antiplaque |

### USES
• helps prevent and reduce plaque that leads to:
  • gingivitis, an early form of gum disease
  • bleeding gums

### WARNINGS

**STOP USE AND ASK A DENTIST IF**
• gingivitis, bleeding, or redness persists for more than 2 weeks
• you have painful or swollen gums, pus from the gum line, loose teeth, or increasing spacing between the teeth. These may be signs or symptoms of periodontitis, a serious form of gum disease

**Keep out of the reach of children under 6 years of age.** If more than used for rinsing is accidentally swallowed, get medical help or contact a Poison Control Center right away.

### DIRECTIONS

| adults and children 12 years of age and older | vigorously swish 20 milliliters of rinse between your teeth twice a day for 30 seconds and then spit out. Do not swallow the rinse |
| --- | --- |
| children 6 years to under 12 years of age | supervise use |
| children under 6 years of age | do not use |

## OTHER INFORMATION
• this rinse is not intended to replace brushing or flossing
• store at room temperature 20-25°C (68-77°F)
• protect from humidity

## INACTIVE INGREDIENTS
purified water, alcohol 14% v/v, glycerin, sodium phosphate dibasic, eucalyptus oil, polysorbate 80, methyl salicylate, cinnamon oil, peppermint oil, saccharin sodium, sodium phosphate monobasic anhydrous, menthol, edetate disodium, FD&C Yellow no. 5

## QUESTIONS OR COMMENTS
Call **1-888-963-3382.** You may also report side effects to this phone number.

## CEPACOL DUAL RELIEF (benzocaine and glycerin) spray
Combe Incorporated

### DRUG FACTS

| Active ingredients | Purpose |
| --- | --- |
| Benzocaine 5.0% | Oral anesthetic |
| Glycerin 33.0% | Oral demulcent |

### USES
• for the temporary relief of:
  • occasional minor irritation, pain, sore mouth and sore throat
  • pain due to canker sores
  • pain due to minor irritation or injury of the mouth and gums
  • minor discomfort and protection of irritated areas in sore mouth and sore throat

### WARNINGS
**Allergy alert**
Do not use this product if you have a history of allergy to local anesthetics such as procaine, butacaine, benzocaine or any other 'caine' anesthetics.

**Sore throat warning**
If sore throat is severe, persists for more than 2 days, is accompanied or followed by fever, headache, rash, swelling, nausea or vomiting, consult a doctor promptly.

**STOP USE AND ASK A DOCTOR IF**
• sore mouth symptoms do not improve in 7 days, or if irritation, pain or redness persists or worsens

**If pregnant or breastfeeding,** ask a health professional before use.

**Keep this and all drugs out of reach of children.** In case of overdose, get medical help or contact a Poison Control Center right away.

Do not exceed recommended dosage.

**Flammable.** Do not use near fire, flame or heat.

### WHEN USING THIS PRODUCT
• do not get into eyes
• if contact occurs, rinse eyes thoroughly with water
• if irritation persists, consult a doctor

### DIRECTIONS
• shake well before use

| adults and children 6 years of age or older | spray into throat or onto affected area with only ONE spray per use |
|---|---|
| | use up to 4 times daily or as directed by a doctor or dentist |
| children 6 to 12 years of age | should be supervised in the use of this product |
| children under 6 years of age | do not use |

## OTHER INFORMATION
- store at room temperature (68-77°F) (20-25°C)
- do not freeze

## INACTIVE INGREDIENTS
deionized water, flavor, neotame, PEG-40 hydrogenated castor oil, potassium acesulfame, PVP, SD alcohol 38B

---

## CEPACOL FIZZLERS (benzocaine) tablet, orally disintegrating
Combe Incorporated

## DRUG FACTS

| Active ingredients | Purpose |
|---|---|
| Benzocaine 6.0 mg | Oral anesthetic |

## USE
- temporarily relieves occasional minor sore throat pain

## WARNINGS
**Allergy alert**
Do not use this product if you have a history of allergy to local anesthetics such as procaine, butacaine, benzocaine or any other 'caine' anesthetics.

**Sore throat warning**
Severe or persistent sore throat or sore throat accompanied by high fever, headache, rash, nausea or vomiting may be serious. Consult a doctor promptly. Do not use for more than 2 days or give to children under 5 years of age.

## STOP USE AND ASK A DOCTOR IF
- symptoms do not improve in 7 days, or if irritation, pain or redness persists or worsens

**If pregnant or breastfeeding,** ask a health professional before use.

**Keep this and all drugs out of reach of children.** In case of overdose, get medical help or contact a Poison Control Center right away.

**Do not exceed recommended dosage**

## DIRECTIONS

| children 5 years of age and older | place tablet on tongue and let dissolve. For best results, do not chew; may be repeated every 2 hours as needed or as directed by a doctor or dentist |
|---|---|
| children under 5 years of age | do not use |

## OTHER INFORMATION
- store at room temperature (68-77°F) (20-25°C)
- protect contents from humidity

## INACTIVE INGREDIENTS
citric acid, colloidal silicon dioxide, crospovidone, D&C red no. 27, FD&C blue no. 1, flavor (corn syrup solids, modified corn starch, natural flavors), magnesium stearate, mannitol, microcrystalline cellulose, sodium bicarbonate, sucralose

---

## CEPACOL SORE THROAT MAXIMUM NUMBING CHERRY (benzocaine and menthol)
lozenge
Combe Incorporated

## DRUG FACTS

| Active ingredients (in each lozenge) | Purpose |
|---|---|
| Benzocaine 15.0 mg | Oral anesthetic |
| Menthol 3.6 mg | Oral analgesic |

## USES
- temporarily relieves occasional:
  - sore throat pain
  - sore mouth
  - minor mouth irritation
  - pain associated with canker sores

## WARNINGS
**Allergy alert**
Do not use this product if you have a history of allergy to local anesthetics such as procaine, butacaine, benzocaine or any other 'caine' anesthetics.

**Sore throat warning**
Severe or persistent sore throat or sore throat accompanied by high fever, headache, nausea, and vomiting may be serious. Consult a doctor promptly. Do not use for more than 2 days or give to children under 5 years of age.

## STOP USE AND ASK A DOCTOR IF
- sore mouth symptoms do not improve in 7 days, or if irritation, pain or redness persists or worsens

**If pregnant or breastfeeding,** ask a health professional before use.

**Keep this and all drugs out of reach of children.** In case of overdose, get medical help or contact a Poison Control Center right away.

**Do not exceed recommended dosage.**

## DIRECTIONS

| adults and children 5 years or older | allow lozenge to dissolve slowly in the mouth; may be repeated every 2 hours as needed or as directed by a doctor or dentist |
|---|---|
| children under 5 years of age | do not use |

## OTHER INFORMATION
- store at room temperature (68-77°F) (20-25°C)
- protect contents from humidity

## INACTIVE INGREDIENTS
cetylpyridinium chloride (ceepryn), flavor, glucose, potassium acesulfame, propylene glycol, D&C red no. 33, D&C red no. 40, sodium bicarbonate, sucrose

# CEPACOL SORE THROAT PLUS COATING
(benzocaine and pectin) lozenge
Combe Incorporated

## DRUG FACTS

| Active ingredients | Purpose |
|---|---|
| Benzocaine 15.0 mg | Oral anesthetic |
| Pectin 5.0 mg | Oral demulcent |

## USES
- temporarily:
  - relieves occasional minor irritation, pain and discomfort of sore throat and sore mouth
  - protects irritated areas in sore throat and sore mouth

## WARNINGS
**Allergy alert**
Do not use this product if you have a history of allergy to local anesthetics such as procaine, butacaine, benzocaine or any other 'caine' anesthetics.

**Sore throat warning**
Severe or persistent sore throat or sore throat accompanied by high fever, headache, nausea, and vomiting may be serious. Consult a doctor promptly. Do not use for more than 2 days unless directed by a doctor.

**STOP USE AND ASK A DOCTOR IF**
- sore mouth symptoms do not improve in 7 days, or if irritation, pain or redness persists or worsens

**If pregnant or breastfeeding,** ask a health professional before use.

**Keep this and all drugs out of reach of children.** In case of overdose, get medical help or contact a Poison Control Center right away.

**Do not exceed recommended dosage.**

## DIRECTIONS

| adults and children 6 years of age and older | allow lozenge to dissolve slowly in the mouth; may be repeated every 2 hours as needed or as directed by a doctor or dentist |
|---|---|
| children under 6 years of age | do not use |

## OTHER INFORMATION
- store at room temperature (68-77°F) (20-25°C)
- protect contents from humidity

## INACTIVE INGREDIENTS
FD&C blue no. 1, cetylpyridinium chloride (Ceepryn), flavor, isomalt, maltitol, potassium acesulfame, propylene glycol, sodium bicarbonate, D&C yellow no. 10

# CEPACOL SORE THROAT PLUS COUGH
(benzocaine and dextromethorphan hydrobromide) lozenge
Combe Incorporated

## DRUG FACTS

| Active ingredients | Purpose |
|---|---|
| Benzocaine 7.5 mg | Oral anesthetic |
| Dextromethorphan hydrobromide 5.0 mg | Cough suppressant |

## USES
- temporarily:
  - relieves occasional minor irritation, pain, sore mouth and sore throat
  - controls cough due to minor throat and bronchial irritation associated with a cold

## WARNINGS
**Allergy alert**
Do not use this product if you have a history of allergy to local anesthetics such as procaine, butacaine, benzocaine or any other 'caine' anesthetics.

**Sore throat warning**
Severe or persistent sore throat or sore throat accompanied by high fever, headache, nausea, and vomiting may be serious. Consult a doctor promptly. Do not use for more than 2 days or give to children under 6 years of age.

## DO NOT USE THIS PRODUCT IF
- you are now taking a prescription monoamine oxidase inhibitor (MAOI) (certain drugs for depression, psychiatric or emotional conditions, or Parkinson's disease), or for 2 weeks after stopping the MAOI drug
- if you do not know if your prescription drug contains an MAOI, ask a doctor or pharmacist before taking the product

## ASK A DOCTOR BEFORE USE IF YOU HAVE
- a cough that is accompanied by excessive phlegm (mucus)
- a persistent or chronic cough such as occurs with smoking, asthma, or emphysema

## STOP USE AND ASK A DOCTOR IF
- sore mouth symptoms do not improve in 7 days, or if irritation, pain or redness persists or worsens
- cough persists for more than 1 week, tends to recur, or is accompanied by fever, rash, or persistent headache. These could be signs of a serious condition

**If pregnant or breastfeeding,** ask a health professional before use.

**Keep this and all drugs out of reach of children.** In case of overdose, get medical help or contact a Poison Control Center right away.

**Do not exceed recommended dosage.**

## DIRECTIONS

| | |
|---|---|
| adults and children 12 years of age and older | take 2 lozenges (one immediately after the other) and allow each lozenge to dissolve slowly in the mouth; may be repeated every 4 hours, not to exceed 12 lozenges in any 24 hour period, or as directed by a doctor |
| children under 6 years of age | do not use |

## OTHER INFORMATION
- store at room temperature (68-77°F) (20-25°C)
- protect contents from humidity

## INACTIVE INGREDIENTS
FD&C blue no. 1, cetylpyridinium chloride (ceepryn), flavor, glucose, potassium acesulfame, propylene glycol, D&C red no. 40, sodium bicarbonate, sucrose

# CEPACOL SORE THROAT REGULAR STRENGTH (menthol) lozenge
Combe Incorporated

## DRUG FACTS

| Active ingredients | Purpose |
|---|---|
| Menthol 3 mg | Oral analgesic |

## USES
- temporarily relieves occasional:
  - sore throat pain
  - sore mouth
  - minor mouth irritation

## WARNINGS
**Sore throat warning**
Severe or persistent sore throat or sore throat accompanied by high fever, headache, nausea, and vomiting may be serious. Consult a doctor promptly.

## DO NOT USE
- for more than 2 days or give to children under 5 years of age

## STOP USE AND ASK A DOCTOR IF
- sore mouth symptoms do not improve in 7 days, or if irritation, pain or redness persists or worsens

**If pregnant or breastfeeding,** ask a health professional before use.

**Keep this and all drugs out of reach of children**. In case of overdose, get medical help or contact a Poison Control Center right away.

**Do not exceed recommended dosage.**

## DIRECTIONS

| | |
|---|---|
| adults and children 5 years or older | allow lozenge to dissolve slowly in the mouth; may be repeated every 2 hours as needed or as directed by a doctor or dentist |
| children under 5 years of age | do not use |

## OTHER INFORMATION
- store at room temperature (68-77°F) (20-25°C)
- protect contents from humidity

## INACTIVE INGREDIENTS
cetylpyridinium chloride (ceepryn), glucose, peppermint (mentha piperita) oil, propylene glycol, sucrose, D&C yellow no. 10

# CEPACOL SORE THROAT MAXIMUM NUMBING SUGAR FREE CHERRY (benzocaine and menthol) lozenge
Combe Incorporated

## DRUG FACTS

| Active ingredients | Purpose |
|---|---|
| Benzocaine 15.0 mg | Oral anesthetic |
| Menthol 4.0 mg | Oral analgesic |

## USES
- temporarily relieves occasional:
  - sore throat pain
  - sore mouth
  - minor mouth irritation
  - pain associated with canker sores

## WARNINGS
**Allergy alert**
Do not use this product if you have a history of allergy to local anesthetics such as procaine, butacaine, benzocaine or any other 'caine' anesthetics.

**Sore throat warning**
Severe or persistent sore throat or sore throat accompanied by high fever, headache, nausea, and vomiting may be serious. Consult a doctor promptly. Do not use for more than 2 days or give to children under 5 years of age.

## STOP USE AND ASK A DOCTOR IF
- sore mouth symptoms do not improve in 7 days, or if irritation, pain or redness persists or worsens

**If pregnant or breastfeeding,** ask a health professional before use.

**Keep this and all drugs out of reach of children**. In case of overdose, get medical help or contact a Poison Control Center right away.

**Do not exceed recommended dosage.**

## DIRECTIONS

| | |
|---|---|
| adults and children 5 years or older | allow lozenge to dissolve slowly in the mouth; may be repeated every 2 hours as needed or as directed by a doctor or dentist |
| children under 5 years of age | do not use |

## OTHER INFORMATION
- store at room temperature (68-77°F) (20-25°C)
- protect contents from humidity

## INACTIVE INGREDIENTS
cetylpyridinium chloride (Ceepryn), flavor, isomalt, maltitol, potassium acesulfame, propylene glycol, D&C red no. 33, D&C red no. 40, sodium bicarbonate

# CEPACOL SORE THROAT MAXIMUM NUMBING CITRUS (benzocaine and menthol) lozenge

Combe Incorporated

## DRUG FACTS

| Active ingredients | Purpose |
|---|---|
| Benzocaine 15.0 mg | Oral anesthetic |
| Menthol 2.1 mg | Oral analgesic |

### USES
- temporarily relieves occasional:
  - sore throat pain
  - sore mouth
  - minor mouth irritation
  - pain associated with canker sores

### WARNINGS
**Allergy alert**
Do not use this product if you have a history of allergy to local anesthetics such as procaine, butacaine, benzocaine or any other 'caine' anesthetics.

**Sore throat warning**
Severe or persistent sore throat or sore throat accompanied by high fever, headache, nausea, and vomiting may be serious. Consult a doctor promptly. Do not use for more than 2 days or give to children under 5 years of age.

### STOP USE AND ASK A DOCTOR IF
- sore mouth symptoms do not improve in 7 days, or if irritation, pain or redness persists or worsens

**If pregnant or breastfeeding,** ask a health professional before use.

**Keep this and all drugs out of reach of children.** In case of overdose, get medical help or contact a Poison Control Center right away.

**Do not exceed recommended dosage.**

### DIRECTIONS

| adults and children 5 years or older | allow lozenge to dissolve slowly in the mouth; may be repeated every 2 hours as needed or as directed by a doctor or dentist |
|---|---|
| children under 5 years of age | do not use |

### OTHER INFORMATION
- store at room temperature (68-77°F) (20-25°C)
- protect contents from humidity

### INACTIVE INGREDIENTS
cetylpyridinium chloride (Ceepryn), flavor, isomalt, maltitol syrup, propylene glycol, sodium bicarbonate, sucralose, D&C yellow no. 6

# CEPACOL SORE THROAT MAXIMUM NUMBING HONEY LEMON (benzocaine and menthol) lozenge

Combe Incorporated

## DRUG FACTS

| Active ingredients | Purpose |
|---|---|
| Benzocaine 15.0 mg | Oral anesthetic |
| Menthol 2.6 mg | Oral analgesic |

### USES
- temporarily relieves occasional:
  - sore throat pain
  - sore mouth
  - minor mouth irritation
  - pain associated with canker sores

### WARNINGS
**Allergy alert**
Do not use this product if you have a history of allergy to local anesthetics such as procaine, butacaine, benzocaine or any other 'caine' anesthetics.

**Sore throat warning**
Severe or persistent sore throat or sore throat accompanied by high fever, headache, nausea, and vomiting may be serious. Consult a doctor promptly. Do not use for more than 2 days or give to children under 5 years of age.

### STOP USE AND ASK A DOCTOR IF
- sore mouth symptoms do not improve in 7 days, or if irritation, pain or redness persists or worsens

**If pregnant or breastfeeding,** ask a health professional before use.

**Keep this and all drugs out of reach of children.** In case of overdose, get medical help or contact a Poison Control Center right away.

**Do not exceed recommended dosage.**

### DIRECTIONS

| adults and children 5 years or older | allow lozenge to dissolve slowly in the mouth; may be repeated every 2 hours as needed or as directed by a doctor or dentist |
|---|---|
| children under 5 years of age | do not use |

### OTHER INFORMATION
- store at room temperature (68-77°F) (20-25°C)
- protect contents from humidity

### INACTIVE INGREDIENTS
cetylpyridinium chloride (Ceepryn), flavor, isomalt, maltitol syrup, propylene glycol, sodium bicarbonate, sucralose, D&C yellow no. 6, D&C yellow no. 10

# CEPACOL SORE THROAT FROM POST NASAL DRIP (menthol) lozenge
Combe Incorporated

## DRUG FACTS

| Active ingredients | Purpose |
|---|---|
| Menthol 4.5 mg | Oral analgesic |

### USES
- temporarily relieves occasional:
  - sore throat pain
  - sore mouth
  - minor mouth irritation

### WARNINGS
**Sore throat warning**
Severe or persistent sore throat or sore throat accompanied by high fever, headache, nausea, and vomiting may be serious. Consult a doctor promptly. Do not use for more than 2 days or give to children under 5 years of age.

### STOP USE AND ASK A DOCTOR IF
- sore mouth symptoms do not improve in 7 days, or if irritation, pain or redness persists or worsens

**If pregnant or breastfeeding,** ask a health professional before use.

**Keep this and all drugs out of reach of children.** In case of overdose, get medical help or contact a Poison Control Center right away.

**Do not exceed recommended dosage.**

### DIRECTIONS

| adults and children 5 years or older | allow lozenge to dissolve slowly in the mouth; may be repeated every 2 hours as needed or as directed by a doctor or dentist |
|---|---|
| children under 5 years of age | do not use |

### OTHER INFORMATION
- store at room temperature (68-77°F) (20-25°C)
- protect contents from humidity

### INACTIVE INGREDIENTS
cetylpyridinium chloride (Ceepryn), flavor, glucose, propylene glycol, D&C red no. 33, D&C red no. 40, sucrose

# CEPACOL SORE THROAT SPRAY (dyclonine hydrochloride and glycerin) spray
Reckitt Benckiser LLC

## DRUG FACTS

| Active ingredients | Purpose |
|---|---|
| Dyclonine hydrochloride 0.1% | Oral pain reliever |
| Glycerin 33% | Oral demulcent |

### USES
- for temporary relief of:
  - occasional minor irritation, pain, sore mouth, and sore throat
  - pain associated with canker sores
  - minor discomfort and protection of irritated areas in sore mouth and sore throat

### WARNINGS
**Sore throat warning**
If sore throat is severe, persists for more than 2 days, is accompanied or followed by fever, headache, rash, swelling, nausea or vomiting, consult a doctor promptly.

### STOP USE AND ASK A DOCTOR OR DENTIST IF
- sore mouth symptoms do not improve in 7 days

### WHEN USING THIS PRODUCT
- try to avoid swallowing spray

**If pregnant or breastfeeding,** ask a health professional before use.

**Keep out of the reach of children.** In case of overdose, get medical help or contact a Poison Control Center right away.

**Do not exceed recommended dosage.**

### DIRECTIONS

| adults and children 4 years of age and older | spray 4 times into throat or affected area. Gargle, swish around or allow to remain in place at least 1 minute and then spit out. Repeat up to 4 times daily or as directed by a dentist or doctor |
|---|---|
| children 4 to under 12 years of age | should be supervised in the use of this product |
| children under 4 years of age | do not use |

### OTHER INFORMATION
- store at room temperature 20-25°C (68-77°F)
- do not freeze

### INACTIVE INGREDIENTS
cetylpyridinium chloride, D&C red no. 33, deionized water, FD&C yellow no. 6, menthol, phosphoric acid, poloxamer 338, potassium sorbate, sodium phosphate dibasic, sorbitol

### QUESTIONS OR COMMENTS
Call **1-888-963-3382.** You may also report side effects to this phone number.

# CETAPHIL (triclosan) soap
Bradford Soap Works, Inc.

## DRUG FACTS

| Active ingredient | Purpose |
|---|---|
| Triclosan 0.3% | Antibacterial |

### USE
- decrease bacteria on the skin

### WARNINGS
**For external use only.**

**Keep out of reach of children.** Except under adult supervision. If swallowed, get help or contact a Poison Control Center right away.

## DIRECTIONS
- apply to skin while bathing or washing
- rinse and repeat

## INACTIVE INGREDIENTS
sodium cocoyl isethionate, stearic acid, sodium tallowate, water, sodium stearate, sodium dodecylbenzene sulfonate, sodium chloride, masking fragrance, sodium isethionate, petrolatum, sodium isostearoyl lactylate, sucrose cocoate, titanium dioxide, pentasodium pentetate, tetrasodium etidronate

# CHLOR-TRIMETON ALLERGY 4 HOUR
(chlorpheniramine maleate) tablet
Schering-Plough

## DRUG FACTS

| Active ingredient (per tablet) | Purpose |
|---|---|
| Chlorpheniramine maleate 4 mg | Antihistamine |

### USES
- Temporarily relieves the following symptoms due to hay fever or other upper respiratory allergies:
  - sneezing
  - runny nose
  - itchy, watery eyes
  - itching of the nose or throat

### WARNINGS

**ASK A DOCTOR BEFORE USE IF YOU HAVE**
- a breathing problem such as emphysema or chronic bronchitis
- glaucoma
- trouble urinating due to an enlarged prostate gland

**ASK A DOCTOR OR PHARMACIST BEFORE USE IF**
- you are taking sedatives or tranquilizers

**WHEN USING THIS PRODUCT**
- excitability may occur, especially in children
- drowsiness may occur
- avoid alcoholic beverages
- alcohol, sedatives and tranquilizers may increase drowsiness
- use caution when driving a motor vehicle or operating machinery

**If pregnant or breastfeeding,** ask a health professional before use.

**Keep out of reach of children.** In case of overdose, get medical help or contact a Poison Control Center immediately.

### DIRECTIONS

| adults and children over 12 years old | 1 tablet every 4-6 hours, not to exceed 6 tablets in 24 hours |
|---|---|
| children over 6 to under 12 years of age | ½ tablet (break tablet in half) every 4 to 6 hours, not to exceed 3 whole tablets in 24 hours |
| children under 6 years of age | ask a doctor |

## OTHER INFORMATION
- store between 15°C-25°C (59°F-77°F)
- protect from excessive moisture
- do not use if foil imprinted with Chlor-Trimeton is torn or missing

## INACTIVE INGREDIENTS:
crosprovidone, D&C yellow 10 (cl74005), lactase monohydrate, magnesium stearate, microcrystalline cellulose, providone, silicon dioxide

# CHLOR-TRIMETON ALLERGY 12 HOUR
(chlorpheniramine maleate) tablet, extended release
Schering Plough

## DRUG FACTS

| Active ingredient | Purpose |
|---|---|
| Chlorpheniramine maleate 12 mg | Antihistamine |

### USES
- temporarily relieves the following symptoms due to hay fever or other upper respiratory allergies:
  - sneezing
  - runny nose
  - itchy, watery eyes
  - itching of the nose or throat

### WARNINGS

**ASK A DOCTOR BEFORE USE IF YOU HAVE**
- a breathing problem such as emphysema or chronic bronchitis
- glaucoma
- trouble urinating due to an enlarged prostate gland

**ASK A DOCTOR OR PHARMACIST BEFORE USE IF YOU ARE**
- taking sedatives or tranquilizers

**WHEN USING THIS PRODUCT**
- excitability may occur, especially in children
- drowsiness may occur
- avoid alcoholic beverages
- alcohol, sedatives and tranquilizers may increase drowsiness
- use caution when driving a motor vehicle or operating machinery

**If pregnant or breastfeeding,** ask a health professional before use.

**Keep out of reach of children.** In case of overdose, get medical help or contact a Poison Control Center right away.

### DIRECTIONS

| adults and children over 12 years of age | 1 tablet every 12 hours; do not exceed 2 tablets in 24 hours |
|---|---|
| children under 12 years of age | ask a doctor |

## OTHER INFORMATION
- each tablet contains: calcium 30 mg
- store between 20°C-25°C (68°F-77°F)

## INACTIVE INGREDIENTS
acacia, calcium phosphate tribasic, calcium sulfate, carnauba wax, corn starch, FD&C yellow no. 6, FD&C yellow no. 6 aluminum lake, lactose monohydrate, magnesium stearate,

neutral soap, oleic acid, pharmaceutical ink, povidone, rosin, sucrose, talc, titanium dioxide, white wax, zein

## QUESTIONS OR COMMENTS
Call **1-800-317-2165** between 8:00 AM and 5:00 PM Central Standard Time, Monday through Friday

# CHLORASEPTIC KIDS SORE THROAT SPRAY GRAPE (phenol) spray

Prestige Brands Inc.

## DRUG FACTS

| Active ingredients | Purpose |
|---|---|
| Phenol 0.5% | Oral anesthetic/analgesic |

## USES
- for the temporary relief of:
  - occasional minor irritation, pain, sore mouth and sore throat

## WARNINGS
**Sore throat warning**
Severe or persistent sore throat or sore throat accompanied by high fever, headache, nausea, and vomiting may be serious. Consult a doctor promptly. Do not use more than 2 days or administer to children under 6 years of age unless directed by a doctor.

## WHEN USING THIS PRODUCT
- do not exceed recommended dosage

## STOP USE AND ASK A DENTIST OR DOCTOR IF
- sore mouth symptoms do not improve in 7 days
- irritation, pain or redness persists or worsens
- swelling, rash or fever develops

**If pregnant or breastfeeding,** ask a health care professional before use.

**Keep out of reach of children.** In case of overdose or accidental poisoning, get medical help or contact a Poison Control Center right away.

## DIRECTIONS
- apply to affected area (one spray)
- allow to remain in place for at least 15 seconds, then spit out
- use every 2 hours or as directed by a doctor or dentist

| children under 12 years of age | should be supervised in use of this product |
|---|---|
| children under 3 years of age | ask a doctor or dentist |

## OTHER INFORMATION
- store at room temperature
- do not use if imprinted neckband is broken or missing
- check expiration date before using

## INACTIVE INGREDIENTS
FD&C blue no. 1, FD&C red no. 40, flavor, glycerin, saccharin sodium, sodium chloride, water

# CHLORASEPTIC TOTAL SORE THROAT WILD CHERRY (menthol, benzocaine and dextromethorphan hydrobromide) lozenge

Prestige Brands Holdings, Inc.

## DRUG FACTS

| Active ingredients (in each lozenge) | Purpose |
|---|---|
| Benzocaine 6 mg | Oral anesthetic/analgesic |
| Dextromethorphan hydrobromide 5 mg | Cough suppressant |
| Menthol 10 mg | Cough suppressant/oral anesthetic/analgesic |

## USES
- temporarily relieves:
  - occasional minor irritation, pain, sore throat and sore mouth
  - cough due to minor throat and bronchial irritation as may occur with the common cold

## WARNINGS
**Allergy alert**
Do not use this product if you have a history of allergy to local anesthetics such as procaine, butacaine, benzocaine or other "caine" anesthetics.

**Sore throat warning**
Severe or persistent sore throat or sore throat accompanied by high fever, headache, nausea, and vomiting may be serious. Consult doctor promptly. Do not use more than 2 days or administer to children under 6 years of age unless directed by a doctor.

## DO NOT USE
- this product if you are now taking a prescription monoamine oxidase inhibitor (MAOI) (certain drugs for depression, psychiatric or emotional conditions, or Parkinson's disease), or for 2 weeks after stopping the MAOI drug. If you are uncertain whether your prescription drug contains an MAOI, consult a health care professional before taking this product
- this product for persistent or chronic cough such as occurs with smoking, asthma, or emphysema, or if cough is accompanied by excessive phlegm (mucus) unless directed by a doctor

**Do not exceed recommended dosage**

## STOP USE AND ASK A DENTIST OR DOCTOR IF
- sore mouth symptoms do not improve in 7 days
- irritation, pain or redness persists or worsens
- swelling, rash or fever develops
- cough persists for more than 1 week, tends to recur, or is accompanied by a high fever, rash, or persistent headache. These could be symptoms of a serious condition

**If pregnant or breastfeeding,** ask a health care professional before use.

**Keep out of reach of children.** In case of overdose or accidental poisoning, get medical help or contact a Poison Control Center right away.

## DIRECTIONS

| adults and children over 12 years of age | 2 lozenges every 4 hours – not to exceed 12 lozenges every 24 hours |
|---|---|
| children 6-12 years of age | 1 lozenge every 4 hours – not to exceed 6 lozenges every 24 hours |
| children under 6 years of age | consult a doctor |

## OTHER INFORMATION
- store between 59°F-86°F (15-30°C)
- protect from moisture
- do not use if blister package with Chloraseptic name has been disturbed or opened
- check expiration date before using

## INACTIVE INGREDIENTS
corn syrup, FD&C blue no. 1, FD&C red no. 40, flavor, glycerine, soy lecithin, sucrose, water

## QUESTIONS OR COMMENTS
Call **1-800-552-7932** or visit www.chloraseptic.com

---

## CHLORASEPTIC SORE THROAT MAX WILD BERRY (menthol and benzocaine) lozenge
Prestige Brands Holdings, Inc.

## DRUG FACTS

| Active ingredients (in each lozenge) | Purpose |
|---|---|
| Benzocaine 15 mg | Oral anesthetic/analgesic |
| Menthol 10 mg | Oral anesthetic/analgesic |

## USES
- temporarily relieves:
  - occasional minor irritation, pain, sore throat and sore mouth

## WARNINGS
**Allergy alert**
Do not use this product if you have a history of allergy to local anesthetics such as procaine, butacaine, benzocaine or other "caine" anesthetics.

**Sore throat warning**
Severe or persistent sore throat or sore throat accompanied by high fever, headache, nausea and vomiting may be serious. Consult a doctor promptly. Do not use more than 2 days or administer to children under 6 years of age unless directed by a doctor.

**Do not exceed recommended dosage**

## STOP USE AND ASK A DENTIST OR DOCTOR IF
- sore mouth symptoms do not improve in 7 days
- irritation, pain or redness persists or worsens
- swelling, rash or fever develops

**If pregnant or breastfeeding,** ask a health care professional before use.

**Keep out of reach of children.** In case of overdose or accidental poisoning, get medical help or contact a Poison Control Center right away.

## DIRECTIONS

| adults and children 6 years of age and over | take 1 lozenge every 2 hours as needed<br><br>allow lozenges to dissolve slowly in the mouth |
|---|---|
| children under 6 years of age | consult a doctor or dentist |

## OTHER INFORMATION
- store between 59°F-86°F (15-30°C)
- protect from moisture
- check expiration date before using
- do not use if blister package with Chloraseptic name has been disturbed or opened

## INACTIVE INGREDIENTS
corn syrup, FD&C blue no. 1, FD&C red no. 40, flavor, glycerine, propylene glycol, soy lecithin, sucrose, water

## QUESTIONS OR COMMENTS
Call **1-800-552-7932** or visit www.chloraseptic.com

---

## CITRUCEL (methylcellulose) powder, for solution
GlaxoSmithKline Consumer Healthcare LP

## DRUG FACTS

| Active ingredient orange and sugar free(in each rounded tablespoon) | Purpose |
|---|---|
| Methylcellulose (a non-allergenic fiber) 2 grams | Bulk-forming fiber laxative |

## USES
- relieves constipation (irregularity)
- helps to restore and maintain regularity
- for constipation associated with other bowel disorders like IBS when recommended by a doctor
- generally produces a bowel movement in 12-72 hours

## WARNINGS
**Choking**
- taking this product without adequate fluid may cause it to swell and block your throat or esophagus and may cause choking

## DO NOT TAKE THIS PRODUCT IF YOU HAVE
- difficulty in swallowing
- if you experience chest pain, vomiting, or difficulty swallowing or breathing after taking this product, seek immediate medical attention

## ASK A DOCTOR BEFORE USE IF YOU HAVE
- a sudden change in bowel habits that persists for two weeks
- abdominal pain, nausea or vomiting

## STOP USE AND ASK A DOCTOR IF
- constipation lasts more than 7 days
- you have rectal bleeding

These could be signs of a serious condition.

**Keep out of reach of children.** In case of overdose, get medical help or contact a Poison Control Center right away.

## DIRECTIONS
- mix this product (child or adult dose) with at least 8 ounces (a full glass) of water or other fluid. Taking this product without enough liquid may cause choking. See choking warning

- use product at the first sign of constipation or irregularity
- put one dose in a full glass of cold water
- stir briskly and drink promptly
- drinking another glass of water is helpful

## CITRUCEL Orange

| Age | Dose |
|---|---|
| adults & children 12 years of age and over | start with 1 heaping tablespoon<br><br>increase as needed, 1 heaping tablespoon at a time, up to 3 times per day |
| children 6–11 years of age | start with 2.5 level teaspoons<br><br>Increase as needed, 2.5 level teaspoons at a time, up to 3 times per day |
| children under 6 years of age | consult a physician |

## CITRUCEL Sugar Free

| Age | Dose |
|---|---|
| adults & children 12 years of age and over | start with 1 rounded tablespoon<br><br>increase as needed, 1 rounded tablespoon at a time, up to 3 times per day |
| children 6–11 years of age | start with 2 level teaspoons<br><br>increase as needed, 2 level teaspoons at a time, up to 3 times per day |
| children under 6 years of age | consult a physician |

## OTHER INFORMATION
### CITRUCEL Orange
- each heaping tablespoon contains: calcium 80 mg and potassium 110 mg
- each heaping tablespoon contributes 60 calories from sucrose and maltodextrin
- store below 77°F (25°C)
- protect contents from humidity
- keep tightly closed

### CITRUCEL Sugar Free
- each rounded tablespoon contains: calcium 85 mg and potassium 125 mg
- each rounded tablespoon contributes 24 calories from maltodextrin
- store below 77°F (25°C)
- protect contents from humidity
- keep tightly closed
- **Phenylketonurics:** contains **phenylalanine 52 mg** per adult dose

## INACTIVE INGREDIENTS
### CITRUCEL Orange
citric acid, dibasic calcium phosphate, FD&C yellow no. 6, maltodextrin, orange flavors (natural and artificial), potassium citrate, riboflavin, sucrose, titanium dioxide, tricalcium phosphate

### CITRUCEL Sugar Free
aspartame, dibasic calcium phosphate, FD&C yellow no. 6, malic acid, maltodextrin, orange flavors (natural and artificial), potassium citrate, riboflavin

## QUESTIONS OR COMMENTS
Call **toll-free 1-800-897-6081** (English/Spanish) weekdays

# CHILDREN'S CLARITIN (loratadine) solution
Schering-Plough HealthCare Products, Inc.

## DRUG FACTS

| Active ingredient (in each 5 mL teaspoonful) | Purpose |
|---|---|
| Loratadine 5 mg | Antihistamine |

## USES
- temporarily relieves these symptoms due to hay fever or other upper respiratory allergies:
  - runny nose
  - sneezing
  - itchy, watery eyes
  - itching of the nose or throat

## WARNINGS
**DO NOT USE**
- if you have ever had an allergic reaction to this product or any of its ingredients

**ASK A DOCTOR BEFORE USE IF YOU HAVE**
- liver or kidney disease. Your doctor should determine if you need a different dose

**WHEN USING THIS PRODUCT**
- do not take more than directed. Taking more than directed may cause drowsiness

**STOP USE AND ASK A DOCTOR IF**
- an allergic reaction to this product occurs. Seek medical help right away

**If pregnant or breastfeeding,** ask a health professional before use.

**Keep out of reach of children.** In case of overdose, get medical help or contact a Poison Control Center right away.

## DIRECTIONS
- use only with enclosed dosing cup

| adults and children 6 years and over | 2 teaspoonfuls (tsp) daily; do not take more than 2 teaspoonfuls (tsp) in 24 hours |
|---|---|
| children 2 to under 6 years of age | 1 teaspoonful (tsp) daily; do not take more than 1 teaspoonful (tsp) in 24 hours |
| children under 2 years of age | ask a doctor |
| consumers with liver or kidney disease | ask a doctor |

## OTHER INFORMATION
- each teaspoonful contains: sodium 5 mg
- do not use if tape imprinted with "SEALED FOR YOUR PROTECTION" on top and bottom flaps of carton is not intact
- store between 20°C-25°C (68°F-77°F)

## INACTIVE INGREDIENTS
edetate disodium, flavor, glycerin, maltitol, monobasic sodium phosphate, phosphoric acid, propylene glycol, sodium benzoate, sorbitol, sucralose, purified water

## QUESTIONS OR COMMENTS
Call **1-800-CLARITIN (1-800-252-7484)** or visit www.claritin.com

# CLARITIN REDITABS 12-HOUR (loratadine)
MSD Consumer Care, Inc

## DRUG FACTS

| Active ingredient (in each tablet) | Purpose |
|---|---|
| Loratadine 5 mg | Antihistamine |

### USES
- temporarily relieves these symptoms due to hay fever or other upper respiratory allergies:
  - runny nose
  - itchy, watery eyes
  - sneezing
  - itching of the nose or throat

### WARNINGS

**DO NOT USE**
- if you have ever had an allergic reaction to this product or any of its ingredients

**ASK A DOCTOR BEFORE USE IF**
- you have liver or kidney disease. Your doctor should determine if you need a different dose

**WHEN USING THIS PRODUCT**
- do not take more than directed. Taking more than directed may cause drowsiness

**STOP USE AND ASK A DOCTOR IF**
- an allergic reaction to this product occurs. Seek medical help right away

**If pregnant or breastfeeding,** ask a health professional before use.

**Keep out of reach of children.** In case of overdose, get medical help or contact a Poison Control Center right away.

### DIRECTIONS
- place 1 tablet on tongue; tablet disintegrates, with or without water

| adults and children 6 years and over | 1 tablet every 12 hours; not more than 2 tablets in 24 hours |
|---|---|
| children under 6 years of age | ask a doctor |
| consumers with liver or kidney disease | ask a doctor |

### OTHER INFORMATION
- safety sealed: do not use if the individual blister unit imprinted with Claritin RediTabs is open or torn
- store between 20°C-25°C (68°F-77°F)
- use tablet immediately after opening individual blister

### INACTIVE INGREDIENTS
anhydrous citric acid, gelatin, mannitol, mint flavor

### QUESTIONS OR COMMENTS
Call **1-800-CLARITIN (1-800-252-7484)** or visit www.claritin.com

# CHILDREN'S CLARITIN GRAPE CHEWABLES
(loratadine)
MSD Consumer Care, Inc

## DRUG FACTS

| Active ingredient (in each tablet) | Purpose |
|---|---|
| Loratadine 5 mg | Antihistamine |

### USES
- temporarily relieves these symptoms use to hay fever or other upper respiratory allergies:
  - runny nose
  - itchy, watery eyes
  - sneezing
  - itching of the nose or throat

### WARNINGS

**DO NOT USE**
- if you have ever had an allergic reaction to this product or any of its ingredients

**ASK A DOCTOR BEFORE USE IF YOU HAVE**
- liver or kidney disease. Your doctor should determine it you need a different dose

**WHEN USING THIS PRODUCT**
- do not take more than directed

Taking more than directed may cause drowsiness

**STOP USE AND ASK A DOCTOR IF**
- an allergic reaction to this product occurs. Seek medical help right away

**If pregnant or breastfeeding,** ask a health professional before use.

Keep out of reach of children. In case of overdose, get medical help or contact a Poison Control Center right away.

### DIRECTIONS

| adults and children 6 years and over | chew 2 tablets daily, not more than 2 tablets in 24 hours |
|---|---|
| children 2 to under 6 years of age | chew 1 tablets daily, not more than 1 tablets in 24 hours |
| children under 2 years of age | ask a doctor |
| consumers with liver or kidney disease | ask a doctor |

### OTHER INFORMATION
- **Phenylketonurics:** contains phenylalanine 1.4 mg per tablet
- safety sealed: do not use if the individual blister unit imprinted with Children's Claritin is open or torn
- store between 20°C-25°C (68°F-77°F)

### INACTIVE INGREDIENTS
aspartame, citric acid anhydrous, colloidal silicon dioxide, D&C red no. 27 aluminum lake, FD&C Blue no. 2 aluminum lake, flavor, magnesium stearate, mannitol, microcrystaline cellulose, sodium starch glycolata, stearic acid

### QUESTIONS OR COMMENTS
Call **1-800-CLARITIN (1-800-252-7484)** or visit www.claritin.com

## CHILDREN'S CLARITIN GRAPE FLAVORED SYRUP (loratadine) liquid

MSD Consumer Care, Inc

### DRUG FACTS

| Active ingredient (in each 5 ml teaspoonful) | Purpose |
|---|---|
| Loratadine 5 mg | Antihistamine |

### USES
- temporarily relieves these symptoms due to hay fever or other upper respiratory allergies:
  - runny nose
  - itchy, watery eyes
  - sneezing
  - itching of the nose or throat

### WARNINGS

### DO NOT USE
- if you have ever had an allergic reaction to this product or any of its ingredients

### ASK A DOCTOR BEFORE USE IF YOU HAVE
- liver or kidney disease. Your doctor should determine if you need a different dose

### WHEN USING THIS PRODUCT
- do not take more than directed. Taking more than directed may cause drowsiness

### STOP USE AND ASK A DOCTOR IF
- an allergic reaction to this product occurs. Seek medical help right away

**If pregnant or breastfeeding,** ask a health professional before use.

**Keep out of reach of children.** In case of overdose, get medical help or contact a Poison Control Center right away.

### DIRECTIONS
- use only with enclosed dosing cup

| adults and children 6 years and over | 2 teaspoonfuls (tsp) daily; do not take more than 2 teaspoonfuls (tsp) in 24 hours |
|---|---|
| children 2 to under 6 years of age | 1 teaspoonful (tsp) daily; do not take more than 1 teaspoonful (tsp) in 24 hours |
| children under 2 years of age | ask a doctor |
| consumers with liver or kidney disease | ask a doctor |

### OTHER INFORMATION
- each teaspoonful contains: sodium 5 mg
- do not use if tape imprinted with "SEALED FOR YOUR PROTECTION" on top and bottom flaps of carton is not intact
- store between 20°C-25°C (68°F-77°F)

### INACTIVE INGREDIENTS
edetate disodium, flavor, glycerin, maltitol, monobasic sodium phosphate, phosphoric acid, propylene glycol, sodium benzoate, sorbitol, sucralose, purified water

### QUESTIONS OR COMMENTS
Call **1-800-CLARITIN (1-800-252-7484)** or visit www.claritin.com

## CLARITIN REDITABS 24-HOUR (loratadine)

MSD Consumer Care, Inc

### DRUG FACTS

| Active ingredient (in each tablet) | Purpose |
|---|---|
| Loratadine 10 mg | Antihistamine |

### USES
- temporarily relieves these symptoms due to hay fever or other upper respiratory allergies:
  - runny nose
  - itchy, watery eyes
  - sneezing
  - itching of the nose or throat

### WARNINGS

### DO NOT USE
- if you have ever had an allergic reaction to this product or any of its ingredients

### ASK A DOCTOR BEFORE USE IF
- you have liver or kidney disease. Your doctor should determine if you need a different dose

### WHEN USING THIS PRODUCT
- do not take more than directed. Taking more than directed may cause drowsiness

### STOP USE AND ASK A DOCTOR IF
- an allergic reaction to this product occurs. Seek medical help right away

**If pregnant or breastfeeding,** ask a health professional before use.

**Keep out of reach of children.** In case of overdose, get medical help or contact a Poison Control Center right away.

### DIRECTIONS
- place 1 tablet on tongue; tablet disintegrates, with or without water

| adults and children 6 years and over | 1 tablet daily: not more than 1 tablets in 24 hours |
|---|---|
| children under 6 years of age | ask a doctor |
| consumers with liver or kidney disease | ask a doctor |

### OTHER INFORMATION
- safety sealed: do not use if the individual blister unit imprinted with Claritin RediTabs is open or torn
- store between 20°C-25°C (68°F-77°F)
- use tablet immediately after opening individual blister

### INACTIVE INGREDIENTS
anhydrous citric acid, gelatin, mannitol, mint flavor

### QUESTIONS OR COMMENTS
Call **1-800-CLARITIN (1-800-252-7484)** or visit www.claritin.com

## CLEAN AND CLEAR CONTINUOUS CONTROL ACNE CLEANSER (benzoyl peroxide) lotion

Johnson & Johnson Consumer Products Co.

### DRUG FACTS

| Active ingredient | Purpose |
|---|---|
| Benzoyl peroxide 10% | Acne medication |

### USE
• for the treatment of acne

### WARNINGS
**For external use only.**

### DO NOT USE
• this medication if you have very sensitive skin or if you are sensitive to benzoyl peroxide

### WHEN USING THIS PRODUCT
• keep away from eyes, lips and mouth
• avoid unnecessary sun exposure and use a sunscreen
• avoid contact with hair or dyed fabric, including carpet and clothing which may be bleached by this product
• skin irritation may occur, characterized by redness, burning, itching, peeling, or possibly swelling. Mild irritation may be reduced by using the product less frequently or in a lower concentration. If irritation becomes severe, discontinue use, if irritation still continues, consult a doctor
• using other topical acne medications at the same time or immediately following the use of this product may increase dryness or irritation of the skin. If this occurs, only one medication should be used unless directed by a doctor

**Keep out of reach of children.** If swallowed, get medical help or contact a Poison Control Center right away.

### DIRECTIONS
• wet face
• gently massage product all over face for 23-30 seconds, avoiding eye area
• rinse thoroughly and pat dry
• recommended for use twice daily
• if going outside, use a sunscreen

### OTHER INFORMATION
• keep tightly closed
• avoid storing at temperatures above 90°F

### INACTIVE INGREDIENTS
acrylates/C10-30 alkyl acrylate crosspolymer, C12-15 alkyl benzoate, carbomer, fragrance, glycerin, menthol, mineral oil, petrolatum, potassium polyphosphate, sodium C14-16 olefin sulfonate, sodium cocoyl isethionate, titanium dioxide, water, zinc lactate

### QUESTIONS OR COMMENTS
Call **1-877-754-6411**

## CLEAN AND CLEAR DEEP CLEANING ASTRINGENT (salicylic acid) liquid

Johnson & Johnson Consumer Products Company

### DRUG FACTS

| Active ingredient | Purpose |
|---|---|
| Salicylic acid (2%) | Acne medication |

### USE
• For the treatment of acne

### WARNINGS
**For external use only.**

**Flammable: Keep away from open fire or flame.**

### WHEN USING THIS PRODUCT
• avoid contact with eyes
• if contact occurs, immediately flush with water
• using other topical acne medications at the same time or immediately following use of this product may increase dryness or irritation of the skin. If this occurs, only one medication should be used unless directed by a doctor

**Keep out of reach of children.** If swallowed, get medical help or contact a Poison Control Center immediately.

### DIRECTIONS
• cleanse skin thoroughly before applying medication
• moisten a cotton ball and cover the entire affected area with a thin layer one to three times daily
• because excessive drying of the skin may occur, start with one application daily, then gradually increase to two or three times daily if needed or as directed by a physician. If bothersome drying or peeling occurs, reduce application to once a day or every other day

### INACTIVE INGREDIENTS
alcohol (41%), benzophenone-4, denatonium benzoate, dimethicone propyl PG-betaine, fragrance, isoceteth-20, water, FD&C red no. 4

### QUESTIONS OR COMMENTS
Call **1-877-754-6411** or visit us at www.cleanandclear.com

## CLEAN AND CLEAR SENSITIVE SKIN DEEP CLEANING ASTRINGENT (salicylic acid) liquid

Johnson & Johnson Consumer Products Company

### DRUG FACTS

| Active ingredient | Purpose |
|---|---|
| Salicylic acid (0.5%) | Acne medication |

### USE
• for the treatment of acne

### WARNINGS
**For external use only.**

**Flammable: Keep away from open fire or flame.**

### WHEN USING THIS PRODUCT
• avoid contact with eyes. If contact occurs, immediately flush with water
• using other topical acne medications at the same time or immediately following use of this product may increase dryness or irritation of the skin. If this occurs, only one medication should be used unless directed by a doctor

**Keep out of reach of children.** If swallowed, get medical help or contact a Poison Control Center immediately.

### DIRECTIONS
• cleanse skin thoroughly before applying medication
• moisten a cotton ball and cover the entire affected area with a thin layer one to three times daily

- because excessive drying of the skin may occur, start with one application daily, then gradually increase to two or three times daily if needed or as directed by a physician
- if bothersome drying or peeling occurs, reduce application to once a day or every other day

## INACTIVE INGREDIENTS
alcohol (24.5%), algae extract, aloe barbadensis leaf extract, benzophenone-4, denatonium benzoate, dimethicone propyl PG-betaine, fragrance, glycerin, isoceteth-20, PEG-32, propylene glycol, sodium citrate, water, FD&C blue no. 1

## QUESTIONS OR COMMENTS
Call **1-877-754-6411**

---

# CLEAN AND CLEAR ADVANTAGE 3-IN-1 EXFOLIATING CLEANSER (benzoyl peroxide) liquid

Johnson & Johnson Consumer Products Company

## DRUG FACTS

| Active ingredient | Purpose |
|---|---|
| Benzoyl peroxide 5% | Acne medication |

## USE
- for the treatment of acne

## WARNINGS
**For external use only.**

## DO NOT USE
- this medication if you have very sensitive skin or if you are sensitive to benzoyl peroxide

## WHEN USING THIS PRODUCT
- avoid unnecessary sun exposure and use a sunscreen
- avoid contact with the eyes, lips and mouth
- avoid contact with hair or dyed fabric, including carpet and clothing which may be bleached by this product
- skin irritation may occur, characterized by redness, burning, itching, peeling, or possibly swelling. Mild irritation may be reduced by using the product less frequently or in lower concentrations. If irritation becomes severe, discontinue use. If irritation still continues, consult a doctor. Using other topical acne medications at the same time or immediately following use of this product may increase dryness or irritation of the skin. If this occurs, only one medication should be used unless directed by a doctor

## STOP USE AND ASK A DOCTOR
- if skin irritation becomes severe

**Keep out of reach of children.** If swallowed, get medical help or contact a Poison Control Center right away.

## DIRECTIONS
- wet face
- gently massage all over face, avoiding eye area
- rinse thoroughly and pat dry. Because excessive drying of the skin may occur, start using once a day, then gradually increase up to 2 times daily if needed or as directed by a doctor
- if bothersome dryness or peeling occurs, reduce use to once a day or every other day
- if going outside, use a sunscreen

## INACTIVE INGREDIENTS
Acrylates/C-10-30 alkyl acrylate crosspolymer, C12-15 Alkyl benzoate, carbomer, fragrance, glycerin, menthol, mineral oil, petrolatum, polyethylene, potassium polyphosphate, sodium C14-16 olefin sulfonate, sodium cocoyl isethionate, sodium sulfate, titanium dioxide, water, zinc lactate

## QUESTIONS OR COMMENTS
Call **1-877-754-6411** or visit www.cleanandclear.com

---

# CLEAN AND CLEAR ADVANTAGE ACNE CONTROL MOISTURIZER (salicylic acid) lotion

Johnson & Johnson Consumer Products Company

## DRUG FACTS

| Active ingredient | Purpose |
|---|---|
| Salicylic acid (0.5%) | Acne medication |

## USES
- for the treatment of acne

## WARNINGS
**For external use only.**

## WHEN USING THIS PRODUCT
- avoid contact with eyes. If contact occurs, immediately flush with water
- other topical acne medications at the same time or immediately following use of this product, may increase dryness or irritation of the skin
- if this occurs, only one medication should be used unless directed by a doctor

**Keep out of reach of children.** If swallowed, get medical help or contact a Poison Control Center right away.

## DIRECTIONS
- cleanse thoroughly before applying medication
- cover the entire affected area with a thin layer one to three times daily
- if bothersome dryness or peeling occurs, reduce application to once a day or even every other day
- sun protection is recommended by dermatologists as an essential part of a healthy skin care regimen

## OTHER INFORMATION
- keep tightly closed
- avoid storing at temperatures above 90°F

## INACTIVE INGREDIENTS
benzalkonium chloride, butylene glycol, C12-15 alkyl benzoate, C12-15 alkyl lactate, C13-14 isoparaffin, capryloyl glycine, cedrus atlantica bark extract, cetearyl alcohol, cetearyl glucoside, cetyl lactate, cinnamomum zeylanicum bark extract, cocamidopropyl PG-dimonium chloride phosphate, dimethicone, disodium EDTA, ethylene/acrylic acid copolymer, fragrance, glycerin, glycine soja (soybean) seed extract, isoceteth-20, laureth-7, methyl gluceth-20, pentaerythrityl tetra-di-butyl hydroxyhydrocinnamate, phenoxyethanol, phenyl trimethicone, polyacrylamide, polysorbate 60, portulaca oleracea extract, PPG-10 cetyl ether, propylene glycol, sarcosine, steareth-21, water

## QUESTIONS OR COMMENTS
Call **1-877-SKIN-411**

## CLEAN AND CLEAR ADVANTAGE MARK TREATMENT (salicylic acid) lotion

Johnson & Johnson Consumer Products Company

### DRUG FACTS

| Active ingredient | Purpose |
|---|---|
| Salicylic acid (2%) | Acne medication |

### USE
- for the treatment of acne

### WARNINGS
**For external use only.**

**Flammable: Keep away from open fire or flame.**

### WHEN USING THIS PRODUCT
- using other topical acne medications at the same time or immediately following use of this product may increase dryness or irritation of the skin. If this occurs, only one medication should be used unless directed by a doctor

**Keep out of reach of children.** If swallowed, get medical help or contact a Poison Control Center right away. Avoid contact with eyes. If contact occurs, flush thoroughly with water.

### DIRECTIONS
- cleanse skin thoroughly before applying medication
- cover the entire affected area with a thin layer one to three times daily
- because excessive drying of the skin may occur, start with one application daily, then gradually increase to two or three times daily if needed or as directed by a doctor
- if bothersome dryness or peeling occurs, reduce application to once a day or even every other day

### INACTIVE INGREDIENTS
alcohol, benzalkonium chloride, bisabolol, butylene glycol, C12-15 alkyl lactate, cetyl lactate, cocamidopropyl pg-dimonium chloride phosphate, cyclopentasiloxane, fragrance, glycerin, glycolic acid, hamamelis virginiana (witch hazel) leaf extract, isodecyl laurate polyquaternium-37, polysorbate 20, portulaca oleracea extract, sodium benzotriazolyl butylphenol sulfonate, sodium hydroxide, water

### QUESTIONS OR COMMENTS
Call **1-877-754-6411** or visit cleanandclear.com

## CLEAN AND CLEAR ADVANTAGE POPPED PIMPLE RELIEF (salicylic acid) lotion

Johnson & Johnson Consumer Products Company

### DRUG FACTS

| Active ingredient | Purpose |
|---|---|
| Salicylic acid (0.5 %) | Acne Medication (Lotion) |

### USE
- for the management of acne

### WARNINGS
**For external use only.**

### WHEN USING THIS PRODUCT
- skin irritation and dryness is more likely to occur if you use another topical acne medication at the same time
- if irritation occurs, only use one topical acne medication at a time
- rinse right away with water if it gets in eyes

**Keep out of reach of children.** If swallowed, get medical help or contact a Poison Control Center right away.

### DIRECTIONS
- clean the skin thoroughly before applying this product
- cover the entire affected area with a thin layer one to three times daily
- because excessive drying of the skin may occur, start with one application daily, then gradually increase to two or three times daily if needed or as directed by a doctor
- if bothersome dryness or peeling occurs, reduce application to once a day or every other day

### OTHER INFORMATION
- dermatologists do not recommend intentionally popping pimples

### INACTIVE INGREDIENTS
water, hydrated silica, C12-15 alkyl benzoate, propylene glycol, glycerin, isoceteth-20, peg-6 caprylic/capric glycerides, titanium dioxide, phenoxyethanol, cocamidopropyl betaine, xanthan gum, sodium citrate, dimethicone propyl pg-betaine, fragrance, menthyl lactate, cocamidopropyl pg-dimonium chloride phosphate, C12-15 alkyl lactate, citric acid, benzalkonium chloride, FD&C blue no. 1

### QUESTIONS OR COMMENTS
Call **1-877-754-6411** or visit www.cleanandclear.com

## CLEAN AND CLEAR BLACKHEAD ERASER CLEANSING MASK (salicylic acid) cream

Johnson & Johnson Consumer Products Company

### DRUG FACTS

| Active ingredient | Purpose |
|---|---|
| Salicylic acid (0.5%) | Acne medication |

### USES
- for the treatment of acne
- clears blackheads

### WARNINGS
**For external use only.**

### WHEN USING THIS PRODUCT
- and other topical acne medications at the same time or immediately following use of this product, dryness or irritation of the skin may be increased
- If this occurs, only one medication should be used unless directed by a doctor

**Keep out of reach of children.** If swallowed, get medical help or contact a Poison Control Center right away. Avoid contact with eyes. If contact occurs, flush thoroughly with water.

### DIRECTIONS
- use 1-2 times per week
- apply a thin layer to face, avoiding mouth and eye areas
- let dry 5 minutes or until mask turns white
- after the mask has dried, rinse thoroughly
- pat dry with towel

## INACTIVE INGREDIENTS

benzalkonium chloride, FD&C blue no. 1, C12-15 alkyl benzoate, C12-15 alkyl lactate, citric acid, cocamidopropyl betaine, cocamidopropyl pg-dimonium chloride phosphate, dimethicone propyl pg-betaine, fragrance, glycerin, hydrated silica, isoceteth-20, menthyl lactate, PEG-6 caprylic/capric glycerides, phenoxyethanol, propylene glycol, sodium citrate, titanium dioxide, water, xanthan gum

## QUESTIONS OR COMMENTS

Call **1-877-754-6411** or visit cleanandclear.com

---

# CLEAN & CLEAR ADVANTAGE MARK ERASING SPOT TREATMENT (salicylic acid)

Johnson & Johnson Consumer Products Co.

## DRUG FACTS

| Active ingredient | Purpose |
|---|---|
| Salicylic acid (2%) | Acne medication |

## USES

• for the treatment of acne

## WARNINGS

**For external use only.**

**Flammable: Keep away from open fire or flame.**

**Sunburn alert**
This product contains an alpha hydroxyl acid (AHA) that may increase your skin's sensitivity to the sun and particularly the possibility of sunburn. Use a sunscreen, wear protective clothing and limit sun exposure while using this product and for a week afterwards.

## USING THIS PRODUCT

• and other topical acne medications at the same time or immediately following use of this product may increase dryness or irritation of the skin
• if this occurs, only one medication should be used unless directed by a doctor
• avoid contact with eyes
• if contact occurs, immediately flush with water

**Keep out of reach of children**. If swallowed, get medical help or contact a Poison Control Center right away.

## DIRECTIONS

• cleanse skin thoroughly before applying medication
• cover the entire affected area with a thin layer one to three times daily
• if bothersome dryness or peeling occurs, reduce application to once a day or even every other day
• recommended for daily use

## INACTIVE INGREDIENTS

alcohol, benzalkonium chloride, bisabolol, butylene glycol, C12-15 alkyl lactate, cetyl lactate, cocamidopropyl pg-dimonium chloride phosphate, cyclopentasiloxane, fragrance, glycerin, glycolic acid, hamamelis virginiana (witch hazel) leaf extract, isodecyl laurate, polyquaternium-37, polysorbate 20, portulaca oleracea extract, sodium benzotriazolyl butylphenol sulfonate, sodium hydroxide, water

---

# CLEAN & CLEAR ADVANTAGE NIGHTLY MARK CLEARING LOTION (salicylic acid) lotion

Johnson & Johnson Consumer Products Co.

## DRUG FACTS

| Active ingredient | Purpose |
|---|---|
| Salicylic acid (2%) | Acne medication |

## USE

• for the treatment of acne

## WARNINGS

**For external use only.**

## WHEN USING THIS PRODUCT

• and other topical acne medications at the same time or immediately following use of this product may increase dryness or irritation of the skin
• if this occurs, only one medication should be used unless directed by a doctor
• avoid contact with eyes
• if contact occurs, immediately flush with water

**Keep out of reach of children**. If swallowed, get medical help or contact a Poison Control Center right away.

## DIRECTIONS

• cleanse face thoroughly before applying medication
• pat dry
• cover the entire affected area with a thin layer at night
• for best results, apply over your entire face
• if bothersome dryness or peeling occurs, reduce application to once a day or even every other day
• recommended for daily use

## INACTIVE INGREDIENTS

ammonium hydroxide, arachidyl alcohol, arachidyl glucoside, behenyl alcohol, benzalkonium chloride, benzyl alcohol, BHT, butyene glycol, C12-15 alkyl benzoate, C13-14 isoparaffin, cetearyl alcohol, cetearyl clucoside, dimethicone, disodium EDTA, ethylene/acrylic acid copolymer, ethylparaben, fragrance, glycerin, glycine soja (soybean) protein, glycine soja (soybean) seed extract, isoceteth-20, laureth-7, methyl gluceth-20, methylparaben, PEG-16 soy sterol, phenoxyethanol, phenyl trimethicone, polyacrylamide, polysorbate 20, PPG-10 cetyl ether, propylparaben, retinol, sodium ascorbyl phosphate, tocopheryl acetate, water

---

# CLEAN & CLEAR ADVANTAGE BREAKOUT ERASING CLEANSER (benzoyl peroxide) lotion

Johnson & Johnson Consumer Products Co.

## DRUG FACTS

| Active ingredient | Purpose |
|---|---|
| Benzoyl peroxide (10%) | Acne medication |

## USE

• for the treatment of acne

## WARNINGS

**For external use only.**

**DO NOT USE**
- if you have very sensitive skin or are sensitive to benzoyl peroxide

**WHEN USING THIS PRODUCT**
- avoid unnecessary sun exposure and use a sunscreen
- avoid contact with the eyes, lips and mouth
- avoid contact with hair or dyed fabrics, including carpet and clothing which may be bleached by this product with other topical acne medications, at the same time or immediately following use of this product may increase dryness or irritation of the skin
- if this occurs, only one medication should be used unless directed by a doctor
- skin irritation may occur, characterized by redness, burning, itching peeling or possibly swelling. More frequent use or higher concentrations may aggravate skin irritation. Mild irritation may be reduced by using the product less frequently or in lower concentrations

**STOP USE AND ASK A DOCTOR IF**
- skin irritation becomes severe

**Keep out of reach of children.** If swallowed, get medical help or contact a Poison Control Center right away.

**DIRECTIONS**
- wet face
- gently massage all over face for 20-30 seconds, avoiding eye area
- rinse thoroughly and pat dry
- because excessive drying of the skin may occur, start with using once a day, then gradually increase to up to two times daily if needed or as directed by a doctor. If bothersome dryness or peeling occurs, reduce use to once a day or every other day
- use to help prevent new pimple from forming
- if going outside, use a sunscreen

**OTHER INFORMATION**
- keep tightly closed
- avoid storing at temperatures above 90°F

**INACTIVE INGREDIENTS**
acrylates/C10-30 alkyl acrylate crosspolymer C12-15 alkyl benzoate, carbomer, fragrance, glycerin, menthol, mineral oil, petrolatum, potassium polyphosphate, sodium C14-16 olefin sulfonate, sodium cocoyl isethionate, titanium dioxide, water, zinc lactate

---

# CLEAN AND CLEAR FINISHES MATTIFYING MOISTURIZER SPF 15 (octinoxate and titanium dioxide) lotion
Johnson & Johnson Consumer Products Company

## DRUG FACTS

| Active ingredients | Purpose |
|---|---|
| Octinoxate (7.5%) | Sunscreen |
| Titanium dioxide (3%) | Sunscreen |

**USES**
- helps prevent sunburn
- higher SPF gives more sunburn protection
- provides moderate protection against sunburn

**WARNINGS**
**For external use only.**

**WHEN USING THIS PRODUCT**
- keep out of eyes. Rinse with water to remove

**STOP USE AND ASK A DOCTOR IF**
- rash or irritation develops and lasts

**Keep out of reach of children.** If swallowed, get medical help or contact a Poison Control Center right away.

**DIRECTIONS**
- apply liberally before sun exposure and as needed
- children under 6 months of age: ask a doctor

**OTHER INFORMATION**
**Sun alert**
Limiting sun exposure, wearing protective clothing, and using sunscreens may reduce the risks of skin aging, skin cancer, and other harmful effects of the sun.

**INACTIVE INGREDIENTS**
water, propylene glycol, cetyl alcohol, isohexadecane, potassium cetyl phosphate, dicaprylyl carbonate, dimethicone, silica, caprylyl glycol, hydroxyethyl acrylate/sodium acryloyldimethyl taurate copolymer, phenoxyethanol, stearic acid, squalane, fragrance, oryza sativa (rice) seed protein, caprylhydroxamic acid, sodium hydroxide, carbomer, polysorbate 60, disodium EDTA, D&C red 33

**QUESTIONS?**
Call **1-877-SKIN-411** or visit www.cleanandclear.com

---

# CLEAN AND CLEAR FINISHES PORE PERFECTING MOISTURIZER (avobenzone, octisalate, oxybenzone and octocrylene) lotion
Johnson & Johnson Consumer Products Co.

## DRUG FACTS

| Active ingredients | Purpose |
|---|---|
| Avobenzone (3%) | Sunscreen |
| Octisalate (5%) | Sunscreen |
| Octocrylene (1.7%) | Sunscreen |
| Oxybenzone (3%) | Sunscreen |

**USES**
- helps prevent sunburn
- higher SPF gives more sunburn protection
- provides moderate protection against sunburn

**WARNINGS**
**For external use only.**

**WHEN USING THIS PRODUCT**
- keep out of eyes
- rinse with water to remove

**STOP USE AND ASK A DOCTOR IF**
- rash or irritation develops and lasts

**Keep out of reach of children.** If swallowed, get medical help or contact a Poison Control Center right away.

**DIRECTIONS**
- after cleansing, smooth evenly over face before sun exposure or as needed
- use daily
- children under 6 months of age, ask a doctor

## OTHER INFORMATION
**Sun Alert**
- Limiting sun exposure, wearing protective clothing, and using sunscreens may reduce the risk of skin aging, skin cancer, and other harmful effects of the sun

## INACTIVE INGREDIENTSW
acer saccharum (sugar maple) extract, alanine, aluminum starch octenylsuccinate, arachidyl alcohol, arachidyl glucoside, arginine, behenyl alcohol, benzalkonium chloride, betaine, boron nitride, C12-15 alkyl benzoate, camellia sinensis leaf extract, cetearyl alcohol, cetearyl glucoside, citrus aurantium dulcis (orange) fruit extract, citrus medica limonum (lemon) fruit extract, diethylhexyl 2,6-naphthalate, dimethicone, disodium edta, ethylparaben, fragrance, glutamic acid, glycerine, glycine, hydroxypropyl methylcellulose, iodopropynyl butylcarbamate, lysine, methyl methacrylate crosspolymer, methylparaben, pca dimethicone, phenoxyethanol, phenyl trimethicone, proline, propylparaben, saccharum officinarum (sugar cane) extract, serine, silica, sodium hydroxide, sodium pca, sodium polyacrylate, sorbitol, steareth-2, steareth-21, threonine, vaccinium myrtillus fruit/leaf extract, water

# CLEAN AND CLEAR PERSA-GEL 10 (benzoyl peroxide) gel
Johnson & Johnson Consumer Products Company

## DRUG FACTS

| Active ingredients | Purpose |
|---|---|
| Benzoyl peroxide (10%) | Acne treatment |

## USE
- for the treatment of acne

## WARNINGS
**For external use only.**

## DO NOT USE IF YOU
- have very sensitive skin
- are sensitive to benzoyl peroxide

## WHEN USING THIS PRODUCT
- skin irritation and dryness is more likely to occur if you use another topical acne medication at the same time
- if irritation occurs, only use one topical acne medication at a time
- avoid unnecessary sun exposure and use a sunscreen
- avoid contact with the eyes, lips and mouth
- avoid contact with hair or dyed fabrics, which may be bleached by this product
- skin irritation may occur, characterized by redness, burning, itching, peeling, or possibly swelling
- irritation may be reduced by using the product less frequently or in a lower concentration

## STOP USE AND ASK A DOCTOR IF
- irritation becomes severe

**Keep out of reach of children.** If swallowed, get medical help or contact a Poison Control Center right away. Avoid contact with eyes. If control occurs, flush thoroughly with water.

## DIRECTIONS
- clean the skin thoroughly before applying this product
- cover the entire affected area with a thin layer one to three times daily

- because excessive drying of the skin may occur, start with one application daily, then gradually increase to two or three times daily if needed or as directed by a doctor
- if bothersome dryness or peeling occurs, reduce application to once a day or every other day
- if going outside, apply sunscreen after using this product. If irritation or sensitivity develops, stop use of both products and ask a doctor

## OTHER INFORMATION
- keep tightly closed
- avoid storing at extreme temperatures (below 40°F-above 100°F)

## INACTIVE INGREDIENTS
carbomer, disodium EDTA, hydroxypropyl methylcellulose, laureth-4, sodium hydroxide, water

## QUESTIONS OR COMMENTS
Call 1-877-754-6411 or visit www.cleanandclear.com

# CLEAR EYES COOLING REDNESS RELIEF
(glycerin and naphazoline hydrochloride) liquid
Prestige Brands Holdings, Inc.

## DRUG FACTS

| Active ingredients | Purpose |
|---|---|
| Glycerin 0.5% | Lubricant |
| Naphazoline hydrochloride 0.03% | Redness reliever |

## USES
- for the relief of redness of the eye due to minor eye irritations
- for the temporary relief of burning and irritation due to dryness of the eye
- for use as a protectant against further irritation or dryness of the eye

## WARNINGS
**For external use only.**

## DO NOT USE IF
- solution changes color or becomes cloudy

## ASK A DOCTOR BEFORE USE IF
- you have narrow angle glaucoma

## WHEN USING THIS PRODUCT
- to avoid contamination, do not touch tip of container to any surface
- replace cap after using
- overuse may produce increased redness of the eye
- pupils may become enlarged temporarily

## STOP USE AND ASK A DOCTOR IF
- you experience eye pain
- you experience changes in vision
- you experience continued redness or irritation of the eye
- the condition worsens or persists for more than 72 hours

**Keep out of reach of children.** If swallowed, get medical help or contact a Poison Control Center (1-800-222-1222) right away.

## DIRECTIONS
- instill 1 to 2 drops in the affected eye(s) up to four times daily

## OTHER INFORMATION
- store at room temperature
- remove contact lenses before using
- Tamper Evident: Do not use if neckband on bottle is broken or missing

## INACTIVE INGREDIENTS
benzalkonium chloride, boric acid, cyclodextrin, edetate disodium, menthol, purified water, sodium borate

## QUESTIONS OR COMMENTS
Call **1-877-274-1787** or visit www.cleareyes.com

# CLEAR EYES MAXIMUM REDNESS RELIEF
(naphazoline hydrochloride and glycerin) liquid
Prestige Brands Holdings, Inc.

## DRUG FACTS

| Active ingredients | Purpose |
|---|---|
| Glycerin 0.5% | Lubricant |
| Naphazoline hydrochloride 0.03% | Redness reliever |

## USES
- for the relief of redness of the eye due to minor eye irritations
- for the temporary relief of burning and irritation due to the dryness of the eye
- for the use as a protectant against further irritation or dryness of the eye

## WARNINGS
**For external use only.**

## DO NOT USE
- if solution changes color or becomes cloudy

## ASK A DOCTOR BEFORE USE IF
- you have narrow angle glaucoma

## WHEN USING THIS PRODUCT
- to avoid contamination, do not touch tip of container to any surface
- replace cap after using
- overuse may produce increased redness of the eye
- pupils may become enlarged temporarily

## STOP USE AND ASK A DOCTOR IF
- you experience eye pain
- you experience changes in vision
- you experience continued redness or irritation of the eye
- the condition worsens or persists for more than 72 hours

**Keep out of reach of children.** If swallowed, get medical help or contact a Poison Control Center (**1-800-222-1222**) right away.

## DIRECTIONS
- instill 1 to 2 drops in the affected eye(s) up to four times daily

## OTHER INFORMATION
- store at room temperature
- remove contact lenses before using
- Tamper Evident: Do not use if neckband on bottle is broken or missing

## INACTIVE INGREDIENTS
benzalkonium chloride, boric acid, edetate disodium, purified water, sodium borate

## QUESTIONS OR COMMENTS
Call **1-877-274-1787** or visit www.cleareyes.com

# CLEARASIL DAILY CLEAR SKIN PERFECT WASH (salicylic acid) solution
Reckitt Benckiser, Inc.

## DRUG FACTS

| Active ingredient | Purpose |
|---|---|
| Salicylic acid 2% | Acne medication |

## USE
- for the treatment of acne

## WARNINGS
**For external use only.**

## WHEN USING THIS PRODUCT
- with other topical acne medications, at the same time or immediately following use of this product, increased dryness or irritation of the skin may occur
- if this occurs, only one acne medication should be used unless directed by a doctor
- avoid contact with the eyes. If product gets into the eyes rinse thoroughly with water

**Keep out of reach of children.** In case of accidental ingestion, get medical help or contact a Poison Control Center immediately.

## DIRECTIONS
- wet face
- dispense product generously and massage over face and neck
- rinse thoroughly and dry
- for best results, use daily

## OTHER INFORMATION
- store in a cool dry place

## INACTIVE INGREDIENTS
water, PPG-15 stearyl ether, glycerin, stearyl alcohol, cetyl betaine, distearyldimonium chloride, sodium lauryl sulfate, oxidized polyethylene, cetyl alcohol, alcohol, steareth-21, sodium chloride, sodium hydroxide, behenyl alcohol, fragrance, PPG-30, steareth-2, dipropylene glycol, disodium EDTA, BHT

## QUESTIONS OR COMMENTS
Call **1-866-25-CLEAR (1-866-252-5327)**. For ingredient information, www.clearasil.us

# CLEARASIL DAILY CLEAR OIL-FREE DAILY FACE WASH SENSITIVE FORMULA (salicylic acid) cream
Reckitt Benckiser LLC

## DRUG FACTS

| Active ingredient | Purpose |
|---|---|
| Salicylic acid 2% | Acne medication |

## USE
- for the treatment of acne

## WARNINGS
**For external use only.**

**WHEN USING THIS PRODUCT**
- avoid contact with the eyes. If product gets into the eyes rinse thoroughly with water
- with other topical acne medications, at the same time or immediately following use of this product, may increase dryness or irritation of the skin. If this occurs, only one acne medication should be used unless directed by your doctor
- limit use to the face and neck

**STOP USE AND ASK A DOCTOR IF**
- skin or eye irritation develops

**Keep out of reach of children.** In case of accidental ingestion, get medical help or contact a Poison Control Center immediately.

**DIRECTIONS**
- wet face
- dispense product into hands, lather and massage over face and neck avoiding eyes
- rinse thoroughly in warm water and gently pat dry
- for best results, use twice daily

**OTHER INFORMATION**
- keep tightly closed
- store in a cool dry place

**INACTIVE INGREDIENTS**
water, glycerin, myristic acid, stearic acid, sodium lauroyl sarcosinate, palmitic acid, potassium hydroxide, lauric acid, polyquaternium 10, phenoxyethanol, tetrasodium EDTA, pentasodium pentetate, tetrasodium etidronate, methylparaben, butylparaben, ethylparaben, isobutylparaben, propylparaben, aloe barbadensis leaf juice, maltodextrin, potassium sorbate, sodium benzoate

**QUESTIONS OR COMMENTS**
Call 1-866-25-CLEAR (1-866-252-5327)

# CLEARASIL DAILY CLEAR TINTED ACNE TREATMENT (benzoyl peroxide) cream

Reckitt Benckiser, Inc.

## DRUG FACTS

| Active ingredient | Purpose |
|---|---|
| Benzoyl peroxide 10% | Acne medication |

**USE**
- for the treatment of acne

**WARNINGS**
**For external use only.**

**DO NOT USE**
- if you have very sensitive skin or are sensitive to benzoyl peroxide

**WHEN USING THIS PRODUCT**
- avoid unnecessary sun exposure and use a sunscreen
- avoid contact with the eyes, lips and mouth
- avoid contact with hair or dyed fabrics, including carpet and clothing which may be bleached by this product
- with other topical acne medications, at the same time or immediately following use of this product, increased dryness or irritation of the skin may occur. If this occurs, only one medication should be used unless directed by a doctor
- skin irritation may occur, characterized by redness, burning, itching, peeling or possibly swelling. More frequent use or higher concentrations may aggravate skin irritation. Mild

irritation may be reduced by using the product less frequently or in a lower concentration

**STOP USE AND ASK A DOCTOR IF**
- skin irritation becomes severe

**Keep out of reach of children.** In case of accidental ingestion, get medical help or contact a Poison Control Center immediately.

**DIRECTIONS**
- cleanse the skin thoroughly before applying medication
- cover the entire affected area with a thin layer one to three times a day
- because excessive drying of the skin may occur, start with one application daily, then gradually increase to two or three times daily if needed or as directed by a doctor. If bothersome dryness or peeling occurs, reduce application to once a day or every other day
- if going outside use a sunscreen. Allow Clearasil Tinted Acne Treatment Cream to dry, then follow directions in sunscreen labeling. If sensitivity develops, discontinue use of both products and consult a doctor

**OTHER INFORMATION**
- keep tightly closed
- keep away from heat

**INACTIVE INGREDIENTS**
water, propylene glycol, glyceryl stearate se, bentonite, aluminum hydroxide, PEG-12, isopropyl myristate, titanium dioxide, iron oxides, simethicone, methylparaben, carbomer, potassium hydroxide, propylparaben

**QUESTIONS OR COMMENTS**
Call **1 866 25 CLEAR (1 866 252 5327)** or visit www.clearasil.com

# CLEARASIL DAILY CLEAR TINTED ADULT TREATMENT (sulfur and resorcinol) cream

Reckitt Benckiser, Inc.

## DRUG FACTS

| Active ingredients | Purpose |
|---|---|
| Resorcinol 2% | Acne medication |
| Sulfur 8% | Acne medication |

**USE**
- for the treatment of acne

**WARNINGS**
**For external use only.**

**DO NOT USE**
- on broken skin
- on large areas of the body

**WHEN USING THIS PRODUCT**
- apply to affected areas only
- avoid contact with the eyes, lips and mouth
- with other topical acne medications, at the same time or immediately following use of this product, increased dryness or irritation of the skin may occur. If this occurs, only one medication should be used unless directed by a doctor

**STOP USE AND ASK A DOCTOR IF**
- excessive skin irritation develops or increases

**Keep out of reach of children.** In case of accidental ingestion, get medical help or contact a Poison Control Center immediately.

## DIRECTIONS
- cleanse the skin thoroughly before applying medication
- cover the entire affected area with a thin layer one to three times a day
- because excessive drying of the skin may occur, start with one application daily, then gradually increase to two or three times daily if needed or as directed by a doctor. If bothersome dryness or peeling occurs, reduce application to once a day or every other day
- if going outside use a sunscreen. Allow Clearasil to dry, then follow direction in sunscreen labeling
- if sensitivity develops, discontinue use of both products and consult a doctor

## OTHER INFORMATION
- keep tightly closed
- keep away from heat

## INACTIVE INGREDIENTS
water, alcohol denat., bentonite, glyceryl stearate se, propylene glycol, isopropyl myristate, potassium stearate, fragrance, simethicone, methylparaben, propylparaben, titanium dioxide, iron oxides

## QUESTIONS OR COMMENTS
Call **1-866-25-CLEAR (1-866-252-5327)** or visit www.clearasil.com

# CLEARASIL ULTRA ACNE PLUS
## MARKS SPOT (salicylic acid) lotion

Reckitt Benckiser, Inc.

### DRUG FACTS

| Active ingredient | Purpose |
|---|---|
| Salicylic acid 2% | Acne medication |

## USE
- for the treatment of acne

## WARNINGS
**For external use only.**

### Sun alert
- because this product may make your skin more sensitive to the sun, be certain you have adequate sunscreen protection while using this product and for a week after you discontinue use

## WHEN USING THIS PRODUCT
- avoid contact with eyes, lips and mouth. If contact occurs, rinse thoroughly with water
- with other topical acne medications, at the same time or immediately following use of this product, may increase dryness or irritation of the skin. If this occurs, only one acne medication should be used unless directed by your doctor
- limit use to the face and neck
- wash hands after use

## STOP USE AND ASK A DOCTOR IF
- skin or eye irritation develops

**Keep out of reach of children.** In case of accidental ingestion, get medical help or contact a Poison Control Center immediately.

## DIRECTIONS
- cleanse the skin thoroughly before applying medication
- cover the entire affected area with a thin layer one to three times a day
- because excessive drying of the skin may occur, start with one application daily, then gradually increase to two or three times daily if needed or as directed by a doctor. If bothersome dryness or peeling occurs, reduce application to once a day or every other day

## OTHER INFORMATION
- keep tightly closed
- store at controlled room temperature 68-77°F (20-25°C)

## INACTIVE INGREDIENTS
water, Alcohol Denat., octyldodecanol, dimethicone, niacinamide, sodium lactate, isohexadecane, polyacrylamide, sodium hydroxide, acrylates/C10-30 alkyl acrylate crosspolymer, xanthan gum, hexyldecanol, C13-14 isoparaffin, magnesium aluminum silicate, fragrance, laureth-7, disodium EDTA, dipotassium glycyrrhizate, bisabolol, cetylhydroxyproline palmitamide, stearic acid, brassica campestris (rapeseed) sterols, titanium dioxide

## QUESTIONS OR COMMENTS
Call **1-866-25-CLEAR** or visit www.clearasil.com

# CLEARASIL ULTRA ACNE PLUS MARKS
## WASH AND MASK (salicylic acid) solution

Reckitt Benckiser, Inc.

### DRUG FACTS

| Active ingredient | Purpose |
|---|---|
| Salicylic acid 2% | Acne medication |

## USE
- For the treatment of acne

## WARNINGS
**For external use only.**

## WHEN USING THIS PRODUCT
- avoid contact with eyes. If product gets into the eyes rinse thoroughly with water
- with other topical acne medications, at the same time or immediately following use of this product, may increase dryness or irritation of the skin. If this occurs, only one acne medication should be used unless directed by your doctor
- limit use to the face and neck

## STOP USE AND ASK A DOCTOR IF
- skin or eye irritation develops

**Keep out of reach of children.** In case of accidental ingestion, get medical help or contact a Poison Control Center immediately.

## DIRECTIONS
- as a daily wash - wet face. Dispense product into hands, lather and massage gently into face and neck, avoiding the eye area
- because excessive drying of the skin may occur, start with one application daily, then gradually increase to two or three times daily if needed or directed by a doctor. If bothersome dryness or peeling occurs, reduce the application to once a day or every other day
- rinse thoroughly with warm water and gently pat dry. For best results, use twice daily
- as a mask – use up to 3 times a week for a deeper treatment – wet face, apply on to damp skin. Leave on for 1 minute. Rinse off thoroughly with warm water. Gently pat dry

**OTHER INFORMATION**
- keep tightly closed
- store in a cool dry place

**INACTIVE INGREDIENTS**
water, sodium cocoyl isethionate, cetearyl alcohol, laureth-3, glycerin, coconut acid, sodium isethionate, sodium hydroxide, fragrance, lavandula stoechas extract, helichrysum italicum extract, cistus monspeliensis extract, disodium edta, PEG-40 hydrogenated castor oil, phenoxyethanol, methylparaben, butylparaben, ethylparaben, isobutylparaben, propylparaben

**QUESTIONS OR COMMENTS**
Call **1-866-25-CLEAR (1-866-252-5327)** or visit www.clearasil.com

## CLEARASIL ULTRA RAPID ACTION SEAL-TO-CLEAR (salicylic acid) gel

Reckitt Benckiser LLC

### DRUG FACTS

| Active ingredient | Purpose |
|---|---|
| Salicylic acid 2% | Acne medication |

**USE**
- for the treatment of acne

**WARNINGS**
**For external use only.**

**Flammable: Keep away from open fire or flame.**

**WHEN USING THIS PRODUCT**
- avoid contact with the eyes, lips and mouth. If product gets into the eyes rinse thoroughly with water
- with other topical acne medications, at the same time or immediately following use of this product, may increase dryness or irritation of the skin. If this occurs, only one acne medication should be used unless directed by your doctor
- limit use to the face and neck
- wash hands after use

**STOP USE AND ASK A DOCTOR IF**
- skin or eye irritation develops

**Keep out of reach of children.** In case of accidental ingestion, get medical help or contact a Poison Control Center immediately.

**DIRECTIONS**
- cleanse the skin thoroughly, as needed, before applying medication cover the affected area with a thin layer and allow to dry one to three times a day
- because excessive drying of the skin may occur, start with one application daily, then gradually increase to two or three times daily if needed or as directed by a doctor
- if bothersome dryness or peeling occurs, reduce application to once a day or every other day

**OTHER INFORMATION**
- keep tightly closed
- store in a cool dry place
- cap may pose choking hazard

**INACTIVE INGREDIENTS**
water, alcohol denat., sodium gluconate, propylene glycol, hydroxyethylcellulose, isoceteth-20, dimethylacrylamide/acrylic acid/polystyrene ethyl methacrylate copolymer, sodium hydroxide, disodium EDTA, phenoxyethanol, sodium benzoate, oryza sativa (rice) extract, denatonium benzoate

**QUESTIONS OR COMMENTS**
Call **1-866-25-CLEAR (1-866-252-5327)**

## CLEARASIL ULTRA TINTED RAPID ACTION TREATMENT (salicylic acid) gel

Reckitt Benckiser, Inc.

### DRUG FACTS

| Active ingredient | Purpose |
|---|---|
| Salicylic acid 2% | Acne medication |

**USE**
- for the treatment of acne

**WARNINGS**
**For external use only.**

**Flammable: Keep away from extreme heat or open flame.**

**WHEN USING THIS PRODUCT**
- avoid contact with the eyes. If product gets into the eyes rinse thoroughly with water
- with other topical acne medications, at the same time or immediately following use of this product, may increase dryness or irritation of the skin. If this occurs, only one acne medication should be used unless directed by your doctor
- limit use to the face and neck

**STOP USE AND ASK A DOCTOR IF**
- skin or eye irritation develops

**Keep out of reach of children.** In case of accidental ingestion, get medical help or contact a Poison Control Center immediately.

**DIRECTIONS**
- cleanse the skin thoroughly before applying medication
- cover the entire affected area with a thin layer one to three times daily
- because excessive drying of the skin may occur, start with one application daily, then gradually increase to 2 or 3 applications daily if needed or as directed by a doctor
- if bothersome dryness or peeling occurs, reduce application to once a day or every other day

**OTHER INFORMATION**
- store in a cool dry place
- keep outer packaging for precautions and directions

**INACTIVE INGREDIENTS**
water, alcohol, sorbitol, polysorbate 20, hydroxyethylcellulose, sodium hydroxide, menthol, fragrance, lavandula stoechas extract, helichrysum italicum extract, cistus monspeliensis extract, disodium EDTA, PEG-40 hydrogenated castor oil, phenoxyethanol, methylparaben, butylparaben, ethylparaben, isobutylparaben, propylparaben

**QUESTIONS OR COMMENTS**
Call **1-866-25-CLEAR (1-866-252-5327)** or visit us at www.clearasil.com

## COLACE (docusate sodium) capsule
Purdue Products LP

### DRUG FACTS

| Active ingredient (in each capsule) | Purpose |
|---|---|
| Docusate sodium 50 mg | Stool softener |

### USES
- relieves occasional constipation (irregularity)
- generally produces a bowel movement in 12 to 72 hours

### WARNINGS

**DO NOT USE**
- if you are presently taking mineral oil, unless told to do so by a doctor

**ASK A DOCTOR BEFORE USE IF YOU HAVE**
- stomach pain
- nausea
- vomiting
- noticed a sudden change in bowel movements that continues over a period of 2 weeks

**STOP USE AND ASK A DOCTOR IF**
- you have rectal bleeding or fail to have a bowel movement after use of a laxative. These could be signs of a serious condition
- you need to use a stool softener laxative for more than 1 week

**If pregnant or breastfeeding,** ask a health professional before use.

**Keep out of reach of children.** In case of overdose, get medical help or contact a Poison Control Center right away.

### DIRECTIONS
- take only by mouth
- doses may be taken as a single daily dose or in divided doses

| adults and children 12 years and over | take 1-6 capsules daily |
|---|---|
| children 2 to under 12 years of age | take 1-3 capsules daily |
| children under 2 years | ask a doctor |

### OTHER INFORMATION
- each tablet contains: sodium 3 mg (very low sodium)
- store at 25°C (77°F); excursions permitted between 15-30°C (59-86°F)
- keep tightly closed

### INACTIVE INGREDIENTS
D&C red no. 33, FD&C red no. 40, gelatin, glycerin, PEG 400, propylene glycol, sorbitol

### QUESTIONS OR COMMENTS
1-800-726-7535 (8AM-5PM, EST, M-F) or visit www.colacecapsules.com

## COLD-EEZE COLD REMEDY (zinc gluconate glycine) lozenge
ProPhase Labs, Inc.

### DRUG FACTS

| Active ingredient (per lozenge) | Purpose |
|---|---|
| Zincum gluconicum 2× (13.3 mg) | Cold remedy |

### USES
- to reduce the duration of the common cold
- reduces the severity of cold symptoms:
  - cough
  - sore throat
  - stuffy nose
  - sneezing
  - post nasal drip and/or hoarseness

### WARNINGS

**ASK A DOCTOR BEFORE USE IF YOU**
- are taking minocycline, doxycycline, tetracycline or are on coumadin therapy, zinc treatment may inhibit the absorption of these medicines

**Diabetic warning**
Sugar replacements may affect blood sugar levels.

**STOP USE AND ASK A DOCTOR**
- if symptoms persist beyond 7 days

**If pregnant or breastfeeding,** ask a health professional before use.

**Keep out of reach of children.**

### DIRECTIONS

| adults and children 12 years and over | for best results, begin treatment at start of symptoms (within 24-48 hours of onset) |
|---|---|
| | repeat every 2-4 hours as needed until all symptoms subside |
| | completely dissolve a COLD-EEZE lozenge in mouth (do not chew) |
| | recommended daily dosage is 6 lozenges for adults and 4 lozenges for ages 12-17 |
| children under 12 years of age | should consult a health professional prior to use |

### OTHER INFORMATION
- avoid minor stomach upset do not dissolve COLD-EEZE lozenges on an empty stomach
- avoid citrus fruits or juices and products containing citric acid ½ hour before or after taking COLD-EEZE lozenges as they may diminish product effectiveness, otherwise, drink plenty of fluids
- store in a cool dry place after opening
- gluten-free
- product may produce a laxative effect

### INACTIVE INGREDIENTS
acesulfame-k, glycine, isomalt, natural flavors, no artificial colors or preservatives

# COLD EEZE KID-EEZE SORE THROAT POPS
(zincum gluconicum 2)

Quigley Corporation

## DRUG FACTS

| Active ingredient (per lozenge) | Purpose |
|---|---|
| Zincum gluconicum 2 (13.3 mg) | Cold remedy |

## USES
- to reduce the duration of the common cold
- reduces the severity of cold symptoms:
  - cough sore throat
  - stuffy nose
  - sneezing
  - post nasal drip
  - hoarseness

## WARNINGS

### ASK A DOCTOR BEFORE USE IF
- you are taking minocycline, doxycycline, tetracycline or are on coumadin therapy, zinc treatment may inhibit the absorption of these medicines

### STOP USE AND ASK A DOCTOR
- if symptoms persist beyond 7 days

**If pregnant or breastfeeding,** ask a health professional before use.

**Keep out of reach of children.**

## DIRECTIONS

| adults and children 12 years and over | for best results, begin treatment at start of symptoms (within 24-48 hours of onset) |
|---|---|
| | repeat every 2-4 hours as needed until all symptoms subside |
| | completely dissolve a COLD-EEZE lozenge in mouth (do not chew) |
| | recommended daily dosage is 6 lozenges for adults and 4 lozenges for ages 12-17 |
| children under 12 years of age | should consult a health professional prior to use |

## OTHER INFORMATION
- avoid minor stomach upset
- do not dissolve COLD-EEZE lozenges on an empty stomach
- avoid citrus fruits or juices and products containing citric acid ½ hour before or after taking COLD-EEZE lozenges as they may diminish product effectiveness, otherwise, drink plenty of fluids
- store in a cool dry place after opening
- gluten-free

# COLGATE ORABASE MAXIMUM STRENGTH ORAL PAIN RELIEVER (benzocaine) paste
Colgate Oral Pharmaceuticals, Inc.

## DRUG FACTS

| Active ingredient | Purpose |
|---|---|
| Benzocaine 20% | Oral pain reliever |

## USE
- for the temporary relief of pain associated with canker sores, due to minor irritation or injury of the mouth and gums, or due to minor irritation of the mouth and gums caused by dentures or orthodontic appliances

## WARNINGS

### DO NOT USE
- for more than 7 days unless directed by a dentist or physician
- if you have a history of allergy to local anesthetics such as procaine, butacaine, benzocaine, or other "caine" anesthetics

### WHEN USING THIS PRODUCT
- do not exceed recommended dosage
- avoid contact with eyes
- localized allergic reactions may occur after prolonged or repeated use

### STOP USE AND ASK A DOCTOR IF
- sore mouth symptoms do not improve in 7 days
- swelling, rash or fever develops
- irritation, pain or redness persists or worsens

**Keep out of reach of children.** If more than used for pain relief is accidentally swallowed, get medical help or contact a Poison Control Center immediately.

## DIRECTIONS

| adults and children 2 years and older | gently dab paste on the site of irritation with a cotton swab or fingertip |
|---|---|
| | allow to remain in place at least 1 minute and then spit out |
| | use up to 4 times daily or as directed by a dentist or physician |
| children under 12 years of age | should be supervised in the use of the product |
| children under 2 years of age | consult a dentist or physician |

## OTHER INFORMATION
- store at controlled room temperature, 68-77°F (20-25°C)

## INACTIVE INGREDIENTS
butylparaben, cellulose gum, ethylparaben, flavor, methylparaben, mineral oil, pectin, polyethylene, propylparaben, xanthan gum

## QUESTIONS OR COMMENTS
Call toll-free **1-800-962-2345**

## COLLYRIUM EYE WASH (purified water) solution
Bausch & Lomb Incorporated

### DRUG FACTS

| Active ingredient | Purpose |
|---|---|
| Purified water (99.05%) | Eyewash |

### USES
- washes the eye to help relieve:
  - irritation
  - discomfort
  - stinging
  - itching
- by removing:
  - loose foreign material
  - air pollutants (smog or pollen)
  - chlorinated water

### WARNINGS

#### DO NOT USE
- if you have open wounds in or near the eyes, and get medical help right away
- if solution changes color or becomes cloudy

#### WHEN USING THIS PRODUCT
- do not touch tip of container to any surface to avoid contamination
- remove contact lenses before using
- replace cap after use

#### STOP USE AND ASK A DOCTOR IF
- you experience eye pain, changes in vision, continued redness or irritation of the eye
- condition worsens or persists

**Keep out of reach of children.** If swallowed, get medical help or contact a Poison Control Center right away.

### DIRECTIONS
- bottle tip permits use with or without cup
- flush the affected eye(s) as needed
- control the rate of flow of solution by pressure on the bottle

#### WHEN USING AN EYE CUP
- rinse the cup with Collyrium Eye Wash immediately before each use
- avoid contamination of the rim and inside surfaces of cup
- fill the cup half full with Collyrium Eye Wash and apply the cup to the affected eye(s), pressing tightly to prevent spillage
- tilt the head backward. Open eyelids wide and rotate eyeball to thoroughly wash the eye
- rinse cup with clean water after each use
- replace cap after use

### OTHER INFORMATION
- store at 15-30°C (59-86°F)
- keep tightly closed
- does not contain thimerosal
- enclosed eyecup is sterile if packaging is intact
- use before expiration date marked on the carton or bottle

### INACTIVE INGREDIENTS
boric acid, sodium borate and sodium chloride, preservative added: benzalkonium chloride (0.01%)

### QUESTIONS OR COMMENTS
Toll-free product information or to report a serious side effect associated with use of the product Call **1-800-553-5340**

## COMMIT (nicotine) lozenge
GlaxoSmithKline Consumer Healthcare LP

### DRUG FACTS

| Active ingredient (in each lozenge) | Purpose |
|---|---|
| Nicotine polacrilex, 4 mg | Stop smoking aid |
| Nicotine polacrilex, 2 mg | Stop smoking aid |

### USES
- reduces withdrawal symptoms, including nicotine craving, associated with quitting smoking

### WARNINGS
- if you are pregnant or breastfeeding, only use this medicine on the advice of your health care provider
- smoking can seriously harm your child. Try to stop smoking without using any nicotine replacement medicine. This medicine is believed to be safer than smoking. However, the risks to your child from this medicine are not fully known

#### DO NOT USE
- if you continue to smoke, chew tobacco, use snuff, or use a nicotine patch or other nicotine containing product

#### ASK A DOCTOR BEFORE USE IF YOU HAVE
- a sodium-restricted diet
- heart disease, recent heart attack, or irregular heartbeat. Nicotine can increase your heart rate
- high blood pressure not controlled with medication. Nicotine can increase your blood pressure
- stomach ulcer or diabetes

#### ASK A DOCTOR OR PHARMACIST BEFORE USE IF YOU ARE
- using a non-nicotine stop smoking drug
- taking prescription medicine for depression or asthma. Your prescription dose may need to be adjusted

#### STOP USE AND ASK A DOCTOR IF
- mouth problems occur
- persistent indigestion or severe sore throat occurs
- irregular heartbeat or palpitations occur
- you get symptoms of nicotine overdose such as nausea, vomiting, dizziness, diarrhea, weakness and rapid heartbeat

**Keep out of reach of children and pets.** Nicotine lozenges may have enough nicotine to make children and pets sick. If you need to remove the lozenge, wrap it in paper and throw away in the trash. In case of overdose, get medical help or contact a Poison Control Center right away.

### DIRECTIONS (4 MG LOZENGE)
- if you are under 18 years of age, ask a doctor before use
- before using this product, read the enclosed User's Guide for complete directions and other important information
- stop smoking completely when you begin using the lozenge
- if you smoke your first cigarette more than 30 minutes after waking up, use 2 mg nicotine lozenge
- if you smoke your first cigarette within 30 minutes of waking up, use 4 mg nicotine lozenge according to the following 12 week schedule:

| Weeks 1 to 6 | Weeks 7 to 9 | Weeks 10 to 12 |
|---|---|---|
| 1 lozenge every 1 to 2 hours | 1 lozenge every 2 to 4 hours | 1 lozenge every 4 to 8 hours |

- nicotine lozenge is a medicine and must be used a certain way to get the best results

- place the lozenge in your mouth and allow the lozenge to slowly dissolve (about 20 – 30 minutes). Minimize swallowing
- do not chew or swallow lozenge
- you may feel a warm or tingling sensation
- occasionally move the lozenge from one side of your mouth to the other until completely dissolved (about 20 – 30 minutes)
- do not eat or drink 15 minutes before using or while the lozenge is in your mouth
- to improve your chances of quitting, use at least 9 lozenges per day for the first 6 weeks
- do not use more than one lozenge at a time or continuously use one lozenge after another since this may cause you hiccups, heartburn, nausea or other side effects
- do not use more than 5 lozenges in 6 hours
- do not use more than 20 lozenges per day
- stop using the nicotine lozenge at the end of 12 weeks. If you still feel the need to use nicotine lozenges, talk to your doctor

## DIRECTIONS (2 MG LOZENGE)
- if you are under 18 years of age, ask a doctor before use
- before using this product, read the enclosed User's Guide for complete directions and other important information
- stop smoking completely when you begin using the lozenge
- if you smoke your first cigarette within 30 minutes of waking up, use 4 mg nicotine lozenge
- if you smoke your first cigarette more than 30 minutes after waking up, use 2 mg nicotine lozenge according to the following 12 week schedule:

| Weeks 1 to 6 | Weeks 7 to 9 | Weeks 10 to 12 |
|---|---|---|
| 1 lozenge every 1 to 2 hours | 1 lozenge every 2 to 4 hours | 1 lozenge every 4 to 8 hours |

- nicotine lozenge is a medicine and must be used a certain way to get the best results
- place the lozenge in your mouth and allow the lozenge to slowly dissolve (about 20 – 30 minutes). Minimize swallowing
- do not chew or swallow lozenge
- you may feel a warm or tingling sensation
- occasionally move the lozenge from one side of your mouth to the other until completely dissolved (about 20 – 30 minutes)
- do not eat or drink 15 minutes before using or while the lozenge is in your mouth
- to improve your chances of quitting, use at least 9 lozenges per day for the first 6 weeks
- do not use more than one lozenge at a time or continuously use one lozenge after another since this may cause you hiccups, heartburn, nausea or other side effects
- do not use more than 5 lozenges in 6 hours
- do not use more than 20 lozenges per day
- stop using the nicotine lozenge at the end of 12 weeks. If you still feel the need to use nicotine lozenges, talk to your doctor

## OTHER INFORMATION
- Each lozenge contains: sodium, 18 mg
- **Phenylketonurics:** contains phenylalanine 3.4 mg per lozenge
- store at 20-25°C (68-77°F)
- keep POPPAC tightly closed and protect from light

## INACTIVE INGREDIENTS
acacia, aspartame, calcium polycarbophil, corn syrup solids, flavors, lactose, magnesium stearate, maltodextrin, mannitol, potassium bicarbonate, sodium alginate, sodium carbonate, soy protein, triethyl citrate, xanthan gum

## QUESTIONS OR COMMENTS
Call toll-free **1-888-569-1743** (English/Spanish)
(9:00 AM-4:30 PM ET) weekdays

# COMPOUND W (salicylic acid) liquid
Medtech Products, Inc.

## DRUG FACTS

| Active ingredients | Purpose |
|---|---|
| Salicylic Acid 17 % | Wart remover |

### USES
- for the removal of common warts. The common wart is easily recognized by the rough 'cauliflower like' appearance on the surface
- for the removal of plantar warts on the bottom of the foot. The plantar wart is recognized by its location only on the bottom of the foot, its tenderness, and the interruption of the footprint pattern

### WARNINGS
**For external use only.**
- avoid inhaling vapors

**Extremely flammable. Keep away from fire or flame.**

### DO NOT USE
- on irritated skin
- on any area that is infected or reddened
- on moles
- on birthmarks
- warts with hair growing from them
- genital warts
- warts on the face
- on warts on mucous membranes such as inside the mouth, nose, anus, genitals, lips

### ASK A DOCTOR BEFORE USE IF YOU HAVE
- diabetes
- poor blood circulation

### WHEN USING THIS PRODUCT
- avoid contact with eyes
- if product gets into the eye, flush with water for 15 minutes
- avoid inhaling vapors

### STOP USE AND ASK A DOCTOR IF
- discomfort persists

**Keep out of reach of children.** If swallowed, get medical help or contact a Poison Control Center right away.

### DIRECTIONS
- wash affected area
- may soak wart in warm water for 5 minutes
- dry area thoroughly
- using applicator, apply one drop at a time to sufficiently cover each wart
- let dry
- repeat this procedure once or twice daily as needed (until wart is removed) for up to 12 weeks

### OTHER INFORMATION
- cap bottle tightly and store at room temperature away from heat

### INACTIVE INGREDIENTS
alcohol (21.2% v/v), camphor, castor oil, collodion, ether (63.6%), ethylcellulose, hypophosphorous acid, menthol, polysorbate 80

## COMTREX MAXIMUM STRENGTH COLD AND COUGH NON-DROWSY (acetaminophen, dextromethorphan hydrobromide, phenylephrine hydrochloride) caplet, coated
Novartis Consumer Health, Inc.

### DRUG FACTS

| Active ingredient | Purpose |
| --- | --- |
| Acetaminophen 325 mg | Pain reliever/fever reducer |
| Dextromethorphan hydrobromide 10 mg | Cough suppressant |
| Phenylephrine hydrochloride 5 mg | Nasal decongestant |

### USES
- temporarily relieve:
  - headache
  - sore throat pain
  - minor aches and pains
  - nasal and sinus congestion
  - cough due to minor throat and bronchial irritation as may occur with a cold
  - temporarily reduces fever

### WARNINGS
**Liver warning**
This product contains acetaminophen. Severe liver damage may occur if you take:
- more than 12 caplets in 24 hours, which is the maximum daily amount
- with other drugs containing acetaminophen
- 3 or more alcoholic drinks every day while using this product

**Sore throat warning**
If sore throat is severe, persists for more than 2 days, is accompanied or followed by fever, headache, rash, nausea, or vomiting consult a doctor promptly.

### DO NOT USE
- in a child under 4 years of age
- if you are allergic to acetaminophen
- with any other drug containing acetaminophen (prescription or nonprescription). If you are not sure whether a drug contains acetaminophen, ask a doctor or pharmacist
- if you are now taking a prescription monoamine oxidase inhibitor (MAOI) (certain drugs for depression, psychiatric, or emotional conditions, or Parkinson's disease), or for 2 weeks after stopping the MAOI drug. If you do not know if your prescription drug contains an MAOI, ask a doctor or pharmacist before taking this product

### ASK A DOCTOR BEFORE USE IF YOU HAVE
- liver disease
- heart disease
- high blood pressure
- diabetes
- cough that occurs with too much phlegm (mucus)
- thyroid disease
- cough that lasts or is chronic such as occurs with smoking, asthma or emphysema
- trouble urinating due to an enlarged prostate gland

### ASK DOCTOR OR PHARMACIST BEFORE USE IF YOU ARE
- taking the blood thinning drug warfarin

### WHEN USING THIS PRODUCT
Do not exceed recommended dosage.

### STOP USE AND ASK A DOCTOR IF
- you get nervous, dizzy, or sleepless
- new symptoms occur
- redness or swelling is present
- symptoms do not get better or worsen
- fever gets worse or lasts more than 3 days
- pain, cough or nasal congestion gets worse or lasts more than 7 days
- cough comes back or occurs with a fever, rash or headache that lasts. These could be signs of a serious condition

**If pregnant or breastfeeding,** ask a health care professional before use.

**Keep out of reach of children.** In case of overdose, get medical help or contact a Poison Control Center right away. Prompt medical attention is critical for adults as well as for children even if you do not notice any signs or symptoms.

### DIRECTIONS
- do not use more than directed
- take every 4 hours, while symptoms persist
- do not take more than 12 caplets in 24 hours

| Age | Dose |
| --- | --- |
| **children under 4 years of age** | **do not use** |
| children 4 to under 12 years of age | do not use unless directed by a doctor |
| adults and children 12 years of age and over | 2 tablets |

### OTHER INFORMATION
- store at controlled room temperature 20-25°C (68-77°F)

### INACTIVE INGREDIENTS
benzoic acid, carnauba wax, D&C yellow no. 10 lake, FD&C red no. 40 lake, hypromellose, magnesium stearate, microcrystalline cellulose, polyethylene glycol, polysorbate 80, pregelatinized starch, stearic acid, titanium dioxide

### QUESTIONS OR COMMENTS
Call **1-800-452-0051**

## CONTAC (acetaminophen and phenylephrine hydrochloride) caplet
GlaxoSmithKline Consumer Healthcare LP

### DRUG FACTS

| Active ingredients (in each caplet) | Purpose |
| --- | --- |
| Acetaminophen 500 mg | Pain reliever/fever reducer |
| Phenylephrine hydrochloride 5 mg | Nasal decongestant |

### USES
- temporarily relieves these symptoms due to the common cold or flu:
  - nasal congestion
  - minor aches and pains
  - sinus congestion and pressure
  - headache
  - stuffy nose
  - sore throat
- temporarily reduces fever

## WARNINGS

### Liver warning

This product contains acetaminophen. Severe liver damage may occur if you take:

- more than 8 caplets in 24 hours, which is the maximum daily amount
- with other drugs containing acetaminophen
- 3 or more alcoholic drinks every day while using this product

### Sore throat warning

If sore throat is severe, persists for more than 2 days, is accompanied or followed by fever, headache, rash, nausea or vomiting, ask a doctor promptly.

### DO NOT USE

- with any other drug containing acetaminophen (prescription or nonprescription). If you are not sure whether a drug contains acetaminophen, ask a doctor or pharmacist
- if you are now taking a prescription monoamine oxidase inhibitor (MAOI) (certain drugs for depression, psychiatric, or emotional conditions, or Parkinson's disease), or for 2 weeks after stopping the MAOI drug. If you do not know if your prescription drug contains an MAOI, ask a doctor or pharmacist before taking this product

### ASK A DOCTOR BEFORE USE IF YOU HAVE

- liver disease
- heart disease
- thyroid disease
- diabetes
- high blood pressure
- trouble urinating due to an enlarged prostate gland

### ASK A DOCTOR OR PHARMACIST BEFORE USE IF YOU ARE

- taking the blood thinning drug warfarin

### WHEN USING THIS PRODUCT

- do not use more than directed

### STOP USE AND ASK A DOCTOR IF

- you get nervous, dizzy or sleepless
- pain or nasal congestion gets worse or last more than 7 days
- fever gets worse or lasts more than 3 days
- redness or swelling is present
- any new symptoms appear

**If pregnant or breastfeeding,** ask a health professional before use.

**Keep out of reach of children.**

### OVERDOSE WARNING

Taking more than the recommended dose can cause serious health problems. In case of overdose, get medical help or contact a Poison Control Center right away. Quick medical attention is critical for adults as well as for children even if you do not notice any signs or symptoms.

### DIRECTIONS

- do not take more than directed (see overdose warning)

| adults and children 12 years of age and over | take 2 caplets every 6 hours as needed |
| | do not take more than 8 caplets in 24 hours |
| children under 12 years of age | ask a doctor |

### OTHER INFORMATION

- store below 25°C (77°F)

### INACTIVE INGREDIENTS

hypromellose, microcrystalline cellulose, polyethylene glycol, potassium sorbate, povidone, pregelatinized starch, sodium lauryl sulfate, starch, stearic acid, talc

### QUESTIONS OR COMMENTS

Call toll-free **1-800-245-1040** (English/Spanish) weekdays

## CORICIDIN (acetaminophen and chlorpheniramine maleate) tablet

Schering-Plough HealthCare Products, Inc.

### DRUG FACTS

| Active ingredients (in each tablet) | Purpose |
|---|---|
| Acetaminophen 325 mg | Pain reliever/fever reducer |
| Chlorpheniramine maleate 2 mg | Antihistamine |

### USES

- temporarily relieves:
  - minor aches and pains
  - sneezing
  - headache
  - runny nose
  - temporarily reduces fever

### WARNING

#### Liver Warning

This product contains acetaminophen. Severe liver damage may occur if:

- adult takes more than 12 tablets in 24 hours
- child takes more than 5 tablets in 24 hours
- taken with other drugs containing acetaminophen
- adult has 3 or more alcoholic drinks everyday while using this product

### DO NOT USE

- with any other drug containing acetaminophen (prescription or non prescription) if you are not sure whether a drug contains acetaminophen, ask a doctor or pharmacist

### ASK A DOCTOR BEFORE USE IF THE USER HAS

- liver disease
- a breathing problem such as emphysema or chronic bronchitis
- glaucoma
- trouble urinating due to an enlarged prostate gland

### ASK A DOCTOR OR PHARMACIST BEFORE USE IF THE USER IS

- taking the blood thinning drug warfarin
- taking sedatives or tranquilizers

### WHEN USING THIS PRODUCT

- excitability may occur, especially in children
- drowsiness may occur
- avoid alcoholic beverages alcohol, sedatives and tranquilizers may increase drowsiness
- use caution when driving a motor vehicle or operating machinery

### STOP USE AND ASK A DOCTOR IF

- pain gets worse or lasts more than 5 days (children 6 to under 12 years) or 10 days (adults)
- fever gets worse or lasts more than 3 days
- redness or swelling is present
- new symptoms occur

**If pregnant or breastfeeding,** ask a health professional before use.

**Keep out of reach of children.**

## OVERDOSE WARNING
Taking more than the recommended dose may cause liver damage. In case of overdose, get medical help or contact a Poison Control Center right away. Quick medical attention is critical for adults as well as children even if you do not notice any signs or symptoms.

## DIRECTIONS
- do not use more than directed (see overdose warning)

| adults and children 12 years and over | 2 tablets every 4 to 6 hours, not more than 12 tablets in 24 hours |
|---|---|
| children 6 to under 12 years of age | 1 tablet every 4 to 6 hours, not more than 5 tablets in 24 hours |

## OTHER INFORMATION
- each tablet contains: magnesium 10 mg
- store between 20°C-25°C (68° to 77°F)
- protect from excessive moisture

## INACTIVE INGREDIENTS
acacia, calcium sulfate, carnauba wax, corn starch, FD&C red no. 40 aluminum lake, FD&C yellow no. 6 aluminum lake, lactose, magnesium stearate, microcrystalline cellulose, pharmaceutical ink, povidone, sugar, talc, titanium dioxide, white wax

---

# CORICIDIN HBP COLD & FLU (acetaminophen and chlorpheniramine maleate) tablet
Schering-Plough HealthCare Products, Inc.

## DRUG FACTS

| Active ingredients (in each tablet) | Purpose |
|---|---|
| Acetaminophen 325 mg | Pain reliever/fever reducer |
| Chlorpheniramine maleate 2 mg | Antihistamine |

## USES
- temporarily relieves:
  - minor aches and pains
  - sneezing
  - headache
  - runny nose
- temporarily reduces fever

## WARNINGS
**Liver Warning**
This product contains acetaminophen. Severe liver damage may occur if:
- adult takes more than 12 tablets in 24 hours
- child takes more than 5 tablets in 24 hours
- taken with other drugs containing acetaminophen
- adult has 3 or more alcoholic drinks everyday while using this product

## DO NOT USE
- with any other drug containing acetaminophen (prescription or nonprescription)
- if you are not sure whether a drug contains acetaminophen, ask a doctor or pharmacist

## ASK A DOCTOR BEFORE USE IF
- the user has:
  - liver disease
  - a breathing problem such as emphysema or chronic bronchitis
  - glaucoma
  - trouble urinating due to an enlarged prostate gland

## ASK A DOCTOR OR PHARMACIST BEFORE USE IF
- the user is:
  - taking the blood thinning drug warfarin
  - taking sedatives or tranquilizers

## WHEN USING THIS PRODUCT
- excitability may occur, especially in children
- drowsiness may occur
- avoid alcoholic beverages alcohol, sedatives and tranquilizers may increase drowsiness
- use caution when driving a motor vehicle or operating machinery

## STOP USE AND ASK A DOCTOR IF
- pain gets worse or lasts more than 5 days (children 6 to under 12 years) or 10 days (adults)
- fever gets worse or lasts more than 3 days
- redness or swelling is present
- new symptoms occur

**If pregnant or breastfeeding,** ask a health professional before use.

**Keep out of reach of children.**

## OVERDOSE WARNING
Taking more than the recommended dose may cause liver damage. In case of overdose, get medical help or contact a Poison Control Center right away. Quick medical attention is critical for adults as well as children even if you do not notice any signs or symptoms.

## DIRECTIONS
- do not use more than directed (see Overdose Warning)

| adults and children 12 years and over | 2 tablets every 4 to 6 hours, not more than 12 tablets in 24 hours |
|---|---|
| children 6 to under 12 years of age | 1 tablet every 4 to 6 hours, not more than 5 tablets in 24 hours |

## OTHER INFORMATION
- each tablet contains: magnesium 10 mg
- store between 20°C-25°C (68°F-77°F)
- protect from excessive moisture

## INACTIVE INGREDIENTS
acacia, calcium sulfate, carnauba wax, corn starch, FD&C red no. 40 aluminum lake, FD&C yellow no. 6 aluminum lake, lactose, magnesium stearate, microcrystalline cellulose, pharmaceutical ink, povidone, sugar, talc, titanium dioxide, white wax

## QUESTIONS OR COMMENTS
For more information, visit www.coricidinhbp.com

# CORTAID ADVANCED ANTI-ITCH CREAM
(hydrocortisone) cream

Johnson & Johnson Consumer Products Company

## DRUG FACTS

| Active ingredient | Purpose |
|---|---|
| Hydrocortisone 1.0% | Anti-itch |

## USES
- temporarily relieves itching associated with minor skin irritation, inflammation, and rashes due to:
  - eczema, insect bites, poison ivy, oak and sumac, soaps, detergents, cosmetics, jewelry, seborrheic dermatitis, psoriasis
  - other uses of this product: ask a doctor

## WARNINGS
**For external use only.**

## DO NOT USE
- in or near eyes, for the treatment of diaper rash, ask a doctor

## ASK A DOCTOR BEFORE USE IF
- you are using any other hydrocortisone product

## STOP USE AND ASK A DOCTOR IF
- condition worsens or if symptoms persist for more than 7 days
- symptoms clear up and return within a few days

**Keep out of reach of children.** If swallowed, get medical help or contact a Poison Control Center right away.

## DIRECTIONS
- apply to affected area not more than 3 to 4 times daily
- children under 2 years of age: do not use; ask a doctor

## OTHER INFORMATION
- store at room temperature

## INACTIVE INGREDIENTS
aloe barbadensis leaf juice, avena sativa (oat) kernel extract, benzyl alcohol, ceteareth-20, cetearyl alcohol, cetyl palmitate, chrysanthemum parthenium (feverfew) extract, citric acid, cyclopentasiloxane, dimethicone/vinyltrimethylsiloxysilicate crosspolymer, dimethyl mea, glycerin, isopropyl myristate, isostearyl neopentanoate, methylparaben, PEG-40 stearage, potassium lactate, sodium hydroxide, water

# CORTAID MAXIMUM STRENGTH
(hydrocortisone) cream

Johnson & Johnson Consumer Products Company

## DRUG FACTS

| Active ingredient | Purpose |
|---|---|
| Hydrocortisone 1% | Anti-itch |

## USES
- temporarily relieves itching associated with minor skin irritations, inflammation, and rashes due to:
  - eczema
  - insect bites
  - poison ivy, oak, or sumac
  - soaps
  - detergents
  - cosmetics
  - jewelry
  - seborrheic dermatitis
  - psoriasis
- temporarily relieves external anal and genital itching
- other uses of this product should only be under the advice and supervision of a doctor

## WARNINGS
**For external use only.**

## DO NOT USE
- in the genital area if you have a vaginal discharge. Consult a doctor
- for the treatment of diaper rash. Ask a doctor

## WHEN USING THIS PRODUCT
- avoid contact with eyes
- do not use more than directed unless told to do so by a doctor
- do not put directly into the rectum by using fingers or any mechanical device or applicator

## STOP USE AND ASK A DOCTOR IF
- condition worsens, symptoms persist for more than 7 days or clear up and occur again within a few days, and do not begin use of any other hydrocortisone product unless you have asked a doctor
- rectal bleeding occurs

**Keep out of reach of children.** If swallowed, get medical help or contact a Poison Control Center right away.

## DIRECTIONS
- for itching of skin irritation, inflammation, and rashes:

| adults and children 2 years of age and older | apply to affected area not more than 3 to 4 times daily |
|---|---|
| children under 2 years of age | ask a doctor |

- for external anal and genital itching:

| adults | when practical, clean the affected area with mild soap and warm water and rinse thoroughly |
|---|---|
| | gently dry by patting or blotting with toilet tissue or a soft cloth before applying |
| | apply to affected area not more than 3 to 4 times daily |
| children under 12 years of age | ask a doctor |

## OTHER INFORMATION
- store at 20°C-25°C (68°F-77°F)
- see end of carton or tube crimp for lot number and expiration date

## INACTIVE INGREDIENTS
water, petrolatum, glycerin, mineral oil, ceteareth-6, dimethicone, VP/eicosene copolymer, phenoxyethanol, stearyl alcohol, ammonium acryloyldimethyltaurate/VP copolymer, cetyl alcohol, carbomer, edetate disodium, methylparaben, sodium citrate, ethylparaben, citric acid, propylparaben, sodium hydroxide

## QUESTIONS OR COMMENTS
Call **1-800-451-5084**

## CORTIZONE 10 (hydrocortisone) ointment
Chattem, Inc.

### DRUG FACTS

| Active ingredient | Purpose |
|---|---|
| Hydrocortisone 1% | Anti-itch |

### USES
- temporarily relieves itching associated with minor skin irritations, inflammation, and rashes due to:
  - eczema
  - psoriasis
  - poison ivy, oak, sumac
  - insect bites
  - detergents
  - jewelry
  - cosmetics
  - soaps
  - seborrheic dermatitis
  - temporarily relieves external anal and genital itching
  - other uses of this product should only be under the advice and supervision of a doctor

### WARNINGS
**For external use only.**

### DO NOT USE
- in the genital area if you have a vaginal discharge. Consult a doctor
- for the treatment of diaper rash. Consult a doctor

### WHEN USING THIS PRODUCT
- avoid contact with eyes
- do not use more than directed unless told to do so by a doctor
- do not put directly into the rectum by using fingers or any mechanical device or applicator

### STOP USE AND ASK A DOCTOR IF
- condition worsens, symptoms persist for more than 7 days or clear up and occur again within a few days, and do not begin use of any other hydrocortisone product unless you have asked a doctor
- rectal bleeding occurs

**Keep out of reach of children.** If swallowed, get medical help or contact a Poison Control Center right away.

### DIRECTIONS
- for itching of skin irritation, inflammation, and rashes:

| adults and children 2 years of age and older | apply to affected area not more than 3 to 4 times daily |
|---|---|
| children under 2 years of age | ask a doctor |

- for external anal and genital itching:

| adults | when practical, clean the affected area with mild soap and warm water and rinse thoroughly |
|---|---|
|  | gently dry by patting or blotting with toilet tissue or a soft cloth before applying |
|  | apply to affected area not more than 3 to 4 times daily |
| children under 12 years of age | ask a doctor |

### OTHER INFORMATION
- contents filled by weight, not volume

### INACTIVE INGREDIENTS
petrolatum

### QUESTIONS OR COMMENTS
visit www.chattem.com

## CORTIZONE 10 PLUS (hydrocortisone) cream
Chattem, Inc.

### DRUG FACTS

| Active ingredient | Purpose |
|---|---|
| Hydrocortisone 1% | Anti-itch |

### USES
- temporarily relieves itching associated with minor skin irritations, inflammation, and rashes due to:
  - eczema
  - psoriasis
  - poison ivy, oak, sumac
  - insect bites
  - detergents
  - jewelry
  - cosmetics
  - soaps
  - seborrheic dermatitis
  - temporarily relieves external anal and genital itching
  - other uses of this product should only be under the advice and supervision of a doctor

### WARNINGS
**For external use only.**

### DO NOT USE
- in the genital area if you have a vaginal discharge. Consult a doctor
- for the treatment of diaper rash. Consult a doctor

### WHEN USING THIS PRODUCT
- avoid contact with eyes
- do not use more than directed unless told to do so by a doctor
- do not put directly into the rectum by using fingers or any mechanical device or applicator

### STOP USE AND ASK A DOCTOR IF
- condition worsens, symptoms persist for more than 7 days or clear up and occur again within a few days, and do not begin use of any other hydrocortisone product unless you have asked a doctor
- rectal bleeding occurs

**Keep out of reach of children.** If swallowed, get medical help or contact a Poison Control Center right away.

### DIRECTIONS
- for itching of skin irritation, inflammation, and rashes:

| adults and children 2 years of age and older | apply to affected area not more than 3 to 4 times daily |
|---|---|
| children under 2 years of age | ask a doctor |

- for external anal and genital itching:

| adults | when practical, clean the affected area with mild soap and warm water and rinse thoroughly |
| | gently dry by patting or blotting with toilet tissue or a soft cloth before applying |
| | apply to affected area not more than 3 to 4 times daily |
| children under 12 years of age | ask a doctor |

## OTHER INFORMATION
- contents filled by weight, not volume

## INACTIVE INGREDIENTS
aloe barbadensis leaf juice, aluminum sulfate, beeswax, calcium acetate, cetearyl alcohol, cetyl alcohol, cholecalciferol, dextrin, glycerin, isopropyl palmitate, maltodextrin, methylparaben, mineral oil, petrolatum, propylene glycol, propylparaben, retinyl palmitate, sodium cetearyl sulfate, sodium lauryl sulfate, tocopheryl acetate, water, zea mays (corn) oil

## QUESTIONS OR COMMENTS
visit www.chattem.com

---

# CROMOLYN SODIUM NASAL SOLUTION
(cromolyn sodium) spray, metered

Bausch & Lomb Incorporated

## DRUG FACTS

| Active ingredient (per spray) | Purpose |
|---|---|
| Cromolyn sodium 5.2 mg | Nasal allergy symptom controller |

## USES
- to prevent and relieve nasal symptoms of hay fever and other nasal allergies:
  - runny/itchy nose
  - sneezing
  - allergic stuffy nose

## WARNINGS
## DO NOT USE
- if you are allergic to any of the ingredients

## ASK A DOCTOR BEFORE USE IF YOU HAVE
- fever
- discolored nasal discharge
- sinus pain
- wheezing

## WHEN USING THIS PRODUCT
- it may take several days of use to notice an effect. Your best effect may not be seen for 1 to 2 weeks
- brief stinging or sneezing may occur right after use
- do not use to treat sinus infection, asthma, or cold symptoms
- do not share bottle with anyone else as this may spread germs

## STOP USE AND ASK A DOCTOR IF
- shortness of breath, wheezing, or chest tightness occurs
- hives or swelling of the mouth or throat occurs
- your symptoms worsen
- you have new symptoms
- your symptoms do not begin to improve within two weeks
- you need to use for more than 12 weeks

**If pregnant or breastfeeding,** ask a health professional before use.

**Keep out of reach of children.** If swallowed, get medical help or contact a Poison Control Center right away.

## DIRECTIONS
- see package insert on how to use pump
- parent or care provider must supervise the use of this product by young children

| adults and children 2 years and older | spray once into each nostril. Repeat 3-4 times a day (every 4-6 hours). If needed, may be used up to 6 times a day |
| | use every day while in contact with the cause of your allergies (pollen, molds, pets, and dust) |
| | to prevent nasal allergy symptoms, use before contact with the cause of your allergies |
| | for best results, start using up to one week before contact |
| | if desired, you can use this product with other medicines, including other allergy medicines |
| children under 2 years | do not use unless directed by a doctor |

## OTHER INFORMATION
- store between 20-25°C (68-77°F)
- protect from light
- keep carton and package insert. They contain important instructions

## INACTIVE INGREDIENTS
benzalkonium chloride, edetate disodium, purified water

## QUESTIONS OR COMMENTS
Call toll-free **1-800-323-0000**

---

# CRUEX (miconazole nitrate) spray

Novartis

## DRUG FACTS

| Active ingredient | Purpose |
|---|---|
| Miconazole nitrate 2% | Antifungal |

## USES
- cures most jock itch (tinea cruris)
- relieves itching, scaling, burning and discomfort that can accompany jock itch

## WARNINGS
**For external use only.**

**Flammability warning**
Contents under pressure. Do not puncture or incinerate. Flammable mixture; do not use near fire or flame, or expose to heat or temperatures above 49°C (120°F). Use only as directed.

Intentional misuse by deliberately concentrating and inhaling contents can be harmful or fatal.

## DO NOT USE
- in or near the mouth or the eyes
- for nail or scalp infections

## WHEN USING THIS PRODUCT
- do not get into the eyes or mouth

## STOP USE AND ASK A DOCTOR IF
- inhalation occurs
- no improvement within 2 weeks

**Keep out of reach of children.** If swallowed, get medical help or contact a poison center right away.

## DIRECTIONS

| adults and children 2 years and older | wash the affected skin with soap and water and dry completely before applying |
| | shake can well, hold can 4" to 6" from skin |
| | spray a thin layer over affected skin area twice a day (morning and night) or as directed by a doctor |
| | use daily for 2 weeks |
| | supervise children in the use of this product |
| children under the age of 2 years | ask a doctor |

## OTHER INFORMATION
- store at room controlled temperature 20-25°C (68-77°F)
- see container bottom for lot number and expiration date
- if clogging occurs, remove button and clean nozzle with a pin

## INACTIVE INGREDIENTS
aloe vera gel, aluminum starch, octenyl succinate, isopropyl myristate, propylene carbonate, SD alchol 40-B (10% w/w), sorbitan monoleate, stearalkonium hectorite. Propellant: isobutene/propane

## QUESTIONS OR COMMENTS
Call **1-800-452-0051** 24 hours a day, 7 days a week

---

# CURAD MEDIPLAST (salicylic acid) pad
Medline Industries, Inc

## DRUG FACTS

| Active ingredient | Purpose |
|---|---|
| Salicylic acid 40% | Corn, callus, and wart remover |

## USES
- for the removal of:
  - corns
  - calluses
  - common warts

## WARNINGS
**For external use only.**
This product contains natural rubber, which may cause allergic reactions.

## DO NOT USE
- if you are diabetic or have poor blood circulation
- on irritated skin or on any area that is infected or reddened
- on moles, birthmarks, or warts with hair growing from them, genital warts, warts on the face, warts on mucous membranes such as warts inside the mouth, nose, anus, genitals or lips

**Keep this and all drugs out of reach of children.** In case of accidental ingestion, seek professional assistance or contact a Poison Control Center immediately.

## STOP USING THIS PRODUCT AND SEE YOUR DOCTOR
- if discomfort persists

## DIRECTIONS
- wash affected area. May soak corn, callus or wart in warm water for 5 minutes.
- dry area thoroughly.
- cut pad to fit corn, callus or wart. Apply medicated pad to area.
- remove medicated pad after 48 hours.
- repeat procedure every 48 hours for up to 14 days for corn/ callus removal and up to 12 weeks for warts, until the problem has cleared

## INACTIVE INGREDIENTS
2, 2'-methylene-bis-(6-tert.-butyl-p-cresol), alpha, alpha'-(propylenedinitrilo)-di-o-cresol, flannel, lanolin, natural rubber, peru balsam, rosin, talcum and terpenephenol resin

---

# DEBROX (carbamide peroxide) liquid
GlaxoSmithKline Consumer Healthcare LP

## DRUG FACTS

| Active ingredient | Purpose |
|---|---|
| Carbamide peroxide 6.5% non USP* | Earwax removal aid |

*pH differs from USP specifications

## USES
- for occasional use as an aid to soften, loosen and remove excessive earwax

## WARNINGS

## ASK A DOCTOR BEFORE USE IF YOU HAVE
- ear drainage or discharge
- irritation or rash in the ear
- an injury or perforation (hole) of the eardrum
- recently had ear surgery
- ear pain
- dizziness

## STOP USE AND ASK A DOCTOR IF
- you need to use for more than four days
- excessive earwax remains after use of this product

## WHEN USING THIS PRODUCT
- avoid contact with the eyes

**Keep this and all drugs out of the reach of children.** If swallowed, get medical help or contact a Poison Control Center right away.

## DIRECTIONS
- for use in the ear only

| adults and children over 12 years of age | tilt head sideways |
|---|---|
| | place 5 to 10 drops into ear |
| | tip of applicator should not enter ear canal |
| | keep drops in ear for several minutes by keeping head tilted or placing cotton in the ear |
| | use twice daily for up to four days if needed, or as directed by a doctor |
| | any wax remaining after treatment may be removed by gently flushing the ear with warm water, using a soft rubber bulb ear syringe |
| children under 12 years | consult a doctor |

## OTHER INFORMATION
- avoid exposing bottle to excessive heat and sunlight
- product foams on contact with earwax due to release of oxygen. There may be an associated "crackling" sound
- keep tip on bottle when not in use

## INACTIVE INGREDIENTS
citric acid, flavor, glycerin, propylene glycol, sodium lauroyl sarcosinate, sodium stannate, water

## QUESTIONS OR COMMENTS
Call **1-800-245-1040** weekdays or visit anytime at www.debrox.com

# DELSYM 12 HOUR COUGH RELIEF
(dextromethorphan polistirex) suspension, extended release

Reckitt Benckiser, Inc.

## DRUG FACTS

| Active ingredient (in each 5 mL teaspoonful) | Purpose |
|---|---|
| Dextromethorphan polistirex equivalent to 30 mg dextromethorphan hydrobromide | Cough suppressant |

## USES
- temporarily relieves cough due to minor throat and bronchial
- irritation as may occur with the common cold or inhaled irritants

## WARNINGS
### DO NOT USE
- if you are now taking a prescription monoamine oxidase inhibitor (MAOI) (certain drugs for depression, psychiatric or emotional conditions, or Parkinson's disease), or for 2 weeks after stopping the MAOI drug
- if you do not know if your prescription drug contains an MAOI, ask a doctor or pharmacist before taking this product

### ASK A DOCTOR BEFORE USE IF YOU HAVE
- chronic cough that lasts as occurs with smoking, asthma or emphysema
- cough that occurs with too much phlegm (mucus)

### STOP USE AND ASK A DOCTOR IF
- cough lasts more than 7 days, cough comes back, or occurs with fever, rash or headache that lasts. These could be signs of a serious condition.

**If pregnant or breastfeeding,** ask a health professional before use.

**Keep out of reach of children.** In case of overdose, get medical help or contact a Poison Control Center right away.

## DIRECTIONS
- shake bottle well before use
- dose as follows or as directed by a doctor

| adults and children 12 years of age and over | 2 teaspoonfuls every 12 hours, not to exceed 4 teaspoonfuls in 24 hours |
|---|---|
| children 6 to under 12 years of age | 1 teaspoonful every 12 hours, not to exceed 2 teaspoonfuls in 24 hours |
| children 4 to under 6 years of age | ½ teaspoonful every 12 hours, not to exceed 1 teaspoonful in 24 hours |
| children under 4 years of age | do not use |

## OTHER INFORMATION
- store at 20-25°C (68-77°F)

## INACTIVE INGREDIENTS
citric acid anhydrous, D&C Red no. 33, edetate disodium, ethylcellulose, FD&C blue no. 1, flavor, high fructose corn syrup, methylparaben, polyethylene glycol 3350, polysorbate 80, propylene glycol, propylparaben, purified water, sucrose, tragacanth, vegetable oil, xanthan gum

## QUESTIONS OR COMMENTS
Call **1-888-963-3382**

# DELSYM NIGHT TIME COUGH AND COLD
(acetaminophen, dextromethorphan hydrobromide, and doxylamine succinate) solution

Reckitt Benckiser, Inc.

## DRUG FACTS

| Active ingredients (in each 15 mL) | Purpose |
|---|---|
| Acetaminophen 500 mg | Pain reliever/fever reducer |
| Dextromethorphan hydrobromide 15 mg | Cough suppressant |
| Doxylamine succinate 6.25 mg | Antihistamine |

## USES
- temporarily relieves these common cold and flu symptoms:
  - cough due to minor throat and bronchial irritation
  - runny nose and sneezing
  - minor aches and pains
  - sore throat
  - headache
  - fever
  - the impulse to cough to help you get to sleep

## WARNINGS

### Liver warning

This product contains acetaminophen. Severe liver damage may occur if you take:

- more than 4 doses in 24 hours, which is the maximum daily amount
- with other drugs containing acetaminophen
- 3 or more alcoholic drinks daily while using this product

### Sore throat warning

If sore throat is severe, persists for more than 2 days, is accompanied or followed by fever, headache, rash, nausea or vomiting, consult a doctor promptly.

### DO NOT USE

- with any other drug containing acetaminophen (prescription or nonprescription)
- if you are not sure whether a drug contains acetaminophen, ask a doctor or pharmacist
- if you are now taking a prescription monoamine oxidase inhibitor (MAOI) (certain drugs for depression, psychiatric, or emotional conditions, or Parkinson's disease), or for 2 weeks after stopping the MAOI drug
- if you do not know if your prescription drug contains an MAOI, ask a doctor or pharmacist before taking this product

### ASK A DOCTOR BEFORE USE IF YOU HAVE

- liver disease
- glaucoma
- trouble urinating due to an enlarged prostate gland
- a breathing problem such as emphysema or chronic bronchitis
- persistent or chronic cough such as occurs with smoking, asthma or emphysema
- cough that occurs with too much phlegm (mucus)
- a sodium restricted diet

### ASK A DOCTOR OR PHARMACIST BEFORE USE IF

- you are taking the blood thinning drug warfarin
- you are taking sedatives or tranquilizers

### WHEN USING THIS PRODUCT

- do not use more than directed
- excitability may occur, especially in children
- marked drowsiness may occur
- alcohol, sedatives and tranquilizers may increase drowsiness
- avoid alcoholic drinks
- be careful when driving a motor vehicle or operating machinery

### STOP USE AND ASK A DOCTOR IF

- pain or cough gets worse or lasts more than 7 days
- fever gets worse or lasts more than 3 days
- redness or swelling is present
- new symptoms occur
- cough comes back or occurs with rash or persistent headache. These could be signs of a serious condition

**If pregnant or breastfeeding,** ask a health professional before use.

**Keep out of reach of children.**

### OVERDOSE WARNING

Taking more than the recommended dose (overdose) may cause liver damage. In case of overdose, get medical help or contact a Poison Control Center right away. Quick medical attention is critical for adults as well as for children even if you do not notice any signs or symptoms.

### DIRECTIONS

- do not take more than directed (see Overdose warning)
- do not take more than 4 doses in any 24-hour period
- measure only with dosing cup provided
- do not use dosing cup with other products
- dose as follows or as directed by a doctor

| adults and children 12 years and older | 30 mL in dosing cup provided every 6 hours |
| --- | --- |
| children under 12 years of age | do not use |

### OTHER INFORMATION

- each 15 mL contains: sodium 23 mg
- tamper evident: do not use if seal under bottle cap printed "SEALED for YOUR PROTECTION" is torn or missing
- dosing cup provided
- store between 15-30°C (59-86°F)
- keep carton for full directions for use

### INACTIVE INGREDIENTS

anhydrous citric acid, anhydrous trisodium citrate, FD&C blue no. 1, FD&C red no. 40, flavors, glycerin, polyethylene glycol, propylene glycol, purified water, saccharin sodium, sodium benzoate, sugar

### QUESTIONS OR COMMENTS

Call **1-888-963-3382.** You may also report side effects to this phone number.

---

# DELSYM CHILDREN'S NIGHT TIME COUGH AND COLD (diphenhydramine hydrochloride and phenylephrine hydrochloride) solution

Reckitt Benckiser, Inc.

## DRUG FACTS

| Active ingredients (in each 5 mL) | Purpose |
| --- | --- |
| Diphenhydramine hydrochloride 12.5 mg | Antihistamine/cough suppressant |
| Phenylephrine hydrochloride 5 mg | Nasal decongestant |

### USES

- temporarily controls cough due to minor throat and bronchial irritation and relieves nasal congestion as may occur with a cold
- temporarily relieves the following symptoms due to hay fever or other upper respiratory allergies:
  - sneezing
  - runny nose
  - itchy, watery eyes
  - itchy nose or throat

## WARNINGS

### DO NOT USE

- to make a child sleepy
- with any other product containing diphenhydramine, even one used on the skin
- if you are now taking a prescription monoamine oxidase inhibitor (MAOI) (certain drugs for depression, psychiatric, or emotional conditions, or Parkinson's disease), or for 2 weeks after stopping the MAOI drug.
- if you do not know if your prescription drug contains an MAOI, ask a doctor or pharmacist before taking this product

### ASK A DOCTOR BEFORE USE IF YOU HAVE

- heart disease
- diabetes
- high blood pressure
- thyroid disease
- glaucoma

- trouble urinating due to an enlarged prostate gland
- a breathing problem such as emphysema or chronic bronchitis
- persistent or chronic cough such as occurs with smoking, asthma or emphysema
- cough that occurs with too much phlegm (mucus)

## ASK A DOCTOR OR PHARMACIST BEFORE USE IF
- you are taking sedatives or tranquilizers

## WHEN USING THIS PRODUCT
- do not use more than directed
- excitability may occur, especially in children
- marked drowsiness may occur
- alcohol, sedatives and tranquilizers may increase drowsiness
- avoid alcoholic drinks
- be careful when driving a motor vehicle or operating machinery

## STOP USE AND ASK A DOCTOR IF
- nervousness, dizziness or sleeplessness occur
- symptoms do not get better within 7 days or occur with fever
- cough lasts more than 7 days, comes back, or occurs with fever, rash or persistent headache. These could be signs of a serious condition

**If pregnant or breastfeeding,** ask a health professional before use.

**Keep out of reach of children.** In case of overdose, get medical help or contact a Poison Control Center right away.

## DIRECTIONS
- do not take more than directed
- do not take more than 6 doses in any 24-hour period
- measure only with dosing cup provided
- do not use dosing cup with other products
- dose as follows or as directed by a doctor

| adults and children 12 years of age and over | 10 mL every 4 hours |
| children 6 to under 12 years of age | 5 mL every 4 hours |
| children 4 to under 6 years of age | do not use unless directed by a doctor |
| children under 4 years of age | do not use |

## OTHER INFORMATION
- each 5 mL contains: sodium 10 mg
- tamper evident: do not use if neckband on bottle cap is broken or missing
- dosing cup provided
- store between 15-30°C (59-86°F)
- keep carton for full directions for use

## INACTIVE INGREDIENTS
anhydrous citric acid, anhydrous trisodium citrate, carboxymethylcellulose sodium, edetate disodium, FD&C blue no. 1, FD&C red no. 40, flavors, glycerin, propyl gallate, propylene glycol, purified water, sodium benzoate, sorbitol, sucralose

## QUESTIONS OR COMMENTS
Call **1-888-963-3382.** You may also report side effects to this phone number.

# DELSYM NIGHT TIME MULTI SYMPTOM
(acetaminophen, dextromethorphan hydrobromide, doxylamine succinate, and phenylephrine hydrochloride) solution

Reckitt Benckiser, Inc.

## DRUG FACTS

| Active ingredients (in each 15 mL) | Purpose |
| --- | --- |
| Acetaminophen 325 mg | Pain reliever/fever reducer |
| Dextromethorphan hydrobromide 10 mg | Cough suppressant |
| Doxylamine succinate 6.25 mg | Antihistamine |
| Phenylephrine hydrochloride 5 mg | Nasal decongestant |

## USES
- temporarily relieves these common cold and flu symptoms:
  - nasal congestion
  - cough due to minor throat and bronchial irritation
  - runny nose and sneezing
  - minor aches and pains
  - sore throat
  - headache
  - fever
  - the impulse to cough to help you get to sleep

## WARNINGS
### Liver warning
This product contains acetaminophen. Severe liver damage may occur if you take:
- more than 6 doses in 24 hours, which is the maximum daily amount
- with other drugs containing acetaminophen
- 3 or more alcoholic drinks daily while using this product

### Sore throat warning
If sore throat is severe, persists for more than 2 days, is accompanied or followed by fever, headache, rash, nausea or vomiting, consult a doctor promptly.

### DO NOT USE
- with any other drug containing acetaminophen (prescription or nonprescription). If you are not sure whether a drug contains acetaminophen, ask a doctor or pharmacist
- if you are now taking a prescription monoamine oxidase inhibitor (MAOI) (certain drugs for depression, psychiatric, or emotional conditions, or Parkinson's disease), or for 2 weeks after stopping the MAOI drug
- if you do not know if your prescription drug contains an MAOI, ask a doctor or pharmacist before taking this product

## ASK A DOCTOR BEFORE USE IF YOU HAVE
- liver disease
- heart disease
- diabetes
- high blood pressure
- thyroid disease
- glaucoma
- trouble urinating due to an enlarged prostate gland
- a breathing problem such as emphysema or chronic bronchitis
- persistent or chronic cough such as occurs with smoking, asthma or emphysema
- cough that occurs with too much phlegm (mucus)

## ASK A DOCTOR OR PHARMACIST BEFORE USE IF
- you are taking the blood thinning drug warfarin
- you are taking sedatives or tranquilizers

## WHEN USING THIS PRODUCT
- do not use more than directed
- excitability may occur, especially in children
- marked drowsiness may occur
- alcohol, sedatives and tranquilizers may increase drowsiness
- avoid alcoholic drinks
- be careful when driving a motor vehicle or operating machinery

## STOP USE AND ASK A DOCTOR IF
- nervousness, dizziness, or sleeplessness occur
- pain, nasal congestion or cough gets worse or lasts more than 7 days
- fever gets worse or lasts more than 3 days
- redness or swelling is present
- new symptoms occur
- cough comes back, or occurs with rash or persistent headache. These could be signs of a serious condition

**If pregnant or breastfeeding,** ask a health professional before use.

**Keep out of reach of children.**

## OVERDOSE WARNING
Taking more than the recommended dose (overdose) may cause liver damage. In case of overdose, get medical help or contact a Poison Control Center right away. Quick medical attention is critical for adults as well as for children even if you do not notice any signs or symptoms.

## DIRECTIONS
- do not take more than directed (see Overdose warning)
- do not take more than 6 doses in any 24-hour period
- measure only with dosing cup provided
- do not use dosing cup with other products
- dose as follows or as directed by a doctor

| adults and children 12 years and older | 30 mL in dosing cup provided every 4 hours |
| --- | --- |
| children under 12 years of age | do not use |

## OTHER INFORMATION
- each 15 mL contains: sodium 5 mg
- tamper evident: do not use if seal under bottle cap printed "SEALED for YOUR PROTECTION" is torn or missing
- dosing cup provided
- store between 15-30°C (59-86°F)
- keep carton for full directions for use

## INACTIVE INGREDIENTS
anhydrous citric acid, FD&C blue no. 1, FD&C red no. 40, FD&C yellow no. 6, flavors, glycerin, propylene glycol, purified water, sodium benzoate, sorbitol, sucralose

## QUESTIONS OR COMMENTS
Call **1-888-963-3382.** You may also report side effects to this phone number.

## DERMOPLAST (benzocaine USP and menthol USP)
spray

Medtech Products Inc.

### DRUG FACTS

| Active Ingredients | Purpose |
| --- | --- |
| Benzocaine USP (20%) | Fast relief of pain & itching |
| Menthol USP (0.5%) | |

## USES
- for temporary relief of pain and itching associated with:
  - sunburn
  - insect bites
  - minor cuts
  - scrapes
  - minor burns
  - minor skin irritations

## WARNINGS
- avoid contact with leather, fabric and upholstery to prevent possible staining or discoloration

### Allergy alert
Do not use this product if you have a history of allergy to local anesthetics such as procaine, butacaine, benzocaine or other "caine" anesthetics.

**For external use only.**
- avoid contact with eyes, mouth and mucous membranes

**Contents flammable. Keep away from fire, open flame and heat.**

### DO NOT USE
- excessive amounts of this product on broken, blistered, abraded skin or open wounds
- excessive amounts of this product over large areas of the body
- this product while smoking

### WHEN USING THIS PRODUCT
- do not spray in eyes on the face or in the mouth
- do not inhale
- intentional misuse by deliberately concentrating and inhaling the contents can be harmful or fatal
- use only as directed

### STOP USE AND ASK A DOCTOR IF
- condition worsens
- symptoms persist for more than 7 days or clear up and occur again within a few days
- itching, rash or irritation develop

**Keep out of reach of children**. If swallowed get medical help or contact a Poison Control Center right away.

### DIRECTIONS
- safe for children 2 years and older
- to use this product, hold can 6 to 12 inches away from affected area

| adults and children 2 years and older: | apply to affected area not more than 3 to 4 times daily |
| --- | --- |
| children under 2 years of age | consult a doctor |

- direct spray nozzle towards skin and press button to activate spray
- to apply to face, first spray into palm of hand then touch hand to face

## OTHER INFORMATION
- contents under pressure
- do not puncture or incinerate can

## INACTIVE INGREDIENTS
acetylated lanolin alcohol, aloe vera oil, butane, cetyl acetate, hydrofluorocarbon 152A, methylparaben, PEG-8 laurate, polysorbate 85

# DESITIN MULTI-PURPOSE FRAGRANCE FREE (petrolatum) ointment
Johnson & Johnson Consumer Products Company

## DRUG FACTS

| Active ingredient | Purpose |
|---|---|
| Petrolatum 70.3% | Skin protectant |

## USES
- helps treat and prevent diaper rash
- protects chafed skin due to diaper rash and helps seal out wetness
- temporarily protects and helps relieve chapped, or cracked skin
- helps prevent and protect from the drying effects of wind and cold weather
- temporarily protects minor:
  - cuts
  - scrapes
  - burns

## WARNINGS
For external use only.

## WHEN USING THIS PRODUCT
- do not get into eyes

## STOP USE AND ASK A DOCTOR IF
- condition worsens
- symptoms last more than 7 days or clear up and occur again within a few days

## DO NOT USE ON
- deep or puncture wounds
- animal bites
- serious burns

Keep out of reach of children. If swallowed, get medical help or contact a Poison Control Center right away.

## DIRECTIONS
- for diaper rash:
  - change wet or soiled diapers promptly
  - cleanse the diaper area and allow to dry
  - apply ointment liberally as often as necessary, with each diaper change, especially at bedtime or any time when exposure to wet diapers may be prolonged
- for skin irritation:
  - apply as needed

## OTHER INFORMATION
- store between 20-25°C (68-776°F)
- twist off cap, remove quality seal
- do not use if quality seal is broken

## INACTIVE INGREDIENTS
mineral oil, paraffin, theobroma cacao (cocoa) seed butter, tocopheryl acetate, sodium pyruvate, retinyl palmitate, cholecalciferol

## QUESTIONS OR COMMENTS
Call **1-800-720-3843**, weekdays, 9 AM-5 PM EST

# DESITIN RAPID RELIEF CREAMY DIAPER RASH (zinc oxide) cream
Johnson & Johnson Consumer Products Company

## DRUG FACTS

| Active ingredient | Purpose |
|---|---|
| Zinc oxide 13% | Skin protectant |

## USES
- helps treat and prevent diaper rash
- protects chafed skin due to diaper rash
- helps seal out wetness

## WARNINGS
For external use only.

## WHEN USING THIS PRODUCT
- do not get into eyes

## STOP USE AND ASK A DOCTOR IF
- condition worsens
- symptoms last more than 7 days or clear up and occur within a few days

Keep out of reach of children. If swallowed, get medical help or contact a Poison Control Center right away.

## DIRECTIONS
- change wet or soiled diapers promptly
- clean the diaper area
- allow to dry
- apply ointment liberally as often as necessary, with each diaper change, especially at bedtime or any time prolonged exposure to wet diapers may be prolonged

## OTHER INFORMATION
- store at 20°C-25°C (68°F-77°F)

## INACTIVE INGREDIENTS
water, mineral oil, petrolatum, beeswax, dimethicone, sorbitan sesquioleate, microcrystalline wax, PEG-30 dipolyhydroxystearate, magnesium sulfate, phenoxyethanol, methylparaben, fragrance, potassium hydroxide, propylparaben, tocopheryl acetate, aloe barbadensis leaf juice

## QUESTIONS OR COMMENTS
Call **1-800-720-3843**, weekdays, 9 AM-5 PM EST

# DESITIN SOOTHING RASH BATH TREATMENT (colloidal) powder
Johnson & Johnson Consumer Products Company

## DRUG FACTS

| Active ingredient | Purpose |
|---|---|
| Colloidal oatmeal (43%) | Skin protectant |

## USES
- temporary protects and helps relieve minor skin irritation and itching due to:
  - rashes

## WARNINGS
**For external use only.**

### WHEN USING THIS PRODUCT
- do not get into eyes
- to avoid slipping use mat in tub or shower
- in some skin conditions, soaking too long may overdry

### STOP USE AND ASK A DOCTOR IF
- condition worsens
- symptoms last more than 7 days or clear up and occur again within a few days

**Keep out of reach of children.** If swallowed, get medical help or contact a Poison Control Center right away.

### DIRECTIONS
- for dispersal in water:
  - turn warm water faucet on to full force
  - slowly sprinkle packette of colloidal oatmeal directly under faucet into the tub or container
  - stir any colloidal oatmeal settled on the bottom
- for use as a soak in a bath:
  - slowly sprinkle one packette in an infant tub filled with warm water
  - stir any colloidal oatmeal that may have settled on the bottom
  - soak affected area for 15 to 30 minutes as needed, or as directed by a doctor
  - pat dry (do not rub) to keep a thin layer on the skin

### INACTIVE INGREDIENTS
mineral oil, calcium silicate, laureth-4, tocopheryl acetate, aloe barbadensis leaf extract

### QUESTIONS OR COMMENTS
Call **1-800-720-384**3 Weekdays, 8 AM-8 PM EST

---

# CHILDREN'S DIMETAPP COLD AND COUGH (brompheniramine maleate, dextromethorphan hydrobromide, phenylephrine hydrochloride) liquid
Richmond Division of Wyeth

## DRUG FACTS

| Active ingredients (in each 5 ml tsp) | Purpose |
|---|---|
| Brompheniramine maleate, USP 1 mg | Antihistamine |
| Dextromethorphan hydrobromide, USP 5 mg | Cough suppressant |
| Phenylephrine hydrochloride, USP 2.5 mg | Nasal decongestant |

### USES
- temporarily relieves cough due to minor throat and bronchial irritation occurring with a cold, and nasal congestion due to the common cold, hay fever or other upper respiratory allergies
- temporarily relieves these symptoms due to hay fever (allergic rhinitis):
  - runny nose
  - sneezing
  - itchy, watery eyes
  - itching of the nose or throat
- temporarily restores freer breathing through the nose

## WARNINGS
### DO NOT USE
- to sedate a child or to make a child sleepy
- if you are now taking a prescription monoamine oxidase inhibitor (MAOI) (certain drugs for depression, psychiatric, or emotional conditions, or Parkinson's disease), or for 2 weeks after stopping the MAOI drug. If you do not know if your prescription drug contains an MAOI, ask a doctor or pharmacist before taking this product

### ASK A DOCTOR BEFORE USE IF YOU HAVE
- heart disease
- high blood pressure
- thyroid disease
- diabetes
- trouble urinating due to an enlarged prostate gland
- glaucoma
- cough that occurs with too much phlegm (mucus)
- a breathing problem or persistent or chronic cough that lasts such as occurs with smoking, asthma, chronic bronchitis, or emphysema

### ASK A DOCTOR OR PHARMACIST BEFORE USE IF YOU ARE
- taking any other oral nasal decongestant or stimulant
- taking sedatives or tranquilizers

### WHEN USING THIS PRODUCT
- do not use more than directed
- may cause marked drowsiness
- avoid alcoholic beverages
- alcohol, sedatives, and tranquilizers may increase drowsiness
- be careful when driving a motor vehicle or operating machinery
- excitability may occur, especially in children

### STOP USE AND ASK A DOCTOR IF
- you get nervous, dizzy, or sleepless
- symptoms do not get better within 7 days or are accompanied by fever
- cough lasts more than 7 days, comes back, or is accompanied by fever, rash, or persistent headache. These could be signs of a serious condition

**If pregnant or breastfeeding,** ask a health professional before use.

**Keep out of reach of children.** In case of overdose, get medical help or contact a Poison Control Center right away.

### DIRECTIONS
- do not take more than 6 doses in any 24-hour period

| adults and children 12 years and over | 4 tsp every 4 hours |
|---|---|
| children 6 to under 12 years | 2 tsp every 4 hours |
| children under 6 years | do not use |

### OTHER INFORMATION
- each teaspoon contains: sodium 3 mg
- store at 20-25°C (68-77°F)
- dosage cup provided

### INACTIVE INGREDIENTS
anhydrous citric acid, artificial flavor, FD&C blue no. 1, FD&C red no. 40, glycerin, propylene glycol, purified water, sodium benzoate, sodium citrate, sorbitol solution, sucralose

### QUESTIONS OR COMMENTS
Call weekdays from 9 AM to 5 PM EST at **1-800-762-4675**

# CHILDREN'S DIMETAPP COLD AND ALLERGY (brompheniramine maleate, phenylephrine hydrochloride) tablet, chewable

Richmond Division of Wyeth

## DRUG FACTS

| Active ingredients (in each tablet) | Purpose |
|---|---|
| Brompheniramine maleate, USP 1 mg | Antihistamine |
| Phenylephrine hydrochloride, USP 2.5 mg | Nasal decongestant |

## USES
- temporarily relieves nasal congestion due to the common cold, hay fever or other upper respiratory allergies
- temporarily relieves these symptoms due to hay fever (allergic rhinitis) or other upper respiratory allergies:
  - runny nose
  - sneezing
  - itchy, watery eyes
  - itching of the nose or throat
- temporarily restores freer breathing through the nose

## WARNINGS

### DO NOT USE
- to sedate a child or to make a child sleepy
- if you are now taking a prescription monoamine oxidase inhibitor (MAOI) (certain drugs for depression, psychiatric, or emotional conditions, or Parkinson's disease), or for 2 weeks after stopping the MAOI drug. If you do not know if your prescription drug contains an MAOI, ask a doctor or pharmacist before taking this product

### ASK A DOCTOR BEFORE USE IF YOU HAVE
- heart disease
- high blood pressure
- thyroid disease
- diabetes
- trouble urinating due to an enlarged prostate gland
- glaucoma
- a breathing problem such as emphysema, asthma or chronic bronchitis

### ASK A DOCTOR OR PHARMACIST BEFORE USE IF YOU ARE
- taking any other oral nasal decongestant or stimulant
- taking sedatives or tranquilizers

### WHEN USING THIS PRODUCT
- do not use more than directed
- drowsiness may occur
- avoid alcoholic beverages
- alcohol, sedatives and tranquilizers may increase drowsiness
- be careful when driving a motor vehicle or operating machinery
- excitability may occur, especially in children

### STOP USE AND ASK A DOCTOR IF
- you get nervous, dizzy, or sleepless
- symptoms do not get better within 7 days or are accompanied by fever

**If pregnant or breastfeeding,** ask a health professional before use.

**Keep out of reach of children.** In case of overdose, get medical help or contact a Poison Control Center right away.

## DIRECTIONS
- do not take more than 6 doses in any 24-hour period

| adults and children 12 years and over | 4 tablets every 4 hours |
|---|---|
| children 6 to under 12 years | 2 tablets every 4 hours |
| children under 6 years | do not use |

## OTHER INFORMATION
- store at 20-25°C (68-77°F)

## INACTIVE INGREDIENTS
carmine, carrageenan, croscarmellose sodium, fructose, fumaric acid, glycine, magnesium stearate, maltodextrin, mannitol, microcrystalline cellulose, modified starch, natural and artificial flavor, polyethylene oxide, silicon dioxide, sorbitol, sucralose, tribasic calcium phosphate

## QUESTIONS OR COMMENTS
Call weekdays from 9 AM to 5 PM EST at **1-800-762-4675**

# CHILDREN'S DIMETAPP LONG ACTING COUGH PLUS COLD (chlorpheniramine maleate, dextromethorphan hydrobromide) liquid

Richmond Division of Wyeth

## DRUG FACTS

| Active ingredients (in each 5 ml teaspoon) | Purpose |
|---|---|
| Chlorpheniramine maleate, USP 1.0 mg | Antihistamine |
| Dextromethorphan hydrobromide, USP 7.5 mg | Cough suppressant |

## USES
- temporarily relieves cough due to minor throat and bronchial irritation as may occur with a cold
- temporarily relieves these symptoms due to hay fever or other upper respiratory allergies:
  - runny nose
  - sneezing
  - itchy, watery eyes
  - itching of the nose or throat

## WARNINGS

### DO NOT USE
- to sedate a child or to make a child sleepy
- if you are now taking a prescription monoamine oxidase inhibitor (MAOI) (certain drugs for depression, psychiatric, or emotional conditions, or Parkinson's disease), or for 2 weeks after stopping the MAOI drug. If you do not know if your prescription drug contains an MAOI, ask a doctor or pharmacist before taking this product

### ASK A DOCTOR BEFORE USE IF YOU HAVE
- trouble urinating due to an enlarged prostate gland
- glaucoma
- a cough that occurs with too much phlegm (mucus)
- a breathing problem or chronic cough that lasts or as occurs with smoking, asthma, chronic bronchitis or emphysema

### ASK A DOCTOR OR PHARMACIST BEFORE USE IF YOU ARE
- taking sedatives or tranquilizers

### WHEN USING THIS PRODUCT
- do not use more than directed
- marked drowsiness may occur
- avoid alcoholic drinks

- alcohol, sedatives, and tranquilizers may increase drowsiness
- be careful when driving a motor vehicle or operating machinery
- excitability may occur, especially in children

## STOP USE AND ASK A DOCTOR IF
- cough lasts more than 7 days, comes back, or is accompanied by fever, rash, or persistent headache. These could be signs of a serious condition

**If pregnant or breastfeeding,** ask a health professional before use.

**Keep out of reach of children.** In case of overdose, get medical help or contact a Poison Control Center right away.

## DIRECTIONS
- do not take more than 4 doses in any 24-hour period

| 12 years and over | 4 tsp every 6 hours |
| 6 to under 12 years | 2 tsp every 6 hours |
| under 6 years | do not use |

## OTHER INFORMATION
- each teaspoon contains: sodium 3 mg
- store at 20-25°C (68-77°F)
- dosage cup provided

## INACTIVE INGREDIENTS
anhydrous citric acid, artificial flavor, FD&C blue no. 1, FD&C red no. 40, glycerin, propylene glycol, purified water, sodium benzoate, sodium citrate, sorbitol solution, sucralose

## QUESTIONS OR COMMENTS
Call weekdays from 9 AM to 5 PM EST at **1-800-762-4675**

---

# CHILDREN'S DIMETAPP MULTI-SYMPTOM COLD AND FLU (acetaminophen, chlorpheniramine maleate, dextromethorphan hydrobromide, phenylephrine hydrochloride) liquid

Richmond Division of Wyeth

## DRUG FACTS

| Active ingredients (in each 5 ml tsp) | Purpose |
| --- | --- |
| Acetaminophen, USP 160 mg | Pain reliever/fever reducer |
| Chlorpheniramine maleate, USP 1 mg | Antihistamine |
| Dextromethorphan hydrobromide, USP 5 mg | Cough suppressant |
| Phenylephrine hydrochloride, USP 2.5 mg | Nasal decongestant |

## USES
- temporarily relieves these symptoms associated with a cold, or flu:
  - headache
  - sore throat
  - fever
  - minor aches and pains
- temporarily relieves nasal congestion, and cough due to minor throat and bronchial irritation occurring with a cold
- temporarily relieves these symptoms due to hay fever or other upper respiratory allergies:
  - sneezing

- itching of the nose or throat
- itchy, watery eyes
- runny nose
- temporarily restores freer breathing through the nose

## WARNINGS
### Liver warning
This product contains acetaminophen. Severe liver damage may occur if user takes:
- more than 5 doses in any 24-hour period, which is the maximum daily amount
- with other drugs containing acetaminophen
- 3 or more alcoholic drinks every day while using this product

### Sore throat warning
If sore throat is severe, persists for more than 2 days, is accompanied or followed by fever, headache, rash, nausea, or vomiting, consult a doctor promptly.

## DO NOT USE
- to sedate a child or to make a child sleepy
- in a child under 6 years of age
- if user is now taking a prescription monoamine oxidase inhibitor (MAOI) (certain drugs for depression, psychiatric, or emotional conditions, or Parkinson's disease), or for 2 weeks after stopping the MAOI drug. If you do not know if your prescription drug contains an MAOI, ask a doctor or pharmacist before taking this product
- with any other drug containing acetaminophen (prescription or nonprescription). If you are not sure whether a drug contains acetaminophen ask a doctor or pharmacist

## ASK A DOCTOR BEFORE USE IF USER HAS
- liver disease
- heart disease
- high blood pressure
- thyroid disease
- diabetes
- trouble urinating due to an enlarged prostate gland
- glaucoma
- cough that occurs with too much phlegm (mucus)
- a breathing problem or chronic cough that lasts or as occurs with smoking, asthma, chronic bronchitis, or emphysema

## ASK A DOCTOR OR PHARMACIST BEFORE USE IF USER IS
- taking the blood thinning drug warfarin
- taking any other oral nasal decongestant or stimulant
- taking any other pain reliever/fever reducer
- taking sedatives or tranquilizers

## WHEN USING THIS PRODUCT
- do not use more than directed
- marked drowsiness may occur
- avoid alcoholic drinks
- alcohol, sedatives, and tranquilizers may increase drowsiness
- be careful when driving a motor vehicle or operating machinery
- excitability may occur, especially in children

## STOP USE AND ASK A DOCTOR IF
- user gets nervous, dizzy, or sleepless
- pain, cough, or nasal congestion gets worse or lasts more than 5 days (children) or 7 days (adults)
- fever gets worse or lasts more than 3 days
- redness or swelling is present
- cough comes back or occurs with rash or headache that lasts. These could be signs of a serious condition
- new symptoms occur

**If pregnant or breastfeeding,** ask a health professional before use.

**Keep out of reach of children.** In case of overdose, get medical help or contact a Poison Control Center right away. Prompt medical attention is critical for adults as well as for children, even if you do not notice any signs or symptoms.

## DIRECTIONS
- do not take more than 5 doses in any 24-hour period
- do not exceed recommended dosage. Taking more than the recommended dose (overdose) may cause serious liver damage

| adults and children 12 years and over | 4 teaspoons every 4 hours |
| children 6 to 12 years | 2 teaspoons every 4 hours |
| children under 6 years | do not use |

## OTHER INFORMATION
- each teaspoon contains: sodium 2 mg
- store at 20-25°C (68-77°F)
- dosage cup provided

## INACTIVE INGREDIENTS
anhydrous citric acid, artificial flavor, FD&C red no. 40, glycerin, menthol, polyethylene glycol, propyl gallate, propylene glycol, purified water, sodium benzoate, sodium citrate, sorbitol solution, sucralose

## QUESTIONS OR COMMENTS
Call weekdays from 9 AM to 5 PM EST at **1-800-762-4675**

## CHILDREN'S DIMETAPP NIGHTTIME COLD AND CONGESTION (diphenhydramine hydrochloride, phenylephrine hydrochloride) liquid
Richmond Division of Wyeth

### DRUG FACTS

| Active ingredients (in each 5 ml tsp) | Purpose |
|---|---|
| Diphenhydramine hydrochloride, USP 6.25 mg | Antihistamine/cough suppressant |
| Phenylephrine hydrochloride, USP 2.5 mg | Nasal decongestant |

## USES
- temporarily relieves these symptoms occurring with a cold, hay fever, or other upper respiratory allergies:
  - nasal congestion
  - cough
  - runny nose
  - sneezing
  - itchy, watery eyes
  - itching of the nose or throat

## WARNINGS

### DO NOT USE
- to sedate a child or to make a child sleepy
- if you are now taking a prescription monoamine oxidase inhibitor (MAOI) (certain drugs for depression, psychiatric, or emotional conditions, or Parkinson's disease), or for 2 weeks after stopping the MAOI drug. If you do not know if your prescription drug contains an MAOI, ask a doctor or pharmacist before taking this product

- with any other product containing diphenhydramine, even one used on skin

### ASK A DOCTOR BEFORE USE IF YOU HAVE
- heart disease
- high blood pressure
- thyroid disease
- diabetes
- trouble urinating due to an enlarged prostate gland
- glaucoma
- cough that occurs with too much phlegm (mucus)
- a breathing problem or chronic cough that lasts or as occurs with smoking, asthma, chronic bronchitis, or emphysema

### ASK A DOCTOR OR PHARMACIST BEFORE USE IF YOU ARE
- taking any other oral nasal decongestant or stimulant
- taking sedatives or tranquilizers

### WHEN USING THIS PRODUCT
- do not use more than directed
- marked drowsiness may occur
- avoid alcoholic drinks
- alcohol, sedatives, and tranquilizers may increase drowsiness
- be careful when driving a motor vehicle or operating machinery
- excitability may occur, especially in children

### STOP USE AND ASK A DOCTOR IF
- you get nervous, dizzy, or sleepless
- symptoms do not get better within 7 days or are accompanied by fever
- cough lasts more than 7 days, comes back, or is accompanied by fever, rash or persistent headache. These could be signs of a serious condition

**If pregnant or breastfeeding,** ask a health professional before use.

**Keep out of reach of children.** In case of overdose, get medical help or contact a Poison Control Center right away.

### DIRECTIONS
- do not take more than 6 doses in any 24-hour period
- do not exceed recommended dosage

| adults and children 12 years and over | 4 tsp every 4 hours |
| children 6 to under 12 years | 2 tsp every 4 hours |
| children under 6 years | do not use |

### OTHER INFORMATION
- each teaspoon contains: sodium 4 mg
- store at 20-25°C (68-77°F)
- dosage cup provided

### INACTIVE INGREDIENTS
anhydrous citric acid, artificial flavor, FD&C blue no.1, FD&C red no. 40, glycerin, propyl gallate, propylene glycol, purified water, sodium benzoate, sodium citrate, sorbitol solution, sucralose

### QUESTIONS OR COMMENTS
Call weekdays from 9 AM to 5 PM EST at **1-800-762-4675**

# DR. SCHOLL'S CLEAR AWAY WART REMOVER (salicylic acid) liquid
Schering-Plough HealthCare Products, Inc.

## DRUG FACTS

| Active ingredient | Purpose |
|---|---|
| Salicylic acid 17% | Wart remover |

### USES
- for removal of common and plantar warts
- common warts can be easily recognized by the rough cauliflower-like appearance of the surface
- plantar warts can be recognized by its location only on the bottom of the foot, its tenderness, and the interruption of the footprint pattern

### WARNINGS
**For external use only.**

**Flammable: Keep away from fire or flame.**

### DO NOT USE
- if you are a diabetic
- if you have poor blood circulation
- on irritated skin or any area that is infected or reddened
- on moles, birthmarks, warts with hair growing from them, genital warts, or warts on the face or mucous membranes

### WHEN USING THIS PRODUCT
- if product gets in eyes, flush with water for 15 minutes
- do not inhale vapors
- cap bottle tightly when not in use and store at room temperature away from heat

### STOP USE AND ASK A DOCTOR IF
- discomfort lasts

**Keep out of reach of children.** If swallowed, get medical help or contact a Poison Control Center right away.

### DIRECTIONS
- wash affected area
- may soak wart in warm water for 5 minutes
- dry thoroughly
- apply one drop at a time with applicator to sufficiently cover each wart
- let dry
- self-adhesive cover-up discs may be used to conceal wart
- repeat procedure once or twice daily as needed (until wart is removed) for up to 12 weeks

### OTHER INFORMATION
- store between 20°C-25°C (68°F-77°F)

### INACTIVE INGREDIENTS
castor oil, ethyl lactate, flexible collodion, polybutene. (contains alcohol 18% v/v and ether 53% v/v from the flexible collodion)

# DR. SCHOLL'S CLEAR AWAY WART REMOVER ONE STEP (salicylic acid) plaster
Schering-Plough HealthCare Products, Inc.

## DRUG FACTS

| Active ingredient | Purpose |
|---|---|
| Salicylic acid 40% | Wart remover |

### USES
- for removal of common warts, easily recognized by the rough cauliflower-like appearance of the surface

### WARNINGS
**For external use only.**

### DO NOT USE
- if you are a diabetic
- if you have poor blood circulation
- on irritated skin or any area that is infected or reddened
- on moles, birthmarks, warts with hair growing from them, genital warts, or warts on the face or mucous membranes

### STOP USE AND ASK A DOCTOR IF
- discomfort lasts

**Keep out of reach of children.** If swallowed, get medical help or contact a Poison Control Center right away.

### DIRECTIONS
- wash affected area
- may soak wart in warm water for 5 minutes
- dry area thoroughly
- apply medicated strip, positioning medicated disc directly over wart
- secure adhesive strips firmly to skin
- repeat procedure every 48 hours as needed (until wart is removed) for up to 12 weeks

### OTHER INFORMATION
- store between 20°C-25°C (68°F-77°F)

### INACTIVE INGREDIENTS
antioxidant (CAS 991-84-4), iron oxides, mineral oil, petroleum hydrocarbon resin, silicon dioxide, synthetic polyisoprene rubber, talc

# DR. SCHOLL'S INGROWN TOENAIL PAIN RELIEVER (sodium sulfide) gel
MSD Consumer Care, Inc.

## DRUG FACTS

| Active ingredient (in each 5 mL*) | Purpose |
|---|---|
| Sodium sulfide 1 % | Ingrown toenail reliever |

\* 5 mL = one teaspoonful

### USE
- for temporary relief of pain and discomfort from ingrown toenails

### WARNINGS:
**For external use only.**

### DO NOT USE
- on open sores

### ASK A DOCTOR BEFORE USE IF YOU HAVE
- diabetes
- poor blood circulation
- gout

### WHEN USING THIS PRODUCT
- use with a retainer ring
- avoid contact with the eyes. If product gets in eyes, flush with water for 15 minutes and get medical help right away

## STOP USE AND ASK A DOCTOR IF
- redness or swelling of your toe increases
- discharge is present around the nail
- symptoms last more than 7 days or clear up and occur again within a few days

**Keep out of reach of children.** If swallowed, get medical help right away or contact a Poison Control Center right away.

## DIRECTIONS

| adults and children 12 years and over | wash affected area and dry thoroughly |
| --- | --- |
| | place retainer ring on toe with slot over the area where the ingrown nail and skin meet. Smooth ring down firmly |
| | apply enough gel product to fill slot in the ring. Immediately replace the cap on tube. |
| | place round center section of bandage directly over the gel-filled ring to seal the gel in place. Smooth ends of bandage around the toe. (purpose of the bandage is to keep everything in place) |
| | repeat twice daily (morning and night) for up to 7 days until pain and discomfort is relieved or until the nail can be lifted out of the nail groove and easily trimmed |
| children under 12 years | ask a doctor |

## OTHER INFORMATION
- retain carton for future reference on warnings, directions and labeling
- keep tube tightly closed when not in use
- store between 20°C-25°C (68°F-77°F)

## INACTIVE INGREDIENTS
edetate disodium, hydroxyethyl cellulose, potassium acetate, purified water.

# DRAMAMINE ORIGINAL FORMULA
(dimenhydrinate) tablet
McNeil Consumer Healthcare, Division of McNeil-PPC, Inc.

## DRUG FACTS

| Active ingredient (in each tablet) | Purpose |
| --- | --- |
| Dimenhydrinate 50 mg | Antiemetic |

## USE
- for prevention and treatment of these symptoms associated with motion sickness:
  - nausea
  - vomiting
  - dizziness

## WARNINGS

## DO NOT USE
- for children under 2 years of age unless directed by a doctor

## ASK A DOCTOR BEFORE USE IF YOU HAVE
- a breathing problem such as emphysema or chronic bronchitis
- glaucoma
- trouble urinating due to an enlarged prostate gland

## ASK A DOCTOR OR PHARMACIST BEFORE USE IF YOU ARE
- taking sedatives or tranquilizers

## WHEN USING THIS PRODUCT
- marked drowsiness may occur
- avoid alcoholic drinks
- alcohol, sedatives, and tranquilizers may increase drowsiness
- be careful when driving a motor vehicle or operating machinery

**If pregnant or breastfeeding,** ask a health professional before use.

**Keep out of reach of children.** In case of overdose, get medical help or contact a Poison Control Center right away. (1-800-222-1222)

## DIRECTIONS
- to prevent motion sickness, the first dose should be taken ½ to 1 hour before starting activity
- to prevent or treat motion sickness, see below:

| adults and children 12 years and over | take 1 to 2 tablets every 4-6 hours |
| --- | --- |
| | do not take more than 8 tablets in 24 hours, or as directed by a doctor |
| children 6 to under 12 years | give ½ to 1 tablet every 6-8 hours |
| | do not give more than 3 tablets in 24 hours, or as directed by a doctor |
| children 2 to under 6 years | give ½ tablet every 6-8 hours |
| | do not give more than 1-½ tablets in 24 hours, or as directed by a doctor |

## OTHER INFORMATION
- store between 20-25°C (68-77°F)
- do not use if carton is opened or if blister unit is broken or torn
- see side panel for lot number and expiration date

## INACTIVE INGREDIENTS
anhydrous lactose, colloidal silicon dioxide, croscarmellose sodium, magnesium stearate, microcrystalline cellulose

## QUESTIONS OR COMMENTS
Call **1-800-382-7219**

# DRAMAMINE CHEWABLE FORMULA
(dimenhydrinate) tablet, chewable
McNeil Consumer Healthcare, Division of McNeil-PPC, Inc.

## DRUG FACTS

| Active ingredient (in each tablet) | Purpose |
| --- | --- |
| Dimenhydrinate 50 mg | Antiemetic |

## USE
- for prevention and treatment of these symptoms associated with motion sickness:
  - nausea
  - vomiting
  - dizziness

## WARNINGS

### DO NOT USE
- for children under 2 years of age unless directed by a doctor

### ASK A DOCTOR BEFORE USE IF YOU HAVE
- a breathing problem such as emphysema or chronic bronchitis
- glaucoma
- trouble urinating due to an enlarged prostate gland

### ASK A DOCTOR OR PHARMACIST BEFORE USE IF YOU ARE
- taking sedatives or tranquilizers

### WHEN USING THIS PRODUCT
- marked drowsiness may occur
- avoid alcoholic drinks
- alcohol, sedatives, and tranquilizers may increase drowsiness
- be careful when driving a motor vehicle or operating machinery

**If pregnant or breastfeeding,** ask a health professional before use.

**Keep out of reach of children.** In case of overdose, get medical help or contact a Poison Control Center right away. (**1-800-222-1222**)

## DIRECTIONS
- to prevent motion sickness, the first dose should be taken ½ to 1 hour before starting activity
- to prevent or treat motion sickness, see below:

| adults and children 12 years and over | take 1 to 2 chewable tablets every 4-6 hours |
| | do not take more than 8 chewable tablets in 24 hours, or as directed by a doctor |
| children 6 to under 12 years | give ½ to 1 chewable tablet every 6-8 hours |
| | do not give more than 3 chewable tablets in 24 hours, or as directed by a doctor |
| children 2 to under 6 years | give ½ chewable tablet every 6-8 hours |
| | do not give more than 1½ chewable tablets in 24 hours, or as directed by a doctor |

## OTHER INFORMATION
- **Phenylketonurics:** contains phenylalanine 0.84 mg per tablet
- store between 20-25°C (68-77°F)
- do not use if carton is opened or if blister unit is broken or torn
- see side panel for lot number and expiration date

## INACTIVE INGREDIENTS
anhydrous citric acid, aspartame, FD&C yellow no. 6 aluminum lake, flavors, magnesium stearate, maltodextrin, methacrylic acid copolymer, modified starch, sorbitol

## QUESTIONS OR COMMENTS
Call **1-800-382-7219**

# DRAMAMINE LESS DROWSY FORMULA
(meclizine hydrochloride) tablet
McNeil Consumer Healthcare, Division of McNeil-PPC, Inc.

## DRUG FACTS

| Active ingredient (in each tablet) | Purpose |
| --- | --- |
| Meclizine hydrochloride 25 mg | Antiemetic |

## USE
- for prevention and treatment of these symptoms associated with motion sickness:
  - nausea
  - vomiting
  - dizziness

## WARNINGS

### DO NOT USE
- for children under 12 years of age unless directed by a doctor

### ASK A DOCTOR BEFORE USE IF YOU HAVE
- a breathing problem such as emphysema or chronic bronchitis
- glaucoma
- trouble urinating due to enlarged prostate gland

### ASK A DOCTOR OR PHARMACIST BEFORE USE IF YOU ARE
- taking sedatives or tranquilizers

### WHEN USING THIS PRODUCT
- drowsiness may occur
- avoid alcoholic drinks
- alcohol, sedatives, and tranquilizers may increase drowsiness
- be careful when driving a motor vehicle or operating machinery

**If pregnant or breastfeeding,** ask a health professional before use.

**Keep out of reach of children.** In case of overdose, get medical help or contact a Poison Control Center right away. (**1-800-222-1222**)

## DIRECTIONS
- take first dose one hour before starting activity

| adults and children 12 years and over | 1 to 2 tablets once daily, or as directed by a doctor |
| --- | --- |

## OTHER INFORMATION
- store between 20-25°C (68-77°F)
- do not use if blister is broken or torn

## INACTIVE INGREDIENTS
anhydrous lactose, corn starch, colloidal silicon dioxide, D&C yellow no. 10 aluminum lake, magnesium stearate, microcrystalline cellulose

## QUESTIONS OR COMMENTS
Call **1-800-382-7219**

# DRISTAN 12 HR NASAL SPRAY (oxymetazoline hydrochloride) spray
Wyeth Consumer Healthcare

## DRUG FACTS

| Active ingredient | Purpose |
|---|---|
| Oxymetazoline hydrochloride 0.05% | Nasal decongestant |

## USE
- temporarily relieves nasal congestion due to a cold, hay fever or other upper respiratory allergies

## WARNINGS
**For intranasal use only.**

## ASK A DOCTOR BEFORE USE IF YOU HAVE
- heart disease
- high blood pressure
- thyroid disease
- diabetes
- difficulty in urination due to enlargement of the prostate gland

## WHEN USING THIS PRODUCT
- do not exceed recommended dosage
- do not use for more than 3 days
- use only as directed
- frequent or prolonged use may cause nasal congestion to recur or worsen
- you may experience temporary discomfort such as burning, stinging, sneezing or an increase in nasal discharge
- the use of this container by more than one person may spread infection

## STOP USE AND ASK A DOCTOR IF
- symptoms persist

**If pregnant or breastfeeding,** ask a health professional before use.

**Keep out of reach of children.** If swallowed, get medical help or contact a Poison Control Center right away.

## DIRECTIONS

| adults and children 12 years and over | with head upright, insert nozzle in nostril. Spray quickly, firmly and sniff deeply |
|---|---|
| | spray 2 or 3 times into each nostril not more often than every 10-12 hours |
| | do not exceed 2 doses in any 24-hour period |
| children under 12 years | ask a doctor |

## OTHER INFORMATION
- store at 20-25°C (68-77°F)
- container is filled to proper level for correct spray action

## INACTIVE INGREDIENTS
benzalkonium chloride, benzyl alcohol, dibasic sodium phosphate, edetate disodium, hypromellose, phosphoric acid, purified water, sodium chloride

## QUESTIONS OR COMMENTS
Call weekdays from 9 AM to 5 PM EST at **1-800-535-0026**

# DRISTAN COLD MULTI-SYMPTOM
(acetaminophen, chlorpheniramine maleate, phenylephrine hydrochloride) tablet
Pfizer Consumer Healthcare

## DRUG FACTS

| Active ingredients (in each tablet) | Purpose |
|---|---|
| Acetaminophen, USP 325 mg | Pain reliever/fever reducer |
| Chlorpheniramine maleate, USP 2 mg | Antihistamine |
| Phenylephrine hydrochloride, USP 5 mg | Nasal decongestant |

## USES
- temporarily relieves these symptoms associated with a cold, or flu:
  - headache
  - nasal congestion
  - sore throat
  - fever
  - minor aches and pains
- temporarily relieves minor aches, pains and headache as well as these symptoms of hay fever or other upper respiratory allergies:
  - runny nose
  - sneezing
  - nasal congestion
  - itching of the nose or throat
  - itchy, watery eyes
- temporarily relieves minor aches, pains, headache and nasal congestion as well as sinus congestion and pressure, and reduces swelling of nasal passages

## WARNINGS
**Liver warning**
This product contains acetaminophen. Severe liver damage may occur if you take:
- more than 12 tablets in any 24-hour period, which is the maximum daily amount
- with other drugs containing acetaminophen
- 3 or more alcoholic drinks every day while using this product

**Sore throat warning**
If sore throat is severe, persists for more than 2 days, is accompanied or followed by fever, headache, rash, nausea, or vomiting, consult a doctor promptly.

## DO NOT USE
- to sedate a child or to make a child sleepy
- if you are now taking a prescription monoamine oxidase inhibitor (MAOI) (certain drugs for depression, psychiatric, or emotional conditions, or Parkinson's disease), or for 2 weeks after stopping the MAOI drug. If you do not know if your prescription drug contains an MAOI, ask a doctor or pharmacist before taking this product
- with any other drug containing acetaminophen (prescription or nonprescription). If you are not sure whether a drug contains acetaminophen ask a doctor or pharmacist

## ASK A DOCTOR BEFORE USE IF YOU HAVE
- liver disease
- heart disease
- high blood pressure
- thyroid disease
- diabetes
- trouble urinating due to an enlarged prostate gland

- glaucoma
- a breathing problem such as emphysema, asthma, or chronic bronchitis

## ASK A DOCTOR OR PHARMACIST BEFORE USE IF YOU ARE

- taking the blood thinning drug warfarin
- taking any other oral nasal decongestant or stimulant
- taking any other pain reliever/fever reducer
- taking sedatives or tranquilizers

## WHEN USING THIS PRODUCT

- do not use more than directed
- drowsiness may occur
- avoid alcoholic drinks
- alcohol, sedatives, and tranquilizers may increase drowsiness
- be careful when driving a motor vehicle or operating machinery
- excitability may occur, especially in children

## STOP USE AND ASK A DOCTOR IF

- you get nervous, dizzy, or sleepless
- pain or nasal congestion gets worse or lasts more than 7 days
- fever gets worse or lasts more than 3 days
- redness or swelling is present
- new symptoms occur

**If pregnant or breastfeeding,** ask a health professional before use.

**Keep out of reach of children.** In case of overdose, get medical help or contact a Poison Control Center right away. Prompt medical attention is critical for adults as well as for children, even if you do not notice any signs or symptoms.

## DIRECTIONS

- do not use more than 12 tablets in any 24-hour period
- do not exceed recommended dosage. Taking more than the recommended dose (overdose) may cause serious liver damage
- this adult product is not intended for use in children under 12 years of age

| adults and children 12 years and over | 2 tablets every 4 hours |
| children under 12 years | do not use |

## OTHER INFORMATION

- store at 20-25°C (68-77°F)
- tamper-evident individual blisters

## INACTIVE INGREDIENTS

calcium stearate, croscarmellose sodium, crospovidone, D&C yellow no. 10 aluminum lake, FD&C yellow no. 6 aluminum lake, hypromellose, microcrystalline cellulose, polyethylene glycol, povidone, pregelatinized starch, stearic acid

## QUESTIONS OR COMMENTS

Call weekdays from 9 AM to 5 PM EST at **1-800-535-0026**

---

# DULCOLAX (bisacodyl) tablet, coated
Boehringer Ingelheim Pharmaceuticals, Inc.

## DRUG FACTS

| Active ingredient (in each tablet) | Purpose |
|---|---|
| Bisacodyl USP 5 mg | Stimulant laxative |

## USES

- for temporary relief of occasional constipation and irregularity
- this product generally produces bowel movement in 6 to 12 hours

## WARNINGS

### DO NOT USE

- if you cannot swallow without chewing

### ASK A DOCTOR BEFORE USE IF YOU HAVE

- stomach pain, nausea or vomiting
- a sudden change in bowel habits that lasts more than 2 weeks

### WHEN USING THIS PRODUCT

- do not chew or crush tablet(s)
- it may cause stomach discomfort, faintness and cramps
- do not use within 1 hour after taking an antacid or milk

### STOP USE AND ASK A DOCTOR IF

- you have rectal bleeding or no bowel movement after using this product. These could be signs of a serious condition
- you need to use a laxative for more than 1 week

**If pregnant or breastfeeding,** ask a health professional before use.

**Keep out of reach of children.** In case of overdose, get medical help or contact a Poison Control Center right away.

## DIRECTIONS

- take with a glass of water

| adults and children 12 years of age and over | 1 to 3 tablets in a single daily dose |
| children 6 to under 12 years of age | 1 tablet in a single daily dose |
| children under 2 years of age | ask a doctor |

## OTHER INFORMATION

- store at 20-25°C (68-77°F)
- protect from excessive humidity

## INACTIVE INGREDIENTS

acacia, acetylated monoglyceride, carnauba wax, cellulose acetate phthalate, corn starch, dibutyl phthalate, docusate sodium, gelatin, glycerin, iron oxides, kaolin, lactose, magnesium stearate, methylparaben, pharmaceutical glaze, polyethylene glycol, povidone, propylparaben, red no. 30 lake, sodium benzoate, sorbitan monooleate, sucrose, talc, titanium dioxide, white wax, yellow no. 10 lake

---

# DULCOLAX BALANCE (polyethylene glycol 3350)
powder, for solution
Boehringer Ingelheim Pharmaceuticals Inc

## DRUG FACTS

| Active ingredient (in each dose) | Purpose |
|---|---|
| **Pouches Only**<br>Polyethylene Glycol 3350, 17 g | Laxative |
| **Bottle Only**<br>Polyethylene Glycol 3350, 17 g (cap filled to line) | |

## USES

- relieves occasional constipation (irregularity)
- generally produces a bowel movement in 1 to 3 days

## WARNINGS
**Allergy alert**
Do not use if you are allergic to polyethylene glycol

## DO NOT USE
- if you have kidney disease, except under the advice and supervision of a doctor

## ASK A DOCTOR BEFORE USE IF YOU HAVE
- nausea, vomiting or abdominal pain
- a sudden change in bowel habits that lasts over 2 weeks
- irritable bowel syndrome

## ASK A DOCTOR OR PHARMACIST BEFORE USE IF YOU ARE
- taking a prescription drug

## WHEN USING THIS PRODUCT
- you may have loose, watery, more frequent stools

## STOP USE AND ASK A DOCTOR IF
- you have rectal bleeding or your nausea, bloating, cramping or abdominal pain gets worse. These may be signs of a serious condition
- you get diarrhea
- you need to use a laxative for longer than 1 week

**If pregnant or breastfeeding,** ask a health professional before use.

**Keep out of reach of children.** In case of overdose, get medical help or contact a Poison Control Center right away.

## DIRECTIONS (POUCHES ONLY)
- do not take more than directed unless advised by your doctor

| adults and children 17 years of age and older | stir and dissolve one packet of powder (17 g) in any 4 to 8 ounces of beverage (cold, hot or room temperature) then drink |
| | use once a day |
| | use no more than 7 days |
| children 16 years of age or under | ask a doctor |

## DIRECTIONS (BOTTLE ONLY)
- do not take more than directed unless advised by your doctor
- the bottle top is a measuring cap marked to contain 17 grams of powder when filled to the indicated line (white section in cap)

| adults and children 17 years of age or older | fill to top of white section in cap which is marked to indicate the correct dose (17 g) |
| | stir and dissolve in any 4 to 8 ounces of beverage (cold, hot or room temperature) then drink |
| | use once a day |
| | use no more than 7 days |
| children 16 years of age or under | ask a doctor |

## OTHER INFORMATION
- store at 20-25°C (68-77°F)
- tamper-evident: do not use if printed foil pouch is open or broken (pouches only)
- tamper-evident: do not use if printed foil seal under cap is missing, open or broken (bottle only)

## INACTIVE INGREDIENTS
none

## QUESTIONS OR COMMENTS
**1-888-285-9159** (English/Spanish) or visit www.Dulcolax.com

# DUOFILM WART REMOVER (salicylic acid) liquid
Schering-Plough HealthCare Products, Inc.

## DRUG FACTS

| Active ingredient | Purpose |
|---|---|
| Salicylic acid 17% | Wart remover |

## USES
- for removal of common and plantar warts
- common warts can be easily recognized by the rough cauliflower-like appearance of the surface
- plantar warts can be recognized by its location only on the bottom of the foot, its tenderness, and the interruption of the footprint pattern

## WARNINGS
**For external use only.**

**Flammable: Keep away from fire or flame.**

## DO NOT USE
- if you have diabetes
- if you have poor blood circulation
- on irritated skin or any area that is infected or reddened
- on moles, birthmarks, warts with hair growing from them, genital warts, or warts on the face or mucous membranes

## WHEN USING THIS PRODUCT
- if product gets in eyes, flush with water for 15 minutes
- do not inhale vapors
- cap bottle tightly when not in use and store at room temperature away from heat

## STOP USE AND ASK A DOCTOR IF
- discomfort lasts

**Keep out of reach of children.** If swallowed, get medical help or contact a Poison Control Center right away.

## DIRECTIONS
- wash affected area
- may soak wart in warm water for 5 minutes
- dry thoroughly
- apply one drop at a time with applicator to sufficiently cover each wart
- let dry
- self-adhesive cover-up discs may be used to conceal wart
- repeat procedure once or twice daily as needed (until wart is removed) for up to 12 weeks

## OTHER INFORMATION
- store between 20°C-25°C (68°F-77°F)

## INACTIVE INGREDIENTS
castor oil, ethyl lactate, flexible collodion, polybutene. (contains alcohol 18% v/v and ether 53%v/v from the flexible collodion)

# ECOTRIN (aspirin) tablet, coated
## GlaxoSmithKline Consumer Healthcare LP

## DRUG FACTS

| Active ingredient (in each tablet) | Purpose |
|---|---|
| Low Strength Aspirin (NSAID)* 81 mg Regular Strength Aspirin (NSAID)* 325 mg | Pain reliever |

*nonsteroidal anti-inflammatory drug

## USES
- temporarily relieves minor aches and pains due to:
  - headache
  - menstrual pain
  - minor arthritis pain
  - muscle pain
  - toothache
  - colds
- or as recommended by a doctor

## WARNINGS
### Reye's syndrome
Children and teenagers who have or are recovering from chicken pox or flu-like symptoms should not use this product. When using this product, if changes in behavior with nausea and vomiting occur, consult a doctor because these symptoms could be an early sign of Reye's syndrome, a rare but serious illness.

### Allergy alert
Aspirin may cause a severe allergic reaction with may include:
- hives
- facial swelling
- shock
- asthma (wheezing)

### Stomach bleeding warning
This product contains an NSAID, which may cause severe stomach bleeding. The chance is higher if you:
- are age 60 or older
- have had stomach ulcers or bleeding problems
- take a blood thinning (anticoagulant) or steroid drug
- take other drugs containing prescription or nonprescription NSAIDs (aspirin, ibuprofen, naproxen, or others)
- have 3 or more alcoholic drinks every day while using this product
- take more or for a longer time than directed

## DO NOT USE
- if you have ever had an allergic reaction to aspirin or any other pain reliever/fever reducer

## ASK A DOCTOR BEFORE USE IF
- stomach bleeding warnings applies to you
- you have a history of stomach problems, such as heartburn
- you have high blood pressure, heart disease, liver cirrhosis, or kidney disease
- you are taking a diuretic
- you have asthma

## ASK A DOCTOR OR PHARMACIST BEFORE USE IF YOU ARE
- taking a prescription drug for
  - diabetes
  - gout
  - arthritis

## STOP USE AND ASK A DOCTOR IF
- allergic reaction occurs. Seek medical help right away
- you experience any of the following signs of stomach bleeding:
  - feel faint
  - vomit blood
  - have bloody or black stools
  - have stomach pain that does not get better
- pain gets worse or lasts more than 10 days
- redness or swelling is present
- any new symptoms appear
- ringing in the ears or a loss of hearing occurs. These could be signs of a serious condition

**If pregnant or breastfeeding,** ask a health professional before use.

It is especially important not to use aspirin during the last 3 months of pregnancy unless definitely directed to do so by a doctor because it may cause problems in the unborn child or complications during delivery.

**Keep out of reach of children.** In case of overdose, get medical help or contact a Poison Control Center right away.

## DIRECTIONS (LOW STRENGTH)

| adults and children 12 years of age or over | take 4 to 8 tablets every 4 hours, while symptoms persist. Drink a full glass of water with each dose. |
| | do not take more than 48 tablets in 24 hours unless directed by a doctor |
|---|---|
| children under 12 years of age | ask a doctor |

## DIRECTIONS (REGULAR STRENGTH)

| adults and children 12 years of age or over: | take 1 to 2 tablets every 4 hours, while symptoms persist. Drink a full glass of water with each dose |
| | do not take more than 12 tablets in 24 hours unless directed by a doctor |
|---|---|
| children under 12 years of age | ask a doctor |

## OTHER INFORMATION
- tamper evident feature: do not use if printed inner-seal beneath cap is missing or broken
- store below 25°C (77°F)

## INACTIVE INGREDIENTS (LOW STRENGTH)
carnauba wax, colloidal silicon dioxide, EDTA, FD&C yellow no. 6, glyceryl monostearate, hypromellose, methacrylic acid copolymer, methylparaben, microcrystalline cellulose, polysorbate 80, propylparaben, starch, stearic acid, talc, titanium dioxide, triethyl citrate, printed with edible black ink

## INACTIVE INGREDIENTS (REGULAR STRENGTH)
carnauba wax, colloidal silicon dioxide, EDTA, FD&C yellow no. 6, glyceryl monostearate, hypromellose, methacrylic acid copolymer, methylparaben, microcrystalline cellulose, polysorbate 80, pregelatinized starch, propylparaben, sodium starch glycolate, stearic acid, talc, titanium dioxide, triethyl citrate, printed with edible ink

## QUESTIONS OR COMMENTS
Call toll-free **1-800-245-1040** (English/Spanish) weekdays or visit www.ecotrin.com

## EMETROL CHERRY (phosphorated carbohydrate) solution

WellSpring Pharmaceutical Corporation

### DRUG FACTS

| Active ingredient | Purpose |
|---|---|
| Phosphorated carbohydrate solution* | Upset stomach reliever |

*each 5 mL contains:
- 3.74 g total sugar
- 21.5 mg phosphoric acid

### USES
- for relief of upset stomach associated with nausea due to overindulgence in food and drink

### WARNINGS
- this product contains fructose and should not be taken by persons with hereditary fructose intolerance (HFI)

### DO NOT USE IF YOU HAVE
- allergic reactions to any of the ingredients in this product

### ASK A DOCTOR BEFORE USE IF YOU HAVE
- diabetes

### STOP USE AND ASK A DOCTOR IF
- symptoms persist, return or get worse

**If pregnant or breastfeeding,** ask a health professional before use.

**Keep out of reach of children.** In case of overdose, get medical help or contact a Poison Control Center right away. (**1-800-222-1222**)

### DIRECTIONS
- for maximum effectiveness never dilute or drink fluids of any kind immediately before or after taking this product

| adults and children 12 years of age and over | one to two tablespoons |
|---|---|
| children 2 to under 12 | one or two teaspoons |
| | repeat dose every 15 minutes or until distress subsides |
| | do not take more than 5 doses in 1 hour without consulting a doctor |

### OTHER INFORMATION
- store between 20-25°C (68-77°F) away from heat and direct light; keep from freezing
- do not use if printed foil seal under bottle cap is broken or missing

### INACTIVE INGREDIENTS
FD&C red no. 40, flavors, glycerin, methylparaben, purified water

### QUESTIONS OR COMMENTS
Call **1-866-337-4500**

## EUCERIN CALMING ITCH RELIEF TREATMENT (menthol) lotion

Beiersdorf Inc

### DRUG FACTS

| Active ingredient | Purpose |
|---|---|
| Menthol 0.1% | External analgesic lotion |

### USE
- for the temporary relief of itching associated with minor skin irritations

**For external use only.**

### WHEN USING THIS PRODUCT
- avoid contact with eyes

### STOP USE AND ASK A DOCTOR IF
- condition worsens
- symptoms last more than 7 days or clear up and occur again within a few days
- irritation occurs

**Keep out of reach of children.** If swallowed, get medical help or contact a Poison Control Center right away.

### INACTIVE INGREDIENTS
water, glycerin, octyldodecanol, caprylic/capric triglyceride, isopropyl stearate, myristyl myristate, cetyl alcohol, colloidal oatmeal, cetearyl alcohol, dimethicone, glyceryl stearate SE, oenothera biennis (evening primrose) oil, benzyl alcohol, phenoxyethanol, DMDM hydantoin, PEG-40 castor oil, caprylyl glycol, acrylates/C10-30 alkyl acrylate crosspolymer, sodium cetearyl sulfate, sodium citrate, polyglyceryl-3 methyl glucose distearate, potassium sorbate, citric acid

### DIRECTIONS

| adults and children 2 years of age and older | apply to affected area not more than 3 to 4 times daily |
|---|---|
| children under 2 years of age | consult a doctor |

### QUESTIONS OR COMMENTS
Call **1-800-227-4703**

## EUCERIN EVERYDAY PROTECTION BODY
(homosalate, octinoxate, octisalate, titanium dioxide) lotion

Beiersdorf Inc

### DRUG FACTS

| Active ingredients | Purpose |
|---|---|
| Homosalate | External body lotion |
| Octinoxate | |
| Octisalate | |
| Titanium dioxide | |

### USES
- provides broad spectrum sunscreen UVA UVB protection to help prevent skin aging, long term skin damage and skin cancer

## WARNINGS
**For external use only.**

**Keep out of eyes**

**STOP USE AND CONSULT A DOCTOR IF**
• irritation develops

**Keep out of reach of children**

## DIRECTIONS
• apply generously to hands and body daily
• re-apply as needed

## OTHER INFORMATION
• anti-oxidant enriched with Vitamin E to help protect from free radical damage
• non-greasy, moisturizing formula is clinically proven to relieve dry skin for 24 hours

## INACTIVE INGREDIENTS
water, glycerin, butylene glycol, cetearyl alcohol, urea, C18-36 acid triglyceride, caprylic/capric triglyceride, dimethicone, octyldodecanol, sodium lactate, arginine hydrochloride, tocopheryl acetate, glyceryl stearate SE, chondrus crispus (carrageenan), PEG-40 castor oil, sodium cetearyl sulfate, disodium EDTA, sodium citrate, lactic acid, carbomer, citric acid, trimethoxycaprylylsilane, benzyl alcohol, phenoxyethanol, methylparaben, propylparaben, potassium sorbate

## QUESTIONS OR COMMENTS
Call **1-800-227-4703**

# EUCERIN EVERYDAY PROTECTION FACE
(octinoxate, zinc oxide, octisalate, ensulizole, titanium dioxide) lotion
Beiersdorf Inc

## DRUG FACTS

| Active ingredients | Purpose |
|---|---|
| Octinoxate | Sunscreen |
| Zinc oxide | |
| Octisalate | |
| Ensulizole | |
| Titanium dioxide | |

## WARNINGS
**For external use only.**

**Keep out of eyes**

**STOP USE AND CONSULT A DOCTOR IF**
• irritation develops

**Keep out of reach of children.**

## DIRECTIONS
• after cleansing apply to face and neck every morning

## INACTIVE INGREDIENTS
water, glycerin, C12-15 alkyl benzoate, dimethicone, cyclomethicone, cetyl alcohol, cetearyl alcohol, ceteareth-20, glyceryl stearate se, sodium lactate, lactic acid, hydrogenated coco-glycerides, vp/hexadecene copolymer, PEG-40 castor oil, sodium cetearyl sulfate, xanthan gum, trisodium EDTA, sodium hydroxide, alumina, simethicone, phenoxyethanol, dmdm hydantoin

## QUESTIONS OR COMMENTS
Call **1-800-227-4703**

# EUCERIN Q10 ANTI-WRINKLE SENSITIVE SKIN (octinoxate, octisalate, oxybenzone) lotion
Beiersdorf Inc

## DRUG FACTS

| Active ingredients | Purpose |
|---|---|
| Octinoxate | Anti-wrinkle/Sunscreen |
| Octisalate | |
| Oxybenzone | |

## USES
• reduces the appearance of fine lines and wrinkles within 5 weeks
• firms and moisturizes for softer, smoother skin
• SPF 15 helps prevent fine lines and wrinkles caused by sun exposure
• can be used alone or under make-up
• is fragrance-free, non-comedogenic and won´t irritate sensitive skin
• recommended by the Skin Cancer Foundation as an effective UV sunscreen

## WARNINGS
**For external use only.**

**STOP USE AND CONSULT A DOCTOR IF**
• irritation develops

**Keep out of reach of children.**

## DIRECTIONS
• after cleansing with Eucerin Gentle Hydrating Cleanser apply to face and neck every morning

## OTHER INFORMATION
• the Skin Cancer Foundation recommends this product as an effective UV sunscreen
• the light yellow color is due to the natural color of the ingredients

## INACTIVE INGREDIENTS
water, glycerin, stearic acid, cetyl alcohol, cetearyl isononanoate, cyclopentasiloxane, glyceryl stearate SE, alcohol denat., cyclohexasiloxane, caprylic/capric triglyceride, octyldodecanol, ubiquinone, tocopheryl acetate, panthenol, carbomer, EDTA, sodium hydroxide, phenoxyethanol, methylparaben, ethylparaben, propylparaben, butylparaben, isobutylparaben

## QUESTIONS OR COMMENTS
Call **1-800-227-4703**

# EX-LAX REGULAR STRENGTH (sennosides) pill
Novartis Consumer Healthcare, Inc.

## DRUG FACTS

| Active ingredient(in each pill) | Purpose |
|---|---|
| Sennosides, USP, 15 mg | Stimulant laxative |

## USES
• relieves occasional constipation (irregularity)
• generally produces bowel movement in 6 to 12 hours

## WARNINGS

### DO NOT USE
- laxative products when abdominal pain, nausea, or vomiting are present unless directed by a doctor

### ASK A DOCTOR BEFORE USE IF YOU HAVE
- noticed a sudden change in bowel habits that persists over a period of 2 weeks

### ASK A DOCTOR OR PHARMACIST BEFORE USE IF YOU
- are taking a prescription drug. Laxatives may affect how other drugs work. Take this product 2 or more hours before or after other drugs

### WHEN USING THIS PRODUCT
- do not use for a period longer than 1 week

### STOP USE AND ASK A DOCTOR IF
- rectal bleeding or failure to have a bowel movement occur after use of a laxative. These may be signs of a serious condition

**If pregnant or breastfeeding,** ask a health professional before use.

**Keep out of reach of children.** In case of overdose, get medical help or contact a Poison Control Center right away.

## DIRECTIONS
- swallow pill(s) with a glass of water
- swallow pill(s) whole, do not crush, break, or chew

| adults and children 12 years of age and older | 2 pills once or twice daily |
|---|---|
| children 6 to under 12 years of age | 1 pill once or twice daily |
| children under 6 years of age | ask a doctor |

## OTHER INFORMATION
- each pill contains: calcium 50 mg
- sodium free
- store at controlled room temperature 20-25°C (68-77°F)

## INACTIVE INGREDIENTS
acacia, alginic acid, carnauba wax, colloidal silicon dioxide, dibasic calcium phosphate, iron oxides, magnesium stearate, microcrystalline cellulose, sodium benzoate, sodium lauryl sulfate, starch, stearic acid, sucrose, talc, titanium dioxide

## QUESTIONS OR COMMENTS
Call **1-800-452-0051**

---

# EX-LAX REGULAR STRENGTH CHOCOLATE
(sennosides)

Novartis Consumer Healthcare, Inc.

## DRUG FACTS

| Active ingredient (in each piece) | Purpose |
|---|---|
| Sennosides, USP, 15 mg | Stimulant laxative |

## USES
- relieves occasional constipation (irregularity)
- generally produces bowel movement in 6 to 12 hours

## WARNINGS

### DO NOT USE
- laxative products when abdominal pain, nausea, or vomiting are present unless directed by a doctor

### ASK A DOCTOR BEFORE USE IF YOU HAVE
- noticed a sudden change in bowel habits that persists over a period of 2 weeks Ask a doctor or pharmacist before use if you are taking a prescription drug. Laxatives may affect how other drugs work. Take this product 2 or more hours before or after other drugs

### WHEN USING THIS PRODUCT
- do not use for a period longer than 1 week

### STOP USE AND ASK A DOCTOR IF
- rectal bleeding or failure to have a bowel movement occur after use of a laxative. These may be signs of a serious condition

**If pregnant or breastfeeding,** ask a health professional before use.

**Keep out of reach of children.** In case of overdose, get medical help or contact a Poison Control Center right away.

## DIRECTIONS

| adults and children 12 years of age and older | chew 2 chocolated pieces once or twice daily |
|---|---|
| children 6 to under 12 years of age | chew 1 chocolated piece once or twice daily |
| children under 6 years of age | ask a doctor |

## OTHER INFORMATION
- each piece contains: potassium 10 mg
- sodium free
- store at controlled room temperature 20-25°C (68-77°F)

## INACTIVE INGREDIENTS
cocoa, confectioners sugar, hydrogenated palm kernel oil, lecithin, non-fat dry milk, vanillin

## QUESTIONS OR COMMENTS
Call **1-800-452-0051**

---

# EXCEDRIN EXTRA STRENGTH (acetaminophen, aspirin [NSAID], and caffeine) tablet, film coated

Novartis Consumer Health, Inc.

## DRUG FACTS

| Active ingredient (in each tablet) | Purpose |
|---|---|
| Acetaminophen 250 mg | Pain reliever |
| Aspirin 250 mg (NSAID)* | Pain reliever |
| Caffeine 65 mg | Pain reliever aid |

*nonsteroidal anti-inflammatory drug

## USES
- temporarily relieves minor aches and pains due to:
  - headache
  - a cold
  - arthritis
  - muscular aches
  - sinusitis
  - toothache
  - premenstrual & menstrual cramps

## WARNINGS
**Reye's syndrome**
Children and teenagers who have or are recovering from chicken pox or flu-like symptoms should not use this product. When

using this product, if changes in behavior with nausea and vomiting occur, consult a doctor because these symptoms could be an early sign of Reye's syndrome, a rare but serious illness.

**Allergy alert**
Aspirin may cause a severe allergic reaction which may include:
- hives
- facial swelling
- asthma (wheezing)
- shock

**Liver warning**
This product contains acetaminophen. Severe liver damage may occur if you take:
- more than 8 tables in 24 hours, which is the maximum daily amount
- with other drugs containing acetaminophen
- 3 or more alcoholic drinks every day while using this product

**Stomach bleeding warning**
This product contains a nonsteroidal anti-inflammatory drug (NSAID), which may cause stomach bleeding. The chance is higher if you:
- are age 60 or older
- have had stomach ulcers or bleeding problems
- take a blood thinning (anticoagulant) or steroid drug
- take other drugs containing an NSAID (aspirin, ibuprofen, naproxen, or others
- have 3 or more alcoholic drinks every day while using this product
- take more or for a longer time than directed

**Caffeine warning**
The recommended dose of this product contains about as much caffeine as a cup of coffee. Limit the use of caffeine-containing medications, foods, or beverages while taking this product because too much caffeine may cause nervousness, irritability, sleeplessness, and, occasionally, rapid heart beat.

**DO NOT USE**
- if you have ever had an allergic reaction to aspirin or any other pain reliever/fever reducer
- with any other drug containing acetaminophen (prescription or nonprescription). If you are not sure whether a drug contains acetaminophen, ask a doctor or pharmacist

**ASK DOCTOR BEFORE USE IF**
- you have liver disease
- stomach bleeding warning applies to you
- you have a history of stomach problems, such as heartburn
- you have high blood pressure, heart disease, liver cirrhosis. or kidney disease
- you are taking a diuretic
- you have asthma

**ASK A DOCTOR OR PHARMACIST BEFORE USE**
- any other drug containing an NSAID (prescription or nonprescription)
- a blood thinning (anticoagulant) or steroid drug
- a prescription drug for diabetes, gout, or arthritis
- any other drug, or are under a doctor's care for any serious condition

**STOP USE AND ASK DOCTOR IF**
- an allergic reaction occurs. Seek medical help right away
- you experience any of the following signs of stomach bleeding:
  - feel faint
  - vomit blood
  - have bloody or black stools
  - have stomach pain that does not get better
- ringing in the ears or loss of hearing occurs
- painful area is red or swollen
- pain gets worse or lasts for more than 10 days

- fever gets worse or lasts for more than 3 days
- any new symptoms appear

**If pregnant or breastfeeding,** ask a health professional before use.

It is especially important not to use aspirin during the last 3 months of pregnancy unless definitely directed to do so by a doctor because it may cause problems in the unborn child or complications during delivery.

**Keep out of reach of children.**

**OVERDOSE WARNING**
In case of overdose, get medical help or contact a Poison Control Center right away. Quick medical attention is critical for adults as well as for children even if you do not notice any signs or symptoms.

**DIRECTIONS**
- do not use more than directed (see Overdose Warning)
- drink a full glass of water with each dose

| adults and children 12 years and over | take 2 tablets every 6 hours; not more than 8 tablets in 24 hours |
|---|---|
| children under 12 years | ask a doctor |

**OTHER INFORMATION**
- store at controlled room temperature 20-25°C (68-77°F)
- read all product information before using
- keep this box for important information

**INACTIVE INGREDIENTS**
benzoic acid, carnauba wax, FD&C blue no. 1, hydroxypropyl cellulose, hypromellose, light mineral oil, microcrystalline cellulose, polysorbate 20, povidone, propylene glycol, simethicone emulsion, sorbitan monolaurate, stearic acid, titanium dioxide

---

# EXCEDRIN EXTRA STRENGTH EXPRESS GELS (acetaminophen, aspirin, and caffeine) [NSAID]
Novartis

## DRUG FACTS

| Active ingredients (in each gelcap) | Purpose |
|---|---|
| Acetaminophen 250 mg | Pain reliever |
| Aspirin 250 mg (NSAID)* | Pain reliever |
| Caffeine 65 mg | Pain reliever aid |

*nonsteroidal anti-inflammatory drug

**USES**
- temporarily relieves minor aches and pains due to:
  - headache
  - a cold
  - arthritis
  - muscular aches
  - sinusitis
  - toothache
  - premenstrual & menstrual cramps

**WARNINGS**
**Reye's syndrome**
Children and teenagers who have or are recovering from chicken pox or flu-like symptoms should not use this product. When using this product, if changes in behavior with nausea and vomiting occur, consult a doctor because these symptoms could be an early sign of Reye's syndrome, a rare but serious illness.

**Allergy alert**

Aspirin may cause a severe allergic reaction which may include:
- hives
- facial swelling
- asthma (wheezing)
- shock

**Liver warning**

This product contains acetaminophen. Severe liver damage may occur if you take:
- more than 8 gelcaps in 24 hours, which is the maximum daily amount
- with other drugs containing acetaminophen
- 3 or more alcoholic drinks every day while using this product

**Stomach bleeding warning**

This product contains an NSAID which may cause severe stomach bleeding. The chance is higher if you:
- are age 60 or older
- have had stomach ulcers or bleeding problems
- take a blood thinning (anticoagulant) or steroid drug
- take other drugs containing prescription or nonprescription NSAIDs (aspirin, ibuprofen, naproxen, or others)
- have 3 or more alcoholic drinks every day while using this product
- take more or for a longer time than directed

**Caffeine warning**

The recommended dose of this product contains about as much caffeine as a cup of coffee. Limit the use of caffeine-containing medications, foods, or beverages while taking this product because too much caffeine may cause nervousness, irritability, sleeplessness, and occasionally, rapid heart beat.

**DO NOT USE**
- if you have ever had an allergic reaction to acetaminophen, aspirin or any other pain reliever/fever reducer
- with any other drug containing acetaminophen (prescription or nonprescription). If you are not sure whether a drug contains acetaminophen, ask a doctor or pharmacist

**ASK A DOCTOR BEFORE USE IF**
- you have liver disease
- stomach bleeding warning applies to you
- you have a history of stomach problems, such as heartburn
- you have high blood pressure, heart disease, liver cirrhosis, or kidney disease
- you are taking a diuretic
- you have asthma

**ASK A DOCTOR OR PHARMACIST BEFORE USE IF YOU ARE TAKING**
- any other drug containing an NSAID (prescription or nonprescription)
- a blood thinning (anticoagulant) or steroid drug
- a prescription drug for diabetes, gout, or arthritis
- any other drug, or are under a doctor's care for any serious condition

**STOP USE AND ASK A DOCTOR IF**
- an allergic reaction occurs. Seek medical help right away
- you experience any of the following signs of stomach bleeding:
  - feel faint
  - vomit blood
  - have bloody or black stools
  - have stomach pain that does not get better
- ringing in the ears or loss of hearing occurs
- painful area is red or swollen
- pain gets worse or lasts for more than 10 days
- fever gets worse or lasts for more than 3 days
- any new symptoms appear

**If pregnant or breastfeeding,** ask a health professional before use.

It is especially important not to use aspirin during the last 3 months of pregnancy unless definitely directed to do so by a doctor because it may cause problems in the unborn child or complications during delivery.

**Keep out of reach of children.** In case of overdose, get medical help or contact a Poison Control Center right away. Quick medical attention is critical for adults as well as for children even if you do not notice any signs or symptoms.

**DIRECTIONS**
- do not use more than directed
- drink a full glass of water with each dose

| adults and children 12 years and over | take 2 gelcaps every 6 hours; not more than 8 gelcaps in 24 hours |
|---|---|
| children under 12 years | ask a doctor |

**OTHER INFORMATION**
- store at controlled room temperature 20-25°C (68-77°F)
- read all product information before using

**INACTIVE INGREDIENTS**

benzoic acid, D&C red no. 28, D&C yellow no. 10, FD&C green no. 3, gelatin, hydroxypropyl cellulose, hypromellose, light mineral oil, microcrystalline cellulose, pepsin, polysorbate 20, povidone, propylene glycol, simethicone emulsion, sorbitan monolaurate, stearic acid, titanium dioxide

**QUESTIONS OR COMMENTS**

Call **1-800-468-7746**

# EXCEDRIN EXTRA STRENGTH GELTABS
(acetaminophen, aspirin, and caffeine)

Novartis

## DRUG FACTS

| Active ingredients (in each geltab) | Purpose |
|---|---|
| Acetaminophen 250 mg | Pain reliever |
| Aspirin 250 mg (NSAID)* | Pain reliever |
| Caffeine 65 mg | Pain reliever aid |

*nonsteroidal anti-inflammatory drug

## USES
- temporarily relieves minor aches and pains due to:
  - headache
  - a cold
  - arthritis
  - muscular aches
  - sinusitis
  - toothache
  - premenstrual & menstrual cramps

## WARNINGS
**Reye's syndrome**

Children and teenagers who have or are recovering from chicken pox or flu-like symptoms should not use this product. When using this product, if changes in behavior with nausea and vomiting occur, consult a doctor because these symptoms could be an early sign of Reye's syndrome, a rare but serious illness.

## Allergy alert

Aspirin may cause a severe allergic reaction which may include:
- hives
- facial swelling
- asthma (wheezing)
- shock

## Liver warning

This product contains acetaminophen. Severe liver damage may occur if you take:
- more than 8 geltabs in 24 hours, which is the maximum daily amount
- with other drugs containing acetaminophen
- 3 or more alcoholic drinks every day while using this product

## Stomach bleeding warning

This product contents a NSAID, which may cause severe stomach bleeding. The chance is higher if you:
- are age 60 or older
- have had stomach ulcers or bleeding problems
- take a blood thinning (anticoagulant) or steroid drug
- take other drugs containing prescription or nonprescription NSAIDs (aspirin, ibuprofen, naproxen, or others)
- have 3 or more alcoholic drinks every day while using this product
- take more or for a longer time than directed

## Caffeine warning

The recommended dose of this product contains about as much caffeine as a cup of coffee. Limit the use of caffeine-containing medications, foods, or beverages while taking this product because too much caffeine may cause nervousness, irritability, sleeplessness, and, occasionally, rapid heart beat.

## DO NOT USE

- if you have ever had an allergic reaction to acetaminophen, aspirin or any other pain reliever/fever reducer
- with any other drug containing acetaminophen (prescription or nonprescription). If you are not sure whether a drug contains acetaminophen, ask a doctor or pharmacist

## ASK A DOCTOR BEFORE USE IF

- you have liver disease
- stomach bleeding warning applies to you
- you have a history of stomach problems, such as heartburn
- you have high blood pressure, heart disease, liver cirrhosis, or kidney disease
- you are taking a diuretic
- you have asthma

## ASK A DOCTOR OR PHARMACIST BEFORE USE IF YOU ARE TAKING

- any other drug containing an NSAID (prescription or nonprescription)
- a blood thinning (anticoagulant) or steroid drug
- a prescription drug for diabetes, gout, or arthritis
- any other drug, or are under a doctor's care for any serious condition

## STOP USE AND ASK A DOCTOR IF

- an allergic reaction occurs. Seek medical help right away
- you experience any of the following signs of stomach bleeding:
  - feel faint
  - vomit blood
  - have bloody or black stools
  - have stomach pain that does not better
- ringing in the ears or loss of hearing occurs
- painful area is red or swollen
- pain gets worse or lasts for more than 10 days
- fever gets worse or lasts to more than 3 days
- any new symptoms appear

**If pregnant or breastfeeding,** ask a health professional before use.

It is especially important not to use aspirin during the last 3 months of pregnancy unless definitely directed to do so by a doctor because it may cause problems in the unborn child or complications during delivery.

**Keep out of reach of children.** In case of overdose, get medical help of contact a Poison Control Center right away. Quick medical attention is critical for adults as well as for children even if you do not notice any signs or symptoms.

## DIRECTIONS

- do not use more than directed
- drink a full glass of water with each dose

| adults and children 12 years and over | take 2 geltabs every 6 hours; not more than 8 geltabs in 24 hours |
|---|---|
| children under 12 years | ask a doctor |

## OTHER INFORMATION

- store at controlled room temperature 20-25°C (68-77°F)
- read all product information before using

## INACTIVE INGREDIENTS

benzoic acid, D&C red no. 28, D&C yellow no. 10, FD&C green no. 3, gelatin, hydroxypropyl cellulose, hypromellose, light mineral oil, microcrystalline cellulose, pepsin, polysorbate 20, povidone, propylene glycol, simethicone emulsion, sorbitan monolaurate, stearic acid, titanium dioxide

## QUESTIONS OR COMMENTS

Call **1-800-468-7746**

---

# EXCEDRIN EXTRA STRENGTH PAIN RELIEVER (acetaminophen, aspirin [NSAID], and caffeine) tablet, film coated

Novartis Consumer Health, Inc.

## DRUG FACTS

| Active ingredients (in each caplet) | Purpose |
|---|---|
| Acetaminophen 250 mg | Pain reliever |
| Aspirin 250 mg (NSAID)* | Pain reliever |
| Caffeine 65 mg | Pain reliever aid |

*nonsteroidal anti-inflammatory drug

## USES

- temporarily relieves minor aches and pains due to:
  - headache
  - a cold
  - arthritis
  - muscular aches
  - sinusitis
  - toothache
  - premenstrual & menstrual cramps

## WARNINGS

**Reye's syndrome**

Children and teenagers who have or are recovering from chicken pox or flu-like symptoms should not use this product. When using this product, if changes in behavior with nausea and vomiting occur, consult a doctor because these symptoms could be an early sign of Reye's syndrome, a rare but serious illness.

**Allergy alert**
Aspirin may cause a severe allergic reaction which may include:
- hives
- facial swelling
- asthma (wheezing)
- shock

**Liver warning**
This product contains acetaminophen. Severe liver damage may occur if you take:
- more than 8 caplets in 24 hours, which is the maximum daily amount
- with other drugs containing acetaminophen
- 3 or more alcoholic drinks every day while using this product

**Stomach bleeding warning**
This product contains a nonsteroidal anti-inflammatory drug (NSAID), which may cause stomach bleeding. The chance is higher if you:
- are age 60 or older
- have had stomach ulcers or bleeding problems
- take a blood thinning (anticoagulant) or steroid drug
- take other drugs containing a NSAID (aspirin, ibuprofen, naproxen, or others)
- have 3 or more alcoholic drinks every day while using this product
- take more or for a longer time than directed

**Caffeine warning**
The recommended dose of this product contains about as much caffeine as a cup of coffee. Limit the use of caffeine-containing medications, foods, or beverages while taking this product because too much caffeine may cause nervousness, irritability, sleeplessness, and, occasionally, rapid heart beat.

**DO NOT USE**
- if you have ever had an allergic reaction to aspirin or any other pain reliever/fever reducer
- with any other drug containing acetaminophen (prescription or nonprescription). If you are not sure whether a drug contains acetaminophen, ask a doctor or pharmacist

**ASK DOCTOR BEFORE USE IF**
- you have liver disease
- stomach bleeding warning applies to you
- you have a history of stomach problems, such as heartburn
- you have high blood pressure, heart disease, liver cirrhosis, or kidney disease
- you are taking a diuretic
- you have asthma

**ASK A DOCTOR OR PHARMACIST BEFORE USE**
- any other drug containing a NSAID (prescription or nonprescription)
- a blood thinning (anticoagulant) or steroid drug
- a prescription drug for diabetes, gout, or arthritis
- any other drug, or are under a doctor's care for any serious condition

**STOP USE AND ASK DOCTOR IF**
- an allergic reaction occurs. Seek medical help right away
- you experience any of the following signs of stomach bleeding:
  - feel faint
  - vomit blood
  - have bloody or black stools
  - have stomach pain that does not get better
- ringing in the ears or loss of hearing occurs
- painful area is red or swollen
- pain gets worse or lasts for more than 10 days
- fever gets worse or lasts for more than 3 days
- any new symptoms appear

**If pregnant or breastfeeding,** ask a health professional before use.

It is especially important not to use aspirin during the last 3 months of pregnancy unless definitely directed to do so by a doctor because it may cause problems in the unborn child or complications during delivery.

**Keep out of reach of children.**

**OVERDOSE WARNING**
In case of overdose, get medical help or contact a Poison Control Center right away. Quick medical attention is critical for adults as well as for children even if you do not notice any signs or symptoms.

**DIRECTIONS**
- do not use more than directed (see Overdose Warning)
- drink a full glass of water with each dose

| adults and children 12 years and over | take 2 caplets every 6 hours; not more than 8 caplets in 24 hours |
|---|---|
| children under 12 years | ask a doctor |

**OTHER INFORMATION**
- store at controlled room temperature 20-25°C (68-77°F)
- read all product information before using
- keep box for important information

**INACTIVE INGREDIENTS**
benzoic acid, carnauba wax, FD&C blue no. 1, hydroxypropylcellulose, hypromellose, light mineral oil, microcrystalline cellulose, polysorbate 20, povidone, propylene glycol, simethicone emulsion, sorbitan monolaurate, stearic acid, titanium dioxide

---

# EXCEDRIN BACK AND BODY (acetaminophen, aspirin) tablet, film coated
## Novartis Consumer Health, Inc.

### DRUG FACTS

| Active ingredients | Purpose |
|---|---|
| Acetaminophen 250 mg | Pain reliever |
| Buffered aspirin equal to 250 mg aspirin (NSAID)* (buffered with calcium carbonate) | Pain reliever |

*nonsteroidal anti-inflammatory drug

**USES**
- for the temporary relief of minor aches and pains due to:
  - minor pain of arthritis
  - backache
  - muscular aches

**WARNINGS**
**Reye's syndrome**
Children and teenagers who have or are recovering from chicken pox or flu-like symptoms should not use this product. When using this product, if changes in behavior with nausea and vomiting occur, consult a doctor because these symptoms could be an early sign of Reye's syndrome, a rare but serious illness.

**Allergy alert**

Aspirin may cause a severe allergic reaction which may include:
- hives
- facial swelling
- asthma (wheezing)
- shock

**Liver warning**

This product contains acetaminophen. Severe liver damage may occur if you take:
- more than 8 caplets in 24 hours, which is the maximum daily amount
- with other drugs containing acetaminophen
- 3 or more alcoholic drinks every day while using this product

**Stomach bleeding warning**

This product contains an NSAID, which may cause severe stomach bleeding. The chance is higher if you:
- are age 60 or older
- have had stomach ulcers or bleeding problems
- take a blood thinning (anticoagulant) or steroid drug
- take other drugs containing prescription or nonprescription NSAIDs (aspirin, ibuprofen, naproxen, or others)
- have 3 or more alcoholic drinks every day while using this product
- take more or for a longer time than directed

**DO NOT USE**
- if you have ever had an allergic reaction to acetaminophen, aspirin or any other pain reliever/fever reducer
- with any other drug containing acetaminophen (prescription or nonprescription). If you are not sure whether a drug contains acetaminophen, ask a doctor or pharmacist

**ASK DOCTOR BEFORE USE IF**
- you have liver disease
- stomach bleeding warning applies to you
- you have a history of stomach problems, such as heartburn
- you have high blood pressure, heart disease, liver cirrhosis, or kidney disease
- you are taking a diuretic
- you have asthma

**ASK THE DOCTOR OR PHARMACIST BEFORE USE IF YOU ARE TAKING**
- any other drug containing a NSAID (prescription or nonprescription)
- a blood thinning (anticoagulant) or steroid drug
- a prescription drug for diabetes, gout, or arthritis
- any other drug, or are under a doctor's care for any serious condition

**STOP USE AND ASK A DOCTOR IF**
- an allergic reaction occurs. Seek medical help right away
- you experience any of the following signs of stomach bleeding:
  - feel faint
  - vomit blood
  - have bloody or black stools
  - have stomach pain that does not get better
- ringing in the ears or loss of hearing occurs
- painful area is red or swollen
- pain gets worse or lasts for more than 10 days
- fever gets worse or lasts for more than 3 days
- any new symptoms appear

**Pregnancy or breastfeeding,** ask a health professional before use.

It is especially important not to use aspirin during the last 3 months of pregnancy unless definitely directed to do so by a doctor because it may cause problems in the unborn child or complications during delivery.

**Keep out of reach of children.** In case of overdose, get medical help or contact a Poison Control Center right away. Quick medical attention is critical for adults as well as for children even if you do not notice any signs or symptoms.

**DIRECTIONS**
- do not use more than directed
- drink a full glass of water with each dose

| adults and children 12 years and over | take 2 caplets every 6 hours; not more than 8 caplets in 24 hours |
|---|---|
| children under 12 years | ask a doctor |

**OTHER INFORMATION**
- each caplet contains: calcium 80 mg
- store at controlled room temperature 20-25°C (68-77°F)
- read all product information before using
- keep this box for important information
- tamper evident bottle. Do not use if inner seal imprinted with "sealed for your protection" is broken or missing

**QUESTIONS OR COMMENTS**

Call **1-800-468-7746** or visit www.excedrin.com

# EXCEDRIN MENSTRUAL COMPLETE
(acetaminophen, asprin [NSAID], and caffine) capsule, gelatin coated

Novartis Consumer Health, Inc.

## DRUG FACTS

| Active ingredients (in each gelcap) | Purpose |
|---|---|
| Acetaminophen 250 mg | Pain reliever |
| Aspirin 250 mg (NSAID)* | Pain reliever |
| Caffeine 65 mg | Diuretic |

*nonsteroidal anti-inflammatory drug

**USES**
- temporarily relieves minor aches and pains due to:
  - muscular aches
  - headache
  - backache
  - premenstrual & menstrual cramps
- temporarily relieves these symptoms associated with menstrual periods:
  - water-weight gain
  - bloating
  - swelling
  - full feeling
  - fatigue

**WARNINGS**

**Reye's syndrome**

Children and teenagers who have or are recovering from chicken pox or flu-like symptoms should not use this product. When using this product, if changes in behavior with nausea and vomiting occur, consult a doctor because these symptoms could be an early sign of Reye's syndrome, a rare but serious illness.

**Liver warning**

This product contains acetaminophen. Severe liver damage may occur if you take:
- more than 8 gelcaps in 24 hours, which is the maximum daily amount

- with other drugs containing acetaminophen
- 3 or more alcoholic drinks every day while using this product

**Stomach bleeding warning**
This product contains an NSAID, which may cause severe stomach bleeding. The chance is higher if you:
- are age 60 or older
- have had stomach ulcers or bleeding problems
- take a blood thinning (anticoagulant) or steroid drug
- take other drugs containing prescription or nonprescription NSAIDs (aspirin, ibuprofen, naproxen, or others)
- have 3 or more alcoholic drinks every day while using this product
- take more or for a longer time than directed

**Caffeine warning**
The recommended dose of this product contains about as much caffeine as a cup of coffee. Limit the use of caffeine-containing medications, foods, or beverages while taking this product because too much caffeine may cause nervousness, irritability, sleeplessness, and, occasionally, rapid heart beat.

**Allergy alert**
Aspirin may cause a severe allergic reaction which may include:
- hives
- facial swelling
- asthma (wheezing)
- shock

**DO NOT USE**
- if you have ever had an allergic reaction to acetaminophen, aspirin or any other pain reliever/fever reducer
- with any other drug containing acetaminophen (prescription or nonprescription). If you are not sure whether a drug contains acetaminophen, ask a doctor or pharmacist

**ASK A DOCTOR BEFORE USE IF**
- you have liver disease
- stomach bleeding warning applies to you
- you have a history of stomach problems, such as heartburn
- you have high blood pressure, heart disease, liver cirrhosis, or kidney disease
- you are taking a diuretic
- you have asthma

**ASK A DOCTOR OR PHARMACIST BEFORE USE IF YOU ARE TAKING**
- any other drug containing an NSAID (prescription or nonprescription)
- a blood thinning (anticoagulant) or steroid drug
- a prescription drug for diabetes, gout, or arthritis
- any other drug, or are under a doctor's care for any serious condition

**STOP USE AND ASK A DOCTOR IF**
- an allergic reaction occurs. Seek medical help right away
- you experience any of the following signs of stomach bleeding:
  - feel faint
  - vomit blood
  - have bloody or black stools
  - have stomach pain that does not get better
- ringing in the ears or loss of hearing occurs
- painful area is red or swollen
- pain gets worse or lasts for more than 10 days
- fever gets worse or lasts for more than 3 days
- any new symptoms appear

**If pregnant or breastfeeding,** ask a health professional before use.

It is especially important not to use aspirin during the last 3 months of pregnancy unless definitely directed to do so by a doctor because it may cause problems in the unborn child or complications during delivery.

**Keep out of reach of children.**

**OVERDOSE WARNING**
In case of overdose, get medical help or contact a Poison Control Center right away. Quick medical attention is critical for adults as well as for children even if you do not notice any signs or symptoms.

**DIRECTIONS**
- do not use more than directed
- drink a full glass of water with each dose

| adults and children 12 years and over | take 2 gelcaps every 4-6 hours; not more than 8 gelcaps in 24 hours |
|---|---|
| children under 12 years | ask a doctor |

**OTHER INFORMATION**
- store at controlled room temperature 20-25°C (68-77°F)
- read all product information before using
- keep this box for important information

**INACTIVE INGREDIENTS**
benzoic acid, D&C red no. 28, D&C yellow no. 10, FD&C green no. 3, gelatin, hydroxypropyl cellulose, hypromellose, light mineral oil, microcrystalline cellulose, pepsin, polysorbate 20, povidone, propylene glycol, simethicone emulsion, sorbitan monolaurate, stearic acid, titanium dioxide

**QUESTIONS OR COMMENTS**
Call **1-800-468-7746** or visit www.excedrin.com

---

**EXCEDRIN MIGRAINE** (acetaminophen, aspirin and caffeine) tablet, film coated
Novartis Consumer Health, Inc.

| Active ingredient | Purpose |
|---|---|
| Acetaminophen 250 mg | Pain reliever |
| Aspirin 250 mg (NSAID) * | Pain reliever |
| Caffeine 65 mg | Pain reliever aid |

* nonsteroidal anti-inflammatory drug

**USES**
- treats migraine

**WARNINGS**
**Reye's syndrome**
Children and teenagers who have or are recovering from chicken pox or flu-like symptoms should not use this product. When using this product, if changes in behavior with nausea and vomiting occur, consult a doctor because these symptoms could be an early sign of Reye's syndrome, a rare but serious illness.

**Allergy alert**
Aspirin may cause a severe allergic reaction which may include:
- hives
- facial swelling
- asthma (wheezing)
- shock

**Liver warning**
This product contains acetaminophen. Severe liver damage may occur if you take:
- more than 2 tablets in 24 hours, which is the maximum daily amount
- with other drugs containing acetaminophen
- 3 or more alcoholic drinks every day while using this product

**Stomach bleeding warning**
This product contains an NSAID, which may cause severe stomach bleeding. The chance is higher if you:
- are age 60 or older
- have had stomach ulcers or bleeding problems
- take a blood thinning (anticoagulant) or steroid drug
- take other drugs containing prescription or nonprescription NSAIDs (aspirin, ibuprofen, naproxen, or others)
- have 3 or more alcoholic drinks every day while using this product
- take more or for a longer time than directed

**Caffeine warning**
The recommended dose of this product contains about as much caffeine as a cup of coffee. Limit the use of caffeine-containing medications, foods, or beverages while taking this product because too much caffeine may cause nervousness, irritability, sleeplessness, and, occasionally, rapid heart beat.

**DO NOT USE**
- if you have ever had an allergic reaction to acetaminophen, aspirin or any other pain reliever/fever reducer
- with any other drug containing acetaminophen (prescription or nonprescription). If you are not sure whether a drug contains acetaminophen, ask a doctor or pharmacist

**ASK DOCTOR BEFORE USE IF**
- you have never had migraines diagnosed by a health professional
- you have a headache that is different from your usual migraines
- you have the worst headache of your life
- you have fever and stiff neck
- you have headaches beginning after or caused by head injury, exertion, coughing or bending
- you experienced your first headache after the age of 50
- you have daily headaches
- you have a migraine so severe as to require bed rest
- you have liver disease
- stomach bleeding warning applies to you
- you have a history of stomach problems, such as heartburn
- you have high blood pressure, heart disease, liver cirrhosis, or kidney disease
- you are taking a diuretic
- you have asthma
- you have problems or serious side effects from taking pain relievers or fever reducers
- you have vomiting with your migraine headache

**ASK A DOCTOR OR PHARMACIST BEFORE USE IF YOU ARE**
- taking a prescription drug for:
  - anticoagulation (thinning of the blood)
  - diabetes
  - gout
  - arthritis
- under a doctor's care for any serious condition
- taking any other drug
- taking any other product that contains aspirin, acetaminophen, or any other pain reliever/fever reducer

**STOP USE AND ASK A DOCTOR IF**
- an allergic reaction occurs. Seek medical help right away
- you experience any of the following signs of stomach bleeding:
  - feel faint
  - vomit blood
  - have bloody or black stools
  - have stomach pain that does not get better
- your migraine is not relieved or worsens after first dose
- new or unexpected symptoms occur
- ringing in the ears or loss of hearing occurs

**If pregnant or breastfeeding,** ask a health professional before use.

It is especially important not to use aspirin during the last 3 months of pregnancy unless definitely directed to do so by a doctor because it may cause problems in the unborn child or complications during delivery.

**Keep out of reach of children.** In case of overdose, get medical help or contact a Poison Control Center right away. Quick medical attention is critical for adults as well as for children even if you do not notice any signs or symptoms.

**DIRECTIONS**
- do not use more than directed

| adults | take 2 tablets with a glass of water |
| | if symptoms persist or worsen, ask your doctor |
| | do not take more than 2 tablets in 24 hours, unless directed by a doctor |
| under 18 years of age | ask a doctor |

**OTHER INFORMATION**
- store at controlled room temperature 20-25°C (68-77°F)
- read all product information before using
- keep this box for important information

**INACTIVE INGREDIENTS**
benzoic acid, carnauba wax, FD&C blue no. 1, hydroxypropylcellulose, hypromellose, light mineral oil, microcrystalline cellulose, polysorbate 20, povidone, propylene glycol, simethicone emulsion, sorbitan monolaurate, stearic acid, titanium dioxide

**QUESTIONS OR COMMENTS**
Call **1-800-468-7746**

---

**EXCEDRIN PM** (acetaminophen, diphenhydramine citrate) tablet, film coated
Novartis Consumer Health, Inc.

**DRUG FACTS**

| Active ingredients | Purpose |
| --- | --- |
| Acetaminophen 500 mg | Pain reliever |
| Diphenhydramine citrate 38 mg | Nighttime sleep-aid |

**USES**
- for the temporary relief of occasional headaches and minor aches and pains with accompanying sleeplessness

**WARNINGS**
**Liver warning**
This product contains acetaminophen. Severe liver damage may occur if you take:
- more than 2 caplets in 24 hours, which is the maximum daily amount
- with other drugs containing acetaminophen
- 3 or more alcoholic drinks every day while using this product

## DO NOT USE
- if you are allergic to acetaminophen
- with any other drug containing acetaminophen (prescription or nonprescription). If you are not sure whether a drug contains acetaminophen, ask a doctor or pharmacist
- with any other product containing diphenhydramine, even one used on skin
- in children under 12 years of age

## ASK A DOCTOR BEFORE USE IF YOU HAVE
- liver disease
- glaucoma
- a breathing problem such as emphysema or chronic bronchitis
- trouble urinating due to an enlarged prostate gland

## ASK A DOCTOR OR PHARMACIST BEFORE USE IF YOU ARE
- taking the blood thinning drug warfarin
- taking sedatives or tranquilizers

## WHEN USING THIS PRODUCT
- avoid alcoholic drinks
- drowsiness may occur
- be careful when driving a motor vehicle or operating machinery

## STOP USE AND ASK A DOCTOR IF
- any new symptoms occur
- sleeplessness lasts continuously for more than 2 weeks. Insomnia may be a symptom of serious underlying medical illness
- pain gets worse or lasts for more than 10 days
- painful area is red or swollen
- fever gets worse or lasts for more than 3 days

**If pregnant or breastfeeding,** ask a health professional before use.

**Keep out of reach of children.**

## OVERDOSE WARNING
In case of overdose, get medical help or contact a Poison Control Center right away. Quick medical attention is critical for adults as well as for children even if you do not notice any signs or symptoms

## DIRECTIONS
- do not use more than directed
- do not use in children under 12 years of age
- adults and children 12 years of age and over:
  - take 2 caplets at bedtime, if needed, or as directed by a doctor

## OTHER INFORMATION
- store at controlled room temperature 20-25°C (68-77°F)
- read all product information before using. Keep box for important information
- tamper evident bottle. Do not use if when foil seal imprinted with "sealed for your protection" is broken or missing

## INACTIVE INGREDIENTS
benzoic acid, carnauba wax, croscarmellose sodium, D&C yellow no. 10 lake, FD&C blue no. 1 lake, hypromellose, light mineral oil, magnesium stearate, microcrystalline cellulose, polysorbate 20, povidone, pregelatinized starch, propylene glycol, simethicone emulsion, sodium citrate, sorbitan monolaurate, stearic acid, titanium dioxide

## QUESTIONS OR COMMENTS
Call **1-800-468-7746** or visit www.excedrin.com

# EXCEDRIN TENSION HEADACHE
(acetaminophen and caffeine) tablet, film coated
Novartis Consumer Health, Inc.

## DRUG FACTS

| Active ingredients | Purpose |
|---|---|
| Acetaminophen 500 mg | Pain reliever |
| Caffeine 65 mg | |

## USES
- temporarily relieves minor aches and pains due to:
  - headache
  - muscular aches

## WARNINGS
**Liver warning**
This product contains acetaminophen. Severe liver damage may occur if you take:
- more than 8 caplets in 24 hours, which is the maximum daily amount
- with other drugs containing acetaminophen
- 3 or more alcoholic drinks every day while using this product

**Caffeine warning**
The recommended dose of this product contains about as much caffeine as a cup of coffee. Limit the use of caffeine-containing medications, foods, or beverages while taking this product because too much caffeine may cause nervousness, irritability, sleeplessness, and, occasionally, rapid heart beat.

## DO NOT USE
- if you are allergic to acetaminophen
- with any other drug containing acetaminophen (prescription or nonprescription). If you are not sure whether a drug contains acetaminophen, ask a doctor or pharmacist

## ASK A DOCTOR BEFORE USE
- if you have liver disease

## ASK A DOCTOR OR PHARMACIST IF YOU ARE TAKING
- taking the blood thinning drug warfarin

## STOP USE AND ASK A DOCTOR IF
- any new symptoms occur
- painful area is red or swollen
- pain gets worse or lasts for more than 10 days
- fever gets worse or lasts for more than 3 days

**Pregnancy or breastfeeding,** ask a health professional before use.

**Keep out of reach of children.** In case of overdose, get medical help or contact a Poison Control Center right away. Quick medical attention is critical for adults as well as for children even if you do not notice any signs or symptoms.

## DIRECTIONS
- do not use more than directed

| | |
|---|---|
| - adults and children 12 years and over: | - take 2 caplets every 6 hours; not more than 8 caplets in 24 hours |

## OTHER INFORMATION
- store at controlled room temperature 20-25°C (68-77°F)
- read all product information before using
- keep this box for important information

## INACTIVE INGREDIENTS
benzoic acid, carnauba wax, D&C red no. 27 lake, D&C yellow no. 10 lake, FD&C blue no. 1 lake, FD&C red no. 40, hypromellose, light mineral oil, magnesium stearate, microcrystalline cellulose, polysorbate 20, povidone, pregelatinized starch, propylene glycol, simethicone emulsion, sorbitan monolaurate, stearic acid, titanium dioxide

## QUESTIONS OR COMMENTS
Call 1-800-468-7746

---

# EYE WASH (water) solution
Bausch & Lomb Incorporated

## DRUG FACTS

| Active ingredient | Purpose |
|---|---|
| Purified water (99.05%) | Eyewash |

## USES
- washes the eye to help relieve:
  - irritation
  - stinging
  - discomfort
  - itching
- by removing:
  - loose foreign material
  - air pollutants (smog or pollen)
  - chlorinated water

## WARNINGS

### DO NOT USE
- if you have open wounds in or near the eyes, and get medical help right away
- if solution changes color or becomes cloudy

### WHEN USING THIS PRODUCT
- remove contact lenses before using
- do not touch tip of container to any surface to avoid contamination
- replace cap after use

### STOP USE AND ASK A DOCTOR IF
- you experience eye pain, changes in vision, continued redness or irritation of the eye
- condition worsens or persists

**Keep out of reach of children.** If swallowed, get medical help or contact a Poison Control Center right away.

## DIRECTIONS
- for use with nozzle applicator
  - flush the affected eye(s) as needed
  - control the rate of flow of solution by pressure on the bottle

## WHEN USING AN EYE CUP
- rinse the cup with Bausch & Lomb Eye Wash immediately before each use
- avoid contamination of the rim and inside surfaces of the cup
- fill the cup half full with Bausch & Lomb Eye Wash Solution and apply the cup to the affected eye(s), pressing tightly to prevent spillage
- tilt the head backward
- open eyelids wide and rotate eyeball to thoroughly wash the eye
- rinse cup with clean water after each use
- replace cap after use

## OTHER INFORMATION
- store at room temperature
- keep tightly closed
- use before expiration date marked on the carton or bottle

## INACTIVE INGREDIENTS
boric acid, sodium borate and sodium chloride, hydrochloric acid and/or sodium hydroxide may be used to adjust pH, preservative added: edetate disodium 0.025% and sorbic acid 0.1%

## QUESTIONS OR COMMENTS
Toll-free product information or to report a serious side effect associated with use of this product
Call: 1-800-553-5340

---

# CHILDREN'S FEVER ALL (acetaminophen)
suppositories
Actavis

## DRUG FACTS

| Active ingredient (in each rectal suppository) | Purpose |
|---|---|
| Acetaminophen 120 mg | Pain reliever/fever reducer |

## USES
- temporarily:
  - reduces fever
  - relieves minor aches, pains, and headache

## WARNINGS
**Liver warning**
This product contains acetaminophen. Severe liver damage may occur if your child takes:
- more than 5 doses in 24 hours, which is the maximum daily amount
- with other drugs containing acetaminophen

**For rectal use only.**

### DO NOT USE
- if you are allergic to acetaminophen
- with any other drug containing acetaminophen (prescription or nonprescription)
- if you are not sure whether a drug contains acetaminophen, ask a doctor or pharmacist

### ASK A DOCTOR BELORE USE IF
- the child has liver disease
- the child is taking the blood thinning drug warfarin

### STOP USE AND ASK A DOCTOR IF
- fever lasts more than 3 days (72 hours), or recurs
- pain lasts more than 5 days or gets worse
- new symptoms occur
- redness or swelling is present in the painful area
- these may be signs of a serious condition.

**Keep out of reach of children.** If swallowed or in case of overdose, get medical help or contact a Poison Control Center right away. Quick medical attention is critical in case of overdose for adults and for children even if you do not notice any signs or symptoms.

## DIRECTIONS
- this product does not contain directions or warnings for adult use
- do not use more than directed
- remove wrapper
- carefully insert suppository well up into the rectum

| under 3 years | do not use unless directed by a doctor |
|---|---|
| 3 to 6 years | use 1 suppository every 4 to 6 hours (maximum of 5 doses in 24 hours) |

## OTHER INFORMATION
- store at 2-27°C (35-80°F)
- do not use if imprinted suppository wrapper is opened or damaged

## INACTIVE INGREDIENTS
glycerol monostearate, hydrogenated vegetable oil, polyoxyethylene stearate, polysorbate 80

## QUESTIONS OR COMMENTS
Call **1-800-432-8534** (select option no. 2) between 9 am and 4 pm EST, Monday-Friday.

---

# FEVER ALL JR STRENGTH (acetaminophen)
suppositories
Actavis

## DRUG FACTS

| Active ingredient (in each rectal suppository) | Purpose |
|---|---|
| Acetaminophen 325 mg | Pain reliever/fever reducer |

## USES
- temporarily:
  - reduces fever
  - relieves minor aches, pains, and headache

## WARNINGS
**Liver warning**
This product contains acetaminophen. Severe liver damage may occur if:
- a child 6 to 12 years takes more than 5 doses in 24 hours
- an adult or child 12 years and older takes more than 6 doses in 24 hours, which is the maximum daily amount
- taken with other drugs containing acetaminophen
- an adult takes 3 or more alcoholic drinks everyday while using this product

**For rectal use only.**

## DO NOT USE
- in children under 6 years
- if you are allergic to acetaminophen
- with any other drug containing acetaminophen (prescription or nonprescription)
- if you are not sure whether a drug contains acetaminophen, ask a doctor or pharmacist

## ASK A DOCTOR BEFORE USE IF
- you have liver disease
- you are taking the blood thinning drug warfarin

## STOP USE AND ASK A DOCTOR IF
- fever lasts more than 3 days (72 hours), or recurs
- pain gets worse or lasts more than 10 days

- new symptoms occur
- redness or swelling is present in the painful area

These may be signs of a serious condition.

**If pregnant or breastfeeding,** ask a health professional before use.

**Keep out of reach of children.** If swallowed or in case of overdose, get medical help or contact a Poison Control Center right away. Quick medical attention is critical in case of overdose for adults and for children even if you do not notice any signs or symptoms.

## DIRECTIONS
- do not use more than directed
- remove wrapper
- carefully insert suppository well up into the rectum

| under 6 years | do not use |
|---|---|
| 6 to 12 years | use 1 suppository every 4 to 6 hours, (maximum of 5 doses in 24 hours) |
| adults and children 12 years and older | use 2 suppositories every 4 to 6 hours, (maximum of 6 doses) |

## OTHER INFORMATION
- store at 2-27°C (35-80°F)
- do not use if imprinted suppository wrapper is opened or damaged

## INACTIVE INGREDIENTS
glycerol monostearate, hydrogenated vegetable oil, polyoxyethylene stearate, polysorbate 80

## QUESTIONS OR COMMENTS
Call **1-800-432-8534** (select option no. 2) between 9 am and 4 pm EST, Monday-Friday.

---

# FIBERCON (calcium polycarbophil) caplet
Wyeth Pharmaceutical Division of Wyeth Holdings Corporation

## DRUG FACTS

| Active ingredient (in each caplet) | Purpose |
|---|---|
| Calcium polycarbophil 625 mg equivalent to 500 mg polycarbophil | Bulk-forming laxative |

## USES
- relieves occasional constipation to help restore and maintain regularity
- this product generally produces bowel movement in 12 to 72 hours

## WARNINGS
**Choking**
Taking this product without adequate fluid may cause it to swell and block your throat or esophagus and may cause choking. Do not take this product if you have difficulty in swallowing. If you experience chest pain, vomiting, or difficulty in swallowing or breathing after taking this product, seek immediate medical attention.

## ASK A DOCTOR BEFORE USE IF YOU HAVE
- abdominal pain, nausea, or vomiting
- a sudden change in bowel habits that persists over a period of 2 weeks

## ASK A DOCTOR OR PHARMACIST BEFORE USE IF YOU ARE
- taking any other drug. Take this product 2 or more hours before or after other drugs. All laxatives may affect how other drugs work

## WHEN USING THIS PRODUCT
- do not use for more than 7 days unless directed by a doctor
- do not take more than 8 caplets in a 24-hour period unless directed by a doctor

## STOP USE AND ASK A DOCTOR IF
- rectal bleeding occurs or if you fail to have a bowel movement after use of this or any other laxative. These could be signs of a serious condition.

**Keep out of reach of children.** In case of overdose, get medical help or contact a Poison Control Center right away.

## DIRECTIONS
- take each dose of this product with at least 8 ounces (a full glass) of water or other fluid. Taking this product without enough liquid may cause choking. See Choking Warning
- FiberCon works naturally so continued use for one to three days is normally required to provide full benefit. Dosage may vary according to diet, exercise, previous laxative use or severity of constipation

| adults and children 12 years of age and over | 2 caplets once a day | up to 4 times a day |
| --- | --- | --- |
| children under 12 years | consult a physician | |

## OTHER INFORMATION
- each caplet contains: 140 mg calcium and 10 mg magnesium
- protect contents from moisture
- store at 20-25°C (68-77°F)

## INACTIVE INGREDIENTS
caramel, crospovidone, hypromellose, magnesium stearate, microcrystalline cellulose, polyethylene glycol, silicon dioxide, sodium lauryl sulfate

## QUESTIONS OR COMMENTS
Call weekdays from 9 AM to 5 PM EST at **1-800-282-8805**

---

# FISHERMAN'S FRIEND (menthol) lozenge
Lofthouse of Fleetwood Ltd.

## DRUG FACTS

| Active ingredients | Purpose |
| --- | --- |
| Menthol 10 mg | Cough suppressant/oral anesthetic |

## USES
- temporarily relieves
  - cough due to minor throat and bronchial irritation occurring with the common cold or inhaled irritants
  - occasional minor sore throat

## WARNINGS
### Sore throat warning
Severe or persistent sore throat or sore throat that occurs with high fever, headache, nausea and vomiting may be serious. Ask a doctor right away. Do not use more than 2 days or give to children under 2 years of age unless directed by a doctor.

## ASK A DOCTOR BEFORE USE IF YOU HAVE
- cough that occurs with too much phlegm (mucus)
- a persistent or chronic cough that lasts such as occurs with smoking, asthma, or emphysema

## WHEN USING THIS PRODUCT
- do not use more than directed

## STOP USE AND ASK A DOCTOR IF
- cough lasts more than 7 days, comes back, or occurs with fever, rash, or headache that lasts. These could be signs of a serious condition
- sore throat is severe, lasts more than 2 days, is accompanied or followed by fever, headache, rash, swelling, nausea, or vomiting

**If pregnant or breastfeeding,** ask a health professional before use.

**Keep out of reach of children.**

## DIRECTIONS

| adults and children 2 years of age and over | allow 1 lozenge to dissolve slowly in the mouth |
| --- | --- |
| | repeat every 2 hours as needed or as directed by a doctor |
| children under 2 years of age | ask a doctor |

## INACTIVE INGREDIENTS
capsicum, dextrin, eucalyptus oil, natural licorice, sugar, tragacanth

---

# FISHERMAN'S FRIEND MENTHOL COUGH SUPPRESSANT (menthol) lozenge
Lofthouse of Fleetwood, Ltd.

## DRUG FACTS

| Active ingredient (in each lozenge) | Purpose |
| --- | --- |
| Menthol 10 mg | Cough suppressant/oral anesthetic |

## USES
- temporarily relieves
  - cough due to minor throat and bronchial irritation occurring with the common cold or inhaled irritants
  - occasional minor sore throat

## WARNINGS
- do not take this product for persistent or chronic cough such as occurs with smoking, asthma, emphysema, or if cough is accompanied by excessive phlegm (mucus) unless directed by a doctor

### Sore throat warning
If sore throat is severe or persists more than 2 days accompanied by headache, nausea, and vomiting, contact a doctor right away. If sore mouth symptoms do not improve in 7 days, see your dentist or doctor promptly.

**WHEN USING THIS PRODUCT**
- do not use more than directed

**If pregnant or breastfeeding,** ask a health professional before use.

**Keep out of reach of children.**

## DIRECTIONS

| adults and children 2 to under 12 years of age | allow 1 lozenge to dissolve slowly in the mouth |
| --- | --- |
| | may be repeated every hour as needed for cough, or every 2 hours as needed for sore throat, or as directed by a doctor |
| children under 2 years of age | consult a doctor |

## INACTIVE INGREDIENTS

capsicum, dextrin, eucalyptus oil, natural licorice, sugar, tragacanth

---

# FISHERMAN'S FRIEND MENTHOL COUGH SUPPRESSANT SUGAR FREE CHERRY

(menthol) lozenge

Lofthouse of Fleetwood, Ltd.

## DRUG FACTS

| Active ingredient (in each lozenge) | Purpose |
| --- | --- |
| Menthol 6.9 mg | Cough suppressant/oral anesthetic |

## USES
- temporarily relieves:
  - cough due to minor throat and bronchial irritation occurring with the common cold or inhaled irritants
  - occasional minor sore throat

## WARNINGS
**Sore throat warning**
Severe or persistent sore throat or sore throat that occurs with high fever, headache, nausea, and vomiting may be serious. Ask a doctor right away. Do not use more than 2 days or give to children under 2 years of age unless directed by a doctor.

**ASK A DOCTOR BEFORE USE IF YOU HAVE**
- cough that occurs with too much phlegm (mucus)
- a persistent or chronic cough that lasts such as occurs with smoking, asthma, or emphysema

**WHEN USING THIS PRODUCT**
- do not use more than directed

**STOP USE AND ASK A DOCTOR IF**
- cough lasts more than 7 days, comes back, or occurs with fever, rash, or headache that lasts. These could be signs of a serious condition
- sore throat is severe, lasts more than 2 days, is accompanied or followed by fever, headache, rash, swelling, nausea, or vomiting

**If pregnant or breastfeeding,** ask a health professional before use.

**Keep out of reach of children.**

## DIRECTIONS

| adults and children 2 years of age and over | allow 1 lozenge to dissolve slowly in the mouth |
| --- | --- |
| | repeat every 2 hours as needed or as directed by a doctor |
| children under 2 years of age | ask a doctor |

## INACTIVE INGREDIENTS

sorbitol, flavor (including elderberry juice concentrate), magnesium stearate, sucralose, potassium acesulfame

---

# FLEET (mineral oil) enema

C.B. Fleet Company, Inc.

## DRUG FACTS

| Active ingredient (in each 118 mL delivered dose) | Purpose |
| --- | --- |
| Mineral oil 100% | Lubricant laxative |

## USES
- for relief of fecal impaction
- for relief of occasional constipation
- for removal of residue after barium administration

## WARNINGS
**For rectal use only.**

**ASK A DOCTOR BEFORE USING ANY LAXATIVE IF YOU HAVE**
- abdominal pain, nausea or vomiting
- a sudden change in bowel habits lasting more than 2 weeks
- already used a laxative for more than 1 week

**STOP USE AND ASK A DOCTOR IF YOU HAVE**
- rectal bleeding
- no bowel movement after use

These symptoms may indicate a serious condition.

**If pregnant or breastfeeding,** ask a health professional before use.

**Keep out of reach of children.** If swallowed, get medical help or contact a Poison Control Center right away.

## DIRECTIONS
- single daily dose

| adults and children 12 years and over | 1 bottle |
| --- | --- |
| children 2 to under 12 years | one-half bottle |
| children under 2 years | do not use |

## OTHER INFORMATION
- sodium free
- this product generally produces a bowel movement in 2-15 minutes
- carton sealed for safety. If seal with Fleet emblem on top or bottom flap is missing, do not use
- consult Physicians' Desk Reference for complete professional labeling

## QUESTIONS OR COMMENTS
Call **1-866-255-6960** or visit www.fleetlabs.com

## FLEXALL (menthol) gel
Chattem, Inc.

### DRUG FACTS

| Active ingredient | Purpose |
|---|---|
| Menthol 7% | Topical analgesic |

### USES
- temporarily relieves minor pain associated with:
  - arthritis
  - simple backache
  - muscle strains
  - muscle sprains
  - bruises
  - cramps

### WARNINGS
**For external use only.**

**Allergy alert**
**Do not use** if you are allergic to salicylates (including aspirin) unless directed by a doctor.

### WHEN USING THIS PRODUCT
- use only as directed
- do not bandage lightly or use a heating pad
- avoid contact with eyes or mucous membranes
- do not apply to wounds or damaged skin

### STOP USE AND ASK A DOCTOR IF
- condition worsens
- symptoms persist for more than 7 days or clear up and occur again within a few days
- redness is present
- irritation develops

**If pregnant or breastfeeding,** ask a health professional before use.

**Keep out of reach of children.** In case of accidental digestion, get medical help or contact a Poison Control Center right away.

### DIRECTIONS

| adults and children over 12 years | apply generously to affected area<br><br>massage into painful area until thoroughly absorbed into skin<br><br>repeat as necessary, but no more than 4 times daily |
|---|---|
| children 12 years or younger | ask a doctor |

### INACTIVE INGREDIENTS
allantoin, aloe barbadensis leaf juice, carbomer, eucalyptus globulus leaf oil, glycerin, mentha piperita (peppermint) oil, methyl saticylate, SD alcohol 40 (15% w/w). steareth-2, steareth-21 thymus vuigaris (thyme) oil, tocopheryl acetate, triethanolamine, water (234-95)

## FLEXALL MAX PAIN RELIEVING (menthol) gel
Chattem, Inc.

### DRUG FACTS

| Active ingredient | Purpose |
|---|---|
| Menthol 16% | Topical analgesic |

### USES
- temporarily relieves minor pain associated with:
  - arthritis
  - simple backache
  - muscle strains
  - sprains
  - bruises
  - cramps

### WARNINGS
**For external use only.**

**Allergy alert**
Do not use if you are allergic to salicylates (including aspirin) unless directed by a doctor.

### WHEN USING THIS PRODUCT
- use only as directed
- do not bandage tightly or use with a heating pad
- avoid contact with eyes and mucous membranes
- do not apply to wounds or damaged, broken or irritated skin

### STOP USE AND ASK A DOCTOR IF
- condition worsens
- redness is present
- irritation develops
- symptoms persist for more than 7 days or clear up and occur again within a few days

**If pregnant or breastfeeding,** ask a health professional before use.

**Keep out of reach of children.** If swallowed, get medical help or contact a Poison Control Center right away.

### DIRECTIONS

| adults and children over 12 years | apply generously to affected area<br><br>massage into painful area until thoroughly absorbed into skin<br><br>repeat as necessary, but no more than 3 to 4 times daily |
|---|---|
| children 12 years or younger | ask a doctor |

### INACTIVE INGREDIENTS
allantoin, aloe barbadensis leaf juice, carbomer, diisopropyl adipate, eucalyptus globulus leaf oil, glycerin, mentha piperita (peppermint) oil, methyl salicylate, SD alcohol 40 (15% w/w), steareth-2, steareth-21, thymus vulgaris (thyme) oil, tocopheryl acetate, triethanolamine, water (234-166)

# FLEXALL PLUS (menthol, camphor and methyl salicylate) gel
Chattem, Inc.

## DRUG FACTS

| Active ingredients | Purpose |
|---|---|
| Camphor 3.1%<br>Menthol 16%<br>Methyl salicylate 10% | Topical analgesic |

### USES
- temporarily relieves minor pain associated with:
  - arthritis
  - simple backache
  - muscle strains
  - muscle sprains
  - bruises
  - cramps

### WARNINGS
**For external use only.**

**Allergy alert**
Do not use if you are allergic to salicylates (including aspirin) unless directed by a doctor.

### WHEN USING THIS PRODUCT
- use only as directed
- do not bandage tightly
- avoid contact with eyes or mucous membranes
- do not apply to wounds or damaged skin

### STOP USE AND ASK A DOCTOR IF
- condition worsens or if symptoms persist for more than 7 days to clear up and occur again within a few days
- redness is present
- irritation develops

**If pregnant or breastfeeding,** ask a health professional before use.

**Keep out of reach of children.** If swallowed, get medical help or contact a Poison Control Center right away.

### DIRECTIONS

| adults and children over 12 years | apply generously to affected area |
|---|---|
| | massage into painful area until thoroughly absorbed into skin |
| | repeat as necessary, but no more than 4 times daily |
| children 12 years or younger | ask a doctor |

### INACTIVE INGREDIENTS
allantoin, aloe barbadensis leaf juice, carbomer, diisopropyl adipate, eucalyptus globulus leaf oil, glycerin, mentha piperita (peppermint) oil, SD alcohol 40 (15% w/w), steareth-2, steareth-21, thymus vulgaris (thyme) oil, tocopheryl acetate, triethanolamine, water (234-97)

# FUNGI NAIL (undecylenic acid) solution
Kramer Consumer Healthcare

## DRUG FACTS

| Active ingredient | Purpose |
|---|---|
| Undecylenic acid 25% | Anti-fungal |

### USES
- proven effective in the treatment of most athlete's foot (tinea pedis) and ringworm (tinea corporis)
- helps prevent most athlete's foot with daily use
- for effective relief of itching, burning and cracking

### WARNINGS
**For external use only.**

### DO NOT USE
- on children under 2 years of age unless directed by a doctor

### WHEN USING THIS PRODUCT
- avoid contact with eyes

### STOP USE AND ASK A DOCTOR IF
- irritation occurs
- there is no improvement within 4 weeks

**Keep this and all medication out of the reach of children.** In case of accidental ingestion, contact a physician, emergency medical care facility or Poison Control Center immediately for advice.

### DIRECTIONS
- clean affected area with soap and warm water and dry thoroughly
- apply a thin layer of Fungi-Nail Brand Anti-Fungal Solution over affected area twice daily (morning and night) or as directed by a doctor
- the brush application allows for easy application under nails and surrounding cuticle area
- wear well-fitting, ventilated shoes, and change shoes and socks at least once daily
- for athlete's foot pay special attention to spaces between the toes
- for athlete's foot and ringworm, use daily for 4 weeks. If condition persists longer, consult a doctor
- this product is not effective on the scalp or nails
- supervise children in the use of this product

### OTHER INFORMATION
- store at room temperature 15-30°C (59-86°F)
- protect from freezing, if freezing occurs warm to room temperature

### INACTIVE INGREDIENT
isopropyl palmitate

# FUNGICURE (tolnaftate) gel
Alva-Amco Pharmacal Companies, Inc.

## DRUG FACTS

| Active ingredient | Purpose |
|---|---|
| Tolnaftate 1% w/w | Antifungal |

### USES
- for the cure of most:
  - athlete's foot (tinea pedis)
  - ringworm (tinea corporis)
  - jock itch (tinea cruris)
- for the relief of:
  - itching
  - scaling
  - cracking
  - burning
  - redness
  - soreness
  - irritation
  - and discomforts which may accompany these conditions

Proven effective in the prevention of most athlete's foot with daily use. Clears up most athlete's foot infection and with daily use helps keep it from coming back.

### WARNINGS
**For external use only.**

### ASK A DOCTOR BEFORE USE
- on children under 2 years of age

### WHEN USING THIS PRODUCT
- avoid contact with the eyes

### STOP USE AND ASK A DOCTOR IF
- irritation occurs
- there is no improvement within 4 weeks (2 weeks for jock itch)

**Keep out of reach of children.** If swallowed, get medical help or contact a Poison Control Center right away.

### DIRECTIONS
- read all package directions and warnings before using
- use only as directed
- clean the affected area with soap and warm water and dry thoroughly
- apply a thin layer of Fungicure Gel over the affected area twice daily (morning and night), or as directed by a doctor
- for athlete's foot: pay special attention to spaces between toes; wear well fitting, ventilated shoes and change shoes and socks at least once daily
- for athlete's foot and ringworm, use daily for 4 weeks; for jock itch, use daily for 2 weeks
- supervise children in the use of this product
- persons under 18 years of age or those with highly sensitive or allergic skin should use only as directed by a doctor
- this product is not effective on the scalp or nails

### OTHER INFORMATION
- keep container tightly closed when not in use
- store away from excessive heat and cold

### INACTIVE INGREDIENTS
aloe vera gel, hydroxypropyl cellulose, isopropyl alcohol, polyethylene glycol, propylene glycol, vitamin E. tolnaftate in fungicure gel is widely recognized by doctors to be an anti-fungal agent effective against fungi such as e. floccosum, t mentagrophytes and t. rubrum, which are known to cause topical infections of the body, hands and feet

# FUNGICURE (undecylenic acid) liquid
Alva-Amco Pharmacal Companies, Inc.

## DRUG FACTS

| Active ingredient | Purpose |
|---|---|
| Undecylenic acid, 25% w/v | Antifungal |

### USES
- for the cure of most:
  - ringworm (tinea corporis)
  - athlete's foot (tinea pedis)
- for relief of:
  - itching
  - scaling
  - cracking
  - burning
  - redness
  - soreness
  - irritation
  - discomforts which may accompany these conditions

### WARNINGS
**For external use only.**

### ASK A DOCTOR BEFORE USE
- on children under 2 years of age

### WHEN USING THIS PRODUCT
- avoid contact with the eyes

### STOP USE AND ASK A DOCTOR IF
- irritation occurs
- there is no improvement within 4 weeks

**Keep out of reach of children.** If swallowed, get medical help or contact a Poison Control Center right away.

### DIRECTIONS
- read all package directions and warnings before using
- use only as directed
- clean the affected area with soap and warm water and dry thoroughly
- apply a thin layer of Fungicure Liquid over the affected area twice daily (morning and night), or as directed by a doctor
- this product is not effective on scalp or nails
- for athlete's foot, pay special attention to spaces between toes; wear well fitting, ventilated shoes and change shoes and socks at least once daily
- for athlete's foot and ringworm, use daily for 4 weeks. If condition persists longer, consult a doctor
- intended for use by normally healthy adults only
- persons under 18 years of age or those with highly sensitive or allergic skin should use only as directed by a doctor
- supervise children in the use of this product

### OTHER INFORMATION
- may be applied to cuticles, around nail edges and under nail tips where reachable with its applicator brush. This product is not intended to, nor will it, penetrate hard nail surfaces
- while not all finger and toe fungal infections are curable with OTC topical medications, if you see improvement within 4 weeks of use, you may continue to use Fungicure until satisfactory results are obtained
- You may report serious side effects to the phone number provided under "Questions or Comments"

## INACTIVE INGREDIENTS

aloe vera gel, fragrance, hypromellose, isopropyl alcohol (70% v/v), purified water and vitamin E

## QUESTIONS OR COMMENTS

Call **1-800-792-2582**

# FUNGI-NAIL DOUBLE STRENGTH (undecylenic acid ) liquid

Kramer Laboratories

## DRUG FACTS

| Active ingredient | Purpose |
|---|---|
| Undecylenic acid 25% | Antifungal |

## USES

- treatment of most athlete's foot (tinea pedis) and ringworm (tinea corporis)
- helps prevent most athlete's foot with daily use
- effective relief of itching, burning and cracking

## WARNINGS

**For external use only.** In case of accidental ingestion, contact a physician, emergency medical care facility, or Poison Control Center immediately for advice.

## DO NOT USE

- on children under 2 years of age unless directed by a doctor

## WHEN USING THIS PRODUCT

- avoid contact with eyes

## STOP USE AND ASK A DOCTOR IF

- irritation occurs
- there is no improvement within 4 weeks

## DIRECTIONS

- clean affected area with soap and warm water and dry thoroughly
- apply a thin layer of Fungi-Nail Brand Anti-Fungal Solution over affected area twice daily (morning and night) or as directed by a doctor
- the brush applicator allows for easy application under nails and surrounding cuticle area
- wear well-fitting, ventilated shoes, and change shoes and socks at least once daily
- for athlete's foot pay special attention to spaces between the toes
- for athlete's foot and ringworm, use daily for 4 weeks. If condition persists longer, consult a doctor
- this product is not effective on the scalp or nails
- supervise children in the use of this product

## INACTIVE INGREDIENTS

isopropyl palmitate

# FUNGICURE FOR JOCK ITCH (sepia) soap

Alva-Amco Pharmacal Companies, Inc.

## DRUG FACTS

| Active ingredient | Purpose |
|---|---|
| Sepia 12× | Antifungal treatment |

## USES

- for the treatment of most:
  - jock itch (tinea cruris)
  - ringworm (tinea corporis)
  - athlete's foot (tinea pedis)
- for relief of:
  - itching
  - scaling
  - cracking
  - burning
  - redness
  - soreness
  - irritation
  - discomforts which may accompany these conditions.

## WARNINGS
**For external use only.**

## ASK A DOCTOR BEFORE USE

- on children under 2 years of age

## WHEN USING THIS PRODUCT

- avoid contact with the eyes
- if contact occurs rinse thoroughly with water

## STOP USE AND ASK A DOCTOR IF

- irritation occurs
- there is no improvement within 2 weeks (4 weeks for ringworm and athlete's foot)

**Keep out of reach of children.** If swallowed, get medical help or contact a Poison Control Center right away.

## DIRECTIONS

- read all package directions and warnings before using
- use only as directed
- clean the affected area with Fungicure Anti-Fungal Soap for jock itch and ringworm and warm water, rinse and dry thoroughly
- for best results, leave on for 1-2 minutes before rinsing and drying
- use twice daily (morning and night), or as directed by a doctor
- for jock itch, use daily for 2 weeks
- for ringworm and athlete's foot, use daily for 4 weeks
- for athlete's foot: pay special attention to spaces between the toes; wear well-fitting, ventilated shoes, and change shoes and socks at least once daily
- supervise children in the use of this product
- persons under 18 years of age or those with highly sensitive or allergic skin should use only as directed by a doctor
- this product is not effective on the scalp or nails

## OTHER INFORMATION

- You may report serious side effects to the phone number provided under "Questions or Comments"

## INACTIVE INGREDIENTS

lauramidopropyl betaine, panthenol, phospholipid EFA, purified water, sodium chloride, sodium C14 - 16 olefin sulfonate, tea tree oil

## Storage

- keep tightly closed when not in use
- store away from excessive heat or cold

## QUESTIONS OR COMMENTS

Call **1-800-792-2582**

# FUNGICURE MANICURE PEDICURE
(clotrimazole) liquid

Alva-Amco Pharmacal Companies, Inc.

## DRUG FACTS

| Active ingredient | Purpose |
|---|---|
| Clotrimazole, 1% w/v | Antifungal |

## USES
- for the cure of most:
  - ringworm (tinea corporis)
  - athlete's foot (tinea pedis)
- for relief of:
  - itching
  - scaling
  - cracking
  - burning
  - redness
  - soreness
  - irritation
  - discomfort which may accompany these conditions
- inhibits the growth and reproduction of fungal cells

## WARNINGS
**For external use only.**

## ASK A DOCTOR BEFORE USE
- on children under 2 years of age

## WHEN USING THIS PRODUCT
- avoid contact with the eyes

## STOP USE AND ASK A DOCTOR IF
- irritation occurs
- there is no improvement within 4 weeks

**Keep out of reach of children.** If swallowed, get medical help or contact a Poison Control Center right away.

## DIRECTIONS
- read all package directions and warnings before use
- use only as directed
- clean the affected area with soap and warm water and dry thoroughly
- apply a thin layer of Fungicure Manicure & Pedicure Liquid over the affected area twice daily (morning and night), or as directed by a doctor
- this product is not effective on the scalp or nails
- avoid applying to severely cracked or irritated areas
- for athlete's foot: pay special attention to the spaces between toes; wear well fitting, ventilated shoes, and change shoes and socks at least once daily
- for athlete's foot and ringworm, use daily for 4 weeks. If condition persists longer, consult a doctor
- intended for use by normally healthy adults only
- persons under 18 years of age or those with highly sensitive or allergic skin should use only as directed by a doctor
- supervise children in the use of this product

## OTHER INFORMATION
- Fungicure may be applied to cuticles, around nail edges and under nail tips where reachable with its applicator brush. This product is not intended to, nor will it, penetrate hard intact nail surfaces
- while not all finger and toe fungal infections are curable with OTC topical medications, if you see improvement within 4 weeks of use, you may continue to use Fungicure until satisfactory results are obtained

- you may report serious side effects to the phone number provided under "Questions or Comments"

## Storage
- keep tightly closed when not in use
- store away from excessive heat and cold

## INACTIVE INGREDIENT
isopropyl alcohol

## QUESTIONS OR COMMENTS
Call **1-800-792-2582**

# FUNGICURE MAXIMUM STRENGTH
(undecylenic acid) liquid

Alva-Amco Pharmacal Companies, Inc.

## DRUG FACTS

| Active ingredient | Purpose |
|---|---|
| Undecylenic acid 25% w/v | Antifungal |

## USES
- for the cure of most:
  - ringworm (tinea corporis)
  - athlete's foot (tinea pedis)
- for relief of:
  - itching
  - scaling
  - cracking
  - burning
  - redness
  - soreness
  - irritation
  - discomfort which may accompany these conditions

## WARNINGS
**For external use only.**

## ASK A DOCTOR BEFORE USE
- on children under 2 years of age

## WHEN USING THIS PRODUCT
- avoid contact with the eyes

## STOP USE AND ASK A DOCTOR IF
- irritation occurs
- there is no improvement within 4 weeks

**Keep out of reach of children.** If swallowed, get medical help or contact a Poison Control Center right away.

## DIRECTIONS
- read all package directions and warnings before using
- use only as directed
- clean the affected area with soap and warm water and dry thoroughly
- apply a thin layer of Fungicure Liquid over the affected area twice daily (morning and night), or as directed by a doctor
- this product is not effective on scalp or nails
- for athlete's foot, pay special attention to spaces between toes; wear well fitting, ventilated shoes and change shoes and socks at least once daily
- for athlete's foot and ringworm, use daily for 4 weeks. If condition persists longer, consult a doctor
- intended for use by normally healthy adults only
- persons under 18 years of age or those with highly sensitive or allergic skin should use only as directed by a doctor
- supervise children in the use of this product

## OTHER INFORMATION
- Fungicure may be applied to cuticles, around nail edges and under nail tips where reachable with its applicator brush. This product is not intended to, nor will it, penetrate hard nail surfaces
- while not all finger and toe fungal infections are curable with OTC topical medications, if you see improvement within 4 weeks of use, you may continue to use Fungicure until satisfactory results are obtained
- you may report serious side effects to the phone number provided under "Questions or Comments"

## INACTIVE INGREDIENTS
aloe vera gel, fragrance, hypromellose, isopropyl alcohol (70% v/v), purified water and vitamin E

## QUESTIONS OR COMMENTS
Call **1-800-792-2582** or visit fungicure.com

---

## FUNGOID TINCTURE (miconazole nitrate) liquid
Pedinol Pharmacal, Inc.

### DRUG FACTS

| Active ingredient | Purpose |
|---|---|
| Miconazole nitrate 2% USP | Proven to cure fungal infection of the skin around the nail area |

## USE
- cures most athlete's foot (*tinea pedis*), and ringworm (*tinea corporis*).

## WARNINGS

## DO NOT USE
- on children under 2 years of age except under the advice and supervision of a physician.
- avoid contact with eyes.
- if irritation occurs or if there is no improvement within four weeks, discontinue use and consult your physician or pharmacist.
- do not use if you are known to be sensitive to any of the ingredients in this product.

**For external use only.**

**Keep out of the reach of children.** In case of accidental ingestion, seek professional assistance or contact a Poison Control Center immediately.

## DIRECTIONS
- cleanse and dry affected areas
- apply a thin application twice a day (morning and night) on skin under nails and surrounding cuticle area or as recommended by your doctor or pharmacist

## OTHER INFORMATION
- store at controlled room temperature 15-30°C (59-86°F)
- protect from freezing. If freezing occurs, warm to room temperature
- supervise children in the use of this product
- for fungal infection of the skin around the nail area, if condition persists, consult a doctor
- this product is not effective on the scalp or nails

## INACTIVE INGREDIENTS
phenylcarbinol, isopropyl alcohol (30%), water, acetic acid (glacial), laureth-4

---

## GAS X CHEWABLES EXTRA STRENGTH
(simethicone) tablet

Novartis Consumer Healthcare, Inc.

### DRUG FACTS

| Active ingredient (in each tablet) | Purpose |
|---|---|
| Simethicone 125 mg | Antigas |

## USE
- for the relief of:
  - pressure and bloating commonly referred to as gas

## WARNINGS
**Keep out of reach of children.**

## DIRECTIONS

| adults | chew 1 or 2 tablets as needed after meals and at bedtime |
|---|---|
| | do not exceed 4 tablets in 24 hours except under the advice and supervision of a physician |

## OTHER INFORMATION
- each tablet contains: calcium 45 mg
- store at controlled room temperature 20-25°C (68-77°F)
- protect from moisture

## INACTIVE INGREDIENTS
calcium phosphate tribasic, colloidal silicon dioxide, D&C red no. 30 aluminum lake, dextrose, flavors, maltodextrin, propylene glycol, soy protein isolate

## QUESTIONS OR COMMENTS
Call **1-800-452-0051**

---

## GAVISCON (aluminum hydroxide and magnesium carbonate) liquid
GlaxoSmithKline Consumer Healthcare LP

### DRUG FACTS

| Active ingredient | Purpose |
|---|---|
| **(in each 15 mL tablespoonful) Regular Strength** Aluminum hydroxide 95 mg  Magnesium carbonate 358 mg | Antacid |
| **(in each 5 mL teaspoonful) Extra Strength** Aluminum hydroxide 254 mg  Magnesium carbonate 237.5 mg | |

## USES
- relieves:
  - heartburn
  - acid indigestion
  - sour stomach
  - upset stomach associated with these symptoms

## WARNINGS

## DO NOT USE
- if you have kidney disease

## ASK A DOCTOR OR PHARMACIST BEFORE USE IF YOU ARE
- taking a prescription drug. Antacids may interact with certain prescription drugs
- if you are on a sodium-restricted diet

## WHEN USING THIS PRODUCT (REGULAR STRENGTH)
- do not take more than 8 tablespoonfuls in 24 hours
- do not use the maximum dosage for more than 2 weeks
- laxative effect may occur

## WHEN USING THIS PRODUCT (EXTRA STRENGTH)
- do not take more than 16 teaspoonfuls in 24 hours
- do not use the maximum dosage for more than 2 weeks
- laxative effect may occur

**Keep out of reach of children.** In case of overdose, get medical help or contact a Poison Control Center right away.

## DIRECTIONS (REGULAR STRENGTH)
- shake well
- take 1-2 tablespoonfuls four times a day or as directed by a doctor
- take after meals and at bedtime
- dispense product only by spoon or other measuring device

## DIRECTIONS (EXTRA STRENGTH)
- shake well
- take 2-4 teaspoonfuls four times a day or as directed by a doctor
- take after meals and at bedtime
- dispense product only by spoon or other measuring device

## OTHER INFORMATION (REGULAR STRENGTH)
- each tablespoon (15 mL) contains: magnesium 115 mg, sodium 52 mg
- store at up to 25°C (77°F); avoid freezing
- keep tightly closed

## OTHER INFORMATION (EXTRA STRENGTH)
- each teaspoon (5 mL) contains: magnesium 80 mg, sodium 14 mg
- store at up to 25°C (77°F); avoid freezing
- keep tightly closed

## INACTIVE INGREDIENTS (REGULAR STRENGTH)
benzyl alcohol, D&C yellow no. 10, edetate disodium, FD&C blue no. 1, flavor, glycerin, saccharin sodium, sodium alginate, sorbitol solution, water, xanthan gum

## INACTIVE INGREDIENTS (EXTRA STRENGTH)
benzyl alcohol, edetate disodium, flavor, glycerin, saccharin sodium, simethicone emulsion, sodium alginate, sorbitol solution, water, xanthan gum

## QUESTIONS OR COMMENTS
Call toll-free (English/Spanish) **1-888-367-6471** weekdays

---

# GENTEAL MILD (hypromellose) liquid
Novartis Pharmaceuticals Corporation

## DRUG FACTS

| Active ingredient | Purpose |
|---|---|
| Hypromellose (0.2%) | Lubricant |

## USES
- relieves dryness of the eye
- temporarily relieves discomfort due to minor irritations of the eye or from exposure to wind or sun
- as a protectant against further irritation

## WARNINGS

### DO NOT USE
- if solution changes color or becomes cloudy

### WHEN USING THIS PRODUCT
- do not touch tip of container to any surface
- replace cap after using

### STOP USE AND ASK A DOCTOR IF
- you experience any of the following:
  - eye pain
  - changes in vision
  - continued redness or irritation of the eye
  - condition worsens or persists for more than 72 hours

**Keep out of reach of children.** If swallowed, get medical help or contact a Poison Control Center right away.

## DIRECTIONS
- put 1 or 2 drops in the affected eye(s) as needed

## OTHER INFORMATION
- store between 15-30°C (59-86°F)

## INACTIVE INGREDIENTS
boric acid, calcium chloride dihydrate, GenAqua (sodium perborate), phosphonic acid, potassium chloride, purified water, sodium chloride

## QUESTIONS OR COMMENTS
Call toll-free **1-866-393-6336**, weekdays, 8:30 AM-5:00 PM EST. Serious side effects associated with use of this product may be reported to this number.

---

# GENTEAL MILD TO MODERATE (hypromellose) liquid
Novartis Pharmaceuticals Corporation

## DRUG FACTS

| Active ingredient | Purpose |
|---|---|
| Hypromellose (0.3%) | Lubricant |

## USES
- relieves dryness of the eye
- temporarily relieves discomfort due to minor irritations of the eye or from exposure to wind or sun
- as a protectant against further irritation

## WARNINGS

### DO NOT USE
- if solution changes color or becomes cloudy

### WHEN USING THIS PRODUCT
- do not touch tip of container to any surface
- replace cap after using

### STOP USE AND ASK A DOCTOR IF
- you experience any of the following:
  - eye pain
  - changes in vision
  - continued redness or irritation of the eye
  - condition worsens or persists more than 72 hours

**Keep out of reach of children.** If swallowed, get medical help or contact a Poison Control Center right away.

## DIRECTIONS
- put 1 or 2 drops in the affected eye(s) as needed

## OTHER INFORMATION
- store between 15-30°C (59-86°F)

## INACTIVE INGREDIENTS
boric acid, genaqua (sodium perborate), phosphonic acid, potassium chloride, purified water, sodium chloride

## QUESTIONS OR COMMENTS
Call toll-free **1-866-393-6336**, weekdays, 8:30 AM-5:00 PM EST. Serious side effects associated with use of this product may be reported to this number.

---

# GENTEAL MODERATE TO SEVERE GEL DROPS (hypromellose) gel
Novartis Pharmaceuticals Corporation

## DRUG FACTS

| Active ingredients | Purpose |
|---|---|
| Carboxymethylcellulose sodium (0.25%) | Lubricant |
| Hypromellose (0.3%) | |

## USES
- relieves dryness of the eyes
- temporarily relieves discomfort due to minor irritation of the eye or from exposure to wind or sun
- as a protectant against further irritation

## WARNINGS

### DO NOT USE
- if solution changes color or becomes cloudy

### WHEN USING THIS PRODUCT
- do not touch tip of container to any surface
- replace cap after using

### STOP USE AND ASK A DOCTOR IF
- you experience any of the following:
  - eye pain
  - changes in vision
  - continued redness or irritation of the eye
  - condition worsens or persists more than 72 hours

**Keep out of reach of children.** If swallowed, get medical help or contact a Poison Control Center right away.

## DIRECTIONS
- put 1 or 2 drops in the affected eye(s) as needed

## OTHER INFORMATION
- store between 15-30°C (59-86°F)

## INACTIVE INGREDIENTS
boric acid, calcium chloride dihydrate, citric acid monohydrate, genaqua (sodium perborate), magnesium chloride hexahydrate, phosphonic acid, potassium chloride, purified water, sodium chloride

## QUESTIONS OR COMMENTS
Call toll-free **1-866-393-6336**, weekdays, 8:30 AM-5:00 PM EST. Serious side effects associated with use of this product may be reported to this number.

---

# GENTEAL NIGHT-TIME PM (mineral oil, white petrolatum) ointment
Novartis Pharmaceuticals Corporation

## DRUG FACTS

| Active ingredients | Purpose |
|---|---|
| Mineral oil (15%) | Lubricant |
| White petrolatum (85%) | |

## USES
- relieves dryness of the eye
- temporarily relieves discomfort due to minor irritations of the eye or from exposure to wind or sun
- as a protectant against further irritation

## WARNINGS

### WHEN USING THIS PRODUCT
- do not touch tip of container to any surface
- replace cap after using

### STOP USE AND ASK A DOCTOR IF
- you experience any of the following:
  - eye pain
  - changes in vision
  - continued redness or irritation of the eye
  - condition worsens or persists for more than 72 hours

**Keep out of reach of children.** If swallowed, get medical help or contact a Poison Control Center right away.

## DIRECTIONS
- pull down the lower lid of the affected eye(s) and apply a small amount (¼ inch) of ointment to the inside of the eyelid(s)
- apply one or more times daily or as directed by a doctor

## OTHER INFORMATION
- store between 15-30°C (59-86°F)
- keep tightly closed

## QUESTIONS OR COMMENTS
Call toll-free **1-866-393-6336,** weekdays, 8:30 AM-5:00 PM EST. Serious side effects associated with use of this product may be reported to this number.

---

# GENTEAL SEVERE (hypromellose) gel
Novartis Pharmaceuticals Corporation

## DRUG FACTS

| Active ingredient | Purpose |
|---|---|
| Hypromellose (0.3%) | Lubricant |

## USES
- relieves dryness of the eye
- temporarily relieves discomfort due to minor irritations of the eye or from exposure to wind or sun
- as a protectant against further irritations

## WARNINGS

### DO NOT USE IF
- gel changes color or becomes cloudy

## WHEN USING THIS PRODUCT
- do not touch tip of container to any surface
- replace cap after using

## STOP USE AND ASK A DOCTOR IF
- you experience any of the following
  - eye pain
  - changes in vision
  - continued redness or irritation of the eye
  - condition worsens or persists for more than 72 hours

**Keep out of reach of children.** If swallowed, get medical help or contact a Poison Control Center right away.

## DIRECTIONS
- put 1 or 2 drops in the affected eye(s) as needed

## OTHER INFORMATION
- store between 15-30°C (59-86°F)

## INACTIVE INGREDIENTS
carbopol 980, GenAqua (sodium perborate), phosphonic acid, purified water, sodium hydroxide, sorbitol

## QUESTIONS OR COMMENTS
Call toll-free **1-866-393-6336**, weekdays, 8:30 AM-5:00 PM EST. Serious side effects associated with the use of this product may be reported to this number.

---

# GLY-OXIDE (carbamide peroxide) liquid
GlaxoSmithKline Consumer Healthcare LP

## DRUG FACTS

| Active ingredient | Purpose |
|---|---|
| Carbamide peroxide 10% | Oral debriding agent<br>Oral wound cleanser |

## USES
- temporary use in cleansing:
  - canker sore
  - minor wounds or gum inflammation resulting from minor dental procedures, dentures, orthodontic appliances, accidental injury, or other irritations of the mouth and gums
  - aids in the removal of phlegm, mucus, or other secretions associated with occasional sore mouth

## WARNINGS

## DO NOT USE THIS PRODUCT
- for more than 7 days unless directed by a dentist or doctor

## WHEN USING THIS PRODUCT:
- do not swallow
- avoid contact with eyes

## STOP USE AND ASK A DOCTOR IF
- swelling, rash or fever develops
- irritation, pain, or redness persists or worsens
- sore mouth symptoms do not improve in 7 days

**Keep out of the reach of children.** If an excessive amount of product is accidentally swallowed, get medical help or contact a Poison Control Center right away.

## DIRECTIONS
- replace tip on bottle when not in use

| adults and children 2 years and older | use up to 4 times daily after meals and at bedtime or as directed by dentist or doctor |
|---|---|
| For direct application | do not dilute<br>apply several drops directly from bottle onto affected area<br>spit out after 2 to 3 minutes |
| As a mouthwash | place 10 to 20 drops onto tongue<br>mix with saliva<br>swish around in the mouth over the affected area for at least 1 minute and spit out |
| children under 12 years | should be supervised in the use of this product |
| children under 2 years | consult a dentist or physician |

## OTHER INFORMATION
- protect from excessive heat and direct sunlight

## INACTIVE INGREDIENTS
citric acid, flavor, glycerin, propylene glycol, sodium lauroyl sarcosinate, sodium stannate, water

## QUESTIONS OR COMMENTS
Call toll-free **1-866-844-2797** (English/Spanish) weekdays or visit www.glyoxide.com

---

# GOLD BOND ANTI ITCH (menthol and pramoxine hydrochloride) cream
Chattem, Inc.

## DRUG FACTS

| Active ingredients | Purpose |
|---|---|
| Menthol 1% | Anti-itch |
| Pramoxine hydrochloride 1% | Pain relief |

## USES
- for temporary relief of pain and itching associated with:
  - minor skin irritations
  - minor cuts
  - minor burns
  - minor sunburns
  - rashes due to poison ivy, poison oak or poison sumac
  - scrapes
  - insect bites

## WARNINGS
**For external use only.**

## DO NOT USE ON
- deep or puncture wounds
- animals bites
- serious burns
- large areas of the body

## WHEN USING THIS PRODUCT
- do not get into eyes or nose
- not for prolonged use

## STOP USE AND ASK A DOCTOR IF
- condition worsens

- symptoms last more than 7 days or clear up and occur again within a few days
- if redness, irritation, swelling or pain persists or increases

**Keep out of reach of children.** If swallowed, get medical help or contact a Poison Control Center immediately.

## DIRECTIONS

| adults and children 2 years and older | apply to affected area up to 3 or 4 times daily |
|---|---|
| children under 2 years | consult a doctor |

## INACTIVE INGREDIENTS

water, propylene glycol, petrolatum, stearyl alcohol, aloe barbadensis leaf juice, sodium acrylates copolymer, steareth-21, mineral oil, steareth-2, tocopheryl acetate, thymol, eucalyptol, methyl salicylate, PPG-1 trideceth-6, diazolidinyl urea, disodium EDTA, triethanolamine, iodopropynyl butylcarbamate (240-022)

---

# GOLD BOND INTENSIVE HEALING ANTI ITCH SKIN PROTECTANT (dimethicone and pramoxine hydrochloride) cream

Chattem, Inc.

## DRUG FACTS

| Active ingredient | Purpose |
|---|---|
| Dimethicone 6% | Skin protectant |
| Pramoxine hydrochloride 1% | Anti-itch |

## USES

- for temporary relief of pain and itching associated with:
  - minor skin irritations
  - minor cuts
  - minor burns
  - minor sunburns
  - rashes due to poison ivy, poison oak or poison sumac
  - scrapes
  - insect bites
  - temporarily protects and helps relieve chapped or cracked skin

## WARNINGS
**For external use only.**

## DO NOT USE ON
- deep or puncture wounds
- animal bites
- serious burns
- large areas of the body

## WHEN USING THIS PRODUCT
- do not get into eyes or nose
- not for prolonged use

## STOP USE AND ASK A DOCTOR IF
- condition worsens
- symptoms last for more than 7 days or clear up and occur again within a few days
- if redness, irritation, swelling or pain persists or increases

**Keep out of reach of children.** If swallowed, get medical help or contact a Poison Control Center immediately.

## DIRECTIONS

| adults and children 2 years and older | apply to affected area up to 3 or 4 times daily |
|---|---|
| children under 2 years | consult a doctor |

## INACTIVE INGREDIENTS

water, glycerin, petrolatum, jojoba esters, cetyl alcohol, aloe barbadensis leaf juice, stearyl alcohol, distearyldimonium chloride, cetearyl alcohol, steareth-21, steareth-2, propylene glycol, chamomilla recutita (matricaria) flower extract, polysorbate 60, stearamidopropyl PG-dimonium chloride phosphate, methyl gluceth-20, tocopheryl acetate, magnesium ascorbyl phosphate, panthenol, retinyl palmitate, EDTA, potassium hydroxide, diazolidinyl urea, methylparaben, propylparaben, hydrolyzed jojoba esters, glyceryl stearate (283-069)

## QUESTIONS OR COMMENTS
visit www.goldbond.com

---

# GOLD BOND MEDICATED FOOT (menthol) spray

Chattem, Inc.

## DRUG FACTS

| Active ingredient | Purpose |
|---|---|
| Menthol (to deliver 1% concentration) | Anti-itch |

## USES

- temporarily relieves the pain and itch associated with minor skin irritations on the foot
- provides maximum strength itch relief
- absorbs excess moisture
- helps control foot odor and odor-causing bacteria
- cools and soothes irritated skin

## WARNINGS
**For external use only.**
- avoid spraying in eyes or on mucous membranes

**Flammable mixture**
- contents under pressure
- do not puncture or incinerate
- do not use near fire or flame
- do not expose to heat or temperatures above 49°C (120°F)
- use only as directed

## STOP USE AND ASK A DOCTOR IF
- condition worsens
- symptoms do not get better within 7 days

**Keep out of reach of children.**

## DIRECTIONS

| adults and children 2 years and older | apply freely up to 3 to 4 times daily |
| | thoroughly wash and dry feet |
| | shake well |
| | hold 6 inches from feet and spray generously over feet, between toes, on bottoms of feet, and in socks and shoes |
| | use daily |
| children under 2 years | ask a doctor |

## OTHER INFORMATION
• store at room temperature 15-30°C (59-86°F)

## INACTIVE INGREDIENTS
isobutane, propane, alcohol SD-40B (12% w/w), aluminum starch octenylsuccinate, talc, sodium bicarbonate, benzethonium chloride, eucalyptus globules leaf oil, isopropyl myristate, menthe piperita (peppermint) oil, propylene carbonate, sorbitan oleate, stearylkonium hectorite. (227-078)

---

# GOLD BOND PAIN RELIEVING FOOT ROLL-ON (menthol) liquid
Chattem, Inc.

## DRUG FACTS

| Active ingredient | Purpose |
| --- | --- |
| Menthol 16% | Topical analgesic |

## USES
• temporarily relieves minor foot and ankle aches and pains associated with:
  • arthritis
  • muscle aches
  • strains
  • sprains
  • muscle and joint pain

## WARNINGS
For external use only.

## WHEN USING THIS PRODUCT
• use only as directed
• do not bandage tightly or use with a heating pad
• avoid contact with eyes and mucous membranes
• do not apply to wounds or damaged, broken or irritated skin
• a transient burning sensation may occur upon application but generally disappears in several days

## STOP USE AND ASK A DOCTOR IF
• condition worsens
• symptoms persist for more than 7 days or clear up and occur again within a few days
• redness is present
• irritation develops

---

**Flammable. Keep away from fire or flame.**

**If pregnant or breastfeeding,** ask a health professional before use.

**Keep out of reach of children.** If swallowed, get medical help or contact a Poison Control Center right away.

## DIRECTIONS

| adults and children over 12 years | apply generously to affected area not more than 3 to 4 times daily |
| | massage gently for 30 seconds or until fully absorbed |
| | if product comes into contact with hands, wash with soap and water |
| children under 12 years | ask a doctor |

## INACTIVE INGREDIENTS
acrylates/C10-30 alkyl acrylate crosspolymer, capsaicin, glycerin, isopropyl myristate, propylene glycol, SD alcohol 40 (30%), triethanolamine, water (245-256)

---

# GOLD BOND ULTIMATE HAND SANITIZER MOISTURIZER (benzethonium chloride) lotion
Chattem, Inc.

## DRUG FACTS

| Active ingredient | Purpose |
| --- | --- |
| Benzethonium chloride 0.2% | Antimicrobial |

## USES
• hand sanitizer to decrease bacteria on the skin
• recommended for repeated use

## WARNINGS
For external use only.

## WHEN USING THIS PRODUCT
• do not use in or near eyes. In case of contact, rinse eyes thoroughly with water

## STOP USE AND ASK A DOCTOR IF
• irritation or redness develops and persists for more than 72 hours

**Keep out of reach of children.** If swallowed, get medical help or contact a Poison Control Center right away.

## DIRECTIONS
• wet hands thoroughly with product
• briskly rub hands together until absorbed
• apply to hands as needed
• supervise children under 6 years of age in the use of this product

## INACTIVE INGREDIENTS
water, glycerin, hydroxyethyl urea, behenyl alcohol, dimethicone, distearyldimonium chloride, jojoba esters, petrolatum, aloe barbadensis leaf juice, methyl gluceth-20, glyceryl laurate, behentrimonium methosulfate, cocamidopropyl PG-dimonium chloride phosphate, cetyl alcohol, tocopheryl acetate, butyrospermum parkii (shea butter) extract, cholecalciferol, phytonadione, ascorbic acid, zea mays (corn) oil, panthenol, chamomilla recutita (matricaria) flower extract, butylene glycol, potassium chloride, ethylhexylglycerin, steareth-21, DMDM

hydantoin, hydrolyzed jojoba esters, EDTA, methylparaben, fragrance, propylparaben, potassium hydroxide, PEG-8 dimethicone, benzyl alcohol, sodium propoxyhydroxypropyl, thiosulfate, silica, ethylhexyl palmitate, silica, octyldodecanol (283-009)

---

## GOLD BOND ULTIMATE HAND SANITIZER SHEER MOISTURE (benzethonium chloride) lotion

Chattem, Inc.

### DRUG FACTS

| Active ingredient | Purpose |
|---|---|
| Benzethonium chloride 0.2% | Antimicrobial |

### USES
- hand sanitizer to decrease bacteria on the skin
- recommended for repeated use

### WARNINGS
**For external use only.**

### WHEN USING THIS PRODUCT
- do not use in or near eyes. In case of contact, rinse eyes thoroughly with water

### STOP USE AND ASK A DOCTOR IF
- irritation or redness develops and persists for more than 72 hours

**Keep out of reach of children.** If swallowed, get medical help or contact a Poison Control Center right away.

### DIRECTIONS
- wet hands thoroughly with product
- briskly rub hands together until absorbed
- apply to hands as needed
- supervise children under 6 years of age in the use of this product

### INACTIVE INGREDIENTS
water, glycerin, propanediol, polyacrylate-1 crosspolymer, dimethicone, distearyldimonium chloride, aloe barbadensis leaf juice, jojoba esters, petrolatum, behenyl alcohol, steareth-21, methylgluceth-20, cocamidopropyl PG-dimonium chloride phosphate, behentrimonium methosulfate, glyceryl laurate, tocopheryl acetate, butyrospermum parkii (shea) butter extract, cholecalciferol, phytonadione, ascorbic acid, zea mays (corn) oil, panthenol, chamomilla recutita (matricaria) flower extract, cetyl alcohol, ethylhexylglycerin, DMDM hydantoin, hydrolyzed jojoba esters, EDTA, methylparaben, fragrance, hydroxyethylcellulose, propylparaben, potassium hydroxide, PEG-8 dimethicone, benzyl alcohol, sodium propoxyhydroxypropyl thiosulfate silica, citric acid, ethylhexyl palmitate, silica, octyldodecanol (283-081)

---

## GOLD BOND ULTIMATE HEALING CONCENTRATED THERAPY CREAM

(dimethicone and white petrolatum) cream

Chattem, Inc.

### DRUG FACTS

| Active ingredients | Purpose |
|---|---|
| Dimethicone 3% | Skin protectant |
| White petrolatum 30% | |

### USES
- helps relieve, prevent and temporarily protect chafed, chapped, cracked or windburned skin and lips
- temporarily protects minor burns, cuts and scrapes
- helps protect from the drying effects of wind and cold weather

### WARNINGS
**For external use only.**

### DO NOT USE ON
- deep or puncture wounds
- animal bites
- serious burns

### WHEN USING THIS PRODUCT
- avoid contact with eyes

### STOP USE AND ASK A DOCTOR IF
- condition worsens
- symptoms last for more than 7 days or clear up and occur again within a few days

**Keep out of reach of children.** If swallowed, get medical help or contact a Poison Control Center immediately.

### DIRECTIONS
- apply generously to affected area as needed

### INACTIVE INGREDIENTS
water, glycerin, glyceryl stearate, distearyldimonium chloride, aloe barbadensis leaf juice, polyethylene, stearyl alcohol, cetearyl alcohol, methyl gluceth-20, behentrimonium methosulfate, steareth-21, steareth-2, cetyl alcohol, allantoin, ceramide 2, tocopheryl acetate, butyrospermum parkii (shea butter) extract, hydrolyzed collagen, palmitoyl oligopeptide, PEG-10 rapeseed sterol, magnesium ascorbyl phosphate, cocodimonium hydroxypropyl hydrolyzed rice protein, retinyl palmitate, polysorbate 60, stearamidopropyl PG-dimonium chloride phosphate, jojoba esters, propylene glycol, DMDM hydantoin, butylene glycol, methylparaben, hydrolyzed jojoba esters, C12-15 alkyl benzoate, propylparaben, potassium hydroxide, EDTA, tribehenin (283-001)

### QUESTIONS OR COMMENTS
visit www.goldbondultimate.com

---

## GOLD BOND ULTIMATE HEALING CONCENTRATED THERAPY OINTMENT

(white petrolatum) ointment

Chattem, Inc.

### DRUG FACTS

| Active ingredient | Purpose |
|---|---|
| White petrolatum 45% | Skin protectant |

### USES
- helps relieve, prevent and temporarily protect chafed, chapped, cracked or windburned skin and lips
- helps protect from the drying effects of wind and cold weather
- temporarily protects minor burns, cuts and scrapes

### WARNINGS
**For external use only.**

### DO NOT USE ON
- deep or puncture wounds
- animal bites
- serious burns

**WHEN USING THIS PRODUCT**
- avoid contact with eyes

**STOP USE AND ASK A DOCTOR IF**
- condition worsens
- symptoms last for more than 7 days or clear up and occur again within a few days

**Keep out of reach of children.** If swallowed, get medical help or contact a Poison Control Center immediately.

**DIRECTIONS**
- apply generously to affected area as needed

**INACTIVE INGREDIENTS**
cyclomethicone, dimethicone, butyrospermum parkii (shea butter) extract, glyceryl stearate, polyethylene, silica, persea gratissima (avocado) butter, tocopheryl acetate, aloe barbadensis leaf extract, ceramide 2, C10-30 cholesterol/lanosterol esters, lavandula angustifolia (lavender) extract, ascorbic acid, phytonadione, cholecalciferol, rosmarinus officinalis (rosemary) leaf extract, chamomilla recutita (matricaria) flower extract, palmitoyl oligopeptide, acacia farnesiana flower extract, C12-15 alkyl benzoate, retinyl palmitate, PEG-10 rapeseed sterol, tribehenin, isopropyl palmitate, isopropyl myristate, PEG-8 dimethicone, octyldodecanol, zea mays (corn) oil, sodium propoxyhydroxypropyl thiosulfate silica, jojoba esters, hydrolyzed jojoba esters, ethylhexyl palmitate (245-304)

**QUESTIONS OR COMMENTS**
visit www.goldbondultimate.com

---

# GOLD BOND ULTIMATE PROTECTION
(avobenzone, homosalate, octisalate, octocrylene) lotion
Chattem, Inc.

## DRUG FACTS

| Active Ingredients | Purpose |
|---|---|
| Avobenzone 3% | Sunscreen/moisturizer |
| Homosalate 5% | |
| Octisalate 4% | |
| Octocrylene 2% | |

**WARNINGS**
**For external use only.**
- avoid contact with eyes

**STOP USE AND ASK A DOCTOR**
- if rash or irritation develops
- If swallowed, get medical help or contact a Poison Control Center immediately

**Keep out of reach of children.**

**DIRECTIONS**
- apply liberally before sun exposure to help prevent sunburn or as often as needed to moisturize extremely dry skin

**INACTIVE INGREDIENTS**
water, glycerin, glyceryl stearate, cyclopentasiloxane, cetyl dimethicone, methyl gluceth-20, cetyl alcohol, nylon-12, steareth-21, steareth-2, polyacrylamide, aloe barbadensis leaf juice, C13-14 isoparafin, jojoba esters, dimethicone, tocopheryl acetate, laureth-7, butyrospermum parkii (shea butter) extract, titanium dioxide, dimethicone/vinyl dimethicone crosspolymer, panthenol, magnesium ascorbyl phosphate, retinyl palmitate, saccharum officinarum (sugar cane) extract, citrus medica limonum (lemon)

extract, citrus aurantium dulcis (orange) fruit extract, pyrus malus (apple) extract, camellia sinensis (green tea) extract, camellia oleifera (green tea) extract, lavandula angustifolia (lavender) extract, chamomilla recutita (matricaria) flower extract, rosmarinus officinalis (rosemary) leaf extract, acacia farnesiana extract, phenoxyethanol, methylparaben, benzyl alcohol, fragrance, propylparaben, potassium hydroxide, EDTA, propylene glycol, isopropyl myristate (245-246)

---

# GOODYS (acetaminophen, aspirin, and caffeine) powder
GlaxoSmithKline Consumer Healthcare LP

## DRUG FACTS

| Active ingredients (in each powder) | Purpose |
|---|---|
| Acetaminophen 260 mg Aspirin (NSAID*) 520 mg | Pain reliever/fever reducer |
| Caffeine 32.5 mg | Pain reliever aid |

*nonsteroidal anti-inflammatory drug

**USES**
- temporarily relieves minor aches and pains due to:
  - headache
  - muscular aches
  - minor arthritis pain
  - colds
- temporarily reduces fever

**WARNINGS**
**Reye's syndrome**
Children and teenagers who have or are recovering from chicken pox or flu-like symptoms should not use this product. When using this product, if changes in behavior with nausea and vomiting occur, consult a doctor because these symptoms could be an early sign of Reye's syndrome, a rare but serious illness.

**Allergy alert**
Aspirin may cause a severe allergic reaction which may include:
- hives
- facial swelling
- shock
- asthma (wheezing)

**Liver warning**
This product contains acetaminophen. Severe liver damage may occur if you take:
- more than 4 powders in 24 hours, which is the maximum daily amount
- with other drugs containing acetaminophen
- 3 or more alcoholic drinks every day while using this product

**Stomach bleeding warning**
This product contains an NSAID, which may cause severe stomach bleeding. The chance is higher if you:
- are age 60 or older
- have had stomach ulcers or bleeding problems
- take a blood thinning (anticoagulant) or steroid drug
- take other drugs containing prescription or nonprescription NSAIDs (aspirin, ibuprofen, naproxen, or others)
- have 3 or more alcoholic drinks every day while using this product
- take more or for a longer time than directed

**DO NOT USE**
- if you have ever had an allergic reaction to aspirin or any other pain reliever/fever reducer

- with any other drug containing acetaminophen (prescription or nonprescription). If you are not sure whether a drug contains acetaminophen, ask a doctor or pharmacist

**ASK A DOCTOR BEFORE USE IF**
- you have liver disease
- stomach bleeding warning applies to you
- you have a history of stomach problems, such as heartburn
- you have high blood pressure, heart disease, liver cirrhosis, or kidney disease
- you are taking a diuretic
- you have asthma

**ASK A DOCTOR OR PHARMACIST BEFORE USE IF YOU ARE**
- taking a prescription drug for diabetes, gout, or arthritis

**WHEN USING THIS PRODUCT**
- limit the use of caffeine-containing drugs, foods, or drinks because too much caffeine may cause nervousness, irritability, sleeplessness, and, occasionally, rapid heart beat
- the recommended dose of this product contains about as much caffeine as a cup of coffee

**STOP USE AND ASK A DOCTOR IF**
- an allergic reaction occurs. Seek medical help right away
- you experience any of the following signs of stomach bleeding:
  - feel faint
  - vomit blood
  - have bloody or black stools
  - have stomach pain that does not get better
- pain gets worse or lasts more than 10 days
- fever gets worse or lasts more than 3 days
- redness or swelling is present
- any new symptoms appear
- ringing in the ears or a loss of hearing occurs

These could be signs of a serious condition.

**If pregnant or breastfeeding,** ask a health professional before use.

It is especially important not to use aspirin during the last 3 months of pregnancy unless definitely directed to do so by a doctor because it may cause problems in the unborn child or complications during delivery.

**Keep out of reach of children.**

**OVERDOSE WARNING**
Taking more than the recommended dose can cause serious health problems. In case of overdose, get medical help or contact a Poison Control Center right away. Quick medical attention is critical for adults as well as for children even if you do not notice any signs or symptoms.

**DIRECTIONS**
- do not take more than directed (see Overdose Warning)

| adults and children 12 years of age and over | place 1 powder on tongue every 6 hours, while symptoms persist |
| | drink a full glass of water with each dose, or may stir powder into a glass of water or other liquid |
| | do not take more than 4 powders in 24 hours unless directed by a doctor |
| children under 12 years of age | ask a doctor |

**OTHER INFORMATION**
- each powder contains: potassium 60 mg
- store below 25°C (77°F)

**INACTIVE INGREDIENTS**
lactose monohydrate, potassium chloride

**QUESTIONS OR COMMENTS**
Call **1-866-255-5197** (English/Spanish) weekdays

# GYNE-LOTRIMIN 3 VAGINAL CREAM
(clotrimazole) cream
Schering-Plough

## DRUG FACTS

| Active Ingredient | Purpose |
|---|---|
| Clotrimazole (2%) (100 mg per applicator) | Vaginal/antifungal |

**USE**
- for the treatment of vaginal yeast infections (*candidiasis*)

**WARNINGS**
**For vaginal use only.**
- do not use in eyes or take by mouth
- do not use if you have any of the following signs and symptoms:
  - fever (higher than 100°F)
  - pain in the lower abdomen, back, or either shoulder
  - a foul-smelling vaginal discharge
- while using, if you get a fever, abdominal pain, or a foul-smelling vaginal discharge, stop using the product and contact your doctor right away. You may have a more serious illness
- if your symptoms do not improve in 3 days, or you still have symptoms after 7 days, you should call your doctor
- if your symptoms return within 2 months, you should consult your doctor. You could be pregnant or there could be a serious underlying medical cause for your symptoms, including diabetes or a weakened immune system (which may be due to HIV - the virus that causes AIDS)
- contact your doctor if you get hives or a skin rash while using this product
- do not use tampons, douches, or spermicides while using this product
- do not rely on condoms or diaphragms to prevent sexually transmitted diseases or pregnancy. This product may damage condoms and diaphragms and cause them to fail

**DO NOT USE**
- in girls less than 12 years of age

**If pregnant or breastfeeding,** ask a health professional before use.

**Keep this and all drugs out of the reach of children.** If swallowed, get medical help or contact a Poison Control Center right away.

**DIRECTIONS**
- applicator and instructions are enclosed
- before using, read the enclosed brochure for complete instructions
- to open: use cap to puncture seal
- insert one applicatorful of cream into the vagina at bedtime for 3 days in a row

## OTHER INFORMATION

- store at room temperature 15-30°C (59-86°F)
- avoid heat over 30°C or 86°F
- see end flap of carton and end of tube for lot number and expiration date
- do not purchase if carton is opened. The tube opening should be sealed. If seal has been punctured or the embossed "SP" is not visible, do not use the product. Return the product to the store where you bought it

## INACTIVE INGREDIENTS

benzyl alcohol, cetearyl alcohol, cetyi esters wax, octyldodecanol polysorbate 60, purified water, sorbitan monostearate

---

## GYNE-LOTRIMIN (Clotrimazole) Cream

Schering-Plough HealthCare Products, Inc.

### DRUG FACTS

| Active ingredients | Purpose |
| --- | --- |
| Clotrimazole 1% (50 mg in each applicatorful) | Vaginal antifungal |
| Clotrimazole 1% (external cream) | Vaginal antifungal |

### USES

- treats vaginal yeast infections
- relieves external itching and irritation due to a vaginal yeast infection

### WARNINGS
**For vaginal use only.**

### DO NOT USE IF

- you have never had a vaginal yeast infection diagnosed by a doctor

### ASK A DOCTOR BEFORE USE IF YOU HAVE

- vaginal itching and discomfort for the first time
- lower abdominal, back or shoulder pain, fever, chills, nausea, vomiting, or foul-smelling vaginal discharge. You may have a more serious condition
- vaginal yeast infections often (such as once a month or 3 in 6 months). You could be pregnant or have a serious underlying medical cause for your symptoms, including diabetes or a weakened immune system
- been exposed to the human immunodeficiency virus (HIV) that causes AIDS

### WHEN USING THIS PRODUCT

- do not use tampons, douches, spermicides, or other vaginal products. Condoms and diaphragms may be damaged and fail to prevent pregnancy or sexually transmitted diseases (STDs)
- do not have vaginal intercourse
- mild increase in vaginal burning, itching or irritation may occur
- if you do not get complete relief ask a doctor before using another product

### STOP USE AND ASK A DOCTOR IF

- symptoms do not get better in 3 days
- symptoms last more than 7 days
- you get a rash or hives, abdominal pain, fever, chills, nausea, vomiting, or a foul-smelling vaginal discharge

**If pregnant or breastfeeding,** ask a health professional before use.

**Keep out of reach of children.** If swallowed, get medical help or contact a Poison Control Center right away.

## DIRECTIONS

- before using this product read the enclosed educational brochure for complete directions and information

| adults and children 12 years of age and over | vaginal cream: insert one applicatorful of cream into the vagina at bedtime for 7 days in a row |
| --- | --- |
| | wash applicator after each use |
| | external cream: use the same tube of cream if you have itching and irritation on the skin outside the vagina |
| | squeeze a small amount of cream onto your fingertip |
| | apply to itchy, irritated skin outside the vagina |
| | use 2 times daily for up to 7 days as needed |
| children under 12 years of age | ask a doctor |

## OTHER INFORMATION

- store between 20°C-25°C (68°F-77°F)
- see end panel of carton and tube crimp for lot number and expiration date
- tamper-evident: do not use if seal embossed with "S" over tube opening is missing, open or broken

## INACTIVE INGREDIENTS

benzyl alcohol, cetostearyl alcohol, cetyl esters wax, 2-octyldodecanol, polysorbate 60, purified water, sorbitan monostearate

## QUESTIONS OR COMMENTS

If you have questions or need more information on this product, Call toll-free **1-800-317-2165** between 8:00 AM and 5:00 PM Central Standard Time, Monday through Friday.

---

## HABITROL PATCH NICOTINE TRANSDERMAL SYSTEM, STEP 1 (nicotine)
patch

Novartis Consumer Health, Inc.

### DRUG FACTS

| Active ingredient | Purpose |
| --- | --- |
| Nicotine, 21 mg delivered over 24 hours | Stop smoking aid |

### USES

- reduces withdrawal symptoms, including nicotine craving, associated with quitting smoking

### WARNINGS

- if you are pregnant or breastfeeding, only use this medicine on the advice of your health care provider
- smoking can seriously harm your child. Try to stop smoking without using any nicotine replacement medicine
- this medicine is believed to be safer than smoking
- however, the risks to your child from this medicine are not fully known

## DO NOT USE
- if you continue to smoke, chew tobacco, use snuff, use nicotine gum, or use another nicotine patch or other nicotine containing products

## ASK A DOCTOR BEFORE USE IF YOU HAVE
- heart disease, recent heart attack, or irregular heartbeat. Nicotine can increase your heart rate
- high blood pressure not controlled with medication. Nicotine can increase your blood pressure
- an allergy to adhesive tape or have skin problems, because you are more likely to get rashes

## ASK A DOCTOR OR A PHARMACIST BEFORE USE IF YOU ARE
- using a non-nicotine stop smoking drug
- taking a prescription medicine for depression or asthma. Your prescription dose may need to be adjusted

## WHEN USING THIS PRODUCT
- do not smoke even when not wearing the patch. The nicotine in your skin will still be entering your bloodstream for several hours after you take off the patch
- if you have vivid dreams or other sleep disturbances remove this patch at bedtime

## STOP USE AND ASK A DOCTOR IF
- skin redness caused by the patch does not go away after four days, or if your skin swells, or you get a rash
- irregular heartbeat or palpitations occur
- you get symptoms of nicotine overdose, such as nausea, vomiting, dizziness, weakness and rapid heartbeat

**Keep out of reach of children and pets.** Used patches have enough nicotine to poison children and pets. If swallowed, get medical help or contact a Poison Control Center right away. Save pouch to use for patch disposal. Dispose of the used patches by folding sticky ends together and putting in pouch.

## DIRECTIONS
- if you are under 18 years of age, ask a doctor before use
- before using this product, read the enclosed self-help guide for complete directions and other information
- stop smoking completely when you begin using the patch
- if you smoke more than 10 cigarettes per day, use the following schedule below:

| Weeks 1-4 | Weeks 5 & 6 | Weeks 7 & 8 |
|---|---|---|
| Step1: use one 21-mg patch/day | Step2: use one 14-mg patch/day | Step3: Use one 7-mg patch/day |

- if you smoke 10 or less cigarettes per day, start with Step 2 for 6 weeks, then Step 3 for 2 weeks and then stop
- apply one new patch every 24 hours on skin that is dry, clean and hairless
- remove backing from patch and immediately press onto skin. Hold for 10 seconds
- wash hands after applying or removing patch. Save pouch to use for patch disposal. Dispose of the used patches by folding sticky ends together and putting in pouch
- the used patch should be removed and a new one applied to a different skin site at the same time each day
- if you have vivid dreams, you may remove the patch at bedtime and apply a new one in the morning
- do not wear more than one patch at a time
- do not cut patch in half or into smaller pieces
- do not leave patch on for more than 24 hours because it may irritate your skin and loses strength after 24 hours
- to avoid possible burns, remove patch before undergoing any MRI (magnetic resonance imaging) procedures
- stop using the patch at the end of 8 weeks. If you still feel the need to use the patch talk to your doctor. Steps 1, 2, 3

## OTHER INFORMATION
- store at 20-25°C (68-77°F)18 YO Warning

## INACTIVE INGREDIENTS
acrylate adhesive, aluminized polyester, cellulose paper, methacrylic acid copolymer

## COMMENTS OR QUESTIONS
Call **1-800-585-8682**

---

# HABITROL PATCH NICOTINE TRANSDERMAL SYSTEM, STEP 2 (nicotine)
patch
Novartis Consumer Health, Inc.

## DRUG FACTS

| Active ingredient | Purpose |
|---|---|
| Nicotine, 14 mg delivered over 24 hours | Stop smoking aid |

## USES
- reduces withdrawal symptoms, including nicotine craving, associated with quitting smoking

## WARNINGS
- if you are pregnant or breastfeeding, only use this medicine on the advice of your health care provider
- smoking can seriously harm your child. Try to stop smoking without using any nicotine replacement medicine
- this medicine is believed to be safer than smoking
- however, the risks to your child from this medicine are not fully known

## DO NOT USE
- if you continue to smoke, chew tobacco, use snuff, use nicotine gum, or use another nicotine patch or other nicotine containing products

## ASK A DOCTOR BEFORE USE IF YOU HAVE
- heart disease, recent heart attack, or irregular heartbeat. Nicotine can increase your heart rate
- high blood pressure not controlled with medication. Nicotine can increase your blood pressure
- an allergy to adhesive tape or have skin problems, because you are more likely to get rashes

## ASK A DOCTOR OR A PHARMACIST BEFORE USE IF YOU ARE
- using a non-nicotine stop smoking drug
- taking a prescription medicine for depression or asthma. Your prescription dose may need to be adjusted

## WHEN USING THIS PRODUCT
- do not smoke even when not wearing the patch. The nicotine in your skin will still be entering your bloodstream for several hours after you take off the patch
- if you have vivid dreams or other sleep disturbances remove this patch at bedtime

## STOP USE AND ASK A DOCTOR IF
- skin redness caused by the patch does not go away after four days, or if your skin swells, or you get a rash
- irregular heartbeat or palpitations occur
- you get symptoms of nicotine overdose, such as nausea, vomiting, dizziness, weakness and rapid heartbeat

**Keep out of reach of children and pets.** Used patches have enough nicotine to poison children and pets. If swallowed, get medical help or contact a Poison Control Center right away. Save pouch to use for patch disposal. Dispose of the used patches by folding sticky ends together and putting in pouch.

## DIRECTIONS

- if you are under 18 years of age, ask a doctor before use
- before using this product, read the enclosed self-help guide for complete directions and other information
- stop smoking completely when you begin using the patch
- if you smoke more than 10 cigarettes per day, use the following schedule below:

| Weeks 1-4 | Weeks 5 & 6 | Weeks 7 & 8 |
|---|---|---|
| Step 1: use one 21-mg patch/day | Step 2: use one 14-mg patch/day | Step 3: Use one 7-mg patch/day |

- if you smoke 10 or less cigarettes per day, start with Step 2 for 6 weeks, then Step 3 for 2 weeks and then stop
- apply one new patch every 24 hours on skin that is dry, clean and hairless
- remove backing from patch and immediately press onto skin. Hold for 10 seconds
- wash hands after applying or removing patch. Save pouch to use for patch disposal. Dispose of the used patches by folding sticky ends together and putting in pouch
- the used patch should be removed and a new one applied to a different skin site at the same time each day
- if you have vivid dreams, you may remove the patch at bedtime and apply a new one in the morning
- do not wear more than one patch at a time
- do not cut patch in half or into smaller pieces
- do not leave patch on for more than 24 hours because it may irritate your skin and loses strength after 24 hours
- to avoid possible burns, remove patch before undergoing any MRI (magnetic resonance imaging) procedures
- stop using the patch at the end of 8 weeks. If you still feel the need to use the patch talk to your doctor. Steps 1, 2, 3

## OTHER INFORMATION

- store at 20-25°C (68-77°F)18 YO Warning

## INACTIVE INGREDIENTS

acrylate adhesive, aluminized polyester, cellulose paper, methacrylic acid copolymer

## COMMENTS OR QUESTIONS

Call **1-800-585-8682**

---

## HABITROL PATCH NICOTINE TRANSDERMAL SYSTEM, STEP 3 (nicotine)

patch

Novartis Consumer Health, Inc.

## DRUG FACTS

| Active ingredient | Purpose |
|---|---|
| Nicotine, 7 mg delivered over 24 hours | Stop smoking aid |

## USES

- reduces withdrawal symptoms, including nicotine craving, associated with quitting smoking

## WARNINGS

- if you are pregnant or breastfeeding, only use this medicine on the advice of your health care provider
- smoking can seriously harm your child. Try to stop smoking without using any nicotine replacement medicine

- this medicine is believed to be safer than smoking
- however, the risks to your child from this medicine are not fully known

## DO NOT USE

- if you continue to smoke, chew tobacco, use snuff, use nicotine gum, or use another nicotine patch or other nicotine containing products

## ASK A DOCTOR BEFORE USE IF YOU HAVE

- heart disease, recent heart attack, or irregular heartbeat. Nicotine can increase your heart rate
- high blood pressure not controlled with medication. Nicotine can increase your blood pressure
- an allergy to adhesive tape or have skin problems, because you are more likely to get rashes

## ASK A DOCTOR OR A PHARMACIST BEFORE USE IF YOU ARE

- using a non-nicotine stop smoking drug
- taking a prescription medicine for depression or asthma. Your prescription dose may need to be adjusted

## WHEN USING THIS PRODUCT

- do not smoke even when not wearing the patch. The nicotine in your skin will still be entering your bloodstream for several hours after you take off the patch
- if you have vivid dreams or other sleep disturbances remove this patch at bedtime

## STOP USE AND ASK A DOCTOR IF

- skin redness caused by the patch does not go away after four days, or if your skin swells, or you get a rash
- irregular heartbeat or palpitations occur
- you get symptoms of nicotine overdose, such as nausea, vomiting, dizziness, weakness and rapid heartbeat

**Keep out of reach of children and pets.** Used patches have enough nicotine to poison children and pets. If swallowed, get medical help or contact a Poison Control Center right away. Save pouch to use for patch disposal. Dispose of the used patches by folding sticky ends together and putting in pouch.

## DIRECTIONS

- if you are under 18 years of age, ask a doctor before use
- before using this product, read the enclosed self-help guide for complete directions and other information
- stop smoking completely when you begin using the patch
- if you smoke more than 10 cigarettes per day, use the following schedule below:

| Weeks 1-4 | Weeks 5 & 6 | Weeks 7 & 8 |
|---|---|---|
| Step 1: use one 21-mg patch/day | Step 2: use one 14-mg patch/day | Step 3: Use one 7-mg patch/day |

- apply one new patch every 24 hours on skin that is dry, clean and hairless
- remove backing from patch and immediately press onto skin. Hold for 10 seconds
- wash hands after applying or removing patch. Save pouch to use for patch disposal. Dispose of the used patches by folding sticky ends together and putting in pouch
- the used patch should be removed and a new one applied to a different skin site at the same time each day
- if you have vivid dreams, you may remove the patch at bedtime and apply a new one in the morning
- do not wear more than one patch at a time
- do not cut patch in half or into smaller pieces
- do not leave patch on for more than 24 hours because it may irritate your skin and loses strength after 24 hours
- to avoid possible burns, remove patch before undergoing any MRI (magnetic resonance imaging) procedures

- stop using the patch at the end of 8 weeks. If you still feel the need to use the patch talk to your doctor. Steps 1, 2, 3

**OTHER INFORMATION**
- store at 20-25°C (68-77°F)

**INACTIVE INGREDIENTS**
acrylate adhesive, aluminized polyester, cellulose paper, methacrylic acid copolymer

**COMMENTS OR QUESTIONS**
Call **1-800-585-8682**

# HALFPRIN (aspirin) tablet
Kramer Inc.

## DRUG FACTS

| Active ingredient (in each tablet) | Purpose |
|---|---|
| Aspirin 162 mg (NSAID)* | Pain reliever |

*nonsteroidal anti-inflammatory drug

### USES
- for the temporary relief of minor aches and pains or as recommended by your doctor
- if immediate relief is needed, chew the tablet for quicker absorption

### WARNINGS
**Reye's syndrome**
Children and teenagers who have or are recovering from chicken pox or flu-like symptoms should not use this product. When using this product, if changes in behavior with nausea and vomiting occur, consult a doctor because these symptoms could be an early sign of Reye's syndrome, a rare but serious illness.

**Allergy alert**
Aspirin may cause a severe allergic reaction which may include:
- hives
- facial swelling
- asthma (wheezing)
- shock

**Stomach bleeding warning**
This product contains an NSAID, which may cause severe stomach bleeding. The chance is higher if you:
- are age 60 or older
- have had stomach ulcers or bleeding problems
- take a blood thinning (anticoagulant) or steroid drug
- take other drugs containing prescription or nonprescription NSAIDs (aspirin, ibuprofen, naproxen, or others)
- have 3 or more alcoholic drinks every day while using this product
- take more or for a longer time than directed.

### DO NOT USE
- if you are allergic to aspirin or any other pain reliever/fever reducer

### ASK A DOCTOR BEFORE USE IF
- stomach bleeding warning applies to you
- you have a history of stomach problems, such as heartburn
- you have nigh blood pressure, heart disease, liver cirrhosis, or kidney disease
- you are taking a diuretic

### ASK A DOCTOR OR PHARMACIST BEFORE USE IF YOU ARE
- taking any other drug containing an NSAID (prescription or nonprescription)
- taking a blood thinning (anticoagulant) or steroid drug
- taking a prescription drug for diabetes, gout or arthritis

### STOP USE AND ASK A DOCTOR IF
- you experience any of the following signs of stomach bleeding
- feel faint
- vomit blood
- have bloody or black stools
- have stomach pain that does not get better

**If pregnant or breastfeeding,** ask a health professional before use.

It is especially important not to use aspirin during the last 3 months of pregnancy unless definitely directed to do so by a doctor because it may cause problems in the unborn child or complications during delivery.

**Keep out of reach of children.** In case of overdose, get medical help or contact a Poison Control Center right away.

### DIRECTIONS
- do not exceed recommended dosage
- do not take for pain for more than 10 days unless directed by a doctor
- drink a full glass of water with each dose

| adults and children 12 years and over | take 2 to 4 tablets with water every 4 hours |
| | do not exceed 24 tablets in 24 hours unless directed by a doctor |
| children under 12 years | consult a doctor |

### OTHER INFORMATION
- tamper evident: do not use if imprinted seal under cap is broken or missing
- store at 25°C (77°F) excursions permitted 15-30°C (59-86°F)
- save carton for full directions and warnings
- serious side effects associated with this product may be reported to this number: **1-800-824-4894**

### INACTIVE INGREDIENTS
acetylated monoglycerides, corn starch, croscarmellose sodium, D&C yellow no. 10 aluminum lake, FD&C red no. 40 aluminum lake, FD&C yellow no. 6 aluminum lake, hypromellose, hypromellose phthalate, microcrystalline cellulose, mineral oil, polyethylene glycol (PEG)-400, polysorbate 80, titanium dioxide

### COMMENTS OR QUESTIONS
Call at **1-800-824-4894** or visit www.kramerlabs.com

# HALLS SUGAR FREE BLACK CHERRY
(menthol) lozenge
Kraft Foods Global, Inc.

## DRUG FACTS

| Active ingredient (in each drop) | Purpose |
|---|---|
| Menthol 5.8 mg | Cough suppressant, oral anesthetic |

### USES
- temporarily relieves:
  - cough due to a cold
  - occasional minor irritation or sore throat

## WARNINGS
**Sore throat warning**
If sore throat is severe, persist for more than 2 days, is accompanied or followed by fever, headache, rash, swelling, nausea, or vomiting, consult a doctor promptly. These may be serious.

### ASK A DOCTOR BEFORE USE IF YOU HAVE
- persistent or chronic cough such as occurs with smoking, asthma, or emphysema
- cough accompanied by excessive phlegm (mucus)

### STOP USE AND ASK A DOCTOR IF
- cough persists for more than 1 week, tends to recur, or is accompanied by fever, rash, or persistent headache. These could be signs of a serious condition
- sore mouth does not improve in 7 days
- irritation, pain, or redness persists or worsens

**Keep out of reach of children.**

### DIRECTIONS

| adults and children 5 years and over | dissolve 1 drop slowly in the mouth |
| --- | --- |
| | repeat every 2 hours as needed |
| children under 5 years | ask a doctor |

### OTHER INFORMATION
- **Phenylketonurics:** contains phenylalanine 2 mg per drop
- excessive consumption may have a laxative effect
- 5 calories per drop
- contains soy

### INACTIVE INGREDIENTS
acesulfame potassium, aspartame, eucalyptus oil, FDC blue 1, FDC red 40, flavors, isomalt, sodium carboxymethylcellulose, soy lecithin, water

### COMMENTS OR QUESTIONS
Call **1-800-524-2854**, Monday to Friday, 9 AM-6 PM Eastern Time or visit our website at www.gethalls.com

---

# HERPECIN L (dimethicone, meradimate, octinoxate, octisalate, and oxybenzone)
Chattem

## DRUG FACTS

| Active ingredients | Purpose |
| --- | --- |
| Dimethicone 1% | skin protectant |
| Meradimate 5% | sunscreen |
| Octinoxate 7.5% | sunscreen |
| Octisalate 5% | sunscreen |
| Oxybenzone 6% | sunscreen |

### USES
- relieves dry, chapped lips
- protects lips from the sun
- helps treat and relieve cold sores/fever blisters

### WARNINGS
**For external use only.**

### DO NOT USE IF
- you are allergic to any ingredient in this product

### WHEN USING THIS PRODUCT
- apply only to affected areas
- do not use in or near the eyes
- avoid applying directly inside your mouth
- do not share this product with anyone since this may spread infection

### STOP USE AND ASK A DOCTOR IF
- condition worsens or does not improve within 7 days

**Keep out of reach of children.** If swallowed, get medical help or contact a Poison Control Center right away.

### DIRECTIONS

| adults and children 12 years or over | apply to affected area on lips at first sign of cold sore |
| --- | --- |
| | rub in gently but completely |
| | apply liberally as often as necessary |
| | for cracking or dryness continue to cover lips until absorbed |
| children under 12 years | ask a doctor |

### INACTIVE INGREDIENTS:
helianthus annuus (sunflower) seed oil, petrolatum, ozokerite, mineral oil, microcrystalline wax, talc, titanium dioxide, beeswax, melissa officinalis leaf extract, cetyl lactate, glyceryl laurate, flavor, lysine hydrochloride, ascorbyl palmitate, tocopheryl acetate, pyridoxine hydrochloride, panthenol, BHT (224-014)

---

# HYPO TEARS (polyvinyl alcohol, polyethylene glycol)
Novartis Pharmaceuticals Corporation

## DRUG FACTS

| Active ingredients | Purpose |
| --- | --- |
| Polyvinyl alcohol (1%) | Lubricant |
| Polyethylene glycol 400 (1%) | Lubricant |

### USES
- for use as a lubricant to relieve dryness of the eye
- temporarily relieves burning and irritation due to dryness of the eye or from exposure to wind or sun
- helps protect against further eye irritation

### WARNINGS

### DO NOT USE IF
- solution changes color or becomes cloudy
- you are allergic to any ingredients

### WHEN USING THIS PRODUCT
- do not touch tip of container to any surface to avoid contamination. Replace cap after using

### STOP USE AND ASK A DOCTOR IF
- you experience any of the following:
  - eye pain
  - changes in vision
  - continued redness or irritation of the eye
  - condition worsens or persists for more than 72 hours

**Keep this and all drugs out of the reach of children.** If swallowed, get medical help or contact a Poison Control Center right away.

### DIRECTIONS
• put 1 or 2 drops in the affected eye(s) as needed

### OTHER INFORMATION
• store between 15-30°C (59-86°F)

### INACTIVE INGREDIENTS
Lipiden™ vehicle (dextrose, edetate disodium, purified water) and benzalkonium chloride, 0.1 mg/mL

### QUESTIONS OR COMMENTS
Call toll-tree **1-866-393-6336**, weekdays, 8:30 AM-5:00 PM EST. Serious side effects associated with use of this product may be reported to this number.

---

# ICY HOT MEDICATED SPRAY (menthol) spray
Chattem, Inc.

## DRUG FACTS

| Active ingredient | Purpose |
|---|---|
| Menthol 16% | Topical analgesic |

### USES
• temporarily relieves minor pain associated with:
  • arthritis
  • simple backache
  • muscle strains
  • sprains
  • bruises
  • cramps

### WARNINGS
For external use only.

**Flammable. Do not use near heat or flame or while smoking.**

• avoid long term storage above 104°F (40°C)
• do not puncture or incinerate. Contents under pressure
• do not store at temperatures above 120°F (49°C)

### WHEN USING THIS PRODUCT
• use only as directed
• do not bandage tightly or use with a heating pad
• avoid contact with eyes and mucous membranes
• do not apply to wounds or damaged, broken or irritated skin
• do not spray onto face
• avoid inhaling spray mist and fumes

### STOP USE AND ASK A DOCTOR IF
• condition worsens
• redness is present
• irritation develops
• symptoms persist for more than 7 days or clear up and occur again within a few days

**If pregnant or breastfeeding,** ask a health professional before use.

**Keep out of reach of children.** If swallowed, get medical help or contact a Poison Control Center right away.

---

### DIRECTIONS

| adults and children over 12 years | spray affected area with desired amount of product |
|---|---|
| | product will dry quickly on its own, and does not need to be rubbed in |
| | repeat as necessary, but no more than 3-4 times daily |
| children 12 years or younger | ask a doctor |

### INACTIVE INGREDIENTS
glycerin, propylene glycol, SD alcohol 40-2 (55%), water (283-016)

### QUESTIONS OR COMMENTS
visit www.icyhot.com

---

# ICY HOT MEDICATED NO MESS APPLICATOR (menthol) liquid
Chattem, Inc.

## DRUG FACTS

| Active ingredient | Purpose |
|---|---|
| Menthol 16% | Topical analgesic |

### USES
• temporarily relieves minor pain associated with:
  • arthritis
  • simple backache
  • muscle strains
  • sprains
  • bruises
  • cramps

### WARNINGS
For external use only.

**Flammable. Keep away from fire or flame.**

### WHEN USING THIS PRODUCT
• use only as directed
• do not bandage tightly or use with a heating pad
• avoid contact with eyes and mucous membranes
• do not apply to wounds or damaged, broken or irritated skin
• a transient burning sensation may occur upon application but generally disappears in several days
• if severe burning sensation occurs, discontinue use immediately
• do not expose the area treated with product to heat or direct sunlight

### STOP USE AND ASK A DOCTOR IF
• condition worsens
• redness is present
• irritation develops
• symptoms persist for more than 7 days or clear up and occur again within a few days

**If pregnant or breastfeeding,** ask a health professional before use.

**Keep out of reach of children.** If swallowed, get medical help or contact a Poison Control Center right away.

## DIRECTIONS

| adults and children over 12 years | apply generously to affected area |
| --- | --- |
| | massage into painful area until thoroughly absorbed into skin |
| | repeat as necessary, but no more than 3-4 times daily |
| | if medicine comes in contact with hands, wash with soap and water |
| children 12 years or younger | ask a doctor |

## OTHER INFORMATION
• close cap tightly after use
• keep carton as it contains important information

## INACTIVE INGREDIENTS
acrylates/C10-30 alkyl acrylate crosspolymer, capsaicin, glycerin, isopropyl myristate, propylene glycol, SD alcohol 40 (30%), water (245-256)

## QUESTIONS OR COMMENTS
www.icyhot.com

## ICY HOT NO MESS VAPOR COUGH SUPPRESSANT (camphor, eucalyptus oil and menthol) gel
Chattem, Inc.

### DRUG FACTS

| Active ingredients | Purpose |
| --- | --- |
| Camphor 5.3%<br>Eucalyptus oil 1.3%<br>Menthol 2.8% | Cough suppressant |

## USE
• on chest and throat, to temporarily relieve cough due to the common cold

## WARNINGS
**For external use only.**

## WHEN USING THIS PRODUCT DO NOT
• take this product for persistent or chronic cough such as occurs with smoking, asthma, emphysema, or if cough is accompanied by excessive phlegm (mucus) unless directed by a doctor
• take by mouth
• place in nostrils
• heat
• microwave
• add to hot water or any container where heating water. May cause splattering and result in burns

## STOP USE AND ASK A DOCTOR IF
• cough persists for more than one week, tends to recur, or is accompanied by fever, rash or persistent headache. A persistent cough may be a sign of a serious condition

**If pregnant or breastfeeding,** ask a health professional before use.

**Keep out of reach of children.** If swallowed, get medical help or contact a Poison Control Center right away.

## DIRECTIONS
**See important warnings under "When using this product do not"**

| adults and children 2 years and older | squeeze desired amount of gel onto upper chest and/or throat as a thick layer |
| --- | --- |
| | using the sponge-top applicator, gently massage dispensed gel into skin until thoroughly absorbed |
| | cover with a warm, dry cloth if desired |
| | clothing should be left loose about the throat and chest to help the vapors reach the nose and mouth |
| | use up to 3 times daily or as directed by doctor |
| children under 2 years of age | ask a doctor |

## INACTIVE INGREDIENTS
cyclomethicone, dimethicone, glyceryl stearate, PEG-12 dimethicone, petrolatum, polyethylene, silica (283-083)

## ICY HOT NO MESS VAPOR COUGH SUPPRESSANT FOR KIDS (camphor, eucalyptus oil and menthol) gel
Chattem, Inc.

### DRUG FACTS

| Active ingredients | Purpose |
| --- | --- |
| Camphor 4.7%<br>Eucalyptus oil 1.2%<br>Menthol 2.6% | Cough suppressant |

## USE
• on chest and throat, to temporarily relieve cough due to the common cold

## WARNINGS
**For external use only.**

## WHEN USING THIS PRODUCT DO NOT
• give this product for persistent or chronic cough such as occurs with smoking, asthma, emphysema, or if cough is accompanied by excessive phlegm (mucus) unless directed by a doctor
• take by mouth
• place in nostrils
• heat
• microwave
• add to hot water or any container where heating water. May cause splattering and result in burns

## STOP USE AND ASK A DOCTOR IF
• cough persists for more than one week, tends to recur, or is accompanied by fever, rash or persistent headache. A persistent cough may be a sign of a serious condition

**If pregnant or breastfeeding,** ask a health professional before use.

**Keep out of reach of children.** If swallowed, get medical help or contact a Poison Control Center right away.

## DIRECTIONS
**See important warnings under "When using this product do not"**

| adults and children 2 years and older | squeeze desired amount of gel onto upper chest and/or throat as a thick layer |
| --- | --- |
| | using the sponge-top applicator, gently massage dispensed gel into skin until thoroughly absorbed |
| | cover with a warm, dry cloth if desired |
| | clothing should be left loose about the throat and chest to help the vapors reach the nose and mouth |
| | use up to 3 times daily or as directed by doctor |
| children under 2 years of age | ask a doctor |

## INACTIVE INGREDIENTS
cyclomethicone, dimethicone, glyceryl stearate, PEG-12 dimethicone, petrolatum, polyethylene, silica (283-083)

# ICY HOT MEDICATED PATCH (menthol)
Lead Chemical Co. Ltd.

## DRUG FACTS

| Active ingredient | Purpose |
| --- | --- |
| Menthol 5% | Topical analgesic |

## USES
* temporarily relieves minor aches and pains associated with:
  * arthritis
  * simple backache
  * bursitis
  * tendonitis
  * muscle strains
  * sprains
  * bruises
  * cramps

## WARNINGS
**For external use only.**

## WHEN USING THIS PRODUCT
* use only as directed
* do not bandage tightly or use with a heating pad
* avoid contact with eyes and mucous membranes
* do not apply to wounds or damaged, broken or irritated skin

## STOP USE AND ASK A DOCTOR IF
* condition worsens
* redness is present
* irritation develops
* symptoms persist for more than 7 days or clear up and occur again within a few days

**If pregnant or breastfeeding,** ask a health professional before use.

**Keep out of reach of children.** If swallowed, get medical help or contact a Poison Control Center right away.

## DIRECTIONS

| adults and children over 12 years | remove backing from patch by firmly grasping both ends and gently pulling until backing separates in middle |
| --- | --- |
| | carefully remove smaller portion of backing from patch and apply exposed portion of patch to affected area |
| | once exposed portion of patch is positioned, carefully remove remaining backing to completely apply patch to affected area |
| | wear one Icy Hot Patch up to 8 hours |
| | repeat as necessary, but no more than 3 times daily |
| children 12 years or younger | ask a doctor |

## INACTIVE INGREDIENTS
aluminum hydroxide, carmellose sodium, glycerin, isopropyl myristate, methyl acrylate/2-ethylhexyl acrylate copolymer, nonoxynol-30, polyacrylic acid, polysorbate 80, sodium polyacrylate, sorbitan sesquioleate, starch/acrylic acid graft copolymer sodium salt, talc, tartaric acid, titanium dioxide, water

## QUESTIONS OR COMMENTS
www.icyhot.com

# ICY HOT POWER GEL (menthol)
Chattem, Inc.

## DRUG FACTS

| Active ingredient | Purpose |
| --- | --- |
| Menthol 16% | Topical analgesic |

## USES
* temporarily relieves minor pain associated with:
  * arthritis
  * simple backache
  * muscle strains
  * sprains
  * bruises
  * cramps

## WARNINGS
**For external use only.**

**Flammable. Keep away from fire or flame.**

## WHEN USING THIS PRODUCT
* use only as directed
* do not bandage tightly or use with a heating pad
* avoid contact with eyes and mucous membranes
* do not apply to wounds or damaged, broken or irritated skin

## STOP USE AND ASK A DOCTOR IF
* condition worsens
* redness is present

- irritation develops
- symptoms persist for more than 7 days or clear up and occur again within a few days

**If pregnant or breastfeeding,** ask a health professional before use.

**Keep out of reach of children.** If swallowed, get medical help or contact a Poison Control Center right away.

## DIRECTIONS

| adults and children over 12 years | apply generously to affected area |
| | massage into painful area until thoroughly absorbed into skin |
| | repeat as necessary, but no more than 3-4 times daily |
| | if medicine comes in contact with hands, wash with soap and water |
| children 12 years or younger | ask a doctor |

## INACTIVE INGREDIENTS

acrylates/C10-30 alkyl acrylate crosspolymer, FD&C blue no. 1, glycerin, hydroxypropyl methylcellulose, propylene glycol, SD alcohol 40-2 (30%), triethanolamine, water (283-027)

## QUESTIONS OR COMMENTS

visit www.icyhot.com

---

## ICY HOT PAIN RELIEVING STICK (menthol and methyl salicylate) stick

Chattem, Inc.

### DRUG FACTS

| Active ingredient | Purpose |
|---|---|
| Menthol 10% | Topical analgesic |
| Methyl salicylate 30% | |

### USES

- temporarily relieves minor pain associated with:
  - arthritis
  - simple backache
  - muscle strains
  - sprains
  - bruises
  - cramps

### WARNINGS
**For external use only.**

### Allergy alert
If prone to allergic reaction from aspirin or salicylates, consult a doctor before use.

### WHEN USING THIS PRODUCT
- use only as directed
- do not bandage tightly or use with a heating pad
- avoid contact with eyes or mucous membranes
- do not apply to wounds or damaged, broken or irritated skin

### STOP USE AND ASK A DOCTOR IF
- condition worsens
- redness is present
- irritation develops

- symptoms persist for more than 7 days or clear up and occur again within a few days

**If pregnant or breastfeeding,** ask a health care professional before use.

**Keep out of reach of children.** If swallowed, get medical help or contact a Poison Control Center right away.

## DIRECTIONS

| adults and children over 12 years | apply generously to affected area |
| | massage into painful area until thoroughly absorbed into skin |
| | repeat as necessary, but not more than 4 times daily |
| children 12 years or younger | ask a doctor |

## INACTIVE INGREDIENTS

ceresin, cyclomethicone, hydrogenated castor oil, microcrystalline wax, paraffin, PEG-150 disstearate, propylene glycol, stearic acid, stearyl alcohol (245-111)

---

## ICY HOT PAIN RELIEVING BALM (menthol and methyl salicylate) ointment

Chattem, Inc.

### DRUG FACTS

| Active ingredients | Purpose |
|---|---|
| Menthol 7.6% | Topical analgesic |
| Methyl salicylate 29% | |

### USES

- temporarily relieves minor pain associated with:
  - arthritis
  - simple backache
  - muscle strains
  - sprains
  - bruises
  - cramps

### WARNINGS
**For external use only.**

### Allergy alert
If prone to allergic reaction from aspirin or salicylates, consult a doctor before use.

### WHEN USING THIS PRODUCT
- use only as directed
- avoid contact with eyes or mucous membranes
- do not bandage tightly or use with a heating pad
- do not apply to wounds or damaged, broken or irritated skin

### STOP USE AND ASK A DOCTOR IF
- condition worsens
- redness is present
- irritation develops
- symptoms persist for more than 7 days or clear up and occur again within a few days

**If pregnant or breastfeeding,** ask a health care professional before use.

**Keep out of reach of children.** If case of accidental ingestion, get medical help or contact a Poison Control Center right away.

## DIRECTIONS

| adults and children over 12 years | apply generously to affected area |
|---|---|
| | massage into painful area until thoroughly absorbed into skin |
| | repeat as necessary, but not more than 4 times daily |
| children 12 years or younger | ask a doctor |

## INACTIVE INGREDIENTS
paraffin, white petrolatum (245-109)

# ICY HOT PAIN RELIEVING CREAM (menthol
and methyl salicylate) cream
Chattem, Inc.

## DRUG FACTS

| Active ingredients | Purpose |
|---|---|
| Menthol 10% | Topical analgesic |
| Methyl salicylate 30% | |

## USES
- temporarily relieves minor pain associated with:
  - arthritis
  - simple backache
  - muscle strains
  - sprains
  - bruises
  - cramps

## WARNINGS
For external use only.

### Allergy alert
If prone to allergic reaction from aspirin or salicylates, consult a doctor before use.

### WHEN USING THIS PRODUCT
- use only as directed
- do not bandage tightly or use with a heating pad
- avoid contact with eyes or mucous membranes
- do not apply to wounds or damaged, broken or irritated skin
- close cap tightly after use

### STOP USE AND ASK A DOCTOR IF
- condition worsens
- symptoms persist for more than 7 days or clear up and occur again within a few days
- redness is present
- irritation develops

If pregnant or breastfeeding, ask a health care professional before use.

Keep out of reach of children. If case of accidental ingestion, get medical help or contact a Poison Control Center right away.

## DIRECTIONS

| adults and children over 12 years | apply generously to affected area |
|---|---|
| | massage into painful area until thoroughly absorbed into skin |
| | repeat as necessary, but not more than 4 times daily |
| children 12 years or younger | ask a doctor |

## INACTIVE INGREDIENTS
carbomer, cetyl esters, emulsifying wax, oleth-3 phosphate, stearic acid, triethanolamine, water (245-110)

# ICY HOT VANISHING SCENT (menthol) gel
Chattem, Inc.

## DRUG FACTS

| Active ingredient | Purpose |
|---|---|
| Menthol 2.5% | Topical analgesic |

## USES
- temporarily relieves minor pain associated with:
  - arthritis
  - simple backache
  - muscle strains
  - sprains
  - bruises
  - cramps

## WARNINGS
For external use only.

### WHEN USING THIS PRODUCT
- use only as directed
- do not bandage tightly or use with a heating pad
- avoid contact with eyes or mucous membranes
- do not apply to wounds or damaged, broken or irritated skin

### STOP USE AND ASK A DOCTOR IF
- condition worsens
- symptoms persist for more than 7 days or clear up and occur again within a few days
- redness is present
- irritation develops

If pregnant or breastfeeding, ask a health care professional before use.

Keep out of reach of children. If swallowed, get medical help or contact a Poison Control Center right away.

## DIRECTIONS

| adults and children over 12 years | apply generously to affected area |
| | squeeze desired amount of Icy Hot pain relieving gel onto affected area |
| | using the sponge-top applicator, massage dispensed gel into painful area until thoroughly absorbed |
| | repeat as necessary, but not more than 4 times daily |
| children 12 years or younger | ask a doctor |

## OTHER INFORMATION
- keep carton as it contains important information
- close cap tightly after use

## INACTIVE INGREDIENTS
allantoin, aloe barbadensis leaf juice, carbomer, DMDM hydantoin, glycerin, methylparaben, phenoxyethanol, propylparaben, SD alcohol 40-2 (15.47%), steareth-2, steareth-21, triethanolamine, water (245-135)

---

# IMODIUM (loperamide hydrochloride and simethicone)
McNeil Consumer Healthcare, Div. McNeil-PPC, Inc

## DRUG FACTS

| Active ingredients (in each chewable tablet and caplet) | Purpose |
|---|---|
| Loperamide hydrochloride 2 mg<br>Simethicone 125 mg | Multi-symptom relief |

## USES
- Controls symptoms of diarrhea plus bloating, pressure, and cramps commonly referred to as gas

## WARNINGS
**Allergy alert**
Do not use if you have ever had a rash or other allergic reaction to loperamide hydrochloride.

## DO NOT USE
- if you have bloody or black stool

## ASK A DOCTOR BEFORE USE IF YOU HAVE:
- a fever
- mucus in the stool
- a history of liver disease

## ASK A DOCTOR OR PHARMACIST BEFORE USE IF
- you are taking antibiotics

## WHEN USING THIS PRODUCT
- tiredness, drowsiness, or dizziness may occur
- be careful when driving or operating machinery

## STOP USE AND ASK A DOCTOR IF
- symptoms get worse
- diarrhea lasts for more than 2 days
- you get abdominal swelling or bulging. These may be signs of a serious condition

**Each caplet contains:** calcium 65 mg, sodium 4 mg.
**Each tablet contains:** calcium 50 mg.

**If pregnant or breastfeeding,** ask a health professional before use.

**Keep out of the reach of children.** In case of overdose, get medical help or contact a Poison Control Center right away. (1-800-222-1222)

## DIRECTIONS
- drink plenty of clear fluids to help prevent dehydration caused by diarrhea
- find right dose on chart. If possible, use weight to dose; otherwise, use age

| Age/Weight | Chewable Tablets | Caplets |
|---|---|---|
| adults & children 12 years & over | chew 2 tablets and take with 4-8 ounces of water after the first loose stool; chew 1 tablet and take with 4-8 ounces of water after each subsequent loose stool; but no more than 4 tablets in 24 hours | 2 caplets after the first loose stool; 1 caplet after each subsequent loose stool; but no more than 4 caplets in 24 hours |
| children 9-11 years (60-95 lbs) | chew 1 tablet and take with 4-8 ounces of water after the first loose stool; chew ½ tablet and take with 4-8 ounces of water after each subsequent loose stool; but no more than 3 tablets in 24 hours | 1 caplet after the first loose stool; ½ caplet after each subsequent loose stool; but no more than 3 caplets in 24 hours |
| children 6-8 years (48-59 lbs) | chew 1 tablet and take with 4-8 ounces of water after the first loose stool; chew ½ tablet and take with 4-8 ounces of water after each subsequent loose stool; but no more than 2 tablets in 24 hours | 1 caplet after the first loose stool; ½ caplet after each subsequent loose stool; but no more than 2 caplets in 24 hours |
| children under 6 years (up to 47 lbs) | ask a doctor | ask a doctor |

## OTHER INFORMATION
- store between 20°C-25°C (68-77°F)
- do not use if carton or if blister unit is open or torn, or if pouch is opened
- see side panel for lot number and expiration date
- (caplets) protect from light

## INACTIVE INGREDIENTS (TABLETS)
cellulose acetate, confectioners' sugar, D&C yellow no.10, aluminum lake, dextrates, FD&C blue no. 1 aluminum lake, flavor, microcrystalline cellulose, polymethactylates, saccharin sodium, sorbitol, stearic acid, sucrose, tribasic calcium phosphate

## INACTIVE INGREDIENTS (CAPLETS)
acesulfame potassium, cross carmellose sodium, dibasic calcium phosphate, flavor, microcrystalline, cellulose, stearic acid

## IMODIUM A-D (loperamide hydrochloride) liquid
McNeil Consumer Healthcare, Division of McNeil-PPC, Inc

### DRUG FACTS

| Active ingredient (in each 7.5 mL) | Purpose |
|---|---|
| Loperamide hydrochloride 1 mg | Anti-diarrheal |

### USE
- controls symptoms of diarrhea, including travelers' diarrhea

### WARNINGS
**Allergy alert**
Do not use if you have ever had a rash or other allergic reaction to loperamide hydrochloride.

### DO NOT USE
- if you have bloody or black stool

### ASK A DOCTOR BEFORE USE IF YOU HAVE
- fever
- mucus in the stool
- a history of liver disease

### ASK A DOCTOR OR PHARMACIST BEFORE USE IF YOU ARE
- taking antibiotics

### WHEN USING THIS PRODUCT
- tiredness, drowsiness or dizziness may occur
- be careful when driving or operating machinery

### STOP USE AND ASK A DOCTOR IF
- symptoms get worse
- diarrhea lasts for more than 2 days
- you get abdominal swelling or bulging. These may be signs of a serious condition

**If pregnant or breastfeeding,** ask a health professional before use.

**Keep out of reach of children.** In case of overdose, get medical help or contact a Poison Control Center right away. (1-800-222-1222)

## DIRECTIONS
- drink plenty of clear fluids to help prevent dehydration caused by diarrhea
- find right dose on chart. If possible, use weight to dose; otherwise use age
- shake well before using
- only use attached measuring cup to dose product

| adults and children 12 years and over | 30 mL (6 tsp) after the first loose stool; 15 mL (3 tsp) after each subsequent loose stool; but no more than 60 mL (12 tsp) in 24 hours |
|---|---|
| children 9-11 years (60-95 lbs) | 15 mL (3 tsp) after first loose stool; 7.5 mL (1 ½ tsp) after each subsequent loose stool; but no more than 45 mL (9 tsp) in 24 hours |
| children 6-8 years (48-59 lbs) | 15 mL (3 tsp) after first loose stool; 7.5 mL (1 ½ tsp) after each subsequent loose stool; but no more than 30 mL (6 tsp) in 24 hours |
| children under 6 years (up to 47 lbs) | ask a doctor |

## OTHER INFORMATION
- each 30 mL (6 tsp) contains: sodium 16 mg
- store between 20-25°C (68-77°F)
- do not use if printed inner or outer neckband is broken or missing
- see side panel for lot number and expiration date

## INACTIVE INGREDIENTS
carboxymethylcellulose sodium, citric acid, D&C yellow no. 10, FD&C blue no. 1, glycerin, flavor, microcrystalline cellulose, propylene glycol, purified water, simethicone emulsion, sodium benzoate, sucralose, titanium dioxide, xanthan gum

### QUESTIONS OR COMMENTS
Call **1-877-895-3665**

## IMODIUM A-D (loperamide hydrochloride) tablet, chewable
McNeil Consumer Healthcare, Div. McNeil-PPC, Inc

### DRUG FACTS

| Active ingredient (in each tablet) | Purpose |
|---|---|
| Loperamide hydrochloride 2 mg | Anti-diarrheal |

### USE
- controls symptoms of diarrhea, including travelers' diarrhea

### WARNINGS
**Allergy alert**
Do not use if you have ever had a rash or other allergic reaction to loperamide hydrochloride.

### DO NOT USE
- if you have bloody or black stool

## ASK A DOCTOR BEFORE USE IF YOU HAVE
- fever
- mucus in the stool
- a history of liver disease

## ASK A DOCTOR OR PHARMACIST BEFORE USE IF YOU ARE
- taking antibiotics

## WHEN USING THIS PRODUCT
- tiredness, drowsiness or dizziness may occur
- be careful when driving or operating machinery

## STOP USE AND ASK A DOCTOR IF
- symptoms get worse
- diarrhea lasts for more than 2 days
- you get abdominal swelling or bulging. These may be signs of a serious condition

**If pregnant or breastfeeding,** ask a health professional before use.

**Keep out of reach of children.** In case of overdose, get medical help or contact a Poison Control Center right away. (1-800-222-1222)

## DIRECTIONS
- drink plenty of clear fluids to help prevent dehydration caused by diarrhea
- take only on an empty stomach (1 hour before or 2 hours after a meal)
- find right dose on chart. If possible, use weight to dose; otherwise, use age

| adults and children 12 years and over | chew 2 tablets after the first loose stool; chew 1 tablet after each subsequent loose stool; but no more than 4 tablets in 24 hours |
|---|---|
| children 9-11 years (60-95 lbs) | chew 1 tablet after the first loose stool; chew ½ tablet after each subsequent loose stool; but no more than 3 tablets in 24 hours |
| children 6-8 years (48-59 lbs) | chew 1 tablet after the first loose stool; chew ½ tablet after each subsequent loose stool; but no more than 2 tablets in 24 hours |
| children under 6 years (up to 47 lbs) | ask a doctor |

## OTHER INFORMATION
- contains milk
- store between 20-25°C (68-77°F)
- do not use if carton is open or if printed foil seal under bottle cap is open or torn
- see bottom panel for lot number and expiration date

## INACTIVE INGREDIENTS
acesulfame potassium, basic polymethacrylate, cellulose acetate, confectioner's sugar, crospovidone, D&C yellow no. 10 aluminum lake, dextrose excipient, FD&C blue no. 1 aluminum lake, flavors, magnesium stearate, microcrystalline cellulose, milk powder, sucralose

## QUESTIONS OR COMMENTS
Call **1-877-895-3665**

# IVAREST MAXIMUM STRENGTH (calamine, benzyl alcohol and diphenhydramine hydrochloride) cream
Blistex Inc.

## DRUG FACTS

| Active ingredients | Purpose |
|---|---|
| Calamine 14.0% (w/w) | Skin protectant |
| Benzyl alcohol 10.5% (w/w) | External analgesic |
| Diphenhydramine hydrochloride 2.0% (w/w) | External analgesic |

## USES
- for the temporary relief of pain and itching associated with poison ivy, poison oak, poison sumac, insect bites or minor skin irritations
- dries the oozing and weeping of poison:
  - ivy
  - oak
  - sumac

## WARNINGS
**For external use only.**

## DO NOT USE
- on large areas of the body
- with any other product containing diphenhydramine, even one taken by mouth

## ASK A DOCTOR BEFORE USE
- on chicken pox
- on measles

## WHEN USING THIS PRODUCT
- do not get into eyes

## STOP USE AND ASK A DOCTOR IF
- condition worsens
- symptoms last for more than 7 days or clear up and occur again within a few days

**Keep out of reach of children.** If swallowed, get medical help or contact a Poison Control Center right away.

## DIRECTIONS
- do not use more often than directed
- as soon as possible after exposure, wash affected area with soap and water (or Ivarest Poison Ivy Cleansing Foam). Gently pat dry
- apply Ivarest liberally to form a layer you can not see through

| adults and children 2 years and older | apply to affected area not more than 3 to 4 times daily |
|---|---|
| children under 2 years of age | consult a doctor |

## OTHER INFORMATION
- avoid contact with clothing
- Ivarest may stain certain fabrics

## INACTIVE INGREDIENTS
bentonite, benzethonium chloride, camphor, hydroxyethyl acrylate/sodium acryloyldimethyltaurate copolymer, hydroxyethylcellulose, lanolin alcohol, lanolin oil, magnesium aluminum silicate, menthol, petrolatum, PEG-4, polyglyceryl-3 diisostearate, polysorbate 60, propylene glycol, purified water, PVP, red no. 33, sorbitan stearate, squalane, yellow no. 5, yellow no. 6

## IVAREST MEDICATED POISON IVY CLEANSING FORMULA (menthol) foam

Blistex Inc.

### DRUG FACTS

| Active ingredient | Purpose |
|---|---|
| Menthol 1.0% (w/w) | External analgesic |

### USES
- for the temporary relief of pain and itching
- soothes and cools skin

### WARNINGS
**For external use only.**
- keep out of reach of children
- avoid contact with eyes
- if condition worsens, or if symptoms persist for more than 7 days or clear up and occur again within a few days, discontinue use of this product and consult a physician
- if swallowed, get medical help or contact a Poison Control Center right away

### DIRECTIONS
- apply to affected area, gently rubbing to remove urushiol (toxic plant oil). Rinse under running water

| for use by adults and children 2 years of age and older | apply to affected area not more than 3 to 4 times daily |
|---|---|
| children under 2 years of age | consult a physician |

### OTHER INFORMATION
- to prevent recontamination or cross-contamination, clean any tools or other equipment which may have come in contact with urushiol. Wash all clothing, bedding, etc. that may have come into contact with urushiol. Also, pets which may have come in contact with toxic plants should be bathed to prevent cross-contamination
- for up to 8 hour relief from itching associated with poison plant rash, try Ivarest Maximum Strength Cream with 2 proven itch fighting ingredients

### INACTIVE INGREDIENTS
acetamide MEA, cocamidopropyl betaine, disodium EDTA, DMDM hydantoin, glycerin, lactamide MEA, phenoxyethanol, PEG-4, PEG-40 hydrogenated castor oil, purified water, sodium lauroyl sarcosinate, triclosan

### QUESTIONS OR COMMENTS
For more information on Ivarest products visit www.blistex.com/ivarest.htm.

## IVY BLOCK (bentoquatam) lotion

Hyland's Inc.

### DRUG FACTS

| Active ingredient | Purpose |
|---|---|
| Bentoquatam 5 % | Skin protectant |

### USES
- helps prevent poison ivy, oak and sumac rash when applied before exposure

### WARNINGS
**For external use only.**

**Flammable. Keep away from fire or flame.**

### DO NOT USE
- if you are allergic to any ingredients
- on open rash

### WHEN USING THIS PRODUCT
- do not get into eyes. If contact occurs, rinse eyes thoroughly with water

**Keep out of reach of children.** If swallowed, get medical help or contact a Poison Control Center right away.

### DIRECTIONS
- shake well before use
- apply 15 minutes before risk of exposure
- avoid intentional contact with poison ivy, oak, and sumac
- remove with soap and water after risk of exposure

| adults and children 6 and older | apply every 4 hours for continued protection or sooner if needed |
|---|---|
| children under 6 years | ask a doctor |

### OTHER INFORMATION
- store at 15-30°C (59-86°F)

### INACTIVE INGREDIENTS
bentonite, benzyl alcohol, diisopropyl adipate, methylparaben, purified water, SDA 40 denatured alcohol (25% by weight)

## IVY-DRY CREAM (benzyl alcohol, zinc acetate, camphor and menthol) cream

Ivy-Dry Inc.

### DRUG FACTS

| Active ingredients | Purpose |
|---|---|
| Benzyl alcohol 10% | Anti-itch |
| Zinc acetate 2.0% | Rash treatment |
| Camphor 0.6% | External analgesic |
| Menthol 0.4% | External analgesic |

### USES
- temporarily relieves the itching, oozing and weeping associated with minor skin irritations and rashes due to poison ivy, poison oak, poison sumac and insect bites

### WARNINGS
**For external use only.**
- test product on a small patch of skin before applying to the entire body
- do not use on face or genital areas
- avoid contact with eyes
- not to be used on areas of blistered or broken skin
- do not cover the affected area with a compress after application
- if condition does not improve or persists past 7 days, or clear up and occur again in a couple of days, discontinue use and consult a physician
- severe reactions to urushiol (the chemical released by the plant, which causes the irritation) can look like chemical burns and have a thick leathery appearance. Additional applications may be necessary

**Keep this and all drugs out of reach of children.** If ingested, contact a physician or Poison Control Center immediately.

### DIRECTIONS

| adults and children 2 years of age or older | apply to effected area not more than 3 times daily |
|---|---|
| children under 2 years of age | do not use, consult a physician |

### OTHER INFORMATION
• store at room temperature

### INACTIVE INGREDIENTS
deionized water, glyceryl stearate, hydroxypropyl starch phosphate, cetearyl alcohol (and) cetearath-20, PEG-40 hydrogenated castor oil, zinc stearate, butylene glycol, steareth-2, steareth-20, PEG-100 stearate, isostearyl linoleate, zinc gluconate, isopropyl myristate, ethtylhexyl palmitate, dimethicone, tocopheryl acetate, alanloln, dmdm hydantoin (and) lodopropynyl butylcarbamate.

### QUESTIONS OR COMMENTS
www.ivydry.com

---

## IVY-DRY SUPER (benzyl alcohol, zinc acetate, camphor, and menthol)

Ivy-Dry, Inc.

### DRUG FACTS

| Active ingredients | Purpose |
|---|---|
| Benzyl alcohol 10% | Anti-itch |
| Zinc acetate 2.0% | Rash treatment |
| Camphor 0.5% | External analgesic |
| Menthol 0.25% | External analgesic |

### USES
• temporarily relieves the itching, oozing and weeping associated with minor skin irritations and rashes due to poison ivy, oak, sumac and insect bites

### WARNINGS
**For external use only.**
• test product on a small patch of skin before applying to the entire body
• do not use on face or genital areas
• avoid contact with eyes
• not to be used on areas of blistered or broken skin. Do not cover the affected area with a compress after application
• if condition does not improve or persists past 7 days, or clear up and occur again in a couple of days, discontinue use and consult a physician
• severe reactions to urushlol (the chemical released by the plant, which causes the irritation) can look like chemical burns and have a thick leathery appearance
• additional applications may be necessary

**Pregnant women should contact a doctor before use.**

**Keep this and all drugs out of reach of children.** If ingested, contact a physician or Poison Control Center immediately.

### DIRECTIONS
• shake well before using

| adults and children 6 years of age or older | apply to affected area not more than 3 times daily |
|---|---|
| children under 6 years of age | do not use, consult a physician |

### OTHER INFORMATION
• store at room temperature

### INACTIVE INGREDIENTS
water, isopropyl alcohol, isoceteth-20, zinc lactate, zinc gluconate

### QUESTIONS OR COMMENTS
visit www.ivydry.com

---

## KAOPECTATE REGULAR STRENGTH CHERRY (bismuth subsalicylate) liquid

Chattem, Inc.

### DRUG FACTS

| Active ingredient (per 15 mL) | Purpose |
|---|---|
| Bismuth subsalicylate 262 mg | Anti-diarrheal |
|  | Upset stomach reliever |

### USES
• relieves diarrhea
• relieves nausea and upset stomach associated with this symptom

### WARNINGS
**Reye's Syndrome**
Children and teenagers who have or are recovering from chicken pox or flu-like symptoms should not use this product. When using this product, if changes in behavior with nausea and vomiting occur, consult a doctor because these symptoms could be an early sign of Reye's syndrome, a rare but serious illness.

**Allergy alert**
**Contains salicylate.**

### DO NOT TAKE IF YOU ARE
• allergic to salicylates (including aspirin)
• taking other salicylate products

### DO NOT USE IF YOU HAVE
• an ulcer
• a bleeding problem
• bloody or black stool

### ASK A DOCTOR BEFORE USE IF YOU HAVE
• fever
• mucus in the stool

### ASK A DOCTOR OR PHARMACIST BEFORE USE IF YOU ARE TAKING ANY DRUG FOR
• diabetes
• gout
• arthritis
• anticoagulation (thinning the blood)

### WHEN USING THIS PRODUCT
• a temporary, but harmless, darkening of the stool and/or tongue may occur

## STOP USE AND ASK A DOCTOR IF
- symptoms get worse
- ringing in the ears or loss of hearing occurs
- diarrhea lasts more than 2 days

**If pregnant or breastfeeding,** ask a health professional before use.

**Keep out of reach of children.** In case of overdose, get medical help or contact a Poison Control Center right away.

## DIRECTIONS
- shake well immediately before each use
- drink plenty of clear fluids to help prevent dehydration caused by diarrhea

| | |
|---|---|
| adults and children 12 years of age and older | 30 mL or 2 tablespoonfuls |
| | for accurate dosing, use convenient pre-measured dose cup |
| | repeat dose every ½ hour to 1 hour as needed |
| | do not exceed 8 doses in 24 hours |
| | use until diarrhea stops but not more than 2 days |
| children under 12 years | ask a doctor |

## OTHER INFORMATION
- each 15 mL tablespoonful contains: sodium 4 mg
- each 15 mL tablespoonful contains: total salicylates 130 mg
- do not use if inner seal is broken or missing
- low sodium

## INACTIVE INGREDIENTS
caramel, carboxymethylcellulose sodium, flavor, microcrystalline cellulose, FD&C red no. 40, sodium salicylate, sorbic acid, sucrose, water, xanthan gum (245-240)

## QUESTIONS OR COMMENTS
www.chattem.com

---

# KERASAL (natural menthol) lotion
Alterna, LLC

## DRUG FACTS

| Active ingredient | Purpose |
|---|---|
| Menthol 8.5 mg | Topical analgesic |

## USES
- temporarily relieves minor foot, ankle, and leg pain associated with:
  - arthritis
  - muscle aches
  - muscle strains
  - muscle sprains
  - joint pain

## WARNINGS
**For external use only.**

**Flammable:** Keep away from excessive heat or open flame.

## ASK A DOCTOR BEFORE USE IF YOU HAVE
- sensitive skin

## WHEN USING THIS PRODUCT
- do not use on wounds or irritated skin
- do not bandage tightly or use with a heating pad
- wash hands after use with cool water
- avoid contact with eyes or mucous membranes

## STOP USE AND ASK A DOCTOR IF
- condition worsens or
- if pain persists for more than 7 days, or clears up, then reoccurs within a few days, or
- if excessive skin irritation occurs

**If pregnant or breastfeeding,** ask a health professional before use.

**Keep out of reach of children.** If accidentally swallowed, contact a doctor or Poison Control Center immediately.

## DIRECTIONS
- use only as directed
- do not use on children under 12 years of age
- roll onto affected area no more than four times daily

## OTHER INFORMATION
- store in a cool dry place with the cap tightly closed

Note: Because this product contains natural ingredients, color may vary.

## INACTIVE INGREDIENTS
aloe barbadensis leaf extract, arnica montana extract, boswellia, serrata extract, camphor, carbomer, chondroitin sulfate, glucosamine sulfate, glycerin, ilex paraguarensis extract, isopropyl alcohol, methyl paraben, methylsulfonylmethane, peppermint oil, polysorbate 20, propylene glycol, triethanolamine, purified water

## QUESTIONS OR COMMENTS
Visit our website at www.jointflex.com or Call **(888) 464-3336.**

---

# KONSYL 100% NATURAL PSYLLIUM FIBER
(psyllium husk) capsule
Konsyl Pharmaceuticals, Inc.

## DRUG FACTS

| Active ingredient (in each dose) | Purpose |
|---|---|
| Psyllium husk approx. 520 mg | Bulk-forming laxative |

## USES
- for relief of occasional constipation (irregularity)
- this product generally produces bowel movement in 12 to 72 hours

## WARNINGS
**Allergy alert**
This product may cause an allergic reaction in people sensitive to inhaled or ingested psyllium.

**Choking**
Taking this product without adequate fluid may cause it to swell and block your throat or esophagus and may cause choking.

## DO NOT TAKE THIS PRODUCT IF YOU HAVE
- difficulty in swallowing
- if you experience chest pain, vomiting, or difficulty in swallowing or breathing after taking this product, seek immediate medical attention
- difficulty swallowing

### ASK A DOCTOR BEFORE USE IF YOU HAVE
- stomach pain, nausea, or vomiting
- a sudden change in bowel habits that persists over 2 weeks

### STOP USE AND ASK A DOCTOR IF
- you fail to have a bowel movement or have rectal bleeding. These could be sings of a serious condition
- you need to use a laxative for more than 1 week

**If pregnant or breastfeeding,** ask a health professional before use.

**Keep out of reach of children.** In case of overdose, get medical help or contact a Poison Control Center right away.

### DIRECTIONS
- take this product (child or adult dose) with at least 8 ounces (a full glass of water or other fluid. Taking this product without enough liquid may cause choking. See Choking Warning
- follow dosage below or use as directed by a doctor
- drink a full glass (8 ounces ) of water or other liquid with each dose
- continued use for 1 to 3 days is normally required to provide full benefit

| adults and children 12 years and over | 5 capsules one to three times daily |
|---|---|
| children under 12 years | consult a doctor |

### OTHER INFORMATION
- keep tightly closed
- store at room temperature
- contains a 100% natural therapeutic fiber

### INACTIVE INGREDIENTS
FD&C yellow no. 6, gelatin, polyethylene glycol, polysorbate 80

### QUESTIONS OR COMMENTS
Call **1-800-356-6795** 8:30 AM to 5 PM ET
www.konsyl.com

---

## KONSYL EASY MIX FORMULA
**PSYLLIUM FIBER** (psyllium husk) granule

Konsyl Pharmaceuticals, Inc.

### DRUG FACTS

| Active ingredient (in each dose) | Purpose |
|---|---|
| Psyllium hydrophilic mucilloid 4.3 grams | Bulk-forming laxative |

### USE
- for relief of occasional constipation and to induce regularity. This product generally produces bowel movements within 12 to 72 hours

### WARNINGS
**Allergy alert**
As with any natural grain product, inhaled or ingested psyllium powder may cause an allergic reaction in people sensitive to psyllium.

**Choking**
Taking this product without adequate fluid may cause it to swell and block your throat or esophagus and may cause choking.

### DO NOT TAKE THIS PRODUCT IF YOU HAVE
- difficulty in swallowing
- if you experience chest pain, vomiting or difficulty in swallowing or breathing after taking this product, seek immediate medical attention

### DO NOT USE
- laxative products when abdominal pain, nausea or vomiting are present unless directed by a doctor

### ASK A DOCTOR BEFORE USE IF YOU HAVE
- a sudden change in bowel habits that persists over a period of two weeks

### STOP USE AND ASK A DOCTOR IF
- you experience rectal bleeding
- you fail to have a bowel movement

**Keep out of reach of children.** In case of overdose, get medical help or contact a Poison Control Center right away.

### DIRECTIONS
- mix this product (child or adult dose) with at least 8 ounces (a full glass) of water or other fluid
- taking this product without enough fluid may cause choking. See Choking Warning

| adults and children 12 years and older | sprinkle one teaspoonful into a glass with 8 ounces of juice, water or other fluid; stir briskly 3-5 seconds; drink promptly; if mixture thickens, add more fluid, stir; follow with additional fluid to aid product action; take 1-3 times daily |
|---|---|
| children 6 years to under 12 years | ½ adult dose, in 8 ounces of fluid; 1-3 times daily |
| children under 6 years | ask a doctor |

### OTHER INFORMATION
- each 6 g dose contains: calcium 8 mg, potassium 37 mg, sodium 7 mg
- laxatives, including bulk fibers, may affect how other medicines work, wait 1-2 hours before or after taking other medicines
- tamper-evident bottle mouth sealed for your protection
- do not use if imprinted inner seal is broken or missing
- store below 86°F (30°C)
- keep container tightly closed
- protect from moisture
- heart-healthy diets low in saturated fat and cholesterol that include 7 grams of soluble fiber per day from psyllium husk may reduce the risk of coronary heart disease (CHD) by lowering cholesterol; one adult dose of this product contains 2 grams of this soluble fiber

### INACTIVE INGREDIENTS
maltodextrin, silicon dioxide

### QUESTIONS OR COMMENTS
Konsyl Pharmaceuticals, Inc. at **1-800-356-6795** 8:30 AM to 5 PM EST. or visit www.konsyl.com

# KONSYL NATURALLY SWEETENED PSYLLIUM FIBER (psyllium husk) granule
Konsyl Pharmaceuticals, Inc.

## DRUG FACTS

| Active ingredient (in each dose) | Purpose |
|---|---|
| Psyllium hydrophilic mucilloid 3.4 grams | Bulk-forming laxative |

## USE
- for relief of occasional costipation
- generally produces effect in 12-72 hours
- natural bulk producing fiber encourages normal elimination without chemical stimulants

## WARNINGS
### Allergy alert
Inhaled or ingested psyllium powder may cause an allergic reaction in people sensitive to psyllium.

### Choking
Taking this product without adequate fluid may cause it to swell and block your throat or esophagus and may cause choking. Do not take this product if you have difficulty in swallowing. If you experience chest pain, vomiting or difficulty in swallowing or breathing after taking this product, seek immediate medical attention.

### DO NOT USE
- laxative products when abdominal pain, nausea or vomiting are present unless directed by a doctor

### ASK A DOCTOR BEFORE USE IF YOU HAVE
- a sudden change in bowel habits that persists over a period of two weeks

### WHEN USING THIS PRODUCT
- do not take for a period longer than 1 week, unless directed by a doctor

### STOP USE AND ASK A DOCTOR IF
- you experience rectal bleeding
- you fail to have a bowel movement

**Keep out of reach of children.** In case of overdose get medical help or contact a Poison Control Center right away.

## DIRECTIONS
- mix this product (child or adult dose) with at least 8 ounces (a full glass) of water or other fluid
- taking this product without enough liquid may cause choking
- see Choking Warning

| adults and children 12 years and over | 1 rounded teaspoonful (6.5 g) mixed in 8 ounces of liquid, 1-3 times daily |
|---|---|
| children 6 years to under 12 years | ½ the adult dose in 8 ounces of liquid, up to 3 times daily |
| children under 6 years | consult a doctor |

## OTHER INFORMATION
- each 6.5 g dose contains: calcium 6 mg, potassium 31 mg, sodium 3 mg
- store below 86° F (30°C)
- keep container tightly closed
- protect from excessive moisture

- tamper-evident bottle mouth sealed for your protection
- do not use if imprinted inner seal is broken or missing
- laxatives, including bulk fibers, may affect how other medicines work, wait 1-2 hours before or after taking other medicines
- see label for expiration date
- can be taken 1 to 3 times daily, before or after meals, mornings, or evenings
- maximum daily dose (3 teaspoonfuls) is very low sodium - do not discard powder into any plumbing systems
- note to diabetics: this product contains 48% sugar (dextrose)
- no starch, no flavors, no color added
- each dose provides 3 grams total dietary fiber
- each dose contains 14 calories

## INACTIVE INGREDIENTS
dextrose

## QUESTIONS OR COMMENTS
Konsyl Pharmaceuticals, Inc. at **1-800-356-6795** 8:30 AM to 5 PM EST.

# KONSYL ORANGE FLAVOR PSYLLIUM FIBER - ORIGINAL TEXTURE (psyllium husk) granule
Konsyl Pharmaceuticals, Inc.

## DRUG FACTS

| Active ingredient (in each dose) | Purpose |
|---|---|
| Psyllium hydrophilic mucilloid 3.4 g | Bulk forming laxative |

## USES
- for relief of occasional constipation (irregularity)
- generally produces bowel movement in 12-72 hours
- natural bulk producing fiber encourages normal elimination without chemical stimulants

## WARNINGS
### Allergy alert
Inhaled or ingested psyllium powder may cause an allergic reaction in people sensitive to psyllium.

### Choking
Taking this product without adequate fluid may cause it to swell and block your throat or esophagus and may cause choking. Do not take this product if you have difficulty in swallowing. If you experience chest pain, vomiting or difficulty in swallowing or breathing after taking this product, seek immediate medical attention.

### DO NOT USE
- laxative products when abdominal pain, nausea or vomiting are present unless directed by a doctor

### ASK A DOCTOR BEFORE USE IF YOU HAVE
- a sudden change in bowel habits that persists over a period of two weeks

### WHEN USING THIS PRODUCT
- do not take for a period longer than 1 week, unless directed by a doctor

### STOP USE AND ASK A DOCTOR IF
- you experience rectal bleeding
- you fail to have a bowel movement

**Keep out of reach of children.** In case of overdose, get medical help or contact a Poison Control Center right away.

### DIRECTIONS
- mix this product (child or adult dose) with at least 8 ounces (a full glass) of water or other fluid
- taking this product without enough liquid may cause choking
- see Choking Warnings

| adults and children 12 years and over | 1 rounded tablespoonful (11g) mixed in 8 ounces of liquid, 1-3 times daily, at the first sign of irregularity |
|---|---|
| children 6 to under 12 years | ½ the adult dose in 8 ounces of liquid, up to 3 times daily |
| children under 6 years | consult a doctor |

### OTHER INFORMATION
- each 11 g dose contains: calcium 6 mg, potassium 31 mg, sodium 3 mg
- note to diabetics: this product contains sugar (sucrose)
- store below 30°C (86°F)
- keep tightly closed to protect from humidity
- tamper-evident bottle mouth sealed for your protection
- do not use if imprinted inner seal is broken or missing
- maximum daily dose (3 tablespoonfuls) is very low sodium
- each dose provides 3 grams total dietary fiber
- each dose contains 35 calories

### INACTIVE INGREDIENTS:
sucrose, citric acid, FD&C yellow no. 6 (sunset yellow), flavoring

### QUESTIONS OR COMMENTS
Konsyl Pharmaceuticals, Inc. at **1-800-356-6795** 8:30 AM to 5 PM EST.

---

## KONSYL ORANGE FLAVOR PSYLLIUM FIBER - SMOOTH TEXTURE (psyllium husk)
granule

Konsyl Pharmaceuticals, Inc.

### DRUG FACTS

| Active ingredient (in each dose) | Purpose |
|---|---|
| Psyllium hydrophilic mucilloid 3.4 grams | Bulk-forming laxative |

### USE
- for relief of occasional constipation
- generally produces effect in 12-72 hours
- naural bulk producing fiber encourages normal elimination without chemical stimulants

### WARNINGS
**Allergy alert**
Inhaled or ingested psyllium powder may cause an allergic reaction in people sensitive to psyllium.

**Choking**
Taking this product without adequate fluid may cause it to swell and block your throat or esophagus and may cause choking. Do not take this product if you have difficulty in swallowing. If you experience chest pain, vomiting or difficulty in swallowing or breathing after taking this product, seek immediate medical attention.

### DO NOT USE
- laxative products when abdominal pain, nausea or vomiting are present unless directed by a doctor

### ASK A DOCTOR BEFORE USE IF YOU HAVE
- a sudden change in bowel habits that persists over a period of two weeks

### WHEN USING THIS PRODUCT
- do not take for a period longer than 1 week, unless directed by a doctor

### STOP USE AND ASK A DOCTOR IF
- you experience rectal bleeding
- you fail to have a bowel movement

**Keep out of reach of children.** In case of overdose, get medical help or contact a Poison Control Center right away.

### DIRECTIONS
- mix this product (child or adult dose) with at least 8 ounces (a full glass) of water or other fluid
- taking this product without enough liquid may cause choking
- see Choking Warnings

| adults and children 12 years and over | sprinkle one dose, 1 rounded tablespoonful (12g), in 8 ounces of liquid, 1-3 times daily |
|---|---|
| children 6 years to under 12 years | ½ the adult dose in 8 ounces of liquid, up to 3 times daily |
| children under 6 years | consult a doctor |

### OTHER INFORMATION
- each 12 g dose contains: calcium 6 mg, potassium 31 mg, sodium 3 mg
- store below 86°F (30°C)
- keep container tightly closed
- protect from excessive moisture
- tamper-evident bottle mouth sealed for your protection
- do not use if imprinted inner seal is broken or missing
- laxatives, including bulk fibers, may affect how other medicines work, wait 1-2 hours before or after taking other medicines
- can be taken 1 to 3 times daily, before or after meals, mornings, or evenings
- maximum daily dose (3 tablespoonfuls) is very low sodium
- do not discard Konsyl Orange powder into any plumbing systems
- note to diabetics: this product contains 66% sugar (sucrose)
- each dose provides 3 grams total dietary fiber
- each dose contains 35 calories

### INACTIVE INGREDIENTS
citric acid, D&C yellow no. 10 and FD&C yellow no. 6 (sunset yellow), flavoring, sucrose

### QUESTIONS OR COMMENTS
Konsyl Pharmaceuticals, Inc. at **1-800-36-6795** 8:30 AM to 5 PM EST.

## KONSYL ORIGINAL FORMULA PSYLLIUM FIBER (psyllium husk) granule
Konsyl Pharmaceuticals, Inc.

### DRUG FACTS

| Active ingredient (in each dose) | Purpose |
|---|---|
| Psyllium hydrophilic mucilloid 6 grams | Bulk-forming laxative |

### USE
- for relief of occasional constipation and to induce regularity
- this product generally produces bowel movements within 12-72 hours

### WARNINGS
**Allergy alert**
As with any natural grain product, inhaled or ingested psyllium powder may cause an allergic reaction in people sensitive to psyllium.

### DO NOT USE
- laxative products when abdominal pain, nausea or vomiting are present unless directed by a doctor

### ASK A DOCTOR BEFORE USE IF YOU HAVE
- a sudden change in bowel habits that persists over a period of two weeks

### WHEN USING THIS PRODUCT
- physicians recommend a gradual increase in dietary fiber
- if minor gas or bloating occurs, begin with a half-dose of KONSYL and slowly increase the dose over several days
- always follow with 8 ounces of fluid

### STOP USE AND ASK A DOCTOR IF
- you experience rectal bleeding
- you fail to have a bowel movement

**Keep out of reach of children.** In case of overdose, get medical help or contact a Poison Control Center right away.

### DIRECTIONS
- mix this product (child or adult dose) with at least 8 ounces (a full glass) of water or other fluid
- taking this product without enough fluid may cause choking
- see Choking Warnings

| adults and children 12 years and older | sprinkle one dose (one rounded teaspoonful) into a shaker cup or closed container with at least 8 ounces of juice, water or other beverage; shake 3 to 5 seconds; drink promptly; if mixture thickens, add more fluid stir; follow with additional fluid to aid product action; take 1-3 times daily |
|---|---|
| children 6 years to under 12 years | ½ adult dose, in 8 ounces of fluid; 1-3 times daily |
| children under 6 years | ask a doctor |

### OTHER INFORMATION
- each 6.0 gram dose contains: calcium 10 mg, potassium 55 mg, sodium 5 mg
- maximum daily dose (3 teaspoonfuls) is very low in sodium

- do not discard KONSYL powder into any plumbing systems
- laxatives, including bulk fibers, may affect how other medicines work, wait 1-2 hours before or after taking other medicines
- no additives, no sugars, gluten free, no flavors, 100% natural
- safe for diabetics, non habit-forming
- tamper-evident bottle mouth sealed for your protection
- do not use if imprinted inner seal is broken or missing
- store below 86°F (30°C)
- keep container tightly closed protect from excessive moisture
- can be taken 1 to 3 times daily, before or after meals, mornings or evenings

### INACTIVE INGREDIENTS
None

### QUESTIONS OR COMMENTS
Call **1-800-356-6795** 8:30 AM to 5 PM EST.
www.konsyl.com

## KONSYL OVERNIGHT RELIEF SENNA PROMPT (psyllium, sennosides) capsule
Konsyl Pharmaceuticals, Inc.

### DRUG FACTS

| Active ingredients (in each capsule) | Purpose |
|---|---|
| Psyllium 500 mg | Bulk-forming laxative |
| Sennosides 9 mg | Stimulant laxative |

### USES
- for relief of occasional constipation (irregularity)
- this product generally produces bowel movement in 6 to 12 hours

### WARNINGS
**Allergy alert**
This product may cause an allergic reaction in people sensitive to inhaled or ingested psyllium.

**Choking**
Taking this product without adequate fluid may cause it to swell and block your throat or esophagus and may cause choking. Do not take this product if you have difficulty in swallowing. If you experience chest pain, vomiting, or difficulty in swallowing or breathing after taking this product, seek immediate medical attention.

### ASK A DOCTOR BEFORE USE IF YOU HAVE
- abdominal pain, nausea or vomiting
- a sudden change in bowel habits that persists over 2 weeks

### STOP USE AND ASK A DOCTOR IF
- you fail to have a bowel movement or have rectal bleeding. These could be signs of a serious condition
- you need to use a laxative for more than 1 week

**If pregnant or breastfeeding,** ask a health professional before use.

**Keep out of reach of children.** In case of overdose, get medical help or contact a Poison Control Center right away.

### DIRECTIONS
- take this product (child or adult dose) with at least 8 ounces (a full glass) of water or other fluid. Taking this product without enough liquid may cause choking. See Choking Warning
- follow dosage below or use as directed by a doctor

| adults and children 12 years and over | 1-5 capsules one or two times daily |
| children under 12 years | consult a doctor |

## INACTIVE INGREDIENTS
D&C yellow no. 10 aluminum. lake, FD&C blue no. 1 aluminum, lake, gelatin, polyethylene glycol, polysorbate 80

## OTHER INFORMATION
- keep tightly closed
- store at room temperature

## QUESTIONS OR COMMENTS
Call **1-800-356-6795** or visit www.konsyl.com

---

# KONSYL SUGAR FREE ORANGE FLAVOR PSYLLIUM FIBER (psyllium husk) granule
Konsyl Pharmaceuticals, Inc.

## DRUG FACTS

| Active ingredient (in each dose) | Purpose |
|---|---|
| Psyllium hydrophilic mucilloid 3.5 g | Bulk-forming laxative |

## USES
- for relief of occasional constipation (irregularity)
- generally produces bowel movement in 12-72 hours
- natural bulk producing fiber encourages normal elimination without chemical stimulants

## WARNINGS
**Allergy alert**
Inhaled or ingested psyllium powder may cause an allergic reaction in people sensitive to psyllium.

**Choking**
Taking this product without adequate fluid may cause it to swell and block your throat or esophagus and may cause choking. Do not take this product if you have difficulty in swallowing. If you experience chest pain, vomiting or difficulty in swallowing or breathing after taking this product, seek immediate medical attention.

## DO NOT USE
- laxative products when abdominal pain nausea or vomiting are present unless directed by a doctor

## ASK A DOCTOR BEFORE USE IF YOU HAVE
- a sudden change in bowel habits that persists over a period of two weeks

## WHEN USING THIS PRODUCT
- do not take for a period longer than 1 week, unless directed by a doctor

## STOP USE AND ASK A DOCTOR IF
- you experience rectal bleeding
- you fail to have a bowel movement

**Keep out of reach of children.** In case of overdose, get medical help or contact a Poison Control Center right away.

## DIRECTIONS
- mix this product (child or adult dose) with at least 8 ounces (a full glass) of water or other fluid

- taking this product without enough liquid may cause choking. See Choking Warning

| adults and children 12 years and over | 1 rounded tablespoonful (11g) mixed in 8 ounces of liquid, 1-3 times daily, at the first sign of irregularity |
| children 6 to under 12 years | ½ the adult dose in 8 ounces of liquid, up to 3 times daily |
| children under 6 years | Consult a doctor |

## OTHER INFORMATION
- each 11 g dose contains: calcium 6 mg, potassium 31 mg, sodium 3 mg
- note to diabetics: this product contains sugar (sucrose)
- store below 30°C (86°F)
- keep tightly closed to protect from humidity
- tamper-evident bottle mouth sealed for your protection
- do not use if imprinted inner seal is broken or missing
- maximum daily dose (3 tablespoonfuls) is very low sodium
- each dose provides 3 grams total dietary fiber
- each dose contains 35 calories

## INACTIVE INGREDIENTS
aspartame, citric acid, FD&C yellow no. 6 (sunset yellow), flavoring, maltodextrin, silicon dioxide

## QUESTIONS OR COMMENTS
Call Konsyl Pharmaceuticals, Inc. at **1-800-356-6795** 8:30 AM to 5 PM EST. or visit www.konsyl.com

---

# LAMISIL AF DEFENSE (tolnaftate) cream
Novartis Consumer Health, Inc.

## DRUG FACTS

| Active ingredient | Purpose |
|---|---|
| Tolnaftate | Antifungal |

## USES
- treats and prevents most athlete's foot (*tinea pedis*), and ringworm (*tinea corporis*)
- prevents most athlete's foot (*tinea pedis*) with daily use
- relieves itching, burning, cracking and scaling which accompany these conditions

## WARNINGS
**For external use only.**

## DO NOT USE
- on children under 2 years of age unless directed by a doctor
- in or near the mouth or the eyes
- on nails or scalp

## WHEN USING THIS PRODUCT
- do not get into eyes. If eye contact occurs, rinse eyes thoroughly with water

## STOP USE AND ASK A DOCTOR IF
- irritation occurs or gets worse
- no improvement in athlete's foot within 4 weeks

**Keep out of reach of children.** If swallowed, get medical help or contact a Poison Control Center right away.

## DIRECTIONS

| adults and children 2 years of age and over | to open tube, peel off foil seal |
| --- | --- |
| | wash the affected area and dry thoroughly |
| | apply a thin layer over affected area twice daily (morning and night) or as directed by a doctor |
| | for athlete's foot pay special attention to spaces between the toes |
| | wear well-fitting, ventilated shoes |
| | change shoes and socks at least once daily |
| | use daily for 4 weeks; if condition persists longer, consult a doctor |
| | to prevent athlete's foot, apply once or twice daily (morning and/or night) |
| | supervise children in the use of this product |
| | wash hands after each use |
| children under 2 years of age | ask a doctor |

## OTHER INFORMATION
- do not use if seal on tube is broken or is not visible
- store at controlled room temperature 20-25°C (68-77°F)

## INACTIVE INGREDIENTS
acrylates/C10-30 acrylate cross polymer, carbomer, corn starch, cyclomethicone, edetate disodium, ethyl alcohol, fragrance, isopropyl mysristate, propylene glycol, purified water, strong ammonia solution

## QUESTIONS OR COMMENTS
Call 1-800-452-0051

---

# LAMISIL AT (terbinafine) gel
Novartis Consumer Health, Inc.

## DRUG FACTS

| Active ingredient | Purpose |
| --- | --- |
| Terbinafine 1% | Antifungal |

## USES
- cures most athlete's foot (*tinea pedis*) between the toes Effectiveness on the bottom or sides of foot is unknown
- cures most jock itch (*tinea cruris*) and ringworm (*tinea corporis*)
- relieves itching, burning, cracking and scaling which accompany these conditions

## WARNINGS
For external use only.

## DO NOT USE
- on nails or scalp
- in or near the mouth or eyes
- for vaginal yeast infections

## WHEN USING THIS PRODUCT
- do not get into eyes. If eye contact occurs, rinse thoroughly with water

**Keep out of reach of children.** If swallowed, get medical help or contact a Poison Control Center right away.

## DIRECTIONS

| adults and children 12 years and over | use the tip of the cap to break the seal and open the tube |
| --- | --- |
| | wash the affected skin with soap and water and dry completely before applying |
| | for athlete's foot between the toes: apply once a day at bedtime for 1 week or as directed by a doctor. Wear well-fitting, ventilated shoes. Change shoes and socks at least once daily |
| | for jock itch and ringworm: apply once a day (morning or night) for 1 week or as directed by a doctor |
| | wash hands after each use |
| children under 12 years | ask a doctor |

## OTHER INFORMATION
- do not use if seal on tube is broken or is not visible
- store at or below 30°C (86°F)

## INACTIVE INGREDIENTS
benzyl alcohol, butylated hydroxytoluene, carbomer 974 P, ethanol, isopropyl myristate, polysorbate 20, purified water, sodium hydroxide, sorbitan monolaurate

## QUESTIONS OR COMMENTS
Call 1-800-452-0051

---

# LAMISIL AT (terbinafine hydrochloride) spray
Novartis Consumer Health, Inc.

## DRUG FACTS

| Active ingredient | Purpose |
| --- | --- |
| Terbinafine hydrochloride | Antifungal |

## USES
- cures most athlete's foot (*tinea pedis*), between the toes. Effectiveness on the bottom or sides of foot is unknown
- cures most jock itch (*tinea cruris*) and ringworm (*tinea corporis*)
- relieves itching, burning, cracking and scaling which accompany these conditions

## WARNINGS
For external use only.

## DO NOT USE
- on nails or scalp
- in or near the mouth or eyes
- for vaginal yeast infections

## WHEN USING THIS PRODUCT
- do not get into eyes. If eye contact occurs, rinse thoroughly with water

**STOP USE AND ASK DOCTOR IF**
• too much irritation occurs or gets worse

**Keep out of reach of children.** If swallowed, get medical help or contact a Poison Control Center right away.

**DIRECTIONS**

| adults and children 12 years and over | wash the affected skin with soap and water and dry completely before applying |
|---|---|
| | for athlete's foot wear well-fitting, ventilated shoes. Change shoes and socks at least once daily. |
| | between the toes only: spray twice a day (morning and night) for 1 week or as directed by a doctor |
| | for jock itch and ringworm: spray once a day (morning or night) for 1 week or as directed by a doctor |
| | wash hands after each use |
| children under 12 years | ask a doctor |

**OTHER INFORMATION**
• store at 8-25°C (46-77°F)

**INACTIVE INGREDIENTS**
cetomacrogol, ethanol, propylene glycol, purified water

**QUESTIONS OR COMMENTS**
Call **1-800-452-0051**

---

## LAMISIL AT CONTINUOUS SPRAY (terbinafine hydrochloride) liquid

Novartis Consumer Health, Inc.

**DRUG FACTS**

| Active ingredient | Purpose |
|---|---|
| Terbinafine hydrochloride | Antifungal |

**USES**
• cures most jock itch (*tinea cruris*)
• relieves itching, burning, cracking, and scaling which accompany this condition

**WARNINGS**
**For external use only.**

**DO NOT USE**
• on nails or scalp
• in or near the mouth or the eyes
• for vaginal yeast infections

**WHEN USING THIS PRODUCT**
• do not get into eyes. If contact occurs, rinse eyes thoroughly with water

**STOP USE AND ASK A DOCTOR**
• if too much irritation occurs or gets worse

**Keep out of reach of children.** If swallowed, get medical help or contact a Poison Control Center right away.

---

**DIRECTIONS**

| adults and children 12 years and over | wash the affected area with soap and water and dry completely before applying |
|---|---|
| | to open remove clear cap hold can 4" to 6" from skin. Press and hold to spray a thin layer over affected area |
| | spray affected area once a day (morning or night) for 1 week or as directed by a doctor |
| | release to stop spray |
| | wipe excess from spray opening after each use |
| | return cap to can |
| | wash hands after each use |
| children under 12 years | ask a doctor |

**OTHER INFORMATION**
• store at 8-25°C (46-77°F)

**INACTIVE INGREDIENTS**
ethanol, polyoxyl 20 cetostearyl ether, propylene glycol, purified water

**QUESTIONS OR COMMENTS**
Call **1-800-452-0051** or visit us at www.lamisilat.com

---

## LAMISIL AT JOCK ITCH (terbinafine hydrochloride) cream

Novartis Consumer Health, Inc.

**DRUG FACTS**

| Active ingredient | Purpose |
|---|---|
| Terbinafine hydrochloride | Antifungal |

**USES**
• cures most jock itch (*tinea cruris*)
• relieves itching, burning, cracking and scaling which accompany these conditions

**WARNINGS**
**For external use only.**

**DO NOT USE**
• in or near the mouth or eyes
• for vaginal yeast infections

**WHEN USING THIS PRODUCT**
• do not get into eyes. If eye contact occurs, rinse thoroughly with water

**STOP USE AND ASK DOCTOR IF**
• too much irritation occurs or gets worse

**Keep out of reach of children.** If swallowed, get medical help or contact a Poison Control Center right away.

## DIRECTIONS

| adults and children 12 years and over | use the tip of the cap to break the seal and open the tube |
|---|---|
| | wash the affected skin with soap and water and dry completely before applying |
| | apply once a day (morning or night) for 1 week or as directed by a doctor |
| | wash hands after each use |
| children under 12 years | ask a doctor |

## OTHER INFORMATION
* do not use if seal on tube is broken or is not visible
* store at controlled room temperature 20-25°C (68-77°F)

## INACTIVE INGREDIENTS
benzyl alcohol, cetyl alcohol, cetyl palmitate, isopropyl myristate, polysorbate 60, purified water, sodium hydroxide, sorbitan monostearate, stearyl alcohol

## QUESTIONS OR COMMENTS
Call 1-800-452-0051

# LEVONORGESTREL EMERGENCY CONTRACEPTIVE (levonorgestrel) tablet

Perrigo, New York, Inc

## 1 INDICATIONS AND USAGE
* Levonorgestrel tablets, 0.75 mg is a progestin-only emergency contraceptive indicated for prevention of pregnancy following unprotected intercourse or a known or suspected contraceptive failure. To obtain optimal efficacy, the first tablet should be taken as soon as possible within 72 hours of intercourse. The second tablet should be taken 12 hours later
* Levonorgestrel tablets, 0.75 mg is available only by prescription for women younger than age 17 years, and available over the counter for women 17 years and older
* Levonorgestrel tablets, 0.75 mg is not indicated for routine use as a contraceptive
* Levonorgestrel tablets, 0.75 mg is a progestin-only emergency contraceptive, indicated for prevention of pregnancy following unprotected intercourse or a known or suspected contraceptive failure. Levonorgestrel tablets, 0.75 mg is available only by prescription for women younger than age 17 years, and available over the counter for women 17 years and older. Levonorgestrel tablets, 0.75 mg is not intended for routine use as a contraceptive. (1)

## 2 DOSAGE AND ADMINISTRATION
* Take one tablet of Levonorgestrel tablets, 0.75 mg orally as soon as possible within 72 hours after unprotected intercourse or a known or suspected contraceptive failure. Efficacy is better if the tablet is taken as soon as possible after unprotected intercourse. The second tablet should be taken 12 hours after the first dose. Levonorgestrel tablets, 0.75 mg can be used at any time during the menstrual cycle
* If vomiting occurs within two hours of taking either dose of medication, consideration should be given to repeating the dose
* The first tablet is taken orally as soon as possible within 72 hours after unprotected intercourse. The second tablet should be taken 12 hours after the first dose. Efficacy is better if Levonorgestrel tablets, 0.75 mg is taken as soon as possible after unprotected intercourse. (2)

## 3 DOSAGE FORMS AND STRENGTHS
* Each Levonorgestrel tablets, 0.75 mg tablet is supplied as a white to off-white circular, flat beveled, uncoated tablet debossed with "L840" on one side and plain on the other side
* A total of two 0.75 mg tablets taken 12 hours apart as a single course of treatment. (3)

## 4 CONTRAINDICATIONS
* Levonorgestrel tablets, 0.75 mg is contraindicated for use in the case of known or suspected pregnancy
* Known or suspected pregnancy. (4)

## 5 WARNINGS AND PRECAUTIONS
* Ectopic Pregnancy: Women who become pregnant or complain of lower abdominal pain after taking Levonorgestrel tablets, 0.75 mg should be evaluated for ectopic pregnancy. (5.1)
* Levonorgestrel tablets, 0.75 mg is not effective in terminating an existing pregnancy. (5.2)
* Effect on menses: Levonorgestrel tablets, 0.75 mg may alter the next expected menses. If menses is delayed beyond 1 week, pregnancy should be considered. (5.3)
* STI/HIV: Levonorgestrel tablets, 0.75 mg does not protect against STI/HIV. (5.4)

### 5.1 Ectopic Pregnancy
* Ectopic pregnancies account for approximately 2% of all reported pregnancies. Up to 10% of pregnancies reported in clinical studies of routine use of progestin-only contraceptives are ectopic
* A history of ectopic pregnancy is not a contraindication to use of this emergency contraceptive method. Healthcare providers, however, should consider the possibility of an ectopic pregnancy in women who become pregnant or complain of lower abdominal pain after taking Levonorgestrel tablets, 0.75 mg. A follow-up physical or pelvic examination is recommended if there is any doubt concerning the general health or pregnancy status of any woman after taking Levonorgestrel tablets, 0.75 mg

### 5.2 Existing Pregnancy
Levonorgestrel tablets, 0.75 mg is not effective in terminating an existing pregnancy.

### 5.3 Effects on Menses
* Some women may experience spotting a few days after taking Levonorgestrel tablets, 0.75 mg. Menstrual bleeding patterns are often irregular among women using progestin-only oral contraceptives and women using levonorgestrel for postcoital and emergency contraception
* If there is a delay in the onset of expected menses beyond 1 week, consider the possibility of pregnancy

### 5.4 STI/HIV
Levonorgestrel tablets, 0.75 mg does not protect against HIV infection (AIDS) or other sexually transmitted infections (STIs).

### 5.5 Physical Examination and Follow-Up
A physical examination is not required prior to prescribing Levonorgestrel tablets, 0.75 mg. A follow-up physical or pelvic examination is recommended if there is any doubt concerning the general health or pregnancy status of any woman after taking Levonorgestrel tablets, 0.75 mg.

### 5.6 Fertility Following Discontinuation
A rapid return of fertility is likely following treatment with Levonorgestrel tablets, 0.75 mg for emergency contraception; therefore, routine contraception should be continued or initiated as soon as possible following use of Levonorgestrel tablets, 0.75 mg to ensure ongoing prevention of pregnancy.

## 6 ADVERSE REACTIONS

The most common adverse reactions (> 10%) in the clinical trial included menstrual changes (26%), nausea (23%), abdominal pain (18%), fatigue (17%), headache (17%), dizziness (11%), and breast tenderness (11%). (6.1)

**To report SUSPECTED ADVERSE REACTIONS, contact Call 1-800-719-9260, or contact FDA at 1-800-FDA-1088 or www.fda.gov/medwatch**

### 6.1 Clinical Trial Experience

- Because clinical trials are conducted under widely varying conditions, adverse reaction rates observed in the clinical trials of a drug cannot be directly compared to rates in the clinical trials of another drug and may not reflect the rates observed in clinical practice
- A double-blind, controlled clinical trial in 1,955 evaluable women compared the efficacy and safety of levonorgestrel tablets, 0.75 mg (one 0.75 mg tablet of levonorgestrel taken within 72 hours of unprotected intercourse, and one tablet taken 12 hours later) to the Yuzpe regimen (two tablets each containing 0.25 mg levonorgestrel and 0.05 mg ethinyl estradiol, taken within 72 hours of intercourse, and two tablets taken 12 hours later)
- The most common adverse events (> 10%) in the clinical trial for women receiving levonorgestrel tablets, 0.75 mg included menstrual changes (26%), nausea (23%), abdominal pain (18%), fatigue (17%), headache (17%), dizziness (11%), and breast tenderness (11%). Table 1 lists those adverse events that were reported in > 5% of levonorgestrel tablets, 0.75 mg users.Table 1: Adverse Events in ≥ 5% of Women, by % Frequency

| levonorgestrel tablets, 0.75 mgN=977 (%) | |
| --- | --- |
| Nausea | 23.1 |
| Abdominal Pain | 17.6 |
| Fatigue | 16.9 |
| Headache | 16.8 |
| Heavier Menstrual Bleeding | 13.8 |
| Lighter Menstrual Bleeding | 12.5 |
| Dizziness | 11.2 |
| Breast Tenderness | 10.7 |
| Vomiting | 5.6 |
| Diarrhea | 5.0 |

### 6.2 Postmarketing Experience

The following adverse reactions have been identified during post-approval use of levonorgestrel tablets, 0.75 mg. Because these reactions are reported voluntarily from a population of uncertain size, it is not always possible to reliably estimate their frequency or establish a causal relationship to drug exposure.

### Gastrointestinal Disorders

Abdominal Pain, Nausea, Vomiting

### General Disorders and Administration Site Conditions

Fatigue

### Nervous System Disorders

Dizziness, Headache

### Reproductive System and Breast Disorders

Dysmenorrhea, Irregular Menstruation, Oligomenorrhea, Pelvic Pain

## 7 DRUG INTERACTIONS

Drugs or herbal products that induce enzymes, including CYP3A4, that metabolize progestins may decrease the plasma concentrations of progestins, and may decrease the effectiveness of progestin-only pills. Some drugs or herbal products that may decrease the effectiveness of progestin-only pills include:

- barbiturates
- bosentan
- carbamazepine
- felbamate
- griseofulvin
- oxcarbazepine
- phenytoin
- rifampin
- St. John's wort
- topiramate

Significant changes (increase or decrease) in the plasma levels of the progestin have been noted in some cases of co-administration with HIV protease inhibitors or with non-nucleoside transcriptase inhibitors.

Consult the labeling of all concurrently used drugs to obtain further information about interactions with progestin-only pills or the potential for enzyme alterations.

Drugs or herbal products that induce certain enzymes, such as CYP3A4, may decrease the effectiveness of progestin-only pills. (7)

## 8 USE IN SPECIFIC POPULATIONS

- Nursing Mothers: Small amounts of progestin pass into the breast milk of nursing women taking progestin-only pills for long-term contraception, resulting in detectable steroid levels in infant plasma. (8.3)
- Levonorgestrel tablets, 0.75 mg is not intended for use in premenarcheal (8.4) or postmenopausal females. (8.5)
- Clinical trials demonstrated a higher pregnancy rate in the Chinese population. (8.6)

### 8.1 Pregnancy

Many studies have found no harmful effects on fetal development associated with long-term use of contraceptive doses of oral progestins. The few studies of infant growth and development that have been conducted with progestin-only pills have not demonstrated significant adverse effects.

### 8.3 Nursing Mothers

In general, no adverse effects of progestin-only pills have been found on breastfeeding performance or on the health, growth or development of the infant. However, isolated post-marketing cases of decreased milk production have been reported. Small amounts of progestins pass into the breast milk of nursing mothers taking progestins-only pills for long-term contraception, resulting in detectable steroid levels in infant plasma.

### 8.4 Pediatric Use

Safety and efficacy of progestin-only pills for long-term contraception have been established in women of reproductive age. Safety and efficacy are expected to be the same for postpubertal adolescents less than 17 years and for users 17 years and older. Use of Levonorgestrel tablets, 0.75 mg emergency contraception before menarche is not indicated.

### 8.5 Geriatric Use

This product is not intended for use in postmenopausal women.

### 8.6 Race

No formal studies have evaluated the effect of race. However, clinical trials demonstrated a higher pregnancy rate in Chinese women with both levonorgestrel tablets, 0.75 mg and the Yuzpe regimen (another form of emergency contraception). The reason for this apparent increase in the pregnancy rate with emergency contraceptives in Chinese women is unknown.

**8.7 Hepatic Impairment**

No formal studies were conducted to evaluate the effect of hepatic disease on the disposition of levonorgestrel tablets, 0.75 mg.

**8.8 Renal Impairment**

No formal studies were conducted to evaluate the effect of renal disease on the disposition of levonorgestrel tablets, 0.75 mg.

**9 DRUG ABUSE AND DEPENDENCE**

Levonorgestrel is not a controlled substance. There is no information about dependence associated with the use of levonorgestrel tablets, 0.75 mg.

**10 OVERDOSAGE**

There are no data on overdosage of levonorgestrel tablets, 0.75 mg, although the common adverse event of nausea and associated vomiting may be anticipated.

**11 DESCRIPTION**

each levonorgestrel tablet contains 0.75 mg of a single active steroid ingredient, levonorgestrel [18,19-dinorpregn-4-en-20-yn-3-one-13-ethyl-17-hydroxy-, (17α)-(-)-], a totally synthetic progestogen; the inactive ingredients present are colloidal silicon dioxide, corn starch, lactose monohydrate, magnesium stearate, and povidone; levonorgestrel has a molecular weight of 312.45, and the following structural and molecular formulas: $C_{21}H_{28}O_2$ levonorgestre molecular formula

**12 CLINICAL PHARMACOLOGY**

**12.1 Mechanism of Action**

Emergency contraceptive pills are not effective if a woman is already pregnant. Levonorgestrel tablets, 0.75 mg is believed to act as an emergency contraceptive principally by preventing ovulation or fertilization (by altering tubal transport of sperm and/or ova). In addition, it may inhibit implantation (by altering the endometrium). It is not effective once the process of implantation has begun.

**12.3 Pharmacokinetics**

**Absorption**

No specific investigation of the absolute bioavailability of levonorgestrel tablets, 0.75 mg in humans has been conducted. However, literature indicates that levonorgestrel is rapidly and completely absorbed after oral administration (bioavailability about 100%) and is not subject to first pass metabolism.

After a single dose of levonorgestrel tablets, 0.75 mg administered to 16 women under fasting conditions, the mean maximum serum concentration of levonorgestrel was 14.1 ng/mL at an average of 1.6 hours. See Table 2. Table 2: Pharmacokinetic Parameter Values Following Single Dose Administration of Levonorgestrel Tablets, 0.75 mg to Healthy Female Volunteers under Fasting Conditions

| | Mean (± SD) | | | | | |
|---|---|---|---|---|---|---|
| | Cmax (ng/mL) | Tmax (h) | CL(L/h) | Vd (L) | t½ (h) | AUCinf (ng•hr/mL) |
| levonorgestrel | 14.1 (7.7) | 1.6 ( 0.7) | 7.7 (2.7) | 260.0 | 24.4 (5.3) | 123.1 (50.1) |

Cmax = maximum concentration
Tmax = time to maximum concentration
CL = clearance
Vd = volume of distribution
t½ = elimination half life
AUCinf = area under the drug concentration curve from time 0 to infinity

Effect of Food: The effect of food on the rate and the extent of levonorgestrel absorption following single oral administration of levonorgestrel tablets, 0.75 mg has not been evaluated.

**Distribution**

The apparent volume of distribution of levonorgestrel is reported to be approximately 1.8 L/kg. It is about 97.5 to 99% protein-bound, principally to sex hormone binding globulin (SHBG) and, to a lesser extent, serum albumin.

**Metabolism**

Following absorption, levonorgestrel is conjugated at the 17β-OH position to form sulfate conjugates and, to a lesser extent, glucuronide conjugates in plasma. Significant amounts of conjugated and unconjugated 3α, 5β-tetrahydrolevonorgestrel are also present in plasma, along with much smaller amounts of 3α, 5α-tetrahydrolevonorgestrel and 16βhydroxylevonorgestrel. Levonorgestrel and its phase I metabolites are excreted primarily as glucuronide conjugates. Metabolic clearance rates may differ among individuals by several-fold, and this may account in part for the wide variation observed in levonorgestrel concentrations among users.

**Excretion**

About 45% of levonorgestrel and its metabolites are excreted in the urine and about 32% are excreted in feces, mostly as glucuronide conjugates.

**Specific Populations**

Pediatric: This product is not intended for use in the premenarcheal population, and pharmacokinetic data are not available for this population.

Geriatric: This product is not intended for use in postmenopausal women, and pharmacokinetic data are not available for this population.

Race: No formal studies have evaluated the effect of race on pharmacokinetics of levonorgestrel tablets, 0.75 mg. However, clinical trials demonstrated a higher pregnancy rate in Chinese women with both levonorgestrel tablets, 0.75 mg and the Yuzpe regimen (another form of emergency contraception). The reason for this apparent increase in the pregnancy rate with emergency contraceptives in Chinese women is unknown [see USE IN SPECIFIC POPULATIONS(8.6)].

Hepatic Impairment: No formal studies were conducted to evaluate the effect of hepatic disease on the disposition of levonorgestrel tablets, 0.75 mg.

Renal Impairment: No formal studies were conducted to evaluate the effect of renal disease on the disposition of levonorgestrel tablets, 0.75 mg.

**Drug-Drug Interactions**

No formal drug-drug interaction studies were conducted with levonorgestrel tablets, 0.75 mg [see **DRUG INTERACTIONS (7)**].

**13 NONCLINICAL TOXICOLOGY**

**13.1 Carcinogenesis, Mutagenesis, Impairment of Fertility**

- Carcinogenicity: There is no evidence of increased risk of cancer with short-term use of progestins. There was no increase in tumorgenicity following administration of levonorgestrel to rats for 2 years at approximately 5 µg/day, to dogs for 7 years at up to 0.125 mg/kg/day, or to rhesus monkeys for 10 years at up to 250 µg/kg/day. In another 7 year dog study, administration of levonorgestrel at 0.5 mg/kg/day did increase the number of mammary adenomas in treated dogs compared to controls. There were no malignancies

- Genotoxicity: Levonorgestrel was not found to be mutagenic or genotoxic in the Ames Assay, in vitro mammalian culture assays utilizing mouse lymphoma cells and Chinese hamster ovary cells, and in an in vivo micronucleus assay in mice

- Fertility: There are no irreversible effects on fertility following cessation of exposures to levonorgestrel or progestins in general

## 14 CLINICAL STUDIES

- A double-blind, randomized, multinational controlled clinical trial in 1,955 evaluable women (mean age 27) compared the efficacy and safety of levonorgestrel tablets, 0.75 mg (one 0.75 mg tablet of levonorgestrel taken within 72 hours of unprotected intercourse, and one tablet taken 12 hours later) to the Yuzpe regimen (two tablets each containing 0.25 mg levonorgestrel and 0.05 mg ethinyl estradiol, taken within 72 hours of intercourse, and two additional tablets taken 12 hours later). After a single act of intercourse occurring anytime during the menstrual cycle, the expected pregnancy rate of 8% (with no contraceptive use) was reduced to approximately 1% with levonorgestrel tablets, 0.75 mg
- Emergency contraceptives are not as effective as routine hormonal contraception since their failure rate, while low based on a single use, would accumulate over time with repeated use [see INDICATIONS AND USAGE (1)]
- At the time of expected menses, approximately 74% of women using levonorgestrel tablets, 0.75 mg had vaginal bleeding similar to their normal menses, 14% bled more than usual, and 12% bled less than usual. The majority of women (87%) had their next menstrual period at the expected time or within +7 days, while 13% had a delay of more than 7 days beyond the anticipated onset of menses

## 16 HOW SUPPLIED/STORAGE AND HANDLING

- Levonorgestrel tablets, 0.75 mg are available for a single course of treatment in PVC/aluminum foil blister packages of two tablets each. The tablet is white to off-white, circular, flat beveled, uncoated tablet debossed with "L840" on one side and plain on the other side
- Available as: Unit-of-use NDC 45802-840-54
- Store Levonorgestrel tablets, 0.75 mg at controlled room temperature, 20° to 25°C (68° to 77°F); excursions permitted between 15° to 30°C (59° to 86°F) [See USP]

## 17 PATIENT COUNSELING INFORMATION
### 17.1 Information for Patients

- Take Levonorgestrel tablets, 0.75 mg as soon as possible and not more than 72 hours after unprotected intercourse or a known or suspected contraceptive failure
- If you vomit within two hours of taking either tablet, immediately contact your healthcare provider to discuss whether to take another tablet
- Seek medical attention if you experience severe lower abdominal pain 3 to 5 weeks after taking Levonorgestrel tablets, 0.75 mg, in order to be evaluated for an ectopic pregnancy
- After taking Levonorgestrel tablets, 0.75 mg, consider the possibility of pregnancy if your period is delayed more than one week beyond the date you expected your period
- Do not use Levonorgestrel tablets, 0.75 mg as routine contraception
- Levonorgestrel tablets, 0.75 mg is not effective in terminating an existing pregnancy
- Levonorgestrel tablets, 0.75 mg does not protect against HIV-infection (AIDS) and other sexually transmitted diseases/infections
- For women younger than age 17 years, Levonorgestrel tablets, 0.75 mg is available only by prescription

## QUESTIONS OR COMMENTS
Phone: **1-800-719-9260**
Website: www.Levo4U.com

## LICE MD (dimethicone)
Quantum Pharmaceuticals, LLC

### DRUG FACTS

| Active ingredient | Purpose |
| --- | --- |
| Dimethicone | Lice & egg treatment |

### USE
- intended to eliminate lice, eggs and nits from head hair

### WARNINGS
**For external use only.**
- keep out of reach of children
- for children under 2, consult a physician before use
- avoid contact with eyes
- to avoid injury from slips and falls, clean up spills immediately

### DIRECTIONS
- before using, read instruction leaflet inside package for complete directions

### STEP 1
- apply LiceMD to DRY hair and massage until thoroughly wet. Pay attention to behind the ears and the nape of the neck where lice, eggs and nits are more likely to be found
- WAIT 10 minutes

### STEP 2
- while hair and scalp are wet with LiceMD, comb out lice, eggs and nits with the enclosed lice comb

### STEP 3
- after combing the entire head, wash hair thoroughly with your regular shampoo and warm water
- clean home to prevent reinfestation

Inspect hair and scalp each day for lice, eggs and nits for 10 days. Repeat STEPS 1-3 at any time if necessary.

### USAGE GUIDELINES

| Hair Length | Amount |
| --- | --- |
| Short | 1-2 ounces |
| Medium | 2-3 ounces |
| Long | 3-4 ounces |

### OTHER INFORMATION
- store at room temperature

### QUESTIONS OR COMMENTS
Call toll-free **1-800-431-2610** or visit www.LiceMD.com

## LICE-FREE EVERYDAY (sodium chloride) shampoo
Tec Laboratories, Inc.

### DRUG FACTS

| Active ingredient | Purpose |
| --- | --- |
| Natrum muriaticum 1X (sodium chloride, USP) | Pediculosis remedy and prophylactic |

### USES
- for the prevention and treatment of head lice infestations

## WARNINGS
**For external use only.**

**ASK A DOCTOR BEFORE USE IF YOU**
- have infestation of eyebrows or eyelashes
- are pregnant

**WHEN USING THIS PRODUCT**
- do not use on or near the eyes; close eyes while product is being applied
- do not permit contact with mucous membranes, such as inside the nose as irritation or stinging may occur

**STOP USE AND ASK A DOCTOR IF**
- skin irritation or infection is present or develops

**Keep out of reach of children.** If swallowed, get medical help or contact a Poison Control Center right away.

### DIRECTIONS

| adults and children 6 months of age and older | apply a generous amount of shampoo to wet hair, work into a lather while massaging into scalp. Rinse. |
| | repeat, this time leaving the shampoo on the hair for at least 3 minutes |
| | to treat a head lice infestation, use the shampoo daily for at least 2 weeks |
| | for prevention, use daily |
| | for best results on an extreme head lice infestation, use Licefreee! Spray or Gel treatment before using this shampoo |
| children under 6 months of age | do not use, consult a doctor before use |

### OTHER INFORMATION
- store at room temperature 59-86°F (15-30°C)

### INACTIVE INGREDIENTS
benzyl alcohol, cocamidopropyl betaine, caprylic/capric triglycerides, coconut oil, disodium EDTA, fragrances, purified water, sodium laureth sulfate, tea tree oil

### QUESTIONS OR COMMENTS
Call **1-800-ITCHING** or visit www.licefree.com. Serious side effects may also be reported to this number

## LITTLE COLDS SORE THROAT RELIEF MELT AWAYS (benzocaine) granule
Medtech Products Inc.

### DRUG FACTS

| Active ingredient (in each packet) | Purpose |
|---|---|
| Benzocaine 6 mg | Oral anesthetic/analgesic |

### USE
- for the temporary relief of occasional minor irritation, pain, sore throat, and sore mouth

## WARNINGS
**Allergy alert**
Do not use this product if you have a history of allergy to local anesthetics such as procaine, butacaine, benzocaine or other "caine" anesthetics.

**Sore Throat Warning**
Severe or persistent sore throat or sore throat accompanied by high fever, headache, nausea, and vomiting may be serious. Consult a doctor promptly. Do not use more than 2 days or administer to children under (3) years of age unless directed by a doctor.

**WHEN USING THIS PRODUCT**
- do not exceed recommended dosage

**STOP USE AND ASK A DENTIST OR DOCTOR IF**
- sore mouth symptoms do not improve in 7 days
- irritation, pain or redness persists or worsens
- swelling, rash or fever develops

**If pregnant or breastfeeding,** ask a health care professional before use.

**Keep out of reach of children.** In case of overdose or accidental poisoning, get medical help or contact a Poison Control Center right away.

### DIRECTIONS
- empty entire contents of packet onto tongue, allow to dissolve, then swallow
- for best taste, do not chew granules

| under 3 years | consult a doctor |
| 3 to under 6 years | 1 packet every 2 hours as needed |
| 6 years and over | 1 – 2 packets every 2 hours as needed |

### OTHER INFORMATION
- store at 59-77°F (15-25°C)
- Tamper Evident: Do not use if foil packets are broken
- check expiration date before using

### INACTIVE INGREDIENTS
cocoa butter, crospovidone, flavor, glucose, hypromellose, polyethylene glycol, polysorbate 80, sodium lauryl sulfate, sucralose, sucrose, talc

### QUESTIONS OR COMMENTS
For further information you may contact us at: **1-800-7-LITTLE**, or visit us at www.LittleRemedies.com.

## LITTLE NOSES DECONGESTANT NOSE DROPS (phenylephrine hydrochloride) liquid
Medtech Products Inc.

### DRUG FACTS

| Active ingredient | Purpose |
|---|---|
| Phenylephrine hydrochloride USP 0.125% | Nasal decongestant |

### USES
- temporarily relieves nasal congestion due to common cold, hay fever or other upper respiratory allergies
- helps clear nasal passages; shrinks swollen membranes
- temporarily restores freer breathing through the nose
- helps decongest sinus openings and passages; temporarily relieves sinus congestion and pressure

**WARNINGS**
- do not exceed recommended dosage

**DO NOT USE**
- with any other products containing decongestants

**ASK A DOCTOR BEFORE USE IF THE CHILD HAS**
- heart disease
- high blood pressure
- thyroid disease
- diabetes

**WHEN USING THIS PRODUCT**
- temporary discomfort such as burning, stinging, sneezing or an increase in nasal discharge may occur
- the use of this dispenser by more than one person may spread infection
- use only as directed

**STOP USE AND ASK A DOCTOR IF**
- nervousness, dizziness, or sleeplessness occurs
- symptoms persist. Do not use for more than 3 days. Use only as directed. Frequent or prolonged use may cause nasal congestion to recur or worsen

**Keep out of reach of children.** In case of overdose, get medical help or contact a Poison Control Center (**1-800-222-1222**) right away.

**DIRECTIONS**
**(Nasal Use Only)**

| children 2 to under 6 years (with adult supervision) | 2 to 3 drops in each nostril, not more often than every 4 hours |
|---|---|
| children under 2 years of age | consult a doctor |

**OTHER INFORMATION**
- do not use if plastic neck band on cap is broken or missing
- do not use if solution is brown or contains a precipitate
- protect from light
- store at 20-25°C (68-77°F)
- see bottle or box for lot number and expiration date

**INACTIVE INGREDIENTS**
benzalkonium chloride, glycerin, polyethylene glycol, potassium phosphate monobasic, purified water, sodium EDTA, sodium phosphate dibasic

**QUESTIONS OR COMMENTS**
For further information you may contact us at: **1-800-7-LITTLE** Mon.-Fri. 8:00 AM to 8:00 PM EST or visit us online at www.LittleRemedies.com

---

## LMX4 (lidocaine) cream
Ferndale Laboratories, Inc.

### DRUG FACTS

| Active ingredient | Purpose |
|---|---|
| Lidocaine 4% w/w | Topical anesthetic |

**USES**
- temporarily relieves pain and itching due to:
  - minor cuts
  - minor scrapes
  - minor burns
  - sunburn

- minor skin irritations
- insect bites

**WARNINGS**
**For external use only.**

**DO NOT USE**
- in or near the eyes
- in large quantities, particularly over raw surfaces or blistered areas

**STOP USE AND ASK A DOCTOR IF**
- allergic reaction occurs
- condition worsens or does not improve within 7 days
- symptoms clear up and return within a few days
- redness, irritation, swelling, pain or other symptoms begin or increase

**Keep out of reach of children.** If swallowed, get medical help or contact a Poison Control Center right away.

**DIRECTIONS**

| adults and children 2 years and older | apply externally to the affected area up to 3 to 4 times a day |
|---|---|
| children under 2 years | consult a doctor |

**OTHER INFORMATION**
- may be applied under occlusive dressing
- store at 25°C (77°F); excursions permitted to 15-30°C (59-86°F) [see USP Controlled Room Temperature]

**INACTIVE INGREDIENTS**
benzyl alcohol, carbomer 940, cholesterol, hydrogenated lecithin, polysorbate 80, propylene glycol, trolamine, vitamin E acetate, water

**QUESTIONS OR COMMENTS**
Call Toll-free (888) 548-0900 or visit www.ferndalelabs.com

---

## LOTRIMIN AF (clotrimazole)
Schering-Plough Healthcare Products, Inc.

### DRUG FACTS

| Active ingredient | Purpose |
|---|---|
| Clotrimazole 1 % | Antifungal |

**USES**
- cures most athlete's foot, jock itch, and ringworm
- relieves itching, burning, cracking, scaling and discomfort which accompany these conditions

**WARNINGS**
**For external use only.**

**DO NOT USE**
- on children under 2 years of age unless directed by a doctor

**WHEN USING THIS PRODUCT**
- avoid contact with the eyes

**STOP USE AND ASK A DOCTOR IF**
- irritation occurs
- there is no improvement within 4 weeks (for athlete's foot and ringworm) or 2 weeks (for jock itch)

**Keep out of reach of children.** If swallowed, get medical help or contact a Poison Control Center right away.

## DIRECTIONS

- wash affected area and dry thoroughly
- apply a thin layer over affected area twice daily (morning and night)
- supervise children in the use of this product
- for athlete's foot, pay special attention to spaces between the toes, wear well-fitting, ventilated shoes and change shoes and socks at least once daily
- for athlete's foot and ringworm, use daily for 4 weeks; for jock itch, use daily for 2 weeks
- if condition persists longer, ask a doctor
- this product is not effective on the scalp or nails

## OTHER INFORMATION

- store between 20°C-25°C (68°F-77°F)

## INACTIVE INGREDIENTS

benzyl alcohol, cetyl alcohol, cetyl esters wax, octyldodecanol, polysorbate 60, sorbitan monostearate, stearyl alcohol, water

## QUESTIONS OR COMMENTS

Call 1-866-360-3226 Mon.-Fri. 8AM-5PM CST

## LOTRIMIN ULTRA (butenafine hydrochloride)

Schering-Plough Healthcare Products, Inc.

### DRUG FACTS

| Active ingredient | Purpose |
| --- | --- |
| Butenafine Hydrochloride 1 % | Antifungal |

### USES

- cures most jock itch
- relieves itching, burning, cracking, and scaling which accompany this condition
- relieves chafing

### WARNINGS

For external use only.

### DO NOT USE

- on nails or scalp
- in or near the mouth or the eyes
- for vaginal yeast infections

### WHEN USING THIS PRODUCT

- do not get into the eyes. If eye contact occurs, rinse eyes thoroughly with water

### STOP USE AND ASK A DOCTOR IF

- too much irritation occurs or irritation gets worse

Keep out of reach of children. If swallowed, get medical help or contact a Poison Control Center right away.

### DIRECTIONS

| adults and children 12 years and over | use the tip of the cap to break the seal and open the tube |
| --- | --- |
| | wash the affected skin with soap and water and dry completely before applying |
| | apply once a day to affected skin for 2 weeks or as directed by a doctor |
| | wash hands after each use |
| children under 12 years | ask a doctor |

## OTHER INFORMATION

- store between 20°C-25°C (68°F-77°F)

## INACTIVE INGREDIENTS

benzyl alcohol, cetyl alcohol, diethanolamine, glycerin, glyceryl monostearate se, polyoxyethylene (23) cetyl ether, propylene glycol dicaprylate, purified water, sodium benzoate, stearic acid, white petrolatum

## QUESTIONS OR COMMENTS

Call 1-866-360-3226 Mon.-Fri. 8AM-5PM CST

## LUDENS WILD BERRY THROAT DROPS

(pectin) lozenge

Blacksmith Brands, Inc.

### DRUG FACTS

| Active ingredient (in each drop) | Purpose |
| --- | --- |
| Pectin 2.8 mg | Oral demulcent |

### USES

- for temporary relief of minor discomfort and protection of irritated areas in sore mouth and sore throat

### WARNINGS

Sore throat warning

If sore throat is severe, persists for more than 2 days, is accompanied or followed by fever, headache, rash, swelling, nausea or vomiting, consult a doctor promptly. These may be serious.

### STOP USE AND ASK A DOCTOR IF

- sore mouth does not improve in 7 days
- irritation, pain or redness persists or worsens

Keep out of reach of children.

### DIRECTIONS

| adults and children 3 years of age and older | allow one drop to dissolve slowly in mouth |
| --- | --- |
| | may be repeated as needed or as directed by a doctor |
| children under 3 years of age | ask a doctor |

### OTHER INFORMATION

- store at 20-25°C (68-77°F) in a dry place

### INACTIVE INGREDIENTS

ascorbic acid, citric acid, corn syrup, FD&C blue no. 1, FD&C blue no. 2, FD&C red no. 40, flavors, malic acid, sodium acetate, sodium chloride, soybean oil, and sucrose

### QUESTIONS OR COMMENTS

Call 1-866-583-3677

## LUDENS WILD CHERRY THROAT DROPS (pectin) lozenge

Blacksmith Brands, Inc.

BestSweet Inc.

### DRUG FACTS

| Active ingredient (in each drop) | Purpose |
|---|---|
| Pectin 1.7 mg | Oral demulcent |

### USES

- for temporary relief of minor discomfort and protection of irritated areas in sore mouth and sore throat

### WARNINGS

**Sore throat warning**

If sore throat is severe, persists for more than 2 days, is accompanied or followed by fever, headache, rash, swelling, nausea or vomiting, consult a doctor promptly. These may be serious.

### STOP USE AND ASK A DOCTOR IF

- sore mouth does not improve in 7 days
- irritation, pain or redness persists or worsens

**Keep out of reach of children.**

### DIRECTIONS

| adults and children 3 years of age and older | allow one drop to dissolve slowly in mouth |
| | may be repeated as needed or as directed by a doctor. |
| children under 3 years of age | ask a doctor |

### OTHER INFORMATION

- store at 20-25°C (68-77°F) in a dry place

### INACTIVE INGREDIENTS

ascorbic acid, citric acid, corn syrup, FD&C blue no. 2, FD&C red no. 40, flavors, malic acid, sodium acetate, sodium chloride, soybean oil, and sucrose

### QUESTIONS OR COMMENTS

Call **1-866-583-3677**

## LUDENS ORIGINAL MENTHOL THROAT DROPS (menthol) lozenge

Blacksmith Brands, Inc.

### DRUG FACTS

| Active ingredient (in each drop) | Purpose |
|---|---|
| Menthol 2.5 mg | Oral anesthetic |

### USES

- temporarily relieves occasional minor irritation, pain, sore mouth, and sore throat

### WARNINGS

**Sore throat warning**

If sore throat is severe, persists for more than 2 days, is accompanied or followed by fever, headache, rash, swelling, nausea or vomiting, consult a doctor promptly. These may be serious.

### STOP USE AND ASK A DOCTOR IF

- sore mouth does not improve in 7 days
- irritation, pain or redness lasts or worsens

**If pregnant or breastfeeding,** ask a health professional before use.

**Keep out of reach of children.**

### DIRECTIONS

| adults and children 3 years of age and older | allow drop to dissolve slowly in mouth |
| | repeat as necessary every 2 hours, or as directed by doctor |
| children under 3 years of age | ask a doctor |

### OTHER INFORMATION

- store at 20-25°C (68-77°F) in a dry place

### INACTIVE INGREDIENTS

caramel color, corn syrup, flavors, sodium acetate, soybean oil, and sucrose

### QUESTIONS OR COMMENTS

Call **1-866-583-3677**

## LUDENS HONEY LICORICE THROAT DROPS (menthol) lozenge

Blacksmith Brands, Inc.

### DRUG FACTS

| Active ingredient (in each drop) | Purpose |
|---|---|
| Menthol 1.0 mg | Oral anesthetic |

### USES

- temporarily relieves occasional minor irritation, pain, sore mouth, and sore throat

### WARNINGS

**Sore throat warning**

If sore throat is severe, persists for more than 2 days, is accompanied or followed by fever, headache, rash, swelling, nausea or vomiting, consult a doctor promptly. These may be serious.

### STOP USE AND ASK A DOCTOR IF

- sore mouth does not improve in 7 days
- irritation, pain or redness lasts or worsens

**If pregnant or breastfeeding,** ask a health professional before use.

**Keep out of reach of children.**

## DIRECTIONS

| adults and children 3 years of age and older | 2 drops |
| --- | --- |
| | allow 1 drop at a time to dissolve slowly in mouth |
| | repeat as necessary every 2 hours, or as directed by a doctor |
| children under 3 years of age | ask a doctor |

## OTHER INFORMATION
• store at 20-25°C (68-77°F) in a dry place

## INACTIVE INGREDIENTS
caramel color, corn syrup, flavors, glycerin, honey, sodium acetate, soybean oil, and sucrose

## QUESTIONS OR COMMENTS
Call **1-866-583-3677**

# LUDENS HONEY LEMON THROAT DROPS
(menthol) lozenge

Blacksmith Brands, Inc.

## DRUG FACTS

| Active ingredient (in each drop) | Purpose |
| --- | --- |
| Menthol 1.0 mg | Oral anesthetic |

## USES
• temporarily relieves occasional minor irritation, pain, sore mouth, and sore throat

## WARNINGS
**Sore throat warning**
If sore throat is severe, persists for more than 2 days, is accompanied or followed by fever, headache, rash, swelling, nausea or vomiting, consult a doctor promptly. These may be serious.

## STOP USE AND ASK A DOCTOR IF
• sore mouth does not improve in 7 days
• irritation, pain or redness lasts or worsens

**If pregnant or breastfeeding,** ask a health professional before use.

**Keep out of reach of children.**

## DIRECTIONS

| adults and children 3 years of age and older | 2 drops |
| --- | --- |
| | allow 1 drop at a time to dissolve slowly in mouth |
| | repeat as necessary every 2 hours, or as directed by a doctor |
| children under 3 years of age | ask a doctor |

## OTHER INFORMATION
• store at 20-25°C (68-77°F) in a dry place
• contains FD&C yellow no. 5 (tartrazine) as a color additive

## INACTIVE INGREDIENTS
ascorbic acid, citric acid, corn syrup, FD&C yellow no. 5, flavors, honey, sodium acetate, sodium chloride, soybean oil, sucrose

## QUESTIONS OR COMMENTS
Call **1-866-583-3677**

# MAALOX REGULAR STRENGTH WILD BERRY (calcium carbonate) chewable tablet
Novartis Consumer Healthcare, Inc.

## DRUG FACTS

| Active ingredient (in each tablet) | Purpose |
| --- | --- |
| Calcium carbonate 600 mg | Antacid |

## USES
• for the relief of:
  • acid indigestion
  • heartburn
  • sour stomach
  • upset stomach due to these symptoms

## WARNINGS
### ASK A DOCTOR BEFORE USE IF YOU HAVE
• kidney stones
• a calcium-restricted diet

### ASK A DOCTOR OR PHARMACIST BEFORE USE IF YOU ARE
• presently taking a prescription drug
• antacids may interact with certain prescription drugs

### STOP USE AND ASK A DOCTOR IF
• symptoms last more than 2 weeks

**Keep out of reach of children.**

## DIRECTIONS
• chew 1 to 2 tablets as symptoms occur or as directed by a doctor
• do not take more than 12 tablets in 24 hours or use the maximum dosage for more than 2 weeks except under the advice and supervision of a doctor

## OTHER INFORMATION
• each tablet contains: calcium 240 mg
• store at controlled room temperature 20-25°C (68-77°F)
• keep tightly closed and dry

## INACTIVE INGREDIENTS
aspartame, colloidal silicon dioxide, croscarmellose sodium, D&C red no. 30, dextrose, flavors, magnesium stearate, maltodextrin, mannitol, pregelatinized starch

## QUESTIONS OR COMMENTS
Call **1-800-452-0051**

## MAALOX ADVANCED MAXIMUM STRENGTH MINT (aluminum hydroxide, magnesium hydroxide, and simethicone) liquid
Novartis Consumer Health, Inc.

### DRUG FACTS

| Active ingredients (in each 5 ml = 1 teaspoonful) | Purpose |
|---|---|
| Aluminum hydroxide (equiv. to dried gel USP) 400 mg | Antacid |
| Magnesium hydroxide 400 mg | Antacid |
| Simethicone 40 mg | Antigas |

### USES
- for the relief of:
  - acid indigestion
  - heartburn
  - sour stomach
  - upset stomach associated with these symptoms
  - pressure and bloating commonly referred to as gas

### WARNINGS

**DO NOT TAKE**
- more than 8 teaspoonfuls in a 24-hour period or use the maximum dosage for more than 2 weeks except under the advice and supervision of a physician

**ASK A DOCTOR BEFORE USE IF YOU HAVE**
- kidney disease
- a magnesium-restricted diet

**ASK A DOCTOR OR PHARMACIST BEFORE USE IF YOU ARE**
- presently taking a prescription drug. Antacids may interact with certain prescription drugs

**STOP USE AND ASK A DOCTOR IF**
- symptoms last more than 2 weeks

**Keep out of reach of children.**

### DIRECTIONS
- shake well before using

| adults and children 12 years and older | take 2 to 4 teaspoonsful two times a day or as directed by a physician |
| | do not take more than 8 teaspoonsful in 24 hours or use the maximum dosage for more than 2 weeks |
| children under 12 years | consult a physician |

### OTHER INFORMATION
- each tablespoon contains: magnesium 145 mg, potassium 5 mg
- store at controlled room temperature 20-25°C (68-77°F)
- protect from freezing

### INACTIVE INGREDIENTS
butylparaben, carboxymethylcellulose sodium, flavor, glycerin, hypromellose, microcrystalline cellulose, potassium citrate, propylene glycol, propylparaben, purified water, saccharin sodium, sorbitol

### QUESTIONS OR COMMENTS
Call 1-800-452-0051

## MEDERMA (avobenzone, octocrylene, and oxybenzone) cream
Merz Pharmaceuticals, LLC

### DRUG FACTS

| Active ingredients | Purpose |
|---|---|
| Avobenzone 3%<br>Octocrylene 10%<br>Oxybenzone 6% | Scar removal cream |

### WARNINGS
**For external use only.**

**DO NOT USE**
- on open wounds

**WHEN USING THIS PRODUCT**
- keep out of eyes
- rinse with water to remove

**STOP USE AND ASK A DOCTOR IF**
- rash or irritation develops and lasts

**Keep out of reach of children.** If swallowed, get medical help or contact a Poison Control Center right away.

### DIRECTIONS
- Mederma Cream should be evenly applied and gently rubbed into the scar 3 times daily for 8 weeks on new scars, and 3 times daily for 3-6 months on existing scars
- also apply Mederma Cream to the scar before sun exposure
- children under 6 months of age ask a doctor

### OTHER INFORMATION
- store at room temperature

### INACTIVE INGREDIENTS
water, allium cepa (onion) bulb extract, C12-15 alkyl benzoate, dicaprylyl carbonate, hydrogenated lecithin, caprylic/capric triglyceride, panthenol, pentylene glycol, phenoxyethanol, butyrospermum parkii (shea butter), glycerin, ammonium acryloyl-dimethyltaurate/vp copolymer, fragrance, squalane, methylparaben, xanthan gum, disodium EDTA, ceramide 3, sodium hyaluronate, butylparaben, ethylparaben, propylparaben, isobutylparaben

### QUESTIONS OR COMMENTS
For more information Call **1-888-925-8989** or visit www.mederma.com

## MEN'S ROGAINE EXTRA STRENGTH (minoxidil) solution
Johnson & Johnson Healthcare Products, Division of McNeil-PPC, Inc.

### DRUG FACTS

| Active ingredient | Purpose |
|---|---|
| Minoxidil 5% w/v | Hair regrowth treatment for men |

### USE
- to regrow hair on the top of the scalp (vertex only, see pictures on side of carton)

## WARNINGS
**For external use only.**

**For use by men only.**

**Flammable:** keep away from fire or flame

### DO NOT USE IF
- you are a woman
- your amount of hair loss is different than that shown on the side of this carton or your hair loss is on the front of the scalp. 5% minoxidil topical solution is not intended for frontal baldness or receding hairline
- you have no family history of hair loss
- your hair loss is sudden and/or patchy
- you do not know the reason for your hair loss
- you are under 18 years of age. Do not use on babies and children
- your scalp is red, inflamed, infected, irritated, or painful
- you use other medicines on the scalp

### ASK A DOCTOR BEFORE USE IF YOU HAVE
- heart disease

### WHEN USING THIS PRODUCT
- do not apply on other parts of the body
- avoid contact with the eyes. In case of accidental contact, rinse eyes with large amounts of cool tap water
- some people have experienced changes in hair color and/or texture
- it takes time to regrow hair. Results may occur at 2 months with twice a day usage. For some men, you may need to use this product for at least 4 months before you see results
- the amount of hair regrowth is different for each person. This product will not work for all men

### STOP USE AND ASK A DOCTOR IF
- chest pain, rapid heartbeat, faintness, or dizziness occurs
- sudden, unexplained weight gain occurs
- your hands or feet swell
- scalp irritation or redness occurs
- unwanted facial hair growth occurs
- you do not see hair regrowth in 4 months

**May be harmful if used when pregnant or breastfeeding.**

**Keep out of reach of children.** If swallowed, get medical help or contact a Poison Control Center right away.

### DIRECTIONS
- apply one mL with dropper 2 times a day directly onto the scalp in the hair loss area
- using more or more often will not improve results
- continued use is necessary to increase and keep your hair regrowth, or hair loss will begin again

### OTHER INFORMATION
- see hair loss pictures on side of this carton
- before use, read all information on carton and enclosed booklet
- keep the carton. It contains important information
- hair regrowth has not been shown to last longer than 48 weeks in large clinical trials with continuous treatment with 5% minoxidil topical solution for men
- in clinical studies with mostly white men aged 18-49 years with moderate degrees of hair loss, 5% minoxidil topical solution for men provided more hair regrowth than 2% minoxidil topical solution
- store at controlled room temperature 20°C-25°C (68°F-77°F)

### INACTIVE INGREDIENTS
alcohol, propylene glycol, purified water

## QUESTIONS OR COMMENTS
Call us at **1-800-ROGAINE (1-800-764-2463)** or visit rogaine.com

---

## MICATIN (miconazole nitrate) cream
WellSpring Pharmaceutical Corporation

### DRUG FACTS

| Active ingredient | Purpose |
|---|---|
| Miconazole nitrate 2% | Antifungal |

### USES
- proven clinically effective in the treatment of most athlete's foot, jock itch and ringworm
- for effective relief of itching, scaling, burning and discomfort that can accompany these conditions

### WARNINGS
**For external use only.**

### DO NOT USE
- on children less than 2 years of age unless directed by a doctor

### WHEN USING THIS PRODUCT
- avoid contact with the eyes

### STOP USE AND ASK A DOCTOR IF
- irritation occurs
- condition persists
- there is no improvement of athlete's foot or ringworm within 4 weeks or jock itch within 2 weeks

**Keep out of reach of children.** If swallowed, get medical help or contact a Poison Control Center (**1-800-222-1222**) right away. (**1-800-222-1222**)

### DIRECTIONS
- clean the affected area and dry thoroughly
- apply a thin layer of the product over affected area twice daily (morning and night) or as directed by a doctor
- supervise children in the use of this product
- for athlete's foot, pay special attention to the spaces between the toes; wear well-fitting, ventilated shoes, and change shoes and socks at least once daily
- for athlete's foot and ringworm, use daily for 4 weeks
- for jock itch, use daily for 2 weeks
- not effective on the scalp or nails

### OTHER INFORMATION
- do not use if seal on tube is punctured or not visible
- to puncture the seal, reverse the cap and place the puncture-top onto the tube. Push down firmly until the seal is open. To close, screw the top back on the the tube
- store at 20°C-25°C (68°F-77°F)
- see carton back panel and tube crimp for lot number and expiration date

### INACTIVE INGREDIENTS
benzoic acid, butylated hydroxyanisole, mineral oil, peglicol 5 oleate, pegoxol 7 stearate, purified water

### QUESTIONS OR COMMENTS
Call **1-866-337-4500** or visit info@wellspringpharm.com

# MIDOL COMPLETE (acetaminophen, caffeine, and pyrilamine maleate) caplet

Bayer HealthCare

## DRUG FACTS

| Active ingredients (in each caplet) | Purpose |
|---|---|
| Acetaminophen 500 mg | Pain reliever |
| Caffeine 60 mg | Stimulant |
| Pyrilamine maleate 15 mg | Diuretic |

## USES
- for the temporary relief of these symptoms associated with menstrual periods:
  - cramps
  - bloating
  - water-weight gain
  - breast tenderness
  - headache
  - backache
  - muscle aches
  - fatigue

## WARNINGS
### Liver warning
This product contains acetaminophen. Severe liver damage may occur if you take:
- more than 8 caplets in 24 hours, which is the maximum daily amount
- with other drugs containing acetaminophen
- 3 or more alcoholic drinks every day while using this product

### DO NOT USE
- with any other drug containing acetaminophen (prescription or nonprescription)
- if you are not sure whether a drug contains acetaminophen, ask a doctor or pharmacist

### ASK A DOCTOR BEFORE USE IF YOU HAVE
- liver disease
- glaucoma
- difficulty in urination due to enlargement of the prostate gland
- a breathing problem such as emphysema or chronic bronchitis

### ASK A DOCTOR OR PHARMACIST BEFORE USE IF YOU ARE
- taking the blood thinning drug warfarin
- taking sedatives or tranquilizers

### WHEN USING THIS PRODUCT
- you may get drowsy
- avoid alcoholic drinks
- excitability may occur, especially in children
- alcohol, sedatives, and tranquilizers may increase drowsiness
- be careful when driving a motor vehicle or operating machinery
- limit the use of caffeine-containing medications, foods, or beverages because too much caffeine may cause nervousness, irritability, sleeplessness, and, occasionally, rapid heartbeat. The recommended dose of this product contains about as much caffeine as a cup of coffee

### STOP USE AND ASK A DOCTOR IF
- new symptoms occur
- redness or swelling is present
- pain gets worse or lasts more than 10 days

**If pregnant or breastfeeding,** ask a health professional before use.

**Keep out of reach of children.** In case of overdose, get medical help or contact a Poison Control Center right away. Quick medical attention is critical for adults as well as for children even if you do not notice any signs or symptoms.

## DIRECTIONS
- do not take more than the recommended dose

| adults and children 12 years and older | take 2 caplets with water |
| | repeat every 6 hours, as needed |
| | do not exceed 8 caplets per day |
| children under 12 years | consult a doctor |

## OTHER INFORMATION
- store at room temperature

## QUESTIONS OR COMMENTS
Call **1-800-331-4536** (Mon-Fri 9-5 EST) or visit www.midol.com

# MIDOL EXTENDED RELIEF (naproxen sodium) caplet

Bayer HealthCare LLC, Consumer Care

## DRUG FACTS

| Active ingredient (in each caplet) | Purpose |
|---|---|
| Naproxen sodium 220 mg (naproxen 200 mg) (NSAID)* | Pain reliever/fever reducer |

* nonsteroidal anti-inflammatory drug

## USES
- temporarily relieves minor aches and pains due to:
  - menstrual cramps
  - muscle aches
  - headache
  - backache
  - minor pain of arthritis
  - toothache
  - the common cold
- temporarily reduces fever

## WARNINGS
### Allergy alert
Naproxen sodium may cause a severe allergic reaction, especially in people allergic to aspirin. Symptoms may include:

- hives
- facial swelling
- asthma (wheezing)
- shock
- skin reddening
- rash
- blisters

If an allergic reaction occurs, stop use and seek medical help right away.

### Stomach bleeding warning
This product contains an NSAID, which may cause severe stomach bleeding. The chance is higher if you:
- are age 60 or older
- have had stomach ulcers or bleeding problems
- take a blood thinning (anticoagulant) or steroid drug

- take other drugs containing prescription or nonprescription NSAIDs (aspirin, ibuprofen, naproxen, or others)
- have 3 or more alcoholic drinks every day while using this product
- take more or for a longer time than directed

## DO NOT USE
- if you have ever had an allergic reaction to any other pain reliever/fever reducer
- right before or after heart surgery

## ASK A DOCTOR BEFORE USE IF
- the stomach bleeding warning applies to you
- you have a history of stomach problems, such as heartburn
- you have high blood pressure, heart disease, liver cirrhosis, or kidney disease
- you are taking a diuretic
- you have problems or serious side effects from taking pain relievers or fever reducers
- you have asthma

## ASK A DOCTOR OR PHARMACIST BEFORE USE IF YOU ARE
- under a doctor's care for any serious condition
- taking any other drug

## WHEN USING THIS PRODUCT
- take with food or milk if stomach upset occurs
- the risk of heart attack or stroke may increase if you use more than directed or for longer than directed

## STOP USE AND ASK A DOCTOR IF
- you experience any of the following signs of stomach bleeding:
  - feel faint
  - vomit blood
  - have bloody or black stools
  - have stomach pain that does not get better
- pain gets worse or lasts more than 10 days
- fever gets worse or lasts more than 3 days
- you have difficulty swallowing
- it feels like the pill is stuck in your throat
- redness or swelling is present in the painful area
- any new symptoms appear

**If pregnant or breastfeeding,** ask a health professional before use.

It is especially important not to use naproxen sodium during the last 3 months of pregnancy unless definitely directed to do so by a doctor because it may cause problems in the unborn child or complications during delivery.

**Keep out of reach of children.** In case of overdose, get medical help or contact a Poison Control Center right away.

## DIRECTIONS
- do not take more than directed
- the smallest effective dose should be used
- drink a full glass of water with each dose

| under 12 years | ask a doctor |
|---|---|
| adults and children 12 years and older | take 1 caplet every 8 to 12 hours while symptoms last. For the first dose you may take 2 caplets within the first hour |
| | do not exceed 2 caplets in any 8- to 12-hour period |
| | do not exceed 3 caplets in a 24-hour period. |

## OTHER INFORMATION
- each caplet contains: sodium 20 mg
- store at 20-25°C (68-77°F). Avoid high humidity and excessive heat above 40°C (104°F)

## INACTIVE INGREDIENTS
FD&C blue no. 2 lake, hypromellose, magnesium stearate, microcrystalline cellulose, polyethylene glycol, povidone, talc, titanium dioxide

## QUESTIONS OR COMMENTS
Call **1-800-331-4536** (Mon-Fri 9-5 EST) or visit www.midol.com

## MIDOL PM (acetaminophen and diphenhydramine citrate) caplet
Bayer HealthCare LLC

## DRUG FACTS

| Active ingredients (in each caplet) | Purpose |
|---|---|
| Acetaminophen 500 mg | Pain reliever |
| Diphenhydramine citrate 38 mg | Nighttime sleep-aid |

## USE
- for relief of occasional sleeplessness when associated with minor aches and pains from premenstrual and menstrual periods (dysmenorrhea)

## WARNINGS
### Liver warning
This product contains acetaminophen. Severe liver damage may occur if you take:
- more than 8 caplets in 24 hours, which is the maximum daily amount with other drugs containing acetaminophen
- 3 or more alcoholic drinks every day while using this product

## DO NOT USE
- with any other drug containing acetaminophen (prescription or nonprescription)
- if you are not sure whether a drug contains acetaminophen, ask a doctor or pharmacist
- in children under 12 years of age
- with any other product containing diphenhydramine, even one used on skin

## ASK A DOCTOR BEFORE USE IF YOU HAVE
- liver disease
- a breathing problem such as emphysema or chronic bronchitis
- glaucoma
- trouble urinating due to an enlarged prostate gland

## ASK A DOCTOR OR PHARMACIST BEFORE USE IF YOU ARE
- taking the blood thinning drug warfarin
- taking sedatives or tranquilizers

## WHEN USING THIS PRODUCT
- drowsiness will occur
- avoid alcoholic drinks
- do not drive a motor vehicle or operate machinery

## STOP USE AND ASK A DOCTOR IF
- sleeplessness persists continuously for more than 2 weeks. Insomnia may be a symptom of serious underlying medical illness
- pain gets worse or lasts more than 10 days
- new symptoms occur
- redness or swelling is present

**If pregnant or breastfeeding,** ask a health professional before use.

**Keep out of reach of children.** In case of overdose, get medical help or contact a Poison Control Center right away. Quick medical attention is critical for adults as well as for children even if you do not notice any signs or symptoms.

## DIRECTIONS
- do not take more than the recommended dose

| adults and children 12 years and older | take 2 caplets at bedtime if needed, or as directed by a doctor |
|---|---|
| children under 12 years | do not use |

## OTHER INFORMATION
- store at room temperature

## INACTIVE INGREDIENTS
carnauba wax, corn starch, croscarmellose sodium, FD&C blue no. 1 aluminum lake, FD&C blue no. 2 aluminum lake, hypromellose, microcrystalline cellulose, povidone, propylene glycol, shellac, stearic acid, titanium dioxide

## QUESTIONS OR COMMENTS
Call **1-800-331-4536** (Mon-Fri 9 AM-5 PM EST) or visit www.midol.com

---

## MILK OF MAGNESIA ORIGINAL (Phillips milk of magnesia original) suspension
Aaron Industries Inc.

## DRUG FACTS

| Active ingredients | Purpose |
|---|---|
| Magnesium hydroxide 1200 mg | Saline laxative |

## USES
- relieves occasional constipation (irregularity) generally produces bowel movement in ½ to 6 hours

## WARNINGS

### ASK A DOCTOR BEFORE USE IF YOU HAVE
- kidney disease
- a magnesium restricted diet
- stomach pain, nausea or vomiting
- a sudden change in bowel habits that lasts more than 2 weeks

### ASK A DOCTOR OR PHARMACIST BEFORE USE IF YOU ARE
- presently taking a prescription drug
- this product may interact with certain prescription drugs

### STOP USE AND ASK A DOCTOR IF
- you have rectal bleeding or failure to have a
- bowel movement after using this product
- These could be signs of a serious condition
- you need to use a laxative for more than 1 week

**If pregnant or breastfeeding,** ask a health professional before use.

**Keep this and all drugs out of the reach of children.** In case of accidental overdose, seek professional assistance or contact a Poison Control Center immediately.

## DIRECTIONS
- shake well before use

- do not exceed the maximum recommended daily dose in a 24 hour period
- dose may be taken once a day preferably at bedtime, in divided doses, or as directed by a doctor
- follow each dosage with a full glass (8oz) of fluid

| adults and children 12 years and over | 2-4 tablespoons (30-60 mL) |
|---|---|
| children 6 years to 11 years | 1-2 tablespoons (15-30 mL) |
| children under 6 years | ask a doctor |

## OTHER INFORMATION
- do not freeze
- each tablespoon contains: magnesium 501 mg
- store at room temperature tightly closed
- tamper evident: do not use if printed safety seal is broken or missing

---

## MIRALAX (polyethylene glycol 3350) powder
Schering-Plough HealthCare Products, Inc.

## DRUG FACTS

| Active ingredient (in each dose) | Purpose |
|---|---|
| Polyethylene Glycol 3350, 17 g | Osmotic laxative |

## USES
- relieves occasional constipation (irregularity)
- generally produces a bowel movement in 1 to 3 days

## WARNINGS
**Allergy alert**
Do not use if you are allergic to polyethylene glycol.

### DO NOT USE
- if you have kidney disease, except under the advice and supervision of a doctor

### ASK A DOCTOR BEFORE USE IF YOU HAVE
- nausea, vomiting or abdominal pain
- a sudden change in bowel habits that lasts over 2 weeks
- irritable bowel syndrome

### ASK A DOCTOR OF PHARMACIST BEFORE USE IF YOU ARE
- taking a prescription drug

### WHEN USING THIS PRODUCT
- you may have loose, watery, more frequent stools

### STOP USE AND ASK A DOCTOR IF
- you have rectal bleeding, nausea, bloating or cramping or abdominal pain gets worse. These may be signs of a serious condition
- you get diarrhea
- you need to use a laxative for longer than 1 week

**If pregnant or breastfeeding,** ask a health professional before use.

**Keep out of the reach of children.** In case of overdose, get medical help or contact a Poison Control Center right away.

## DIRECTIONS
• do not take more than directed unless advised by your doctor

| adults and children 17 years of age and older | stir and dissolve one packet of powder (17 g) in any 4 to 8 ounces of beverage (cold, hot or room temperature) then drink<br><br>use once a day<br><br>use no more than 7 days |
|---|---|
| children 16 years of age or under | ask a doctor |

## OTHER INFORMATION
• store at 20-25°C (68-77°F)
• tamper-evident: do not use if foil is open or broken

## INACTIVE INGREDIENTS
none

## QUESTIONS OR COMMENTS
Call **1-800-MiraLAX (1-800-647-2529)** or visit www.MiraLAX.com

# MONISTAT 3 COMBINATION PACK
(miconazole nitrate) cream
McNeil-PPC, Inc.

## DRUG FACTS

| Active ingredients | Purpose |
|---|---|
| Miconazole nitrate (200 mg in each suppository) | Vaginal antifungal |
| Miconazole nitrate 2% (external cream) | Vaginal antifungal |

## USES
• treats vaginal yeast infections
• relieves external itching and irritation due to a vaginal yeast infection

## WARNINGS
**For vaginal use only.**

## DO NOT USE
• if you have never had a vaginal yeast infection diagnosed by a doctor

## ASK A DOCTOR BEFORE USE IF YOU HAVE
• vaginal itching and discomfort for the first time
• lower abdominal, back or shoulder pain, fever, chills, nausea, vomiting, or foul-smelling vaginal discharge. You may have a more serious condition
• vaginal yeast infections often (such as once a month or 3 in 6 months). You could be pregnant or have a serious underlying medical cause for your symptoms, including diabetes or a weakened immune system
• been exposed to the human immunodeficiency virus (HIV) that causes AIDS

## ASK A DOCTOR OR PHARMACIST BEFORE USE IF YOU ARE
• taking the prescription blood thinning medicine warfarin, because bleeding or bruising may occur

## WHEN USING THIS PRODUCT
• do not use tampons, douches, spermicides or other vaginal products. Condoms and diaphragms may be damaged and fail to prevent pregnancy or sexually transmitted diseases (STDs)
• do not have vaginal intercourse
• mild increase in vaginal burning, itching or irritation may occur
• if you do not get complete relief ask a doctor before using another product

## STOP USE AND ASK A DOCTOR IF
• symptoms do not get better in 3 days
• symptoms last more than 7 days
• you get a rash or hives, abdominal pain, fever, chills, nausea, vomiting, or foul-smelling vaginal discharge

**If pregnant or breastfeeding,** ask a health professional before use.

**Keep out of reach of children.** If swallowed, get medical help or contact a Poison Control Center right away.

## DIRECTIONS
• before using this product read the enclosed consumer information leaflet for complete directions and information

| adults and children 12 years of age and over | suppositories: insert 1 suppository into the vagina at bedtime for 3 nights in a row. Throw away applicator after use<br><br>external cream: squeeze a small amount of cream onto your fingertip. Apply the cream onto the itchy, irritated skin outside the vagina. Use 2 times daily for up to 7 days, as needed |
|---|---|
| children under 12 years of age | ask a doctor |

## OTHER INFORMATION
• do not use if printed suppository blister is torn, open or incompletely sealed
• do not use if seal over tube opening has been punctured or embossed design is not visible
• do not purchase if carton is open
• store at 20-25°C (68-77°F)

## INACTIVE INGREDIENTS
**suppository:** hydrogenated vegetable oil base
**external cream:** benzoic acid, cetyl alcohol, isopropyl myristate, polysorbate 60, potassium hydroxide, propylene glycol, purified water, stearyl alcohol

## QUESTIONS OR COMMENTS
If you have any questions or comments, please call **1-877-666-4782** or visit www.monistat.com

# MONISTAT 7 7-DAY CREAM (miconazole nitrate)
cream
McNeil-PPC, Inc.

## DRUG FACTS

| Active ingredient | Purpose |
|---|---|
| Miconazole nitrate 2% (100 mg in each applicatorful) | Vaginal antifungal |

## USES
- treats vaginal yeast infections
- relieves external itching and irritation due to a vaginal yeast infection

## WARNINGS
**For vaginal use only.**

## DO NOT USE
- if you have never had a vaginal yeast infection diagnosed by a doctor

## ASK A DOCTOR BEFORE USE IF YOU HAVE
- vaginal itching and discomfort for the first time
- lower abdominal, back or shoulder pain, fever, chills, nausea, vomiting, or foul-smelling vaginal discharge. You may have a more serious condition
- vaginal yeast infections often (such as once a month or 3 in 6 months). You could be pregnant or have a serious underlying medical cause for your symptoms, including diabetes or a weakened immune system
- been exposed to the human immunodeficiency virus (HIV) that causes AIDS

## ASK A DOCTOR OR PHARMACIST BEFORE USE IF YOU ARE
- taking the prescription blood thinning medicine warfarin, because bleeding or bruising may occur

## WHEN USING THIS PRODUCT
- do not use tampons, douches, spermicides or other vaginal products. Condoms and diaphragms may be damaged and fail to prevent pregnancy or sexually transmitted diseases (STDs)
- do not have vaginal intercourse
- mild increase in vaginal burning, itching or irritation may occur
- if you do not get complete relief ask a doctor before using another product

## STOP USE AND ASK A DOCTOR IF
- symptoms do not get better in 3 days
- symptoms last more than 7 days
- you get a rash or hives, abdominal pain, fever, chills, nausea, vomiting, or foul-smelling vaginal discharge

**If pregnant or breastfeeding,** ask a health professional before use.

**Keep out of reach of children.** If swallowed, get medical help or contact a Poison Control Center right away.

## DIRECTIONS
- before using this product, read the enclosed consumer information leaflet for complete directions and information

| adults and children 12 years of age and over | applicator: insert 1 applicatorful into the vagina at bedtime for 7 nights in a row |
| --- | --- |
| | throw away applicator after use |
| | use the same tube of cream if you have itching and irritation on the skin outside the vagina |
| | squeeze a small amount of cream onto your fingertip |
| | apply to itchy, irritated skin outside the vagina (vulva) |
| | use 2 times daily for up to 7 days as needed |
| children under 12 years of age | ask a doctor |

## OTHER INFORMATION
- do not use if seal over tube opening has been punctured or embossed design not visible
- do not purchase if carton is open
- store at 20-25°C (68-77°F)

## INACTIVE INGREDIENTS
benzoic acid, cetyl alcohol, isopropyl myristate, polysorbate 60, potassium hydroxide, propylene glycol, purified water, stearyl alcohol

## QUESTIONS OR COMMENTS
If you have any questions or comments, please Call **1-877-666-4782**

# MONISTAT SOOTHING CARE CHAFING RELIEF (dimethicone) gel
McNeil-PPC, Inc.

## DRUG FACTS

| Active ingredient | Purpose |
| --- | --- |
| Dimethicone 1.2% | Skin protectant |

## USES
- temporarily protects and helps relieved chafed, chapped or cracked skin

## WARNINGS
**For external use only.**

## WHEN USING THIS PRODUCT
- do not get into eyes

## STOP USE AND ASK A DOCTOR IF
- condition worsens
- symptoms last more than 7 days or clear up and occur again within a few days

**Keep out of reach of children.** If swallowed get medical help or contact a Poison Control Center right away.

## DIRECTIONS
- apply as needed

## INACTIVE INGREDIENTS
cyclopentasiloxane, dimethicone, dimethicone/vinyl dimethicone crosspolymer, silica, tocopheryl acetate, trisiloxane

# MOTRIN IB (ibuprofen) tablet, film coated
McNeil Consumer Healthcare, Div. McNeil-PPC, Inc

## DRUG FACTS

| Active ingredient (in each tablet) | Purpose |
| --- | --- |
| Ibuprofen 200 mg (NSAID)* | Pain reliever/fever reducer |

*nonsteroidal anti-inflammatory drug

## USES
- temporarily relieves minor aches and pains due to:
  - headache
  - muscular aches
  - minor pain of arthritis
  - toothache

- backache
- the common cold
- menstrual cramps
- temporarily reduces fever

## WARNINGS
### Allergy alert
Ibuprofen may cause a severe allergic reaction, especially in people allergic to aspirin. Symptoms may include:

- hives
- facial swelling
- asthma (wheezing)
- shock
- skin reddening
- rash
- blisters

If an allergic reaction occurs, stop use and seek medical help right away.

### Stomach bleeding warning
This product contains an NSAID, which may cause severe stomach bleeding. The chance is higher if you:
- are age 60 or older
- have had stomach ulcers or bleeding problems
- take a blood thinning (anticoagulant) or steroid drug
- take other drugs containing prescription or nonprescription NSAIDs (aspirin, ibuprofen, naproxen, or others)
- have 3 or more alcoholic drinks every day while using this product
- take more or for a longer time than directed

### DO NOT USE
- if you have ever had an allergic reaction to any other pain reliever/fever reducer
- right before or after heart surgery

### ASK A DOCTOR BEFORE USE IF
- you have problems or serious side effects from taking pain relievers or fever reducers
- the stomach bleeding warning applies to you
- you have a history of stomach problems, such as heartburn
- you have high blood pressure, heart disease, liver cirrhosis, or kidney disease
- you have asthma
- you are taking a diuretic

### ASK A DOCTOR OR PHARMACIST BEFORE USE IF YOU ARE
- taking aspirin for heart attack or stroke, because ibuprofen may decrease this benefit of aspirin
- under a doctor's care for any serious condition
- taking any other drug

### WHEN USING THIS PRODUCT
- take with food or milk if stomach upset occurs
- the risk of heart attack or stroke may increase if you use more than directed or for longer than directed

### STOP USE AND ASK A DOCTOR IF
- you experience any of the following signs of stomach bleeding:
  - feel faint
  - vomit blood
  - have bloody or black stools
  - have stomach pain that does not get better
- pain gets worse or lasts more than 10 days
- fever gets worse or lasts more than 3 days
- redness or swelling is present in the painful area
- any new symptoms appear

**If pregnant or breastfeeding,** ask a health professional before use.

It is especially important not to use ibuprofen during the last 3 months of pregnancy unless definitely directed to do so by a doctor because it may cause problems in the unborn child or complications during delivery.

**Keep out of reach of children.** In case of overdose, get medical help or contact a Poison Control Center right away. (**1-800-222-1222**)

## DIRECTIONS
- do not take more than directed
- the smallest effective dose should be used

| adults and children 12 years and older | take 1 tablet every 4 to 6 hours while symptoms persist |
| --- | --- |
| | if pain or fever does not respond to 1 tablet, 2 tablets may be used |
| | do not exceed 6 tablets in 24 hours, unless directed by a doctor |
| children under 12 years | ask a doctor |

## OTHER INFORMATION
- store between 20-25°C (68-77°F)
- do not use if neck wrap or foil inner seal imprinted "Safety Seal" is broken or missing
- see end panel for lot number and expiration date

## INACTIVE INGREDIENTS
carnauba wax, colloidal silicon dioxide, corn starch, FD&C yellow no. 6, hypromellose, iron oxide, magnesium stearate, polydextrose, polyethylene glycol, pregelatinized starch, propylene glycol, shellac, stearic acid, titanium dioxide

## QUESTIONS OR COMMENTS
Call **1-877-895-3665**: weekdays 8:00 AM to 8:00 PM EST

---

# MOTRIN INFANTS (ibuprofen) suspension/drops
McNeil Consumer Healthcare, Div. McNeil-PPC, Inc

## DRUG FACTS

| Active ingredient (in each 1.25 mL) | Purpose |
| --- | --- |
| Ibuprofen 50 mg (NSAID)* | Pain reliever/fever reducer |

*nonsteroidal anti-inflammatory drug

## USES
- temporarily:
  - reduces fever
  - relieves minor aches and pains due to:
    - the common cold
    - flu
    - sore throat
    - headaches
    - toothaches

## WARNINGS
### Allergy alert
Ibuprofen may cause a severe allergic reaction, especially in people allergic to aspirin. Symptoms may include:

- hives
- facial swelling
- asthma (wheezing)
- shock
- skin reddening
- rash
- blisters

If an allergic reaction occurs, stop use and seek medical help right away.

**Stomach bleeding warning**
This product contains an NSAID, which may cause severe stomach bleeding. The chance is higher if you:r child:
- has had stomach ulcers or bleeding problems
- takes a blood thinning (anticoagulant) or steroid drug
- takes other drugs containing prescription or nonprescription NSAIDs (aspirin, ibuprofen, naproxen, or others)
- takes more or for a longer time than directed

**Sore throat warning**
Severe or persistent sore throat or sore throat accompanied by high fever, headache, nausea, and vomiting may be serious. Consult doctor promptly. Do not use more than 2 days or administer to children under 3 years of age unless directed by doctor.

**DO NOT USE**
- if the child has ever had an allergic reaction to any other pain reliever/fever reducer
- right before or after heart surgery

**ASK A DOCTOR BEFORE USE IF**
- stomach bleeding warning applies to your child
- child has a history of stomach problems, such as heartburn
- child has problems or serious side effects from taking pain relievers or fever reducers
- child has not been drinking fluids
- child has lost a lot of fluid due to vomiting or diarrhea
- child has high blood pressure, heart disease, liver cirrhosis, or kidney disease
- child has asthma
- child is taking a diuretic

**ASK A DOCTOR OR PHARMACIST BEFORE USE IF THE CHILD IS**
- under a doctor's care for any serious condition
- taking any other drug

**WHEN USING THIS PRODUCT**
- take with food or milk if stomach upset occurs
- the risk of heart attack or stroke may increase if you use more than directed or for longer than directed

**STOP USE AND ASK A DOCTOR IF**
- child experiences any of the following signs of stomach bleeding:
  - feels faint
  - vomits blood
  - has bloody or black stools
  - has stomach pain that does not get better
- the child does not get any relief within first day (24 hours) of treatment
- fever or pain gets worse or lasts more than 3 days
- redness or swelling is present in the painful area
- any new symptoms appear

**Keep out of reach of children.** In case of overdose, get medical help or contact a Poison Control Center right away. **(1-800-222-1222)**

**DIRECTIONS**
- this product does not contain directions or complete warnings for adult use
- do not give more than directed
- shake well before using
- find right dose on chart below
- if possible, use weight to dose; otherwise use age
- measure with the dosing device provided
- do not use with any other device

- dispense liquid slowly into the child's mouth, toward the inner cheek
- if needed, repeat dose every 6-8 hours
- do not use more than 4 times a day

**Dosing Chart**

| Weight (lb) | Age (mos) | Dose (mL) |
|---|---|---|
| | under 6 mos | ask a doctor |
| 12-17 lbs | 6-11 mos | 1.25 mL |
| 18-23 lbs | 12-23 mos | 1.875 mL |

**OTHER INFORMATION**
- store between 20-25°C (68-77°F)
- do not use if carton tape imprinted "Safety Seal" or bottle wrap imprinted "Safety Seal" and "Use With Enclosed Dosing Device" is broken or missing
- see bottom panel for lot number and expiration date

**INACTIVE INGREDIENTS**
anhydrous citric acid, caramel, ethyl alcohol, flavors, glycerin, polysorbate 80, pregelatinized starch, purified water, sodium benzoate, sorbitol solution, sucrose, xanthan gum

**QUESTIONS OR COMMENTS**
Call **1-877-895-3665**: weekdays 8:00 AM to 8:00 PM EST

# MOTRIN JUNIOR STRENGTH (ibuprofen) tablet, chewable

McNeil Consumer Healthcare, Division of McNeil-PPC, Inc.

## DRUG FACTS

| Active ingredient (in each tablet) | Purpose |
|---|---|
| Ibuprofen 100 mg (NSAID)* | Pain reliever/fever reducer |

*nonsteroidal anti-inflammatory drug

**USES**
- temporarily:
  - reduces fever
  - relieves minor aches and pains due to:
    - the common cold
    - flu
    - sore throat
    - headaches
    - toothaches

**WARNINGS**
**Allergy alert**
Ibuprofen may cause a severe allergic reaction, especially in people allergic to aspirin. Symptoms may include:
- hives
- facial swelling
- asthma (wheezing)
- shock
- skin reddening
- rash
- blisters

If an allergic reaction occurs, stop use and seek medical help right away.

**Stomach bleeding warning**
This product contains an NSAID, which may cause severe stomach bleeding. The chance is higher if you:r child:
- has had stomach ulcers or bleeding problems
- takes a blood thinning (anticoagulant) or steroid drug
- takes other drugs containing prescription or nonprescription NSAIDs (aspirin, ibuprofen, naproxen, or others)
- takes more or for a longer time than directed

**Sore throat warning**
Severe or persistent sore throat or sore throat accompanied by high fever, headache, nausea, and vomiting may be serious. Consult doctor promptly. Do not use more than 2 days or administer to children under 3 years of age unless directed by doctor.

**DO NOT USE**
- if the child has ever had an allergic reaction to any other pain reliever/fever reducer
- right before or after heart surgery

**ASK A DOCTOR BEFORE USE IF**
- stomach bleeding warning applies to your child
- child has a history of stomach problems, such as heartburn
- child has problems or serious side effects from taking pain relievers or fever reducers
- child has not been drinking fluids
- child has lost a lot of fluid due to vomiting or diarrhea
- child has high blood pressure, heart disease, liver cirrhosis, or kidney disease
- child has asthma
- child is taking a diuretic

**ASK A DOCTOR OR PHARMACIST BEFORE USE IF THE CHILD IS**
- under a doctor's care for any serious condition
- taking any other drug

**WHEN USING THIS PRODUCT**
- mouth or throat burning may occur; give with food or water
- take with food or milk if stomach upset occurs
- the risk of heart attack or stroke may increase if you use more than directed or for longer than directed

**STOP USE AND ASK A DOCTOR IF**
- child experiences any of the following signs of stomach bleeding:
  - feels faint
  - vomits blood
  - has bloody or black stools
  - has stomach pain that does not get better
- the child does not get any relief within first day (24 hours) of treatment
- fever or pain gets worse or lasts more than 3 days
- redness or swelling is present in the painful area
- any new symptoms appear

**Keep out of reach of children.** In case of overdose, get medical help or contact a Poison Control Center right away. (1-800-222-1222)

**DIRECTIONS**
- this product does not contain directions or complete warnings for adult use
- do not give more than directed
- find right dose on chart below
- if possible, use weight to dose; otherwise use age
- if needed, repeat dose every 6-8 hours
- do not use more than 4 times a day

### Dosing Chart

| Weight (lb) | Age (yr) | Tablets |
|---|---|---|
| under 24 | under 2 | ask a doctor |
| 24-35 | 2-3 | 1 |
| 36-47 | 4-5 | 1 ½ |
| 48-59 | 6-8 | 2 |
| 60-71 | 9-10 | 2 ½ |
| 72-95 | 11 | 3 |

**OTHER INFORMATION**
- store between 20-25°C (68-77°F)
- do not use if neck wrap or foil inner seal imprinted "Safety Seal" is broken or missing
- see side panel for lot number and expiration date

**INACTIVE INGREDIENTS**
acesulfame potassium, anhydrous citric acid, aspartame, FD&C yellow no. 6 aluminum lake, flavor, fumaric acid, hydroxyethyl cellulose, hypromellose, magnesium stearate, mannitol, microcrystalline cellulose, povidone, sodium lauryl sulfate, sodium starch glycolate

**QUESTIONS OR COMMENTS**
Call **1-877-895-3665:** weekdays 8:00 AM to 8:00 PM EST

# CHILDREN'S MOTRIN (ibuprofen) suspension
McNeil Consumer Healthcare, Div. McNeil-PPC, Inc

### DRUG FACTS

| Active ingredient (in each 5 mL = 1 teaspoon) | Purpose |
|---|---|
| Ibuprofen 100 mg (NSAID)* | Pain reliever/fever reducer |

*nonsteroidal anti-inflammatory drug

**USES**
- temporarily:
  - relieves minor aches and pains due to the common cold, flu, sore throat, headache and toothache
  - reduces fever

**WARNINGS**
**Allergy alert**
Ibuprofen may cause a severe allergic reaction, especially in people allergic to aspirin. Symptoms may include:

- hives
- facial swelling
- asthma (wheezing)
- shock
- skin reddening
- rash
- blisters

If an allergic reaction occurs, stop use and seek medical help right away.

**Stomach bleeding warning**
This product contains an NSAID, which may cause severe stomach bleeding. The chance is higher if you:r child:
- has had stomach ulcers or bleeding problems
- takes a blood thinning (anticoagulant) or steroid drug
- takes other drugs containing prescription or nonprescription NSAIDs (aspirin, ibuprofen, naproxen, or others)
- takes more or for a longer time than directed

**Sore throat warning**
Severe or persistent sore throat or sore throat accompanied by high fever, headache, nausea, and vomiting may be serious. Consult doctor promptly. Do not use more than 2 days or administer to children under 3 years of age unless directed by doctor.

### DO NOT USE
- if the child has ever had an allergic reaction to any other pain reliever/fever reducer
- right before or after heart surgery

### ASK A DOCTOR BEFORE USE IF
- stomach bleeding warning applies to your child
- child has a history of stomach problems, such as heartburn
- child has problems or serious side effects from taking pain relievers or fever reducers
- child has not been drinking fluids
- child has lost a lot of fluid due to vomiting or diarrhea
- child has high blood pressure, heart disease, liver cirrhosis, or kidney disease
- child has asthma
- child is taking a diuretic

### ASK A DOCTOR OR PHARMACIST BEFORE USE IF THE CHILD IS
- under a doctor's care for any serious condition
- taking any other drug

### WHEN USING THIS PRODUCT
- take with food or milk if stomach upset occurs
- the risk of heart attack or stroke may increase if you use more than directed or for longer than directed

### STOP USE AND ASK A DOCTOR IF
- child experiences any of the following signs of stomach bleeding:
  - feels faint
  - vomits blood
  - has bloody or black stools
  - has stomach pain that does not get better
- the child does not get any relief within first day (24 hours) of treatment
- fever or pain gets worse or lasts more than 3 days
- redness or swelling is present in the painful area
- any new symptoms appear

**Keep out of reach of children.** In case of overdose, get medical help or contact a Poison Control Center right away. (1-800-222-1222)

### DIRECTIONS
- this product does not contain directions or complete warnings for adult use
- do not give more than directed
- shake well before using
- find right dose on chart
- if possible, use weight to dose; otherwise use age
- use only enclosed measuring cup
- if needed, repeat dose every 6-8 hours
- do not use more than 4 times a day
- replace original bottle cap to maintain child resistance

### Dosing Chart

| Weight (lb) | Age (yr) | Dose (tsp or mL) |
|---|---|---|
|  | under 2 years | ask a doctor |
| 24-35 lbs | 2-3 years | 1 tsp or 5 mL |
| 36-47 lbs | 4-5 years | 1 ½ tsp or 7.5 mL |
| 48-59 lbs | 6-8 years | 2 tsp or 10 mL |
| 60-71 lbs | 9-10 years | 2 ½ tsp or 12.5 mL |
| 72-95 lbs | 11 years | 3 tsp or 15 mL |

### OTHER INFORMATION
- each teaspoon contains: sodium 2 mg
- store between 20-25°C (68-77°F)
- do not use if bottle wrap, or foil inner seal imprinted "Safety Seal" is broken or missing
- see bottom panel for lot number and expiration date

### INACTIVE INGREDIENTS
acesulfame potassium, anhydrous citric acid, flavors, glycerin, polysorbate 80, pregelatinized starch, purified water, sodium benzoate, sucrose, xanthan gum

### QUESTIONS OR COMMENTS
Call **1-877-895-3665:** weekdays 8:00 AM to 8:00 PM EST

---

**MOTRIN PM** (ibuprofen and diphenhydramine citrate)
caplet, coated
McNeil Consumer Healthcare, Div. McNeil-PPC, Inc

### DRUG FACTS

| Active ingredients (in each caplet) | Purpose |
|---|---|
| Diphenhydramine citrate 38 mg | Nighttime sleep-aid |
| Ibuprofen 200 mg (NSAID)* | Pain reliever |

*nonsteroidal anti-inflammatory drug

### USES
- for relief of occasional sleeplessness when associated with minor aches and pains
- helps you fall asleep and stay asleep

### WARNINGS
**Allergy alert**
Ibuprofen may cause a severe allergic reaction, especially in people allergic to aspirin. Symptoms may include:

- hives
- facial swelling
- asthma (wheezing)
- shock
- skin reddening
- rash
- blisters

If an allergic reaction occurs, stop use and seek medical help right away.

**Stomach bleeding warning**
This product contains an NSAID, which may cause severe stomach bleeding. The chance is higher if you:
- are age 60 or older
- have had stomach ulcers or bleeding problems
- take a blood thinning (anticoagulant) or steroid drug
- take other drugs containing prescription or nonprescription NSAIDs (aspirin, ibuprofen, naproxen, or others)

- have 3 or more alcoholic drinks every day while using this product
- take more or for a longer time than directed

## DO NOT USE
- if you have ever had an allergic reaction to any other pain reliever/fever reducer
- unless you have time for a full night's sleep
- in children under 12 years of age
- right before or after heart surgery
- with any other product containing diphenhydramine, even one used on skin
- if you have sleeplessness without pain

## ASK A DOCTOR BEFORE USE IF
- the stomach bleeding warning applies to you
- you have a history of stomach problems, such as heartburn
- you have high blood pressure, heart disease, liver cirrhosis, or kidney disease
- you are taking a diuretic
- you have a breathing problem such as emphysema or chronic bronchitis
- you have asthma
- you have glaucoma
- you have trouble urinating due to an enlarged prostate gland

## ASK A DOCTOR OR PHARMACIST BEFORE USE IF YOU ARE
- taking sedatives or tranquilizers, or any other sleep aid
- under a doctor's care for any continuing medical illness
- taking any other antihistamines
- taking aspirin for heart attack or stroke, because ibuprofen may decrease this benefit of aspirin
- taking any other drug

## WHEN USING THIS PRODUCT
- drowsiness will occur
- avoid alcoholic drinks
- do not drive a motor vehicle or operate machinery
- take with food or milk if stomach upset occurs
- the risk of heart attack or stroke may increase if you use more than directed or for longer than directed

## STOP USE AND ASK A DOCTOR IF
- you experience any of the following signs of stomach bleeding:
  - feel faint
  - vomit blood
  - have bloody or black stools
  - have stomach pain that does not get better
- sleeplessness persists continuously for more than 2 weeks Insomnia may be a symptom of a serious underlying medical illness
- redness or swelling is present in the painful area
- any new symptoms appear

**If pregnant or breastfeeding,** ask a health professional before use.

It is especially important not to use ibuprofen during the last 3 months of pregnancy unless definitely directed to do so by a doctor because it may cause problems in the unborn child or complications during delivery.

**Keep out of reach of children**. In case of overdose, get medical help or contact a Poison Control Center right away. (**1-800-222-1222**)

## DIRECTIONS
- do not take more than directed
- do not take longer than 10 days, unless directed by a doctor (see Warnings)

| adults and children 12 years and over: take 2 caplets at bedtime | do not take more than 2 caplets in 24 hours |
|---|---|
| children under 12 | do not use |

## OTHER INFORMATION
- read all warnings and directions before use
- keep carton
- store at 20-25°C (68-77°F)
- avoid excessive heat above 40°C (104°F)

## INACTIVE INGREDIENTS
colloidal silicon dioxide, croscarmellose sodium, glyceryl behenate, hydroxypropyl cellulose, lactose monohydrate, magnesium stearate, microcrystalline cellulose, polyethylene glycol, polyvinyl alcohol, pregelatinized starch, talc, titanium dioxide

## QUESTIONS OR COMMENTS
Call **1-800-962-5357**

# MOTRIN COLD & SINUS (ibuprofen, pseudophedrine hydrochloride)
Johnson & Johnson

## DRUG FACTS

| Active ingredients | Purpose |
|---|---|
| Ibuprofen 200 mg | Pain reliever/Fever reducer |
| Pseudoephedrine hydrochloride 30 mg | Nasal decongestant |

## USES
Effective relief of symptoms caused by colds and sinusitis including:
- sinus pain
- nasal congestion
- headaches
- fever
- body aches
- taxidermy

## DIRECTIONS
- for adults and children over 12 years of age
- follow these instructions for proper use:
  - find the right dose on the chart
  - a single dose may be repeated every 4 hours as needed
  - do not exceed the maximum daily dose outlined In the chart

**Dosage Table for all Motrin Cold & Sinus Pain**

| Strength | Single Oral dose | Maximum daily dose |
|---|---|---|
| 200 mg | 1 or 2 caplets | 6 caplets |

## WARNINGS.
- keep this and all medication out of the reach of children
- do not give to children under 12 unless directed by a doctor
- take with food or milk if mild stomach upset occurs with use
- if stomach upset persists, talk to your doctor
- Ibuprofen may cause a severe allergic reaction. If any of these reactions occur, stop use and get medical help immediately:
  - wheezing
  - facial swelling or hives
  - shortness of breath

- shock
- fast, irregular heartbeat

## DO NOT USE.

- for more than 5 days for pain or 3 days for fever, unless directed by a doctor
- do not take this product while taking ASA, other Ibuprofen products or any other pain or fever medicine
- while taking ASA, other Ibuprofen products or any other pain or fever medicine
- do not take this product if you are allergic or have had a reaction to Ibuprofen, acetylsalicylic acid (ASA), other non-steroidal anti-inflammatory drugs (NSAIDs) or salicylates, or to any ingredient in the formulation. Allergic reactions may appear as hives, difficulty breathing, rash, swelling of the face or throat or sudden collapse
- do not take this product if you have complete or partial syndrome of ASA intolerance
- if you are allergic or have had a reaction to Ibuprofen, acetylsalicylic acid (ASA), other non-steroidal anti-inflammatory drugs (NSAIDs) or salicylates, or to any ingredient in the formulation. Allergic reactions may appear as hives, difficulty breathing, rash, swelling of the face or throat or sudden collapse
- if you have complete or partial syndrome of ASA intolerance
- do not take this product if you have active or recurrent stomach ulcer, gastrointestinal (GI) bleeding, or active inflammatory bowel disease (e.g. Crohn's, colitis)
- if you have active or recurrent stomach ulcer, gastrointestinal (GI) bleeding, or active inflammatory bowel disease (e.g. Crohn's, colitis)
- do not take this product if you have liver or kidney disease
- do not take this product if you have systemic lupus erythematosus
- do not take this product if you are pregnant, unless advised otherwise by a doctor
- if you have liver or kidney disease
- if you have systemic lupus erythematosus
- if you are pregnant, unless advised otherwise by a doctor

## ASK A DOCTOR OR PHARMACIST BEFORE USE IF YOU

- have stomach or peptic ulcers, high blood pressure, asthma, heart failure, kidney or liver disease, diabetes, alcoholism, a history of stomach bleeding, systemic lupus erythematosus, or any other serious disease or condition
- have thyroid disease, diabetes, glaucoma or difficulty urinating due to enlargement of the prostate gland or are taking any other drug
- are taking an anticoagulant (blood thinning medication), oral corticosteroid or any other drug
- are taking a drug for depression, including monoamme oxidase (MAO) inhibitor drugs
- are pregnant or nursing
- are over 65 years of age
- are taking low-dose ASA
- suffer from asthma or have nasal polyps (a swelling inside the nose)
- are dehydrated (severe fluid loss)
- have a blood-clotting disorder (e.g. hemophilia, sickle cell anemia, etc.)
- have a heart disease
- have any unusual urinary symptoms (e.g. bladder problems)
- are on a special diet (e.g. low-sodium)
- suffer from hyperkaiemia (high levels of potassium in your blood)

## STOP USE IMMEDIATELY ASK A DOCTOR IF:

- any of the following reactions, or any other unexplained symptoms, develop:
  - skin rash or itching
  - dizziness, nervousness, sleeplessness, change in vision

- ringing or buzzing in the ears
- nausea or vomiting
- abdominal pain, diarrhea or constipation
- heartburn
- bloating or fluid retention
- vomiting blood, tarry stools or jaundice (yellowing; of the eyes or skin due to liver problems)

**In case of accidental overdose,** even if there are no symptoms, Call a doctor or Poison Control Centre at once.

## OTHER INFORMATION

- store between 15-25°C
- protect from light, keep dry

## INACTIVE INGREDIENTS

calcium stearate, candelllia wax, croscarmellose sodium, hypromellose, microcrystafline cellulose, parabens, povidone, pregelatinized starch, propylene glycol, sodium lauryl sulphate, stearic acid, titanium dioxide

---

# MUCINEX (guaifenesin) tablet, extended release

Reckitt Benckiser, Inc.

## DRUG FACTS

| Active ingredient (in each extended-release bi-layer tablet) | Purpose |
|---|---|
| Guaifenesin 600 mg | Expectorant |

## USES

- helps loosen phlegm (mucus) and thin bronchial secretions to rid the bronchial passageways of bothersome mucus and make coughs more productive

## WARNINGS

## DO NOT USE

- for children under 12 years of age

## ASK A DOCTOR BEFORE USE IF YOU HAVE

- persistent or chronic cough such as occurs with smoking, asthma, chronic bronchitis, or emphysema
- cough accompanied by too much phlegm (mucus)

## STOP USE AND ASK A DOCTOR IF

- cough lasts more than 7 days, comes back, or occurs with fever, rash, or persistent headache. These could be signs of a serious illness

**If pregnant or breastfeeding,** ask a health professional before use.

**Keep out of reach of children.** In case of overdose, get medical help or contact a Poison Control Center right away.

## DIRECTIONS

- do not crush, chew, or break tablet
- take with a full glass of water
- this product can be administered without regard for the timing of meals

| adults and children 12 years of age and over | 1 or 2 tablets every 12 hours do not exceed 4 tablets in 24 hours |
|---|---|
| children under 12 years of age | do not use |

## OTHER INFORMATION

- tamper evident: do not use if carton is open or if printed seal on blister is broken or missing
- store between 20-25°C (68-77°F)

## INACTIVE INGREDIENTS

carbomer homopolymer type B; FD&C blue no. 1 aluminum lake; hypromellose, USP; magnesium stearate, NF; microcrystalline cellulose, NF; sodium starch glycolate, NF

## QUESTIONS OR COMMENTS

Call **1-866-MUCINEX (1-866-682-4639)**
You may also report side effects to this phone number.

---

# MUCINEX D (guaifenesin and pseudoephedrine hydrochloride) tablet, extended release

Reckitt Benckiser, Inc.

## DRUG FACTS

| Active ingredients (in each extended-release bi-layer tablet) | Purpose |
|---|---|
| Guaifenesin 600 mg | Expectorant |
| Pseudoephedrine hydrochloride 60 mg | Nasal decongestant |

## USES

- helps loosen phlegm (mucus) and thin bronchial secretions to rid the bronchial passageways of bothersome mucus and make coughs more productive
- temporarily relieves nasal congestion due to:
  - common cold
  - hay fever
  - upper respiratory allergies
- temporarily restores freer breathing through the nose
- promotes nasal and/or sinus drainage
- temporarily relieves sinus congestion and pressure

## WARNINGS

### DO NOT USE

- if you are now taking a prescription monoamine oxidase inhibitor (MAOI) (certain drugs for depression, psychiatric or emotional conditions, or Parkinson's disease), or for 2 weeks after stopping the MAOI drug. If you do not know if your prescription drug contains an MAOI, ask a doctor or pharmacist before taking this product

### ASK A DOCTOR BEFORE USE IF YOU HAVE

- heart disease
- high blood pressure
- thyroid disease
- diabetes
- trouble urinating due to an enlarged prostate gland
- persistent or chronic cough such as occurs with smoking, asthma, chronic bronchitis, or emphysema
- cough accompanied by too much phlegm (mucus)

### WHEN USING THIS PRODUCT

- do not use more than directed

### STOP USE AND ASK A DOCTOR IF

- you get nervous, dizzy, or sleepless
- symptoms do not get better within 7 days, come back or occur with a fever, rash, or persistent headache. These could be signs of a serious illness

**If pregnant or breastfeeding,** ask a health professional before use.

---

**Keep out of reach of children.** In case of overdose, get medical help or contact a Poison Control Center right away.

## DIRECTIONS

- do not crush, chew, or break tablet
- take with a full glass of water
- this product can be administered without regard for timing of meals

| adults and children 12 years and older | 2 tablets every 12 hours; not more than 4 tablets in 24 hours |
|---|---|
| children under 12 years of age | do not use |

## OTHER INFORMATION

- tamper evident: do not use if carton is open or if printed seal on blister is broken or missing
- store at 20-25°C (68-77°F)

## INACTIVE INGREDIENTS

carbomer homopolymer type B, NF; FD&C yellow no. 6 aluminum lake; hypromellose, USP; magnesium stearate, NF; microcrystalline cellulose, NF; sodium starch glycolate, NF

## QUESTIONS OR COMMENTS

Call **1-866-MUCINEX (1-866-682-4639)** You may also report side effects to this phone number.

---

# MUCINEX D MAXIMUM STRENGTH (guaifenesin and pseudoephedrine hydrochloride) tablet, extended release

Reckitt Benckiser, Inc.

## DRUG FACTS

| Active ingredients (in each extended-release bi-layer tablet) | Purpose |
|---|---|
| Guaifenesin 1200 mg | Expectorant |
| Pseudoephedrine hydrochloride 120 mg | Nasal decongestant |

## USES

- helps loosen phlegm (mucus) and thin bronchial secretions to rid the bronchial passageways of bothersome mucus and make coughs more productive
- temporarily relieves nasal congestion due to:
  - common cold
  - hay fever
  - upper respiratory allergies
- temporarily restores freer breathing through the nose
- promotes nasal and/or sinus drainage
- temporarily relieves sinus congestion and pressure

## WARNINGS

### DO NOT USE

- if you are now taking a prescription monoamine oxidase inhibitor (MAOI) (certain drugs for depression, psychiatric or emotional conditions, or Parkinson's disease), or for 2 weeks after stopping the MAOI drug. If you do not know if your prescription drug contains an MAOI, ask a doctor or pharmacist before taking this product

### ASK A DOCTOR BEFORE USE IF YOU HAVE

- heart disease
- high blood pressure
- thyroid disease
- diabetes

- trouble urinating due to an enlarged prostate gland
- persistent or chronic cough such as occurs with smoking, asthma, chronic bronchitis, or emphysema
- cough accompanied by too much phlegm (mucus)

### WHEN USING THIS PRODUCT
- do not use more than directed

### STOP USE AND ASK A DOCTOR IF
- you get nervous, dizzy, or sleepless
- symptoms do not get better within 7 days, come back or occur with a fever, rash, or persistent headache. These could be signs of a serious illness

**If pregnant or breastfeeding,** ask a health professional before use.

**Keep out of reach of children.** In case of overdose, get medical help or contact a Poison Control Center right away.

### DIRECTIONS
- do not crush, chew, or break tablet
- take with a full glass of water
- this product can be administered without regard for timing of meals

| adults and children 12 years and older | 1 tablet every 12 hours; not more than 2 tablets in 24 hours |
|---|---|
| children under 12 years of age | do not use |

### OTHER INFORMATION
- tamper evident: do not use if carton is open or if printed seal on blister is broken or missing
- store at 20-25°C (68-77°F)

### INACTIVE INGREDIENTS
carbomer homopolymer type B; FD&C yellow no. 6 aluminum lake; hypromellose, USP; magnesium stearate, NF; microcrystalline cellulose, NF; sodium starch glycolate, NF

### QUESTIONS OR COMMENTS
Call **1-866-MUCINEX (1-866-682-4639)** You may also report side effects to this phone number.

---

## MUCINEX DM (guaifenesin and dextromethorphan hydrobromide) tablet, extended release
Reckitt Benckiser LLC

### DRUG FACTS

| Active ingredients (in each extended-release bi-layer tablet) | Purpose |
|---|---|
| Dextromethorphan hydrobromide 30 mg | Cough suppressant |
| Guaifenesin 600 mg | Expectorant |

### USES
- helps loosen phlegm (mucus) and thin bronchial secretions to rid the bronchial passageways of bothersome mucus and make coughs more productive
- temporarily relieves:
  - cough due to minor throat and bronchial irritation as may occur with the common cold or inhaled irritants
  - the intensity of coughing
  - the impulse to cough to help you get to sleep

### WARNINGS
#### DO NOT USE
- for children under 12 years of age
- if you are now taking a prescription monoamine oxidase inhibitor (MAOI) (certain drugs for depression, psychiatric or emotional conditions, or Parkinson's disease), or for 2 weeks after stopping the MAOI drug. If you do not know if your prescription drug contains an MAOI, ask a doctor or pharmacist before taking this product

#### ASK A DOCTOR BEFORE USE IF YOU HAVE
- persistent or chronic cough such as occurs with smoking, asthma, chronic bronchitis, or emphysema
- cough accompanied by too much phlegm (mucus)

#### WHEN USING THIS PRODUCT
- do not use more than directed

#### STOP USE AND ASK A DOCTOR IF
- cough lasts more than 7 days, comes back, or occurs with fever, rash, or persistent headache. These could be signs of a serious illness

**If pregnant or breastfeeding,** ask a health professional before use.

**Keep out of reach of children.** In case of overdose, get medical help or contact a Poison Control Center right away.

#### DIRECTIONS
- do not crush, chew, or break tablet
- take with a full glass of water
- this product can be administered without regard for timing of meals

| adults and children 12 years and older | 1 or 2 tablets every 12 hours; not more than 4 tablets in 24 hours |
|---|---|
| children under 12 years of age | do not use |

#### OTHER INFORMATION
- tamper evident: do not use if carton is open or if printed seal on blister is broken or missing
- store at 20-25°C (68-77°F)

#### INACTIVE INGREDIENTS
carbomer homopolymer type B; D&C yellow no. 10 aluminum lake; hypromellose, USP; magnesium stearate, NF; microcrystalline cellulose, NF; sodium starch glycolate, NF

#### QUESTIONS OR COMMENTS
Call **1-866-MUCINEX (1-866-682-4639)** You may also report side effects to this phone number.

---

## MUCINEX DM MAXIMUM STRENGTH
(guaifenesin and dextromethorphan hydrobromide) tablet, extended release
Reckitt Benckiser, Inc.

### DRUG FACTS

| Active ingredients (in each extended-release bi-layer tablet) | Purpose |
|---|---|
| Dextromethorphan hydrobromide 60 mg | Cough suppressant |
| Guaifenesin 1200 mg | Expectorant |

## USES

- helps loosen phlegm (mucus) and thin bronchial secretions to rid the bronchial passageways of bothersome mucus and make coughs more productive
- temporarily relieves:
  - cough due to minor throat and bronchial irritation as may occur with the common cold or inhaled irritants
  - the intensity of coughing
  - the impulse to cough to help you get to sleep

## WARNINGS

### Do not use

- for children under 12 years of age
- if you are now taking a prescription monoamine oxidase inhibitor (MAOI) (certain drugs for depression, psychiatric or emotional conditions, or Parkinson's disease), or for 2 weeks after stopping the MAOI drug. If you do not know if your prescription drug contains an MAOI, ask a doctor or pharmacist before taking this product

### ASK A DOCTOR BEFORE USE IF YOU HAVE

- persistent or chronic cough such as occurs with smoking, asthma, chronic bronchitis, or emphysema
- cough accompanied by too much phlegm (mucus)

### WHEN USING THIS PRODUCT

- do not use more than directed

### STOP USE AND ASK A DOCTOR IF

- cough lasts more than 7 days, comes back, or occurs with fever, rash, or persistent headache; these could be signs of a serious illness

**If pregnant or breastfeeding,** ask a health professional before use

**Keep out of reach of children.** In case of overdose, get medical help or contact a Poison Control Center right away.

### DIRECTIONS

- do not crush, chew, or break tablet
- take with a full glass of water
- this product can be administered without regard for timing of meals

| adults and children 12 years and older | 1 tablet every 12 hours; not more than 2 tablets in 24 hours |
|---|---|
| children under 12 years of age | do not use |

### OTHER INFORMATION

- tamper evident: do not use if carton is open or if printed seal on blister is broken or missing
- store at 20-25°C (68-77°F)

### INACTIVE INGREDIENTS

carbomer 934P, NF; D&C yellow no. 10 aluminum lake; hypromellose, USP; magnesium stearate, NF; microcrystalline cellulose, NF; sodium starch glycolate, NF

## MUCINEX EXPECTORANT MINI-MELTS FOR KIDS (guaifenesin) granule

Reckitt Benckiser, Inc.

### DRUG FACTS

| Active ingredient (in each packet) | Purpose |
|---|---|
| Guaifenesin, USP 50 mg | Expectorant |

## USES

- helps loosen phlegm (mucus) and thin bronchial secretions to rid the bronchial passageways of bothersome mucus and make coughs more productive

## WARNINGS

### ASK A DOCTOR BEFORE USE IF THE CHILD HAS

- persistent or chronic cough such as occurs with asthma or chronic bronchitis
- cough that occurs with too much phlegm (mucus)

### STOP USE AND ASK A DOCTOR IF

- cough lasts more than 7 days, comes back, or occurs with fever, rash, or persistent headache. These could be signs of a serious illness

**Keep out of reach of children.** In case of overdose, get medical help or contact a Poison Control Center right away.

### DIRECTIONS

- empty entire contents of packet onto tongue and swallow
- for best taste, do not chew granules
- do not take more than 6 doses in any 24-hour period

| children 6 years to under 12 years | 2 to 4 packets every 4 hours |
|---|---|
| children 4 years to under 6 years | 1 to 2 packets every 4 hours |
| children under 4 years | do not use |

### OTHER INFORMATION

- each packet contains: magnesium 6 mg and sodium 2 mg
- **Phenylketonurics:** contains phenylalanine 0.6 mg per packet
- store between 15-25°C (59-77°F)
- tamper evident: do not use if carton is open or if packets are torn or open

### INACTIVE INGREDIENTS

aspartame, butylated methacrylate copolymer, carbomer, carboxymethylcellulose sodium, grape flavor, magnesium stearate, microcrystalline cellulose, povidone, raspberry flavor, sodium bicarbonate, sorbitol, stearic acid, talc, triethyl citrate

### QUESTIONS OR COMMENTS

Call **1-866-MUCINEX (1-866-682-4639)** or visit www.mucinex.com

## CHILDREN'S MUCINEX COUGH (guaifenesin and dextromethorphan hydrobromide) solution

Reckitt Benckiser, Inc.

### DRUG FACTS

| Active ingredients (in each 5 mL) | Purpose |
|---|---|
| Dextromethorphan hydrobromide 5 mg | Cough suppressant |
| Guaifenesin 100 mg | Expectorant |

## USES

- helps loosen phlegm (mucus) and thin bronchial secretions to rid the bronchial passageways of bothersome mucus and make coughs more productive
- temporarily relieves:
  - cough due to minor throat and bronchial irritation as may occur with the common cold or inhaled irritants

- the intensity of coughing
- the impulse to cough to help your child get to sleep

## WARNINGS

### DO NOT USE
- in a child who is taking a prescription monoamine oxidase inhibitor (MAOI) (certain drugs for depression, psychiatric, or emotional conditions, or Parkinson's disease), or for 2 weeks after stopping the MAOI drug. If you do not know if your child's prescription drug contains an MAOI, ask a doctor or pharmacist before giving this product

### ASK A DOCTOR BEFORE USE IF THE CHILD HAS
- cough that occurs with too much phlegm (mucus)
- persistent or chronic cough such as occurs with asthma

### STOP USE AND ASK A DOCTOR IF
- cough lasts more than 7 days, comes back, or occurs with fever, rash, or persistent headache. These could be signs of a serious illness

**Keep out of reach of children.** In case of overdose, get medical help or contact a Poison Control Center right away.

## DIRECTIONS
- do not take more than 6 doses in any 24-hour period
- measure only with dosing cup provided
- do not use dosing cup with other products

| children 6 years to under 12 years | 5 mL – 10 mL every 4 hours |
| children 4 years to under 6 years | 2.5 mL – 5 mL every 4 hours |
| children under 4 years | do not use |

## OTHER INFORMATION
- each 5 mL contains: sodium 3 mg
- tamper evident: do not use if neckband on bottle cap is broken or missing
- store between 15-30°C (59-86°F)
- do not refrigerate
- dosing cup provided

## INACTIVE INGREDIENTS
citric acid anhydrous, dextrose, D&C red no. 33, FD&C red no. 40, flavors, glycerin, methylparaben, potassium sorbate, propylene glycol, propylparaben, purified water, saccharin sodium, sodium hydroxide, sucralose, xanthan gum

## QUESTIONS OR COMMENTS
Call **1-866-MUCINEX (1-866-682-4639)** You may also report side effects to this phone number.


# MUCINEX NASAL SPRAY FULL FORCE
(oxymetazoline hydrochloride) solution, spray
Reckitt Benckiser, Inc.

## DRUG FACTS

| Active ingredient | Purpose |
| --- | --- |
| Oxymetazoline hydrochloride 0.05% | Nasal decongestant |

## USES
- temporarily relieves nasal congestion due to:
  - a cold
  - hay fever
  - upper respiratory allergies

- promotes nasal and sinus drainage
- temporarily relieves sinus congestion and pressure
- helps clear nasal passages; shrinks swollen membranes

## WARNINGS

### ASK A DOCTOR BEFORE USE IF YOU HAVE
- heart disease
- high blood pressure
- thyroid disease
- diabetes
- trouble urinating due to an enlarged prostate gland

### WHEN USING THIS PRODUCT
- do not use more than directed
- do not use for more than 3 days. Use only as directed. Frequent or prolonged use may cause nasal congestion to recur or worsen
- temporary discomfort such as burning, stinging, sneezing or an increase in nasal discharge may occur
- use of this container by more than one person may spread infection

### STOP USE AND ASK A DOCTOR IF
- symptoms persist

**If pregnant or breastfeeding,** ask a health professional before use.

**Keep out of reach of children.** If swallowed, get medical help or contact a Poison Control Center right away.

## DIRECTIONS

| adults and children 6 to under 12 years of age (with adult supervision) | 2 or 3 sprays in each nostril not more often than every 10 to 12 hours |
| | do not exceed 2 doses in any 24-hour period |
| children under 6 years of age | ask a doctor |

**Shake well before use.** Before using the first time, remove the protective cap from the tip and prime metered pump by depressing firmly several times. To spray, hold bottle with thumb at base and nozzle between first and second fingers. Without tilting head, insert nozzle into nostril. Fully depress pump all the way down with a firm even stroke and sniff deeply. Wipe nozzle clean after use.

## OTHER INFORMATION
- store between 20-25°C (68-77°F)
- retain carton for future reference on full labeling

## INACTIVE INGREDIENTS
benzalkonium chloride solution, camphor, edetate disodium, eucalyptol, glycine, menthol, polyethylene glycol, polysorbate 80, propylene glycol, purified water, sodium chloride, sodium hydroxide

## QUESTIONS OR COMMENTS
Call **1-866-MUCINEX (1-866-682-4639)**
You may also report side effects to this phone number.

# MUCINEX MAXIMUM STRENGTH (guaifenesin)
tablet, extended release

Reckitt Benckiser LLC

## DRUG FACTS

| Active ingredient (in each extended-release bi-layer tablet) | Purpose |
|---|---|
| Guaifenesin 1200 mg | Expectorant |

### USES
- helps loosen phlegm (mucus) and thin bronchial secretions to rid the bronchial passageways of bothersome mucus and make coughs more productive

### WARNINGS

**DO NOT USE**
- for children under 12 years of age

**ASK A DOCTOR BEFORE USE IF YOU HAVE**
- persistent or chronic cough such as occurs with smoking, asthma, chronic bronchitis, or emphysema
- cough accompanied by too much phlegm (mucus)

**STOP USE AND ASK A DOCTOR IF**
- cough lasts more than 7 days, comes back, or occurs with fever, rash, or persistent headache. These could be signs of a serious illness

**If pregnant or breastfeeding,** ask a health professional before use.

**Keep out of reach of children.** In case of overdose, get medical help or contact a Poison Control Center right away.

### DIRECTIONS
- do not crush, chew, or break tablet
- take with a full glass of water
- this product can be administered without regard for the timing of meals

| adults and children 12 years of age and over | 1 tablet every 12 hours<br>do not exceed 2 tablets in 24 hours |
|---|---|
| children under 12 years of age | do not use |

### OTHER INFORMATION
- tamper evident: do not use if carton is open or if printed seal on blister is broken or missing
- store between 20-25°C (68-77°F)

### INACTIVE INGREDIENTS
carbomer homopolymer type B; FD&C blue no. 1 aluminum lake; hypromellose, USP; magnesium stearate, NF; microcrystalline cellulose, NF; sodium starch glycolate, NF

### QUESTIONS OR COMMENTS
Call **1-866-MUCINEX (1-866-682-4639)** You may also report side effects to this phone number.

# MUCINEX NASAL SPRAY MOISTURE SMART (oxymetazoline hydrochloride) spray

Reckitt Benckiser, Inc.

## DRUG FACTS

| Active ingredient | Purpose |
|---|---|
| Oxymetazoline hydrochloride 0.05% | Nasal decongestant |

### USES
- temporarily relieves nasal congestion due to:
  - a cold
  - hay fever
  - upper respiratory allergies
- promotes nasal and sinus drainage
- temporarily relieves sinus congestion and pressure
- helps clear nasal passages; shrinks swollen membranes

### WARNINGS

**ASK A DOCTOR BEFORE USE IF YOU HAVE**
- heart disease
- high blood pressure
- thyroid disease
- diabetes
- trouble urinating due to an enlarged prostate gland

**WHEN USING THIS PRODUCT**
- do not use more than directed
- do not use for more than 3 days. Use only as directed. Frequent or prolonged use may cause nasal congestion to recur or worsen
- temporary discomfort such as burning, stinging, sneezing or an increase in nasal discharge may occur
- use of this container by more than one person may spread infection

**STOP USE AND ASK A DOCTOR IF**
- symptoms persist

**If pregnant or breastfeeding,** ask a health professional before use.

**Keep out of reach of children.** If swallowed, get medical help or contact a Poison Control Center right away.

### DIRECTIONS

| adults and children 6 to under 12 years of age (with adult supervision) | 2 or 3 sprays in each nostril not more often than every 10 to 12 hours<br>do not exceed 2 doses in any 24-hour period |
|---|---|
| children under 6 years of age | ask a doctor |

**Shake well before use.** Before using the first time, remove the protective cap from the tip and prime metered pump by depressing firmly several times. To spray, hold bottle with thumb at base and nozzle between first and second fingers. Without tilting head, insert nozzle into nostril. Fully depress pump all the way down with a firm even stroke and sniff deeply. Wipe nozzle clean after use.

### OTHER INFORMATION
- store between 20-25°C (68-77°F)
- retain carton for future reference on full labeling

### INACTIVE INGREDIENTS
benzalkonium chloride solution, edetate disodium, glycerin, propylene glycol, purified water, sodium phosphate dibasic, sodium phosphate monobasic, sorbitol

### QUESTIONS OR COMMENTS
Call **1-866-MUCINEX (1-866-682-4639)** You may also report side effects to this phone number.

## CHILDREN'S MUCINEX CHEST CONGESTION (guaifenesin) solution

Reckitt Benckiser, Inc.

### DRUG FACTS

| Active ingredient (in each 5 mL) | Purpose |
|---|---|
| Guaifenesin 100 mg | Expectorant |

### USES
- helps loosen phlegm (mucus) and thin bronchial secretions to rid the bronchial passageways of bothersome mucus and make coughs more productive

### WARNINGS

**ASK A DOCTOR BEFORE USE IF THE CHILD HAS**
- cough that occurs with too much phlegm (mucus)
- persistent or chronic cough such as occurs with asthma

**STOP USE AND ASK A DOCTOR IF**
- cough lasts more than 7 days, comes back, or occurs with fever, rash, or persistent headache. These could be signs of a serious illness

**Keep out of reach of children.** In case of overdose, get medical help or contact a Poison Control Center right away.

### DIRECTIONS
- do not take more than 6 doses in any 24-hour period
- measure only with dosing cup provided
- do not use dosing cup with other products

| children 6 years to under 12 years | 5 mL – 10 mL every 4 hours |
|---|---|
| children 4 years to under 6 years | 2.5 mL – 5 mL every 4 hours |
| children under 4 years | do not use |

### OTHER INFORMATION
- each 5 mL contains: sodium 3 mg
- tamper evident: do not use if neckband on bottle cap is broken or missing
- store between 15-30°C (59-86°F)
- do not refrigerate
- dosing cup provided

### INACTIVE INGREDIENTS
citric acid anhydrous, dextrose, FD&C blue no. 1, FD&C red no. 40, flavor, glycerin, methylparaben, potassium sorbate, propylene glycol, propylparaben, purified water, saccharin sodium, sodium hydroxide, sucralose, xanthan gum

### QUESTIONS OR COMMENTS
Call **1-866-MUCINEX (1-866-682-4639)** You may also report side effects to this phone number.

## CHILDREN'S MUCINEX STUFFY NOSE AND COLD (guaifenesin and phenylephrine hydrochloride) solution

Reckitt Benckiser, Inc.

### DRUG FACTS

| Active ingredients (in each 5 mL) | Purpose |
|---|---|
| Guaifensin 100 mg | Expectorant |
| Phenylephrine hydrochloride 2.5 mg | Nasal decongestant |

### USES
- helps loosen phlegm (mucus) and thin bronchial secretions to rid the bronchial passageways of bothersome mucus and make coughs more productive
- temporarily relieves:
  - nasal congestion due to a cold
  - stuffy nose

### WARNINGS

**DO NOT USE**
- in a child who is taking a prescription monoamine oxidase inhibitor (MAOI) (certain drugs for depression, psychiatric, or emotional conditions, or Parkinson's disease), or for 2 weeks after stopping the MAOI drug. If you do not know if your child's prescription drug contains an MAOI, ask a doctor or pharmacist before giving this product

**ASK A DOCTOR BEFORE USE IF THE CHILD HAS**
- heart disease
- high blood pressure
- thyroid disease
- diabetes
- cough that occurs with too much phlegm (mucus)
- persistent or chronic cough such as occurs with asthma

**WHEN USING THIS PRODUCT**
- do not use more than directed

**STOP USE AND ASK A DOCTOR IF**
- your child gets nervous, dizzy or sleepless
- symptoms do not get better within 7 days or occur with fever
- cough lasts more than 7 days, comes back, or occurs with fever, rash, or persistent headache.These could be signs of a serious illness

**Keep out of reach of children.** In case of overdose, get medical help or contact a Poison Control Center right away.

### DIRECTIONS
- do not take more than 6 doses in any 24-hour period
- measure only with dosing cup provided
- do not use dosing cup with other products

| Age | Dose |
|---|---|
| children 6 years to under 12 years | 10 mL every 4 hours |
| children 4 years to under 6 years | 5 mL every 4 hours |
| children under 4 years | do not use |

## OTHER INFORMATION
- each 5 mL contains: sodium 3 mg
- tamper evident: do not use if neckband on bottle cap is broken or missing
- store between 15-30°C (59-86°F)
- do not refrigerate
- dosing cup provided

## INACTIVE INGREDIENTS
citric acid anhydrous, dextrose, D&C red no. 33, FD&C blue no. 1, FD&C red no. 40, flavors, glycerin, methylparaben, potassium sorbate, propyl gallate, propylene glycol, propylparaben, purified water, saccharin sodium, sodium hydroxide, sorbitol solution, sucralose, xanthan gum

## QUESTIONS OR COMMENTS
Call **1-866-MUCINEX (1-866-682-4639)** You may also report side effects to this phone number.

---

# MURINE EAR WAX REMOVAL SYSTEM
(carbamide peroxide) liquid drops

Prestige Brand, Inc.

## DRUG FACTS

| Active ingredient | Purpose |
|---|---|
| Carbamide peroxide 6.5% | earwax removal aid |

## USES
- for occasional use as an aid to soften, loosen and remove excessive ear wax

## WARNINGS
**For external use only.**

## ASK A DOCTOR BEFORE USE
- if you have ear drainage or discharge, ear pain, irritation or a rash in the ear, or are dizzy
- if you have an injury or perforation (hole) of the eardrum, or after ear surgery

## WHEN USING THIS PRODUCT
- avoid contact with the eyes
- never insert cotton swabs, toothpicks, hairpins or other objects into the ear canal to remove earwax

## DO NOT USE
- this product for more than 4 days

## STOP USE AND ASK A DOCTOR IF
- excessive ear wax remains after 4-day treatment with this product

**Keep out of reach of children.** If swallowed, get medical help or contact a Poison Control Center (**1-800-222-1222**) right away. If accidental contact with eyes occurs, flush eyes with water and consult a doctor.

## OTHER INFORMATION
- Murine Ear Drops foam upon being placed in the ear due to the release of oxygen
- this product is not intended to restore hearing loss due to medical reasons. In such cases, consult a doctor
- protect from heat and sunlight. Secure cap tightly on bottle when not in use
- tamper evident: do not use if neckband on bottle is broken or missing

---

# MYCOCIDE NS (tolnoftate) liquid
Woodward Laboratories

## DRUG FACTS

| Active ingredient | Purpose |
|---|---|
| Tolnaftate 1% | Antifungal |

## USES
- to kill germs that can cause fungal skin infections

## WARNINGS
**For external use only.**

## DO NOT USE
- near the mouth or eyes
- with known sensitivities to any listed ingredients
- on children under 2 years of age unless directed by a doctor

## WHEN USING THIS PRODUCT
- avoid eye contact. If accidental eye contact occurs, rinse thoroughly with water for 10-15 minutes

## STOP USE AND ASK A DOCTOR IF
- rash or irritation occurs, or if no improvement is seen after four weeks

**If pregnant/breastfeeding,** consult a health professional before using.

**Keep out of reach of children.** If swallowed, get medical help or contact a Poison Control Center Immediately.

## DIRECTIONS
- clean affected area with soap and warm water and dry thoroughly
- apply a thin layer two times a day (mornings and evenings) to affected area especially the space between and around toes for athlete's foot, use daily for four weeks or as directed by a physician
- allow solution to soak into skin or rub in to dry more quickly before putting on socks
- this product is not effective on scalp or nails
- following a proper foot hygiene regimen along with wearing well fitting, ventilated shoes and clean socks that are changed at least daily is helpful in preventing future infections

## INACTIVE INGREDIENTS
water, caprylic/capric triglycerides, isopropyl palmitate, polyquaternium 37, propylene glycol, dicaperylate dicaprate, PPG-1 trideceth-6, cocamidopropyl betaine, cocamidopropylamine oxide, phemerol chloride, cetrimonium chloride, allantoin, didecyldimonium chloride, quaternium-15

---

# MYLANTA REGULAR STRENGTH (aluminum hydroxide, magnesium hydroxide, and simethicone) liquid
Johnson & Johnson

## DRUG FACTS

| Active ingredients (in each 5 mL teaspoon) | Purpose |
|---|---|
| Aluminum hydroxide 200 mg (equivalent to dried gel, USP) | Antacid |
| Magnesium hydroxide 200 mg | Antacid |
| Simethicone 20 mg | Antigas |

## USES
- use this remedy to relieve the following symptoms:
  - heartburn
  - acid indigestion
  - sour stomach
  - upset stomach due to these symptoms
  - pressure and bloating commonly referred to as gas

## WARNINGS

### ASK A DOCTOR BEFORE USE IF YOU HAVE
- kidney disease

### ASK A DOCTOR OR PHARMACIST BEFORE USE IF YOU ARE TAKING
- a prescription drug. Antacids may interact with certain prescription drugs

### STOP USE AND ASK A DOCTOR IF
- symptoms last for more than 2 weeks

**Keep out of reach of children.**

## DIRECTIONS
- shake well

| adults and children over 12 years | take 2-4 teaspoonfuls between meals, at bedtime, or as directed by a doctor |
| | do not take more than 24 teaspoonfuls in a 24-hour period or use the maximum dosage for more than 2 weeks |
| children under 12 years | ask a doctor |

## OTHER INFORMATION
- do not use if breakaway band on plastic cap is broken or missing
- do not freeze
- see back panel for lot number and expiration date
- does not meet USP requirements for preservative effectiveness

## INACTIVE INGREDIENTS
**Original flavor**
butylparaben, carboxymethylcellulose sodium, flavors, hypromellose, microcrystalline cellulose, propylparaben, purified water, sorbitol

**Mint flavor**
butylparaben, carboxymethlcellulose sodium, flavors, hypromellose, microcrystalline cellulose, propylparaben, purified water, saccharin sodium, sorbitol

---

# MYLANTA GAS MAXIMUM STRENGTH
(simethicone) tablet, chewable

Johnson & Johnson

## DRUG FACTS

| Active ingredients (in each tablet) | Purpose |
|---|---|
| Simethicone 125 mg | Antigas |

## USES
- fast relief for the pressure, bloating, and discomfort of gas
- use this remedy to relieve the following symptoms:
  - bloating
  - pressure
  - gas discomfort or gas pain caused by certain foods (such as beans, bran, and broccoli)

## WARNINGS
- do not exceed 4 tablets per day unless directed by a physician
- keep this and all drugs out of the reach of children

## DIRECTIONS
- thoroughly chew 1-2 tablets as needed after meals and at bedtime

## OTHER INFORMATION
- store at room temperature
- avoid high humidity and excessive heat 40°C (104°F)
- do not use if printed foil inner seal is broken

## INACTIVE INGREDIENTS
**Cherry flavor**
D&C red no. 7 calcium lake, dextrates, flavors, magnesium stearate, silicon dioxide, tribasic calcium phosphate
**Mint flavor**
dextrates, flavors, magnesium stearate, silicon dioxide, tribasic calcium phosphate

## QUESTIONS OR COMMENTS
Call **1-800-4 69-5268**

---

# INFANTS' MYLICON (simethicone)
suspension/ drops

Johnson & Johnson Merck Consumer Pharmaceuticals

## DRUG FACTS

| Active ingredients (in each 0.3 mL) | Purpose |
|---|---|
| Simethicone 20 mg | Antigas |

## USES
- relieves the discomfort of infant gas frequently caused by air swallowing or certain formulas or foods

## WARNINGS

**Keep out of reach of children.** In case of overdose get medical help or contact a Poison Control Center right away. (**1-800-222-1222**)

## DIRECTIONS
- shake well before using
- all dosages may be repeated as needed, after meals and at bedtime or as directed by a physician
- do not exceed 12 doses per day
- fill enclosed dropper to recommended dosage level and dispense liquid slowly into baby's mouth, toward the inner cheek
- dosage can also be mixed with 1 ounces cool water, infant formula or other suitable liquids
- clean dropper well after each use – recap bottle with original cap

| Age (yr) | Weight (lb) | Dose |
|---|---|---|
| Infants under 2 | Under 24 | 0.3 mL |
| Children over 2 | Over 24 | 0.6 mL |

## OTHER INFORMATION
- do not use if printed plastic overwrap or printed neck wrap is missing or broken
- store between 20-25°C (68-77°F)
- do not freeze
- see bottom panel for lot number and expiration date

## INACTIVE INGREDIENTS

benzoic acid, carboxymethylcellulose sodium, citric acid, D&C red 22, D&C red 28, flavors, glycerides (C14-18, mono- and di-), maltitol, methylcellulose, microcrystalline cellulose, polyoxyl 40 stearate, polysorbate 65, purified water, silica gel, sodium benzoate, sodium citrate, xanthan gum

## QUESTIONS OR COMMENTS

Call **1-800-222-9435** (English) or **1-888-466-8746** (Spanish)

---

# INFANTS' MYLICON DYE FREE (simethicone)
suspension/ drops

Johnson & Johnson Merck Consumer
Pharmaceuticals

## DRUG FACTS

| Active ingredients (in each 0.3 mL) | Purpose |
|---|---|
| Simethicone 20 mg | Antigas |

## USES

- relieves the discomfort of infant gas frequently caused by air swallowing or certain formulas or foods

## WARNINGS

**Keep out of reach of children.** In case of overdose get medical help or contact a Poison Control Center right away. (**1-800-222-1222**)

## DIRECTIONS

- shake well before using
- all dosages may be repeated as needed, after meals and at bedtime or as directed by a physician
- do not exceed 12 doses per day
- fill enclosed dropper to recommended dosage level and dispense liquid slowly into baby's mouth, toward the inner cheek
- dosage can also be mixed with 1 ounces cool water, infant formula or other suitable liquids
- clean dropper well after each use – recap bottle with original cap

| Age (yr) | Weight (lb) | Dose |
|---|---|---|
| Infants under 2 | Under 24 | 0.3 mL |
| Children over 2 | Over 24 | 0.6 mL |

## OTHER INFORMATION

- do not use if printed plastic overwrap or printed neck wrap is missing or broken
- store between 20-25°C (68-77°F)
- do not freeze
- see bottom panel for lot number and expiration date

## INACTIVE INGREDIENTS

benzoic acid, carboxymethylcellulose sodium, citric acid, flavors, glycerides (C14-18, mono- and di-), maltitol, methylcellulose, microcrystalline cellulose, polyoxyl 40 stearate, polysorbate 65, purified water, silica gel, sodium benzoate, sodium citrate, xanthan gum

## QUESTIONS OR COMMENTS

Call **1-800-222-9435** (English) or **1-888-466-8746** (Spanish)

---

# MYOFLEX (trolamine salicylate) cream

Novartis Consumer Health, Inc.

## DRUG FACTS

| Active ingredients | Purpose |
|---|---|
| Trolamine salicylate (10%) | Pain relief |

## USES

- for temporary relief of:
- minor aches and pains of muscles and joints associated with:
  - arthritis
  - strains and sprains
  - simple backache

## WARNINGS
**For external use only.**

## DO NOT USE

- on or near eyes
- on irritated skin or if excessive irritation develops

## STOP USE AND ASK A DOCTOR IF

- condition worsens, or if symptoms persist for more than 7 days

**If you are pregnant or breastfeeding,** ask a health professional before use.

**Keep out of the reach of children.** If swallowed, get medical help or contact a Poison Control Center immediately.

## DIRECTIONS

| adults and children 2 years of age and older | apply to affected area not more than three to four times daily. Affected areas may be wrapped loosely with 2 or 3 inch elastic bandage use only as directed |
|---|---|
| children under 2 years of age | ask a doctor |

## OTHER INFORMATION

- store at controlled room temperature 68-77°F
- close cap tightly

## INACTIVE INGREDIENTS

cetyl alcohol, disodium EDTA, fragrance, propylene glycol, purified water, sodium lauryl sulfate, stearyl alcohol, white wax

---

# NAPHCON A (naphazoline hydrochloride and pheniramine maleate) solution/drops

Alcon Laboratories, Inc.

## DRUG FACTS

| Active ingredients | Purpose |
|---|---|
| Naphazoline hydrochloride 0.025% | Relief of itch |
| Pheniramine maleate 0.3% | Relief of itch |

## USES
- for the temporary relief of the minor eye symptoms of itching and redness caused by:
  - ragweed
  - pollen
  - grass
  - animal dander and hair

## WARNINGS
- to avoid contamination, do not touch tip of container to any surface
- replace cap after using
- accidental swallowing by infants and children may lead to coma and marked reduction in body temperature

## DO NOT USE
- if solution changes color or becomes cloudy
- if you have heart disease, high blood pressure, narrow angle glaucoma or trouble urinating unless directed by a physician

## STOP USE AND ASK A DOCTOR IF
- you feel eye pain, changes in vision occur, redness or irritation of the eye(s) gets worse or lasts more than 72 hours

## WHEN USING THIS PRODUCT
- pupils may become enlarged temporarily. Overuse may cause more redness of the eye(s)
- if you are sensitive to any ingredient in this product

**Keep this and all drugs out of the reach of children.** If swallowed, get medical help or contact a Poison Control Center right away. Remove contact lenses before using.

## DIRECTIONS
- remove contact lenses before using
- put 1 or 2 drops in the affected eye(s) up to 4 times every day
- before using in children under 6 years of age, consult your physician

## OTHER INFORMATION
- store at 20-25°C (68-77°F).
- protect from light
- use before the expiration date marked on the carton or bottle

## INACTIVE INGREDIENTS
boric acid, edetate disodium 0.01%, purified water, sodium borate, sodium chloride, sodium hydroxide and/or hydrochloric acid (to adjust ph). the sterile ophthalmic solution has a ph of about 6 and a tonicity of about 270 mOsm/kg, benzalkonium chloride 0.01%.

---

# NASALCROM (cromolyn sodium) spray, metered
Blacksmith Brands, Inc.

## DRUG FACTS

| Active ingredient (per spray) | Purpose |
|---|---|
| Cromolyn sodium 5.2 mg | Nasal allergy symptom controller |

## USES
- to prevent and relieve nasal symptoms of hay fever and other nasal allergies:
  - runny/itchy nose
  - sneezing
  - allergic stuffy nose

## WARNINGS

## DO NOT USE
- if you are allergic to any of the ingredients

## ASK A DOCTOR BEFORE USE IF YOU HAVE
- fever
- discolored nasal discharge
- sinus pain
- wheezing

## WHEN USING THIS PRODUCT
- it may take several days of use to notice an effect. Your best effect may not be seen for 1 to 2 weeks
- brief stinging or sneezing may occur right after use
- do not use it to treat sinus infection, asthma, or cold symptoms
- do not share this bottle with anyone else as this may spread germs

## STOP USE AND ASK A DOCTOR IF
- shortness of breath, wheezing, or chest tightness occurs
- hives or swelling of the mouth or throat occurs
- your symptoms worsen
- you have new symptoms
- your symptoms do not begin to improve within two weeks
- you need to use for more than 12 weeks

**If pregnant or breastfeeding,** ask a health professional before use.

**Keep out of reach of children.** If swallowed, get medical help or contact a Poison Control Center right away. (**1-800-222-1222**)

## DIRECTIONS
- see package insert on how to use pump
- parent or care provider must supervise the use of this product by young children

| adults and children 2 years and older | spray once into each nostril. Repeat 3-4 times a day (every 4-6 hours). If needed, may be used up to 6 times a day |
| | use every day while in contact with the cause of your allergies (pollen, molds, pets, and dust) |
| | to prevent nasal allergy symptoms, use before contact with the cause of your allergies. For best results, start using up to one week before contact |
| | if desired, you can use this product with other medicines, including other allergy medicines |
| children under 2 years | do not use unless directed by a doctor |

## OTHER INFORMATION
- store between 20-25°C (68-77°F)
- protect from light
- keep carton and package insert. They contain important instructions
- do not use if imprinted plastic bottle wrap is broken or missing
- see bottom panel for lot number and expiration date

## INACTIVE INGREDIENTS
benzalkonium chloride, edetate disodium, purified water

QUESTIONS OR COMMENTS
Call **1-877-9**-ALLERGY (**1-877-925-5374**)

## NEO-SYNEPHRINE REGULAR STRENGTH
(phenylephrine hydrochloride) spray
Bayer Consumer Care Products

### DRUG FACTS

| Active ingredient | Purpose |
|---|---|
| Phenylephrine hydrochloride 0.5% | Nasal decongestant |

### USES
- temporarily relieves nasal congestion:
  - due to common cold
  - due to hay fever or other upper respiratory allergies (allergic rhinitis)
- temporarily relieves stuffy nose
- helps clear nasal passages; shrinks swollen membranes
- temporarily restores freer breathing through the nose
- helps decongest sinus openings and passages
- temporarily relieves sinus congestion and pressure

### WARNINGS

### ASK A DOCTOR BEFORE USE IF YOU HAVE
- heart disease
- high blood pressure
- thyroid disease
- diabetes
- difficulty in urination due to enlargement of the prostate gland

### WHEN USING THIS PRODUCT
- do not exceed recommended dosage
- do not use more than 3 days. Use only as directed. Frequent or prolonged use may cause nasal congestion to recur or worsen
- temporary discomfort may occur such as burning, stinging, sneezing, or an increase in nasal discharge
- use of this container by more than one person may spread infection

### STOP USE AND ASK A DOCTOR IF
- symptoms persist for more than 3 days

**If breastfeeding,** ask a health professional before use.

**Keep out of reach of children**. If swallowed, get medical help or contact a Poison Control Center right away.

### DIRECTIONS
- use only as directed
- to spray, squeeze bottle quickly and firmly

| adults and children 12 years and older | 2 or 3 sprays in each nostril not more often than every 4 hours |
|---|---|
| children under 12 years | ask a doctor |

### OTHER INFORMATION
- store at room temperature
- protect from light

### INACTIVE INGREDIENTS
anhydrous citric acid, benzalkonium chloride, purified water, sodium chloride, sodium citrate

QUESTIONS OR COMMENTS
Call **1-800-986-0369** (Mon-Fri 9 AM-5 PM EST)
or visit www.bayercare.com

## NEOSPORIN ORIGINAL (bacitracin, neomycin, and polymyxin B) ointment
Division of Johnson & Johnson Consumer Companies, Inc.

### DRUG FACTS

| Active ingredients (in each gram) | Purpose |
|---|---|
| Bacitracin 400 units | First aid antibiotic |
| Neomycin 3.5 mg | First aid antibiotic |
| Polymyxin B 5000 units | First aid antibiotic |

### USES
- first aid to help prevent infection in minor:
  - cuts
  - scrapes
  - burns

### WARNINGS
**For external use only.**

### DO NOT USE
- if you are allergic to any of the ingredients
- in the eyes
- over large areas of the body

### ASK A DOCTOR BEFORE USE IF YOU HAVE
- deep or puncture wounds
- animal bites
- serious burns

### STOP USE AND ASK A DOCTOR IF
- you need to use longer than 1 week
- condition persists or gets worse
- rash or other allergic reaction develops

**Keep out of reach of children.** If swallowed, get medical help or contact a Poison Control Center right away.

### DIRECTIONS
- clean the affected area
- apply a small amount of this product (an amount equal to the surface area of the tip of a finger) on the area 1 to 3 times daily
- may be covered with a sterile bandage

### OTHER INFORMATION
- store at 20°C-25°C (68°F-77°F)

### INACTIVE INGREDIENTS
cocoa butter, cottonseed oil, olive oil, sodium pyruvate, vitamin E, white petrolatum

QUESTIONS OR COMMENTS
Call **1-800-223-0182**

## NEOSPORIN LIP HEALTH OVERNIGHT RENEWAL THERAPY (petrolatum) ointment

Division of Johnson & Johnson Consumer Companies, Inc.

### DRUG FACTS

| Active ingredient | Purpose |
|---|---|
| White petrolatum 77.4% | Lip protectant |

### USES
• helps prevent and temporarily protects and helps relieve chapped or cracked lips

### WARNINGS
For external use only.

### DO NOT USE ON
• deep or puncture wounds
• animal bites
• serious burns

### WHEN USING THIS PRODUCT
• do not get into eyes

### STOP USE AND ASK A DOCTOR IF
• condition worsens
• symptoms last more than 7 days or clear up and occur again within a few days

**Keep out of reach of children.** If swallowed, get medical help or contact a Poison Control Center right away.

### DIRECTIONS
• apply as needed

### OTHER INFORMATION
• store between 20°C-25°C (68-77°F)

### INACTIVE INGREDIENTS
lanolin, paraffin, cocoa butter, mineral oil, flavor, VP/eicosene copolymer, ethylhexyl palmitate, titanium dioxide, tribehenin, vitamin E (dl-alpha tocopheryl acetate), sorbitan isostearate, sodium pyruvate, vitamin A palmitate, corn oil, cholecalciferol, palmitoyl oligopeptide

### QUESTIONS OR COMMENTS
Call **1-800-223-0182**

## NEOSPORIN PLUS PAIN RELIEF (bacitracin, neomycin, polymyxin B, and pramoxine hydrochloride) ointment

Division of Johnson & Johnson Consumer Companies, Inc.

### DRUG FACTS

| Active ingredients (in each gram) | Purpose |
|---|---|
| Bacitracin 500 units | First aid antibiotic |
| Neomycin 3.5 mg | First aid antibiotic |
| Polymyxin B 10,000 units | First aid antibiotic |
| Pramoxine hydrochloride 10 mg | External analgesic |

### USES
• first aid to help prevent infection and for temporary relief of pain or discomfort in minor:
  • cuts
  • scrapes
  • burns

### WARNINGS
For external use only.

### DO NOT USE
• if you are allergic to any of the ingredients
• in the eyes
• over large areas of the body

### ASK A DOCTOR BEFORE USE IF YOU HAVE
• deep or puncture wounds
• animal bites
• serious burns

### STOP USE AND ASK A DOCTOR IF
• you need to use longer than 1 week
• condition persists or gets worse
• symptoms persist for more than 1 week, or clear up and occur again within a few days
• rash or other allergic reaction develops

**Keep out of reach of children.** If swallowed, get medical help or contact a Poison Control Center right away.

### DIRECTIONS

| adults and children 2 years of age and older | clean the affected area |
| | apply a small amount of this product (an amount equal to the surface area of the tip of a finger) on the area 1 to 3 times daily |
| | may be covered with a sterile bandage |
| children under 2 years of age | ask a doctor |

### OTHER INFORMATION
• store at 20°C-25°C (68°F-77°F)

### INACTIVE INGREDIENT
white petrolatum

### QUESTIONS OR COMMENTS
Call **1-800-223-0182**

## 3M NEXCARE COLD SORE TREATMENT (benzocaine and allantoin) ointment

3M Company

### DRUG FACTS

| Active ingredient | Purpose |
|---|---|
| Benzocaine 5% | External analgesic |
| Allantoin 1% | Skin protectant |

### USES
• temporarily relieves pain and itching associated with cold sores and fever blisters
• relieves dryness and softens cold sores and fever blisters

## WARNINGS
**For external use only.**

### DO NOT USE
- if you are allergic to any ingredient in this product

### WHEN USING THIS PRODUCT
- do not get into eyes

### STOP USE AND ASK A DOCTOR IF
- condition worsens
- symptoms last more than 7 days or clear up and occur again within a few days

**Keep out of reach of children.** If swallowed, get medical help or contact a Poison Control Center immediately.

### DIRECTIONS

| adults and children 2 years of age and older | apply directly to affected area with clean finger at the first sign of cold sore/fever blister (tingle) |
| --- | --- |
| | apply to affected area not more than 3 to 4 times daily |
| children under 2 years of age | consult a doctor |

### OTHER INFORMATION
- store at 20-25°C(68-77°F)

### INACTIVE INGREDIENTS
acrylates/C10-30 alkyl acrylate crosspolymer, butylated hydroxytoluene, cetyl alcohol, edetate disodium, ethyl oleate, ethylparaben, glycerin, melaleuca alternifolia (tea tree) leaf oil, menthol, methylparaben, phenoxyethanol, poloxamer 185, propylparaben, propylene glycol monolaurate (microvex™), sodium ascorbyl phosphate, sodium hydroxide, tocopheryl acetate, water

### QUESTIONS OR COMMENTS
Call 1-800-537-2191 www.nexcare.com

---

## N'ICE CUBES (menthol) lozenge
Insight Pharmaceuticals

### DRUG FACTS

| Active ingredient (in each lozenge) | Purpose |
| --- | --- |
| menthol 5.5 mg | Cough suppressant/oral anesthetic |

### USES
- temporarily relieves:
  - occasional minor irritation, pain and sore throat and sore mouth
  - cough associated with a cold or inhaled irritants

### WARNINGS
**Sore throat warning**
Severe or persistent sore throat or sore throat that occurs with or is followed by high fever, headache, rash, swelling and nausea and vomiting may be serious. Ask doctor right away. Do not use more than 2 days or give to children under 3 years of age unless directed by a doctor.

### ASK A DOCTOR BEFORE USE IF YOU HAVE
- cough that lasts or is chronic such as occurs with smoking, asthma, or emphysema
- cough that occurs with too much phlegm (mucus)

### STOP USE AND ASK A DOCTOR IF
- sore mouth symptoms do not improve in 7 days
- irritation, pain or redness persists or worsens
- cough lasts more than 7 days, comes back, or occurs with fever, rash, or persistent headache. These could be signs of a serious condition
- swelling, rash or fever develops

**Keep out of reach of children.** In case of overdose, get medical help or contact a Poison Control Center right away.

### DIRECTIONS

| adults and children 3 years of age and older | allow lozenge to dissolve slowly in mouth. May be repeated every 2 hours as needed or as directed by a dentist or doctor |
| --- | --- |
| | do not take more than 10 lozenges a day |
| children under 3 years of age | ask a dentist or doctor |

### INACTIVE INGREDIENTS
acesulfame potassium, ascorbic acid, cherry flavor, FD&C red no. 40, isomalt, maltitol, purified water, sodium ascorbate, zinc gluconate

### QUESTIONS OR COMMENTS
Call 1-800-344-7239 or visit www.insightpharma.com

---

## NICODERM CQ (nicotine) patch, extended release
GlaxoSmithKline Consumer Healthcare LP

### DRUG FACTS

| Active ingredient (in each patch)(clear) | Purpose |
| --- | --- |
| Nicotine 21 mg delivered over 24 hours | Stop smoking aid |
| Nicotine 14 mg delivered over 24 hours | |
| Nicotine 7 mg delivered over 24 hours | |

### USES
- reduces withdrawal symptoms, including nicotine craving, associated with quitting smoking

### WARNINGS
Smoking can seriously harm your child. Try to stop smoking without using any nicotine replacement medicine. This medicine is believed to be safer than smoking. However, the risks to your child from this medicine are not fully known.

### DO NOT USE
- if you continue to smoke, chew tobacco, use snuff, or use a nicotine gum or other nicotine containing products

## ASK A DOCTOR BEFORE USE IF YOU HAVE
- heart disease, recent heart attack, or irregular heartbeat. Nicotine can increase your heart rate
- high blood pressure not controlled with medication. Nicotine can increase your blood pressure
- an allergy to adhesive tape or have skin problems because you are more likely to get rashes

## ASK A DOCTOR OR PHARMACIST BEFORE USE IF YOU ARE
- using a non-nicotine stop smoking drug
- taking a prescription medicine for depression or asthma. Your prescription dose may need to be adjusted

## WHEN USING THIS PRODUCT
- do not smoke even when not wearing the patch. The nicotine in your skin will still be entering your blood stream for several hours after you take off the patch
- if you have vivid dreams or other sleep disturbances remove this patch at bedtime

## STOP USE AND ASK A DOCTOR IF
- skin redness caused by the patch does not go away after four days, or if your skin swells, or you get a rash
- irregular heartbeat or palpitations occur
- you get symptoms of nicotine overdose such as nausea, vomiting, dizziness, weakness and rapid heartbeat

**If you are pregnant or breastfeeding,** only use this medicine on the advice of your health care provider.

**Keep out of reach of children and pets.** Used patches have enough nicotine to poison children and pets. If swallowed, get medical help or contact a Posion Control Center right away. Dispose of the used patches by folding sticky ends together. Replace in pouch and discard.

## DIRECTIONS (Clear)
- if you are under 18 years of age, ask a doctor before use
  - before using this product, read the enclosed User's Guide for complete directions and other information
  - stop smoking completely when you begin using the patch
- if you smoke more than 10 cigarettes per day, use according to the following 10-week schedule:

| STEP 1 | STEP 2 | STEP 3 |
|---|---|---|
| Use one 21 mg patch/day | Use one 14 mg patch/day | Use one 7 mg patch/day |
| Weeks 1-6 | Week 7-8 | Week 9-10 |

- if you smoke 10 or less cigarettes per day, do not use STEP 1 (21 mg). Start with STEP 2 (14 mg) for 6 weeks, then STEP 3 (7 mg) for 2 weeks and then stop
- steps 2 and 3 allow you to gradually reduce your level of nicotine. Completing the full program will increase your chances of quitting successfully
- apply one new patch every 24 hours on skin that is dry, clean and hairless. Save pouch for disposing of the patch after use
- remove backing from patch and immediately press onto skin. Hold for 10 seconds
- wash hands after applying or removing patch. Throw away the patch by folding sticky ends together. Replace in its pouch and discard. See enclosed User's Guide for safety and handling
- you may wear the patch for 16 or 24 hours
- if you crave cigarettes when you wake up, wear the patch for 24 hours
- if you have vivid dreams or other sleep disturbances, you may remove the patch at bedtime and apply a new one in the morning
- the used patch should be removed and a new one applied to a different skin site at the same time each day
- do not wear more than one patch at a time
- do not cut patch in half or into smaller pieces

- do not leave patch on for more than 24 hours because it may irritate your skin and loses strength after 24 hours
- stop using the patch at the end of 10 weeks. If you started with STEP 2, stop using the patch at the end of 8 weeks. If you still feel the need to use the patch, talk to your doctor

## OTHER INFORMATION
- store at 20-25°C (68-77°F)

## INACTIVE INGREDIENTS (CLEAR)
ethylene vinyl acetate-copolymer, polyisobutylene and high density polyethylene between clear polyester backings

## QUESTIONS OR COMMENTS
Call toll-free **1-800-834-5895** (English/Spanish) weekdays (9:00 a.m.- 4:30 p.m. EST)

---

# NICORETTE FRUIT CHILL (nicotine polacrilex)
## gum, chewing
### GlaxoSmithKline Consumer Healthcare LP

## DRUG FACTS

| Active ingredient (in each chewing piece) | Purpose |
|---|---|
| Nicotine polacrilex (equal to 2 mg nicotine) | Stop smoking aid |
| Nicotine polacrilex (equal to 4 mg nicotine) | |

## USE
- reduces withdrawal symptoms, including nicotine craving, associated with quitting smoking

## WARNINGS
Smoking can seriously harm your child. Try to stop smoking without using any nicotine replacement medicine. This medicine is believed to be safer than smoking. However, the risks to your child from this medicine are not fully known.

## DO NOT USE
- if you continue to smoke, chew tobacco, use snuff, or use a nicotine patch or other nicotine containing products

## ASK A DOCTOR BEFORE USE IF YOU HAVE
- a sodium-restricted diet
- heart disease, recent heart attack, or irregular heartbeat Nicotine can increase your heart rate
- high blood pressure not controlled with medication. Nicotine can increase blood pressure
- stomach ulcer or diabetes

## ASK A DOCTOR OR A PHARMACIST BEFORE USE IF YOU ARE
- using a non-nicotine stop smoking drug
- taking prescription medicine for depression or asthma. Your prescription dose may need to be adjusted

## STOP USE AND ASK A DOCTOR IF
- mouth, teeth or jaw problems occur
- irregular heartbeat or palpitations occur
- you get symptoms of nicotine overdose such as nausea, vomiting, dizziness, diarrhea, weakness and rapid heartbeat

**If you are pregnant or breastfeeding,** only use this medicine on the advice of your health care provider.

**Keep out of reach of children and pets.** Pieces of nicotine gum may have enough nicotine to make children and pets sick. Wrap used pieces of gum in paper and throw away in the trash. In case of overdose, get medical help or contact a Poison Control Center right away.

## DIRECTIONS (2 MG)
- if you are under 18 years of age, ask a doctor before use
- before using this product, read the enclosed User's Guide for complete directions and other important information
- stop smoking completely when you begin using the gum
- if you smoke 25 or more cigarettes a day; use 4 mg nicotine gum
- if you smoke less than 25 cigarettes a day; use according to the following 12-week schedule:

| Weeks 1 to 6 | Weeks 7 to 9 | Weeks 10 to 12 |
|---|---|---|
| 1 piece every 1 to 2 hours | 1 piece every 2 to 4 hours | 1 piece every 4 to 8 hours |

- nicotine gum is a medicine and must be used a certain way to get the best results
- chew the gum slowly until it tingles. Then park it between your cheek and gum. When the tingle is gone, begin chewing again, until the tingle returns
- repeat this process until most of the tingle is gone (about 30 minutes)
- do not eat or drink for 15 minutes before chewing the nicotine gum, or while chewing a piece
- to improve your chances of quitting, use at least 9 pieces per day for the first 6 weeks
- if you experience strong or frequent cravings, you may use a second piece within the hour. However, do not continuously use one piece after another since this may cause you hiccups, heartburn, nausea or other side effects
- do not use more than 24 pieces a day
- it is important to complete treatment. Stop using the nicotine gum at the end of 12 weeks. If you still feel the need to use nicotine gum, talk to your doctor

## DIRECTIONS (4 MG)
- if you are under 18 years of age, ask a doctor before use
- before using this product, read the enclosed User's Guide for complete directions and other important information
- stop smoking completely when you begin using the gum
- if you smoke less than 25 cigarettes a day; use 2 mg nicotine gum
- if you smoke 25 or more cigarettes a day; use according to the following 12 week schedule:

| Weeks 1 to 6 | Weeks 7 to 9 | Weeks 10 to 12 |
|---|---|---|
| 1 piece every 1 to 2 hours | 1 piece every 2 to 4 hours | 1 piece every 4 to 8 hours |

- nicotine gum is a medicine and must be used a certain way to get the best results
- chew the gum slowly until it tingles. Then park it between your cheek and gum. When the tingle is gone, begin chewing again, until the tingle returns
- repeat this process until most of the tingle is gone (about 30 minutes)
- do not eat or drink for 15 minutes before chewing the nicotine gum, or while chewing a piece
- to improve your chances of quitting, use at least 9 pieces per day for the first 6 weeks
- if you experience strong or frequent cravings, you may use a second piece within the hour. However, do not continuously use one piece after another since this may cause you hiccups, heartburn, nausea or other side effects
- do not use more than 24 pieces a day

- it is important to complete treatment. Stop using the nicotine gum at the end of 12 weeks. If you still feel the need to use nicotine gum, talk to your doctor
- to increase your success in quitting:
  - you must be motivated to quit
  - use Enough – Chew at least 9 pieces of Nicorette per day during the first six weeks
  - use Long Enough – use Nicorette for the full 12 weeks
  - use with a support program as directed in the enclosed User's Guide
  - to remove the gum:
    - tear off single unit
    - peel off backing, starting at corner with loose edge
    - push gum through foil
- not for sale to those under 18 years of age
- proof of age required
- not for sale in vending machines or from any source where proof of age cannot be verified
- This product is protected in sealed blisters

**Do not use if individual blisters or printed backings are broken, open, or torn.**

## OTHER INFORMATION
- each 2 mg piece contains: calcium 94 mg, sodium 11 mg
- each 4 mg piece contains: calcium 94 mg, sodium 13 mg
- store at 20-25°C (68-77°F)
- protect from light

## INACTIVE INGREDIENTS
**each 2 mg piece contains:**
acacia, acesulfame potassium, carnauba wax, edible ink, flavor, gum base, hypromellose, magnesium oxide, menthol, peppermint oil, polysorbate 80, sodium bicarbonate, sodium carbonate, sucralose, titanium dioxide, xylitol

**each 4 mg piece contains:**
acacia, acesulfame potassium, carnauba wax, D&C yellow no. 10 Al. lake, edible ink, flavor, gum base, hypromellose, magnesium oxide, menthol, peppermint oil, polysorbate 80, sodium carbonate, sucralose, titanium dioxide, xylitol

## QUESTIONS OR COMMENTS
Call toll-free **1-800-419-4766** (English/Spanish) weekdays (9:00 AM-4:30 PM EST) or visit www.Nicorette.com

---

# NICORETTE (nicotine polacrilex) gum, chewing
GlaxoSmithKline Consumer Healthcare LP

## DRUG FACTS

| Active ingredient (in each chewing piece) | Purpose |
|---|---|
| Nicotine polacrilex (equal to 2 mg nicotine) | Stop smoking aid |
| Nicotine polacrilex (equal to 4 mg nicotine) | |

## USE
- reduces withdrawal symptoms, including nicotine craving, associated with quitting smoking

## WARNINGS
Smoking can seriously harm your child. Try to stop smoking without using any nicotine replacement medicine. This medicine is believed to be safer than smoking. However, the risks to your child from this medicine are not fully known.

## DO NOT USE
- if you continue to smoke, chew tobacco, use snuff, or use a nicotine patch or other nicotine containing products
- if individual blisters or printed backings are broken, open, or torn

## ASK A DOCTOR BEFORE USE IF YOU HAVE
- a sodium-restricted diet
- heart disease, recent heart attack, or irregular heartbeat. Nicotine can increase your heart rate
- high blood pressure not controlled with medication. Nicotine can increase blood pressure
- stomach ulcer or diabetes

## ASK A DOCTOR OR A PHARMACIST BEFORE USE IF YOU ARE
- using a non-nicotine stop smoking drug
- taking prescription medicine for depression or asthma. Your prescription dose may need to be adjusted

## STOP USE AND ASK A DOCTOR IF
- mouth, teeth or jaw problems occur
- irregular heartbeat or palpitations occur
- you get symptoms of nicotine overdose such as nausea, vomiting, dizziness, diarrhea, weakness and rapid heartbeat

**If you are pregnant or breastfeeding,** only use this medicine on the advice of your health care provider.

**Keep out of reach of children and pets.** Pieces of nicotine gum may have enough nicotine to make children and pets sick. Wrap used pieces of gum in paper and throw away in the trash. In case of overdose, get medical help or contact a Poison Control Center right away.

## DIRECTIONS (2 MG)
- if you are under 18 years of age, ask a doctor before use
- before using this product, read the enclosed User's Guide for complete directions and other important information
- stop smoking completely when you begin using the gum
- if you smoke 25 or more cigarettes a day; use 4 mg nicotine gum
- if you smoke less than 25 cigarettes a day; use according to the following 12 week schedule:

| Weeks 1 to 6 | Weeks 7 to 9 | Weeks 10 to 12 |
|---|---|---|
| 1 piece every 1 to 2 hours | 1 piece every 2 to 4 hours | 1 piece every 4 to 8 hours |

- nicotine gum is a medicine and must be used a certain way to get the best results
- chew the gum slowly until it tingles. Then park it between your cheek and gum. When the tingle is gone, begin chewing again, until the tingle returns
- repeat this process until most of the tingle is gone (about 30 minutes)
- do not eat or drink for 15 minutes before chewing the nicotine gum, or while chewing a piece
- to improve your chances of quitting, use at least 9 pieces per day for the first 6 weeks
- if you experience strong or frequent cravings, you may use a second piece within the hour. However, do not continuously use one piece after another since this may cause you hiccups, heartburn, nausea or other side effects
- do not use more than 24 pieces a day
- it is important to complete treatment. Stop using the nicotine gum at the end of 12 weeks. If you still feel the need to use nicotine gum, talk to your doctor

## DIRECTIONS (4 MG)
- if you are under 18 years of age, ask a doctor before use
- before using this product, read the enclosed User's Guide for complete directions and other important information
- stop smoking completely when you begin using the gum
- if you smoke less than 25 cigarettes a day; use 2 mg nicotine gum
- if you smoke 25 or more cigarettes a day; use according to the following 12 week schedule:

| Weeks 1 to 6 | Weeks 7 to 9 | Weeks 10 to 12 |
|---|---|---|
| 1 piece every 1 to 2 hours | 1 piece every 2 to 4 hours | 1 piece every 4 to 8 hours |

- nicotine gum is a medicine and must be used a certain way to get the best results
- chew the gum slowly until it tingles. Then park it between your cheek and gum. When the tingle is gone, begin chewing again, until the tingle returns
- repeat this process until most of the tingle is gone (about 30 minutes)
- do not eat or drink for 15 minutes before chewing the nicotine gum, or while chewing a piece
- to improve your chances of quitting, use at least 9 pieces per day for the first 6 weeks
- if you experience strong or frequent cravings, you may use a second piece within the hour. However, do not continuously use one piece after another since this may cause you hiccups, heartburn, nausea or other side effects
- do not use more than 24 pieces a day
- it is important to complete treatment. Stop using the nicotine gum at the end of 12 weeks. If you still feel the need to use nicotine gum, talk to your doctor

This product is protected in sealed blisters.

## OTHER INFORMATION
- to increase your success in quitting:
  - you must be motivated to quit
  - use Enough – Chew at least 9 pieces of Nicorette per day during the first six weeks
  - use Long Enough – Use Nicorette for the full 12 weeks
  - use with a support program as directed in the enclosed User's Guide
  - not for sale to those under 18 years of age
  - proof of age required
  - not for sale in vending machines or from any source where proof of age cannot be verified
- each 2 mg piece contains: calcium 94 mg, sodium 11 mg
- each 4 mg piece contains: calcium 94 mg, sodium 13 mg
- store at 20-25°C (68-77°F)
- protect from light

## INACTIVE INGREDIENTS (WHITE ICE MINT)
### each 2 mg piece contains
acesulfame potassium, carnauba wax, edible ink, flavor, gum base, hypromellose, magnesium oxide, menthol, peppermint oil, polysorbate 80, sodium bicarbonate, sodium carbonate, starch, sucralose, titanium dioxide, xylitol

### each 4 mg piece contains
acesulfame potassium, carnauba wax, D&C yellow no. 10 Al. lake, edible ink, flavor, gum base, hypromellose, magnesium oxide, menthol, peppermint oil, polysorbate 80, sodium carbonate, starch, sucralose, titanium dioxide, xylitol

## INACTIVE INGREDIENTS (ORIGINAL)
### each 2 mg piece contains
flavors, glycerin, gum base, sodium bicarbonate, sodium carbonate, sorbitol

**each 4 mg piece contains**
D&C yellow no. 10, flavors, glycerin, gum base, sodium carbonate, sorbitol

**INACTIVE INGREDIENTS (CINNAMON SURGE)**
**each 2 mg piece contains**
acacia, acesulfame potassium, carnauba wax, edible ink, flavor, gum base, hypromellose, magnesium oxide, menthol, peppermint oil, polysorbate 80, sodium bicarbonate, sodium carbonate, sucralose, titanium dioxide, xylitol

**each 4 mg piece contains**
acacia, acesulfame potassium, carnauba wax, D&C yellow no. 10 Al. lake, edible ink, flavor, gum base, hypromellose, magnesium oxide, menthol, peppermint oil, polysorbate 80, sodium carbonate, sucralose, titanium dioxide, xylitol

**INACTIVE INGREDIENTS (FRESH MINT)**
**each 2 mg piece contains**
acacia, acesulfame potassium, carnauba wax, edible ink, gum base, magnesium oxide, menthol, peppermint oil, sodium bicarbonate, sodium carbonate, titanium dioxide, xylitol

**each 4 mg piece contains**
acacia, acesulfame potassium, carnauba wax, D&C yellow no. 10 Al. lake, edible ink, gum base, magnesium oxide, menthol, peppermint oil, sodium carbonate, titanium dioxide, xylitol

**INACTIVE INGREDIENTS (MINT)**
**each 2 mg piece contains**
acesulfame potassium, gum base, magnesium oxide, menthol, peppermint oil, sodium bicarbonate, sodium carbonate, xylitol

**each 4 mg piece contains**
acesulfame potassium, D&C yellow no. 10 Al. lake, gum base, magnesium oxide, menthol, peppermint oil, sodium carbonate, xylitol

**QUESTIONS AND COMMENTS?**
Call toll-free **1-800-419-4766** (English/Spanish) weekdays (9:00 AM-4:30 PM ET) or visit www.Nicorette.com

---

# NICORETTE (nicotine polacrilex) lozenge
GlaxoSmithKline Consumer Healthcare LP

## DRUG FACTS

| Active ingredient (In each lozenge) | Purpose |
|---|---|
| Nicotine polacrilex, 2 mg<br>Nicotine polacrilex, 4 mg | Stop smoking aid |

## USE
- reduces withdrawal symptoms, including nicotine craving, associated with quitting smoking

## WARNINGS
Smoking can seriously harm your child. Try to stop smoking without using any nicotine replacement medicine. This medicine is believed to be safer than smoking. However, the risks to your child from this medicine are not fully known.

## DO NOT USE
- if you continue to smoke, chew tobacco, use snuff, or use a nicotine patch or other nicotine containing products

## ASK A DOCTOR BEFORE USE IF YOU HAVE
- a sodium-restricted diet
- heart disease, recent heart attack, or irregular heartbeat; nicotine can increase your heart rate
- high blood pressure not controlled with medication; nicotine can increase your blood pressure
- stomach ulcer or diabetes

## ASK A DOCTOR OR PHARMACIST BEFORE USE IF YOU ARE
- using a non-nicotine stop smoking drug
- taking prescription medicine for depression or asthma; your prescription dose may need to be adjusted

## STOP USE AND ASK A DOCTOR IF
- mouth problems occur
- persistent indigestion or severe sore throat occurs
- irregular heartbeat or palpitations occur
- you get symptoms of nicotine overdose such as nausea, vomiting, dizziness, diarrhea, weakness and rapid heartbeat

**If you are pregnant or breastfeeding,** only use this medicine on the advice of your health care provider.

**Keep out of reach of children and pets.** Nicotine lozenges may have enough nicotine to make children and pets sick. If you need to remove the lozenge, wrap it in paper and throw away in the trash. In case of overdose, get medical help or contact a Poison Control Center right away.

## DIRECTIONS (2 MG)
- if you are under 18 years of age, ask a doctor before use
- before using this product, read the enclosed User's Guide for complete directions and other important information
- stop smoking completely when you begin using the lozenge
- if you smoke your first cigarette within 30 minutes of waking up, use 4 mg nicotine lozenge
- if you smoke your first cigarette more than 30 minutes after waking up, use 2 mg nicotine lozenge according to the following 12-week schedule:

| Weeks 1 to 6 | Weeks 7 to 9 | Weeks 10 to 12 |
|---|---|---|
| 1 lozenge every 1 to 2 hours | 1 lozenge every 2 to 4 hours | 1 lozenge every 4 to 8 hours |

- nicotine lozenge is a medicine and must be used a certain way to get the best results
- place the lozenge in your mouth and allow the lozenge to slowly dissolve (about 20 - 30 minutes). Minimize swallowing.
- do not chew or swallow lozenge
- you may feel a warm or tingling sensation
- occasionally move the lozenge from one side of your mouth to the other until completely dissolved (about 20 - 30 minutes)
- do not eat or drink 15 minutes before using or while the lozenge is in your mouth
- to improve your chances of quitting, use at least 9 lozenges per day for the first 6 weeks
- do not use more than one lozenge at a time or continuously use one lozenge after another since this may cause you hiccups, heartburn, nausea or other side effects
- do not use more than 5 lozenges in 6 hours
- do not use more than 20 lozenges per day.
- stop using the nicotine lozenge at the end of 12 weeks. If you still feel the need to use nicotine lozenges, talk to your doctor.

## DIRECTIONS (4 MG)
- if you are under 18 years of age, ask a doctor before use
- before using this product, read the enclosed User's Guide for complete directions and other important information
- stop smoking completely when you begin using the lozenge
- if you smoke your first cigarette more than 30 minutes after waking up, use 2 mg nicotine lozenge
- if you smoke your first cigarette within 30 minutes of waking up, use 4 mg nicotine lozenge according to the following 12 week schedule:

| Weeks 1 to 6 | Weeks 7 to 9 | Weeks 10 to 12 |
|---|---|---|
| 1 lozenge every 1 to 2 hours | 1 lozenge every 2 to 4 hours | 1 lozenge every 4 to 8 hours |

- nicotine lozenge is a medicine and must be used a certain way to get the best results
- place the lozenge in your mouth and allow the lozenge to slowly dissolve (about 20 - 30 minutes). Minimize swallowing
- do not chew or swallow lozenge
- you may feel a warm or tingling sensation
- occasionally move the lozenge from one side of your mouth to the other until completely dissolved (about 20 - 30 minutes)
- do not eat or drink 15 minutes before using or while the lozenge is in your mouth
- to improve your chances of quitting, use at least 9 lozenges per day for the first 6 weeks
- do not use more than one lozenge at a time or continuously use one lozenge after another since this may cause you hiccups, heartburn, nausea or other side effects
- do not use more than 5 lozenges in 6 hours
- do not use more than 20 lozenges per day
- stop using the nicotine lozenge at the end of 12 weeks. If you still feel the need to use nicotine lozenges, talk to your doctor

**OTHER INFORMATION (Original)**
- each lozenge contains: sodium, 18 mg
- **Phenylketonurics:** contains phenylalanine 3.4 mg per lozenge
- store at 20-25°C (68-77°F)
- protect from light

**OTHER INFORMATION (Mint)**
- each lozenge contains: sodium, 18 mg
- **Phenylketonurics:** contains phenylalanine 3.4 mg per lozenge
- store at 20-25°C (68-77°F)
- keep POPPAC tightly closed and protect from light

**OTHER INFORMATION (Cherry)**
- each lozenge contains: sodium, 18 mg
- store at 20-25°C (68-77°F)
- keep POPPAC tightly closed and protect from light

**INACTIVE INGREDIENTS (Original)**
aspartame, calcium polycarbophil, flavor, magnesium stearate, mannitol, potassium bicarbonate, sodium alginate, sodium carbonate, xanthan gum

**INACTIVE INGREDIENTS (Mint)**
acacia, aspartame, calcium polycarbophil, corn syrup solids, flavors, lactose, magnesium stearate, maltodextrin, mannitol, potassium bicarbonate, sodium alginate, sodium carbonate, soy protein, triethyl citrate, xanthan gum

**INACTIVE INGREDIENTS (Cherry)**
acesulfame potassium, benzyl alcohol, butylhydroxy toluene, calcium polycarbophil, coconut and/or palm kernel oil, eugenol, flavors, magnesium stearate, maltodextrin, mannitol, modified corn starch, potassium bicarbonate, sodium alginate, sodium carbonate, xanthan gum

**QUESTIONS OR COMMENTS**
Call toll-free **1-888-569-1743** (English/Spanish) weekdays (9:00 A.M - 4:30 P.M EST) or visit www.nicorette.com

# NICOTINE TRANSDERMAL SYSTEM PATCH
## KIT (nicotine) patch
Novartis Consumer Health, Inc.

**DRUG FACTS**

| Active ingredient | Purpose |
|---|---|
| Nicotine, 21 mg delivered over 24 hours | Stop smoking aid |
| Nicotine, 14 mg delivered over 24 hours | |
| Nicotine, 7 mg delivered over 24 hours | |

**USES**
- reduces withdrawal symptoms, including nicotine craving, associated with quitting smoking

**WARNINGS**
Smoking can seriously harm your child. Try to stop smoking without using any nicotine replacement medicine. This medicine is believed to be safer than smoking. However, the risks to your child from this medicine are not fully known.

**DO NOT USE**
- if you continue to smoke, chew tobacco, use snuff, use nicotine gum, or use another nicotine patch or other nicotine containing products

**ASK A DOCTOR BEFORE USE IF YOU HAVE**
- heart disease, recent heart attack, or irregular heartbeat. Nicotine can increase your heart rate
- high blood pressure not controlled with medication. Nicotine can increase your blood pressure
- an allergy to adhesive tape or have skin problems, because you are more likely to get rashes

**ASK A DOCTOR OR PHARMACIST BEFORE USE IF YOU ARE**
- using a non-nicotine stop smoking drug
- taking a prescription medicine for depression or asthma. Your prescription dose may need to be adjusted

**WHEN USING THIS PRODUCT**
- do not smoke even when not wearing the patch. The nicotine in your skin will still be entering your bloodstream for several hours after you take off the patch
- if you have vivid dreams or other sleep disturbances remove this patch at bedtime

**STOP USE AND ASK A DOCTOR IF**
- skin redness caused by the patch does not go away after four days, or if your skin swells, or you get a rash
- irregular heartbeat or palpitations occur
- you get symptoms of nicotine overdose, such as nausea, vomiting, dizziness, weakness and rapid heartbeat

**If you are pregnant or breastfeeding,** only use this medicine on the advice of your health care provider.

**Keep out of reach of children and pets.** Used patches have enough nicotine to poison children and pets. If swallowed, get medical help or contact a Poison Control Center right away. Save pouch to use for patch disposal. Dispose of the used patches by folding sticky ends together and putting in pouch.

## DIRECTIONS

- if you are under 18 years of age, ask a doctor before use
- before using this product, read the enclosed self-help guide for complete directions and other information
- stop smoking completely when you begin using the patch
- if you smoke more than 10 cigarettes per day, use the following schedule below:

| Weeks 1-4 | Weeks 5 & 6 | Weeks 7 & 8 |
|---|---|---|
| Step 1<br><br>use one 21-mg patch/day | Step 2<br><br>use one 14-mg patch/day | Step 3<br><br>use one 7-mg patch/day |

- if you smoke 10 or less cigarettes per day, start with Step 2 for 6 weeks, then Step 3 for 2 weeks and then stop
- apply one new patch every 24 hours on skin that is dry, clean and hairless
- remove backing from patch and immediately press onto skin. Hold for 10 seconds
- wash hands after applying or removing patch. Save pouch to use for patch disposal. Dispose of the used patches by folding sticky ends together and putting in pouch
- the used patch should be removed and a new one applied to a different skin site at the same time each day
- if you have vivid dreams, you may remove the patch at bedtime and apply a new one in the morning
- do not wear more than one patch at a time
- do not cut patch in half or into smaller pieces
- do not leave patch on for more than 24 hours because it may irritate your skin and loses strength after 24 hours
- to avoid possible burns, remove patch before undergoing any MRI (magnetic resonance imaging) procedures
- stop using the patch at the end of 8 weeks. If you still feel the need to use the patch talk to your doctor

## OTHER INFORMATION

- store at 20-25°C (68-77°F)

## INACTIVE INGREDIENTS

acrylate adhesive, aluminized polyester, cellulose paper, methacrylic acid copolymer

## COMMENTS OR QUESTIONS

Call **1-800-585-8682**

## NIX CREME RINSE AND NIT REMOVAL COMB (permethrin)

Insight Pharmaceuticals

### DRUG FACTS

| Active ingredient (in each fluid ounce) | Purpose |
|---|---|
| Permethrin 280 mg (1%) | Lice treatment |

### USE

- treats head lice

### WARNINGS

**For external use only.**

### DO NOT USE

- on children under 2 months of age
- near the eyes
- inside the nose, ear, mouth, or vagina
- on lice in eyebrows or eyelashes. See your doctor

### ASK A DOCTOR BEFORE USE IF YOU ARE

- allergic to ragweed. May cause breathing difficulty or an asthmatic episode

### WHEN USING THIS PRODUCT

- keep eyes tightly closed and protect eyes with a washcloth or towel
- if product gets into the eyes, immediately flush with large amounts of water
- scalp itching or redness may occur

### STOP USE AND SEE A DOCTOR IF

- breathing difficulty occurs
- eye irritation occurs
- skin or scalp irritation continues or infection occurs

**If pregnant or breastfeeding,** ask a health professional before use.

**Keep out of reach of children.** If swallowed, get medical help or contact a Poison Control Center right away.

### DIRECTIONS

**Inspect**

- all household members should be checked by another person for lice and/or nits (eggs)
- use a magnifying glass in bright light to help you see the lice and nits (eggs)
- use a tool, such as a comb or two unsharpened pencils to lift and part the hair
- look for tiny nits near the scalp, beginning at the back of the neck and behind the ears
- small sections of hair (1-2 inches wide) should be examined at a time
- unlike dandruff, nits stick to the hair. Dandruff should move when lightly touched
- if either lice or nits (eggs) are found, treat with Nix Creme Rinse

**Treat**

- wash hair with a shampoo without conditioner. Do not use a shampoo that contains a conditioner or a conditioner alone since this may decrease the activity of Nix. Rinse with water
- towel dry hair so it is damp but not wet
- shake the bottle of Nix well
- completely saturate the hair and scalp with Nix. Begin to apply Nix behind the ears and at the back of the neck
- keep Nix out of the eyes. Protect the eyes with a washcloth or towel
- leave Nix on the hair for 10 minutes, but no longer
- rinse with warm water
- towel dry hair and comb out tangles
- if live lice are seen seven days or more after the first treatment, a second treatment should be given

**Remove Lice/Nits**

- remove nits by combing the hair with the special small tooth comb provided. Remaining nits may be removed by hand (using a throw-away glove), or cutting the nits out
- use the nit comb provided and make sure the hair remains slightly damp while removing nits
- if the hair dries during combing, dampen it slightly with water
- part the hair into 4 sections. Work on one section at a time. Longer hair may take more time (1-2 hours)
- start at the top of the head on the section you have picked
- with one hand, lift a 1-2 inch wide strand of hair. Get the teeth of the comb as close to the scalp as possible and comb with a firm, even motion away from the scalp to the end of the hair
- use clips to pin back each strand of hair after you have combed out the nits
- clean the comb completely as you go. Wipe the nits from the comb with a tissue and throw away the tissue in a sealed plastic bag to prevent the lice from coming back

- after combing, recheck the entire head for nits and repeat combing if necessary
- check the affected head daily to remove any nits that you might have missed

## OTHER INFORMATION
- read all the directions in the Consumer Information Insert and warnings before use
- keep the carton. It contains important information
- store at 20°C-25°C (68°F-77°F)

## INACTIVE INGREDIENTS
balsam canada, cetyl alcohol, citric acid, FD&C yellow no. 6, fragrance, hydrolyzed animal protein, hydroxyethylcellulose, polyoxyethylene 10 cetyl ether, propylene glycol, stearalkonium chloride, water, isopropyl alcohol 5.6 g (20%), methylparaben 56 mg (0.2%), and propylparaben 22 mg (0.08%)

## QUESTIONS OR COMMENTS
Call **1-888-LICE LINE (1-888-542-3546)**, Monday to Friday, 9 AM-5 PM EST

---

# NIZORAL A-D (ketoconazole) shampoo
McNeil Consumer Healthcare, Division of McNeil-PPC, Inc.

## DRUG FACTS

| Active ingredient | Purpose |
|---|---|
| Ketoconazole 1% | Anti-dandruff shampoo |

## USE
- controls flaking, scaling and itching associated with dandruff

## WARNINGS
**For external use only.**

## DO NOT USE
- on scalp that is broken or inflamed
- if you are allergic to ingredients in this product

## WHEN USING THIS PRODUCT
- avoid contact with eyes
- if product gets into eyes, rinse thoroughly with water

## STOP USE AND ASK A DOCTOR IF
- rash appears
- condition worsens or does not improve in 2-4 weeks

**If pregnant or breastfeeding,** ask a doctor before use

**Keep out of reach of children.** If swallowed, get medical help or contact a Poison Control Center right away.

## DIRECTIONS

| adults and children 12 years and over | wet hair thoroughly |
| | apply shampoo, generously lather, rinse thoroughly. Repeat |
| | use every 3-4 days for up to 8 weeks or as directed by a doctor. Then use only as needed to control dandruff. |
| children under 12 years | ask a doctor |

## OTHER INFORMATION
- store between 35°F-86°F (2°C-30°C)
- protect from light
- protect from freezing
- see top panel for lot number and expiration date

## INACTIVE INGREDIENTS
acrylic acid polymer (carbomer 1342), butylated hydroxytoluene, cocamide MEA, FD&C Blue no. 1, fragrance, glycol distearate, polyquaternium-7, quaternium-15, sodium chloride, sodium cocoyl sarcosinate, sodium hydroxide and/or hydrochloric acid, sodium laureth sulfate, tetrasodium EDTA, water

## QUESTIONS OR COMMENTS
Call **1-800-962-5357**

---

# NUPERCAINAL (dibucaine) ointment
Novartis Consumer Health, Inc.

## DRUG FACTS

| Active ingredient | Purpose |
|---|---|
| Dibucaine 1% | Hemorrhoidal/topical analgesic ointment |

## USES
- temporarily relieves pain and itching due to:
  - hemorrhoids or other anorectal disorders
  - sunburn
  - minor burns
  - minor cuts
  - scrapes
  - insect bites
  - minor skin irritation

## WARNINGS
**For external use only.**

**Allergy alert**
certain persons can develop allergic reactions to ingredients in this product.

## DO NOT USE
- in or near the eyes
- in children under 2 years of age
- in large quantities, particularly over raw surfaces or blistered areas

## WHEN USING THIS PRODUCT
- do not use more than directed
- do not get into the eyes
- do not put this product into the rectum by using fingers or any mechanical device

## STOP USE AND ASK A DOCTOR IF
- condition worsens or does not improve within 7 days
- the symptom being treated does not subside or if redness, irritation, swelling, bleeding or other symptoms develop or increase

**If pregnant or breastfeeding,** ask a health care professional before use.

**Keep out of reach of children.** If swallowed, get medical help or contact a poison control center right away.

## DIRECTIONS
- if possible, clean the affected area with mild soap and warm water and rinse thoroughly
- gently dry by patting or blotting with toilet tissue or a soft cloth before applying

| adults and children 12 years and over | apply externally to the affected area up to 3 or 4 times a day |
|---|---|
| children 2-12 years of age | ask a doctor |
| children under 2 years of age | do not use |

## OTHER INFORMATION
- to secure child resistant cap: screw cap tightly. Then turn cap in opposite direction. If clicking sound is not heard, repeat procedure
- see crimp of tube for lot number and expiration date
- store at controlled room temperature 20-25°C (68-77°F)

## INACTIVE INGREDIENTS
acetone sodium bisulfite, lanolin, light mineral oil, purified water, white petrolatum

## QUESTIONS OR COMMENTS
Call 1-800-452-0051

---

# NYTOL QUICKCAPS (diphenhydramine hydrochloride) caplet
GlaxoSmithKline Consumer Healthcare LP

## DRUG FACTS

| Active ingredient (in each caplet) | Purpose |
|---|---|
| Diphenhydramine hydrochloride 25 mg | Nighttime sleep-aid |

## USE
- relieves occasional sleeplessness

## WARNINGS

### DO NOT USE
- in children under 12 years of age
- with any other product containing diphenhydramine, even one used on skin
- with other antihistamines

### ASK A DOCTOR BEFORE USE IF YOU HAVE
- a breathing problem such as emphysema or chronic bronchitis
- glaucoma
- trouble urinating due to enlarged prostate gland

### ASK A DOCTOR OR PHARMACIST BEFORE USE IF YOU ARE
- taking sedatives or tranquilizers

### WHEN USING THIS PRODUCT
- avoid alcoholic beverages
- be careful when driving a motor vehicle or operating machinery

### STOP USE AND ASK A DOCTOR IF
- sleeplessness persists continuously for more than 2 weeks. Insomnia may be a symptom of serious underlying medical illness

**If pregnant or breastfeeding,** ask a health professional before use.

**Keep out of reach of children.** In case of overdose, get medical help or contact a Poison Control Center right away.

## DIRECTIONS

| adults and children 12 years of age and over | take 2 caplets at bedtime if needed, or as directed by a doctor |
|---|---|

## OTHER INFORMATION
- each caplet contains: calcium 70 mg
- store below 25°C (77°F)

## INACTIVE INGREDIENTS
carnauba wax, dibasic calcium phosphate, hydroxypropyl methylcellulose, magnesium stearate, microcrystalline cellulose, polyethylene glycol, silicon dioxide, starch

## QUESTIONS OR COMMENTS
Call 1-866-255-5203 (English/Spanish) weekdays

---

# OCEAN PREMIUM SALINE (sodium chloride)
nasal spray
Fleming Pharmaceuticals St. Louis Co.

## DRUG FACTS

| Active ingredient | Purpose |
|---|---|
| Sodium chloride 0.65% | Nasal spray |

## USES
- for general moisturizing during dry climates and cold temperature, and while spending time in enclosed spaces (e.g., air travel, office buildings, etc.)
- to relieve allergy, cold & flu symptoms
- to help relieve congestion by thinning mucus
- to return moisture caused by drug-induced dryness
- to help reduce nosebleeds from dryness
- to moisturize and irrigate membranes following nasal surgery
- to relieve dryness associated with oxygen treatments and CPAP machines for sleep apnea

## WARNINGS
- sealed with printed neckband for your protection; use only if intact
- the use of this dispenser by more than one person may spread infection

## DIRECTIONS
- for children and adults
  - squeeze bottle twice in each nostril as often as needed or as directed by physician
  - for infants, use drop application
  - hold bottle upright for spray, horizontally for stream, upside down for drop
  - the use of this dispenser by more than one person may spread infection

## INACTIVE INGREDIENTS
- Sodium phosphate/sodium hydroxide, phenylcarbinol, benzalkonium chloride, benzyl alcohol

## OPCON-A (naphazoline hydrochloride and pheniramine maleate) solution/drops
Bausch & Lomb Incorporated
Loba Feinchemie AG

### DRUG FACTS

| Active ingredients | Purpose |
|---|---|
| Naphazoline hydrochloride (0.02675%) | Redness reliever |
| Pheniramine maleate (0.315%) | Antihistamine |

### USES
- temporarily relieves itching and redness caused by pollen, ragweed, grass, animal hair and dander

### WARNINGS
**DO NOT USE**
- if you are sensitive to any ingredient in this product
- if solution changes color or becomes cloudy

**ASK A DOCTOR BEFORE USE IF YOU HAVE**
- heart disease
- high blood pressure
- trouble urinating due to an enlarged prostate gland
- narrow angle glaucoma

**WHEN USING THIS PRODUCT**
- overuse may cause more eye redness
- pupils may become enlarged temporarily
- do not touch tip of container to any surface to avoid contamination
- you may feel a brief tingling after putting drops in eye
- replace cap after use
- remove contact lenses before using

**STOP USE AND ASK A DOCTOR IF**
- you experience:
  - eye pain
  - changes in vision
  - redness or irritation of the eye that worsens or lasts more than 72 hours

**Keep out of reach of children.** If swallowed, get medical help or contact a Poison Control Center right away. Accidental oral ingestion in infants and children may lead to coma and marked reduction in body temperature.

### DIRECTIONS

| Adults and children 6 years of age and older | Instill 1 or 2 drops in the affected eye(s) up to 4 times daily. |
|---|---|
| Children under 6 years | ask a doctor |

### OTHER INFORMATION
- store at 20-25°C (68-77°F)
- protect from light
- use before expiration date marked on the carton or bottle

### INACTIVE INGREDIENTS
benzalkonium chloride, boric acid, edetate disodium, hypromellose, purified water, sodium borate, sodium chloride

### QUESTIONS OR COMMENTS
Call: **1-800-553-5340**

## ORAJEL MOUTH SORE GEL (benzalkonium chloride, benzocaine, zinc chloride) gel
Church & Dwight Co., Inc.

### DRUG FACTS

| Active ingredients | Purpose |
|---|---|
| Benzalkonium chloride 0.02% | Oral antiseptic |
| Benzocaine 20% | Oral pain reliever |
| Zinc chloride 0.1% | Oral astringent |

### USES
- for the temporary relief of pain associated with:
  - canker sores
  - cold sores
  - fever blisters
  - minor irritation or injury of the mouth and gums. To help protect against infection in minor oral irritation.

### WARNINGS
**Allergy alert**
do not use this product if you have a history of allergy to local anesthetics such as procaine, butacaine, benzocaine or other "caine" anesthetics

**DO NOT USE**
- more than directed
- for more than 7 days unless directed by a dentist or doctor

**STOP USE AND ASK A DOCTOR IF**
- sore mouth symptoms do not improve in 7 days
- swelling, rash or fever develops
- irritation, pain or redness persists or worsens

**Keep out of reach of children.** In case of overdose or allergic reaction, get medical help or contact a Poison Control Center right away.

### DIRECTIONS
- cut open tip of tube on score mark
- do not use if tube tip is cut prior to opening

| adults and children 2 years of age and over | apply to affected area up to 4 times daily or as directed by a dentist or doctor |
|---|---|
| children under 12 years of age | should be supervised in the use of this product |
| children under 2 years of age | ask a dentist or doctor |

### INACTIVE INGREDIENTS
allantoin, carbomer, edelate disodium, mentha piperota (peppermint) oil, polyethylene glycol, polysorbate 60, propylene glycol, propyl gallate, water, pvp, sodium saccharin, sorbic acid, stearyl alcohol

### QUESTIONS OR COMMENTS
Call **1-800-952-5080** M-F 9 AM-5 PM EST or visit at www.orajel.com

# PAMPRIN ALL DAY (naproxen sodium) caplet
Chattem, a Sanofi Company

## DRUG FACTS

| Active ingredient (in each caplet) | Purpose |
|---|---|
| Naproxen sodium 220 mg (naproxen 200 mg) (NSAID*) | Pain reliever/fever reducer |

*nonsteroidal anti-inflammatory drug

## USES
- temporarily relieves minor aches and pains due to:
  - minor pain of arthritis
  - muscular aches
  - backache
  - menstrual cramps
  - headache
  - toothache
  - the common cold
  - temporarily reduces fever

## WARNINGS
### Allergy alert
Naproxen sodium may cause a severe allergic reaction, especially in people allergic to aspirin. Symptoms may include:

- hives
- facial swelling
- asthma (wheezing)
- shock
- skin reddening
- rash
- blisters

If an allergic reaction occurs, stop use and seek medical help right away.

### Stomach bleeding warning
This product contains a nonsteroidal anti-inflammatory drug (NSAID), which may cause stomach bleeding. The chance is higher if you:

- are age 60 or older
- have had stomach ulcers or bleeding problems
- take a blood thinning (anticoagulant) or steroid drug
- take other drugs containing an NSAID [aspirin, ibuprofen, naproxen, or others]
- have 3 or more alcoholic drinks every day while using this product
- take more or for a longer time than directed

## DO NOT USE
- if you have ever had an allergic reaction to any pain reliever/fever reducer
- right before or after heart surgery

## ASK A DOCTOR BEFORE USE IF YOU HAVE
- problems or serious side effects from taking pain relievers or fever reducers
- stomach problems that last or come back, such as heartburn, upset stomach, or stomach pain
- ulcers
- bleeding problems
- high blood pressure
- heart or kidney disease
- taken a diuretic
- reached age 60 or older

## ASK A DOCTOR OR PHARMACIST BEFORE USE IF YOU ARE
- taking any other drug containing a NSAID (prescription or nonprescription)
- taking a blood thinning (anticoagulant) or steroid drug
- under a doctor's care for any serious condition
- taking any other drug

## WHEN USING THIS PRODUCT
- take with food or milk if stomach upset occurs
- long term continuous use may increase the risk of heart attack or stroke

## STOP USE AND ASK A DOCTOR IF
- you feel faint, vomit blood, or have bloody or black stools. These are signs of stomach bleeding
- pain gets worse or lasts more than 10 days
- fever gets worse or lasts more than 3 days
- you have difficulty swallowing
- it feels like the pill is stuck in your throat
- you develop heartburn
- stomach pain or upset gets worse and lasts
- redness or swelling is present in the painful area
- any new symptoms appear

**If pregnant or breastfeeding,** ask a health professional before use.

**It is especially important not to use naproxen sodium during the last 3 months of pregnancy unless definitely directed to do so by a doctor because it may cause problems in the unborn child or complications during delivery.**

**Keep out of reach of children.** In case of overdose, get medical help or contact a Poison Control Center right away.

## DIRECTIONS
- do not take more than directed
- the smallest effective dose should be used
- do not take longer than 10 days, unless directed by a doctor (see Warnings)
- drink a full glass of water with each dose

| adults and children 12 years and over | take 1 caplet every 8-12 hours while symptoms last |
|---|---|
| | for the first dose you may take 2 caplets within the first hour |
| | do not exceed 2 caplets in any 8-12 hour period |
| | do not exceed 3 caplets in a 24-hour period |
| children under 12 years | ask a doctor |

## OTHER INFORMATION
- each caplet contains: sodium 20 mg

## INACTIVE INGREDIENTS
carnauba wax, FD&C blue no. 2 aluminum lake, hypromellose, magnesium stearate, microcystalline cellulose, polyethylene glycol, providone, talc, titanium dioxide

## PAMPRIN CRAMP MENSTRUAL PAIN RELIEF (acetaminophen, magnesium salicylate, pamabrom) caplet

Chattem, Inc.

### DRUG FACTS

| Active ingredients (in each caplet) | Purpose |
|---|---|
| Acetaminophen 250 mg | Pain reliever |
| Magnesium salicylate (NSAID*) 250 mg | |
| Pamabrom 25 mg | Diuretic |

*nonsteroidal anti-inflammatory drug

### USES
- for the temporary relief of these symptoms associated with menstrual periods:
  - cramps
  - headache
  - backache
  - water-weight gain
  - bloating
  - muscular aches

### WARNINGS
**Reye's syndrome**
Children and teenagers who have or are recovering from chicken pox or flu-like symptoms should not use this product. When using this product, if changes in behavior with nausea and vomiting occur, consult a doctor because these symptoms could be an early sign of Reye's syndrome, a rare but serious illness.

**Allergy alert**
Magnesium salicylate may cause a severe allergic reaction which may include:

- hives
- facial swelling
- asthma (wheezing)
- shock

**Liver warning**
This product contains acetaminophen. Severe liver damage may occur if you take:
- more than 8 caplets in 24 hours, which is the maximum daily amount
- with other drugs containing acetaminophen
- 3 or more alcoholic drinks every day while using this product

**Stomach bleeding warning**
This product contains an NSAID, which may cause severe stomach bleeding. The chance is higher if you:
- are age 60 or older
- have had stomach ulcers or bleeding problems
- take a blood thinning (anticoagulant) or steroid drug
- take other drugs containing prescription or nonprescription NSAIDs [aspirin, ibuprofen, naproxen, or others]
- have 3 or more alcoholic drinks every day while using this product
- take more or for a longer time than directed

### DO NOT USE
- if you have ever had an allergic reaction to any other pain reliever/fever reducer
- with any other drug containing acetaminophen (prescription or nonprescription). If you are not sure whether a drug contains acetaminophen, ask a doctor or pharmacist

### ASK A DOCTOR BEFORE USE IF
- you have liver disease

- the stomach bleeding warning applies to you
- you have a history of stomach problems, such as heartburn
- you have high blood pressure, heart disease, liver cirrhosis, or kidney disease
- you are taking a diuretic

### ASK A DOCTOR OR PHARMACIST BEFORE USE
- if you are taking a prescription drug for gout, diabetes or arthritis

### STOP USE AND ASK A DOCTOR IF
- an allergic reaction occurs. Seek medical help right away
- you experience any of the following signs of stomach bleeding:
  - feel faint
  - vomit blood
  - have bloody or black stools
  - have stomach pain that does not get better
- redness or swelling is present
- new symptoms occur
- pain gets worse or lasts more than 10 days
- fever gets worse or lasts more than 3 days
- ringing in the ears or loss of hearing occurs

**If pregnant or breastfeeding,** ask a health professional before use.

It is especially important not to use magnesium salicylate during the last 3 months of pregnancy unless definitely directed to do so by a doctor because it may cause problems in the unborn child or complications during delivery.

**Keep out of reach of children.** In case of overdose, get medical help or contact a Poison Control Center right away. Quick medical attention is critical for adults as well as for children even if you do not notice any signs or symptoms.

### DIRECTIONS

| adults and children 12 years and over | take 2 caplets with water every 6 hours as needed |
|---|---|
| | do not exceed 8 caplets in a 24 hour period or as directed by a doctor |
| | do not use more than directed (see warnings) |
| children under 12 years | ask a doctor |

### OTHER INFORMATION
- each caplet contains: magnesium 20 mg

### INACTIVE INGREDIENTS
carnauba wax, corn starch, croscarmellose sodium, crospovidone, FD&C blue no. 1, hypromellose, magnesium stearate, microcrystalline cellulose, polyethylene glycol, polysorbate 80, povidone, propylene glycol, silicon dioxide, stearic acid, titanium dioxide (224-181)

## PAMPRIN MAX MENSTRUAL PAIN RELIEF (acetaminophen, aspirin, caffeine) caplet

Chattem, Inc.

### DRUG FACTS

| Active ingredients (in each caplet) | Purpose |
|---|---|
| Acetaminophen 250 mg | Pain reliever |
| Aspirin 250 mg (NSAID*) | |
| Caffeine 65 mg | Diuretic |

*nonsteroidal anti-inflammatory drug

## USES

- for the temporary relief of these symptoms associated with menstrual periods:
  - cramps
  - headache
  - backache
  - fatigue
  - bloating

## WARNINGS

### Reye's syndrome

Children and teenagers who have or are recovering from chicken pox or flu-like symptoms should not use this product. When using this product, if changes in behavior with nausea and vomiting occur, consult a doctor because these symptoms could be an early sign of Reye's syndrome, a rare but serious illness.

### Allergy alert

Aspirin may cause a severe allergic reaction which may include:
- hives
- facial swelling
- asthma (wheezing)
- shock

### Liver warning

This product contains acetaminophen. Severe liver damage may occur if you take:
- more than 8 caplets in 24 hours, which is the maximum daily amount
- with other drugs containing acetaminophen
- 3 or more alcoholic drinks every day while using this product

### Stomach bleeding warning

This product contains an NSAID, which may cause severe stomach bleeding. The chance is higher if you:
- are age 60 or older
- have had stomach ulcers or bleeding problems
- take a blood thinning (anticoagulant) or steroid drug
- take other drugs containing prescription or nonprescription NSAIDs [aspirin, ibuprofen, naproxen, or others]
- have 3 or more alcoholic drinks every day while using this product
- take more or for a longer time than directed

### Caffeine warning

The recommended dose of this product contains about as much caffeine as a cup of coffee. Limit the use of caffeine-containing medications, foods, or beverages while taking this product because too much caffeine may cause nervousness, irritability, sleeplessness, and occasionally, rapid heartbeat.

## DO NOT USE

- if you are allergic to aspirin or any other pain reliever/fever reducer
- with any other drug containing acetaminophen (prescription or nonprescription). If you are not sure whether a drug contains acetaminophen, ask a doctor or pharmacist

## ASK A DOCTOR BEFORE USE IF

- you have liver disease
- the stomach bleeding warning applies to you
- you have a history of stomach problems, such as heartburn
- you have high blood pressure, heart disease, liver cirrhosis, or kidney disease
- you are taking a diuretic

## ASK A DOCTOR OR PHARMACIST BEFORE USE

- if you are taking a prescription drug for gout, diabetes or arthritis

## STOP USE AND ASK A DOCTOR IF

- an allergic reaction occurs. Seek medical help right away
- you experience any of the following signs of stomach bleeding:
  - feel faint
  - vomit blood
  - have bloody or black stools
  - have stomach pain that does not get better
- redness or swelling is present
- new symptoms occur
- pain gets worse or lasts more than 10 days
- fever gets worse or lasts more than 3 days
- ringing in the ears or loss of hearing occurs

**If pregnant or breastfeeding,** ask a health professional before use.

It is especially important not to use aspirin during the last 3 months of pregnancy unless definitely directed to do so by a doctor because it may cause problems in the unborn child or complications during delivery.

**Keep out of reach of children.** In case of overdose, get medical help or contact a Poison Control Center right away. Quick medical attention is critical for adults as well as for children even if you do not notice any signs or symptoms.

## DIRECTIONS

| adults and children 12 years and over | take 2 caplets with water every 6 hours as needed |
| --- | --- |
|  | do not exceed 8 caplets in a 24 hour period or as directed by a doctor |
|  | do not use more than directed (see warnings) |
| children under 12 years | ask a doctor |

## INACTIVE INGREDIENTS

D&C red no. 27 lake, FD&C red no. 40 lake, fractionated coconut oil, hypromellose, maltodextrin, microcrystalline cellulose, polydextrose, polyvinylpyrrolidone, pregelatinized starch, silica, sodium starch glycolate, starch, stearic acid, talc, titanium dioxide (245-171)

# PAMPRIN MULTISYMPTOM MENSTRUAL PAIN RELIEF (acetaminophen, pamabrom, and pyrilamine maleate) caplet

Chattem, Inc.

## DRUG FACTS

| Active ingredient (in each caplet) | Purpose |
| --- | --- |
| Acetaminophen 500 mg | Pain reliever |
| Pamabrom 25 mg | Diuretic |
| Pyrilamine maleate 15 mg | Antihistamine |

## USES

- for the temporary relief of these symptoms associated with menstrual periods:
  - cramps
  - headache
  - bloating
  - backache
  - water-weight gain
  - muscular aches
  - irritability

## WARNINGS
**Liver warning**
This product contains acetaminophen. Severe liver damage may occur if you take:
- more than 8 caplets in 24 hours, which is the maximum daily amount
- with other drugs containing acetaminophen
- 3 or more alcoholic drinks every day while using this product

## DO NOT USE
- with any other drug containing acetaminophen (prescription or nonprescription). If you are not sure whether a drug contains acetaminophen, ask a doctor or pharmacist

## ASK A DOCTOR BEFORE USE IF YOU HAVE
- liver disease
- glaucoma
- a breathing problem such as emphysema or chronic bronchitis
- difficulty in urination due to enlargement of the prostate gland

## ASK A DOCTOR OR PHARMACIST BEFORE USE IF YOU ARE
- taking the blood thinning drug warfarin
- taking sedatives or tranquilizers

## WHEN USING THIS PRODUCT
- you may get drowsy, avoid alcoholic beverages
- alcohol, sedatives and tranquilizers may increase drowsiness
- use caution when driving or operating machinery
- excitability may occur, especially in children

## STOP USE AND ASK A DOCTOR IF
- pain gets worse or lasts for more than 10 days
- fever gets worse or lasts for more than 3 days
- new symptoms occur
- redness or swelling is present

**If pregnant or breastfeeding,** ask a health professional before use.

**Keep out of reach of children.** In case of overdose, get medical help or contact a Poison Control Center right away. Quick medical attention is critical for adults as well as for children even if you do not notice any signs or symptoms.

## DIRECTIONS

| adults and children 12 years and over | take 2 caplets with water every 6 hours as needed |
| | do not exceed 8 caplets in a 24 hour period or as directed by a doctor |
| | do not use more than directed (see warnings) |
| children under 12 years | ask a doctor |

## INACTIVE INGREDIENTS
crospovidone, magnesium stearate, povidone, pregelatinized starch, sodium starch glycolate, stearic acid (224-186)

## PANOXYL (benzoyl peroxide) cream
Stiefel Laboratories Inc

## DRUG FACTS

| Active ingredient | Purpose |
|---|---|
| **Panoxyl-4** Benzoyl peroxide 4% | Acne medication |
| **Panoxyl-8** Benzoyl peroxide 8% | |
| **Panoxyl** Benzoyl peroxide 10% | |

## USE
- for the treatment of acne

## WARNINGS
**For external use only.**

## DO NOT USE IF YOU
- have very sensitive skin
- are sensitive to benzoyl peroxide

## WHEN USING THIS PRODUCT
- avoid unnecessary sun exposure and use a sunscreen
- avoid contact with the eyes, lips, and mouth
- avoid contact with hair or dyed fabrics, including carpet and clothing which may be bleached by this product
- skin irritation and dryness is more likely to occur if you use another topical acne medication at the same time. If irritation occurs, only use one topical acne medication at a time
- skin irritation may occur, characterized by redness, burning, itching, peeling, or possibly swelling. Irritation may be reduced by using the product less frequently or in a lower concentration

## STOP USE AND ASK A DOCTOR IF
- irritation becomes severe

**Keep out of reach of children.** If swallowed, get medical help or contact a Poison Control Center right away.

## DIRECTIONS
- wet area to be cleansed
- apply acne wash and gently massage area for 1-2 minutes
- rinse thoroughly and pat dry
- because excessive drying of the skin may occur, start with 1 application daily, then gradually increase to 2 or 3 times daily if needed or as directed by a doctor
- if going outside, use a sunscreen. If irritation or sensitivity develops, discontinue use of both products and consult a doctor

## OTHER INFORMATION
- store at room temperature 59°F-86°F (15°C-30°C)

## INACTIVE INGREDIENTS 4%
cetearyl alcohol, cocamidopropyl betaine, dimethyl isosorbide, glycerin, glycolic acid, hydrogenated castor oil, imidurea, lactic acid, methylparaben, mineral oil, PEG-14M, potassium lauryl sulfate, potassium phosphate, purified water, sodium hydroxide, sodium lauryl sulfate, sodium PCA, titanium dioxide, zea mays (corn) starch

**INACTIVE INGREDIENTS 8%**
cetearyl alcohol, cocamidopropyl betaine, dimethyl isosorbide, glycerin, glycolic acid, hydrogenated castor oil, imidurea, lactic acid, methylparaben, mineral oil, PEG-14M, potassium lauryl sulfate, potassium phosphate, purified water, sodium hydroxide, sodium lauryl sulfate, sodium PCA, titanium dioxide, zea mays (corn) starch

**INACTIVE INGREDIENTS 10%**
cetearyl alcohol, cocamidopropyl betaine, glycerin, glycolic acid, hydrogenated castor oil, imidurea, lactic acid, methylparaben, mineral oil, PEG-14M, potassium lauryl sulfate, potassium phosphate, purified water, sodium hydroxide, sodium lauryl sulfate, sodium PCA, titanium dioxide, zea mays (corn) starch

**QUESTIONS OR COMMENTS**
Call **1-888-438-7426**. Side effects should be reported to this number.

---

# PEDIACARE CHILDREN'S DECONGESTANT
(phenylephrine hydrochloride) liquid

Prestige Brands Inc.

## DRUG FACTS

| Active ingredient (in each 5 mL)* | Purpose |
|---|---|
| Phenylephrine hydrochloride 2.5 mg | Nasal decongestant |

*5 mL = one teaspoon

**USE**
- temporarily relieves nasal congestion due to the common cold, hay fever or other upper respiratory allergies

**WARNINGS**

**DO NOT USE**
- in a child who is taking a prescription monoamine oxidase inhibitor (MAOI) (certain drugs for depression, psychiatric, or emotional conditions, or Parkinson's disease), or for 2 weeks after stopping the MAOI drug. If you do not know if your child's prescription drug contains an MAOI, ask a doctor or pharmacist before giving this product

**ASK A DOCTOR BEFORE USE IF YOUR CHILD HAS**
- heart disease
- high blood pressure
- thyroid disease
- diabetes
- a sodium-restricted diet

**WHEN USING THIS PRODUCT**
- do not exceed recommended dose

**STOP USE AND ASK A DOCTOR IF**
- nervousness, dizziness, or sleeplessness occur
- symptoms do not improve within 7 days or occur with a fever

**Keep out of reach of children.** In case of overdose, get medical help or contact a Poison Control Center right away. (**1-800-222-1222**)

**DIRECTIONS**
- find right dose on chart below
- use only enclosed dosing cup designed for use with this product. Do not use any other dosing device
- if needed, repeat dose every 4 hours
- do not give more than 6 times in 24 hours

| under 4 years | do not use |
|---|---|
| 4 to 5 years | 1 teaspoonful (5 mL) |
| 6 to 11 years | 2 teaspoonfuls (10 mL) |

**OTHER INFORMATION**
- each teaspoon contains: sodium 14 mg
- store between 20-25°C (68-77°F). Protect from light. Store in outer carton until contents are used
- do not use if bottle wrap, or foil inner seal imprinted "Safety Seal" is broken or missing
- see bottom panel for lot number and expiration date

**INACTIVE INGREDIENTS**
carboxymethylcellulose sodium, citric acid, edetate disodium, FD&C red no. 40, flavors, glycerin, sodium benzoate, sodium citrate, sorbitol, sucralose, water

**QUESTIONS OR COMMENTS**
Call **1-888-474-3099**

---

# PEDIACARE CHILDREN'S ALLERGY CHERRY FLAVOR (diphenhydramine hydrochloride) liquid

Blacksmith Brands, Inc.

## DRUG FACTS

| Active ingredient (in each 5 mL)* | Purpose |
|---|---|
| Diphenhydramine hydrochloride 12.5 mg | Antihistamine/cough suppressant |

*5 mL = one teaspoon

**USES**
- temporarily relieves these symptoms due to hay fever or other upper respiratory allergies:
  - runny nose
  - sneezing
  - itchy, watery eyes
  - temporarily relieves cough due to inhaled irritants

**WARNINGS**

**DO NOT USE**
- to make a child sleepy
- with any other product containing diphenhydramine, even one used on skin

**ASK A DOCTOR BEFORE USE IF THE CHILD HAS**
- persistent or chronic cough such as occurs with asthma
- cough accompanied by excessive phlegm (mucus)
- a breathing problem such as chronic bronchitis
- glaucoma

**ASK A DOCTOR OR PHARMACIST BEFORE USE**
- if the child is taking sedatives or tranquilizers

**WHEN USING THIS PRODUCT**
- excitability may occur, especially in children
- marked drowsiness may occur
- sedatives and tranquilizers may increase drowsiness

**STOP USE AND ASK A DOCTOR IF**
- cough gets worse or lasts for more than 7 days
- cough tends to come back or occurs with fever, rash or headache that lasts. These could be signs of a serious condition

**Keep out of reach of children.** In case of overdose, get medical help or contact a Poison Control Center right away. (**1-800-222-1222**)

## DIRECTIONS
- find right dose on chart below
- use only enclosed dosing cup designed for use with this product. Do not use any other dosing device
- if needed, repeat dose every 4 hours
- do not use more than 6 times in 24 hours

| Age (yr) | Dose (tsp) |
|---|---|
| under 4 years | do not use |
| 4 to 5 years | do not use unless directed by a doctor |
| 6 to 11 years | 1 teaspoonful |

## OTHER INFORMATION
- each teaspoon contains: sodium 14 mg
- store between 20-25°C (68-77°F). Protect from light. Store in outer carton until contents used
- do not use if bottle wrap, or foil inner seal imprinted "Safety Seal" is broken or missing
- see bottom panel for lot number and expiration date

## INACTIVE INGREDIENTS
anhydrous citric acid, D&C red no. 33, FD&C red no. 40, flavors, glycerin, monoammonium glycyrrhizinate, poloxamer 407, purified water, sodium benzoate, sodium chloride, sodium citrate, sucrose

## QUESTIONS OR COMMENTS
Call **1-888-474-3099**

---

## PEDIACARE CHILDREN'S ALLERGY BUBBLEGUM FLAVOR (diphenhydramine hydrochloride) liquid
Blacksmith Brands, Inc.

## DRUG FACTS

| Active ingredient | Purpose |
|---|---|
| Diphenhydramine hydrochloride 12.5 mg | Antihistamine |

## USES
- temporarily relieves these symptoms due to hay fever or other upper respiratory allergies:
  - runny nose
  - sneezing
  - itchy, watery eyes
  - itching of the nose or throat

## WARNINGS

### DO NOT USE
- to make a child sleepy
- with any other product containing diphenhydramine, even one used on skin

### ASK A DOCTOR BEFORE USE IF THE CHILD HAS
- glaucoma
- a breathing problem such as chronic bronchitis

### ASK A DOCTOR OR PHARMACIST BEFORE USE
- if the child is taking sedatives or tranquilizers

### WHEN USING THIS PRODUCT
- marked drowsiness may occur
- sedatives and tranquilizers may increase drowsiness
- excitability may occur, especially in children

**Keep out of reach of children.** In case of overdose, seek professional assistance or contact a Poison Control Center (**1-800-222-1222**) immediately.

## DIRECTIONS
- use only enclosed dosing cup designed for use with this product. Do not use any other dosing device
- take every 4 to 6 hours
- do not take more than 6 doses in 24 hours
- tsp = teaspoon, mL = milliliter, mg = milligram

| Age (yr) | Dose (tsp) |
|---|---|
| children 6 to 11 years | 1 to 2 teaspoonfuls (5 mL to 10 mL) |
| children 4 to 5 years | do not use unless directed by a doctor |
| children under 4 years | do not use |

## OTHER INFORMATION
- each teaspoon contains: sodium 6 mg
- store at room temperature

## INACTIVE INGREDIENTS
citric acid, flavors, glycerin, poloxamer 407, purified water, D&C red no. 33, red FD&C no. 40, sodium benzoate, sodium chloride, sodium citrate, sugar

## QUESTIONS OR COMMENTS
Call **1-888-474-3099**

---

## PEDIACARE CHILDREN'S COUGH AND CONGESTION (dextromethorphan hydrobromide and guaifenesin) liquid
Blacksmith Brands, Inc.

## DRUG FACTS

| Active ingredients (in each 5 mL, 1 teaspoon) | Purpose |
|---|---|
| Dextromethorphan hydrobromide, USP 5 mg | Cough suppressant |
| Guaifenesin, USP 100 mg | Expectorant |

## USES
- helps loosen phlegm (mucus) and thin bronchial secretions to rid the bronchial passageways of bothersome mucus and make coughs more productive
- temporarily relieves:
  - cough due to minor throat and bronchial irritation as may occur with the common cold or inhaled irritants
  - the intensity of coughing
  - the impulse to cough to help your child get to sleep

## WARNINGS

### DO NOT USE
- for a child who is taking a prescription monoamine oxidase inhibitor (MAOI) (certain drugs for depression, psychiatric or emotional conditions, or Parkinson's disease), or for 2 weeks after stopping the MAOI drug. If you do not know if your child's prescription drug contains an MAOI, ask a doctor or pharmacist before giving this product

## ASK A DOCTOR BEFORE USE IF THE CHILD HAS
- cough that occurs with too much phlegm (mucus)
- persistent or chronic cough such as occurs with asthma or chronic bronchitis

## STOP USE AND ASK A DOCTOR IF
- cough gets worse or lasts more than 7 days
- cough comes back or occurs with fever, rash, or headache that lasts. These could be signs of a serious illness

## WHEN USING THIS PRODUCT
- do not use more than directed

**Keep this and all drugs out of the reach of children.** In case of accidental overdose, seek professional assistance or contact a Poison Control Center immediately.

## DIRECTIONS
- tsp = teaspoon, mL = milliliter
- this product does not contain directions or complete warnings for adult use
- do not exceed 6 doses in a 24-hour period

| Age (yr) | Dose (tsp) |
|---|---|
| children 6 years to under 12 years | 1-2 teaspoonfuls (tsps) every 4 hours |
| children 4 years to 6 years | ½-1 teaspoonful (tsp) every 4 hours |
| children under 4 years | do not use |

## OTHER INFORMATION
- each teaspoon contains: sodium 3 mg
- store at room temperature
- dosage cup provided

## INACTIVE INGREDIENTS
citric acid anhydrous, dextrose, flavors, glycerin, methyl paraben, potassium sorbate, propylene glycol, propyl paraben, purified water, D&C red 33, FD&C red 40, saccharin sodium, sodium hydroxide, sucralose, xanthan gum

## QUESTIONS OR COMMENTS
Call **1-888-474-3099**

---

# PEDIACARE CHILDREN'S MULTISYMPTOM COLD (dextromethorphan hydrobromide and phenylephrine hydrochloride) liquid
Blacksmith Brands, Inc.

## DRUG FACTS

| Active ingredients (in each 5 mL)* | Purpose |
|---|---|
| Dextromethorphan hydrobromide 5 mg | Cough suppressant |
| Phenylephrine hydrochloride 2.5 mg | Nasal decongestant |

*5 mL = one teaspoon

## USES
- temporarily relieves these symptoms due to the common cold hay fever, or other upper respiratory allergies:
  - cough
  - nasal congestion

## WARNINGS
## DO NOT USE
- in a child who is taking a prescription monoamine oxidase inhibitor (MAOI) (certain drugs for depression, psychiatric or emotional conditions, or Parkinson's disease), or for 2 weeks after stopping the MAOI drug. If you do not know if your child's prescription drug contains an MAOI, ask a doctor or pharmacist before giving this product

## ASK A DOCTOR BEFORE USE IF THE CHILD HAS
- heart disease
- high blood pressure
- thyroid disease
- diabetes
- a persistent or chronic cough such as occurs with asthma
- a cough accompanied by excessive phlegm (mucus)
- a sodium-restricted diet

## WHEN USING THIS PRODUCT
- do not exceed recommended dose

## STOP USE AND ASK A DOCTOR IF
- nervousness, dizziness, or sleeplessness occur
- symptoms do not improve within 7 days or occur with a fever
- cough gets worse or lasts for more than 7 days
- cough tends to come back or occurs with fever, rash or headache that lasts. These could be signs of a serious condition

**Keep out of reach of children** In case of overdose, get medical help or contact a Poison Control Center right away. (1-800-222-1222)

## DIRECTIONS
- find right dose on chart below
- use only enclosed dosing cup designed for use with this product
- if needed, repeat dose every 4 hours
- do not give more than 6 times in 24 hours
- do not use any other dosing device

| Age (yr) | Dose (tsp) |
|---|---|
| under 4 years | do not use |
| 4 to 5 years | 1 teaspoonful (5 mL) |
| 6 to 11 years | 2 teaspoonfuls (10 mL) |

## OTHER INFORMATION
- each teaspoon contains: sodium 15 mg
- store between 20-25°C (68-77°F). Protect from light. Store in outer carton until contents are used
- do not use if bottle wrap, or foil inner seal imprinted "Safety Seal" is broken or missing
- see bottom panel for lot number and expiration date

## INACTIVE INGREDIENTS
anhydrous citric acid, carboxymethylcellulose sodium, edetate disodium, FD&C blue no. 1, FD&C red no. 40, flavors, glycerin, purified water, sodium benzoate, sodium citrate, sorbitol solution, sucralose

## QUESTIONS OR COMMENTS
Call **1-888-474-3099**

# PEPCID AC ORIGINAL STRENGTH (famotidine)
tablet, film coated

Johnson & Johnson Merck Consumer
Pharmaceuticals

## DRUG FACTS

| Active ingredients (in each tablet) | Purpose |
| --- | --- |
| Famotidine 10 mg | Acid reducer |

## USES
- relieves heartburn associated with acid indigestion and sour stomach
- prevents heartburn associated with acid indigestion and sour stomach brought on by eating or drinking certain food and beverages

## WARNINGS
**Allergy alert**
Do not use if you are allergic to famotidine or other acid reducers.

## DO NOT USE
- if you have trouble or pain swallowing food
- vomiting with blood
- bloody or black stools. These may be signs of a serious condition. See your doctor
- with other acid reducers

## ASK A DOCTOR BEFORE USE IF YOU HAVE
- had heartburn over 3 months. This may be a sign of a more serious condition
- heartburn with lightheadedness, sweating, or dizziness
- chest pain or shoulder pain with shortness of breath; sweating; pain spreading to arms, neck or shoulders; or lightheadedness
- frequent chest pain
- frequent wheezing, particularly with heartburn
- unexplained weight loss
- nausea or vomiting
- stomach pain

## STOP USE AND ASK A DOCTOR IF
- your heartburn continues or worsens
- you need to take this product for more than 14 days

**If pregnant or breastfeeding,** ask a health professional before use.

**Keep out of reach of children.** In case of overdose, get medical help or contact a Poison Control Center right away.

## DIRECTIONS

| adults and children 12 years and over | to relieve symptoms, swallow 1 tablet with a glass of water. Do not chew. |
| --- | --- |
| | to prevent symptoms, swallow 1 tablet with a glass of water at any time from 15 to 60 minutes before eating food or drinking beverages that cause heartburn |
| | do not use more than 2 tablets in 24 hours |
| children under 12 years | ask a doctor |

## OTHER INFORMATION
- read the directions and warnings before use
- keep the carton. It contains important information
- store at 20-30°C (68-86°F)
- protect from moisture

## INACTIVE INGREDIENTS
hydroxypropyl cellulose, hypromellose, magnesium stearate, microcrystalline cellulose, red iron oxide, starch, talc, titanium dioxide

## QUESTIONS OR COMMENTS
Call **1-800-755-4008** (English) or **1-888-466-8746** (Spanish)

# PEPCID AC MAXIMUM STRENGTH (famotidine)
tablet, film coated

Johnson & Johnson Merck Consumer
Pharmaceuticals

## DRUG FACTS

| Active ingredients (in each tablet) | Purpose |
| --- | --- |
| Famotidine 20 mg | Acid reducer |

## USES
- relieves heartburn associated with acid indigestion and sour stomach
- prevents heartburn associated with acid indigestion and sour stomach brought on by eating or drinking certain food and beverages

## WARNINGS
**Allergy alert**
Do not use if you are allergic to famotidine or other acid reducers.

## DO NOT USE
- if you have trouble or pain swallowing food
- vomiting with blood
- bloody or black stools. These may be signs of a serious condition. See your doctor
- if you have kidney disease, except under the advice and supervision of a doctor
- with other acid reducers

## ASK A DOCTOR BEFORE USE IF YOU HAVE
- had heartburn over 3 months. This may be a sign of a more serious condition
- heartburn with lightheadedness, sweating, or dizziness
- chest pain or shoulder pain with shortness of breath; sweating; pain spreading to arms, neck or shoulders; or lightheadedness
- frequent chest pain
- frequent wheezing, particularly with heartburn
- unexplained weight loss
- nausea or vomiting
- stomach pain

## STOP USE AND ASK A DOCTOR IF
- your heartburn continues or worsens
- you need to take this product for more than 14 days

**If pregnant or breastfeeding,** ask a health professional before use.

**Keep out of reach of children.** In case of overdose, get medical help or contact a Poison Control Center right away.

## DIRECTIONS

| adults and children 12 years and over | to relieve symptoms, swallow 1 tablet with a glass of water. Do not chew. <br><br> to prevent symptoms, swallow 1 tablet with a glass of water at any time from 10 to 60 minutes before eating food or drinking beverages that cause heartburn <br><br> do not use more than 2 tablets in 24 hours |
|---|---|
| children under 12 years | ask a doctor |

## OTHER INFORMATION
- read the directions and warnings before use
- keep the carton. It contains important information
- store at 20-30°C (68-86°F)
- protect from moisture

## INACTIVE INGREDIENTS
carnauba wax, hydroxypropyl cellulose, hypromellose, magnesium stearate, microcrystalline cellulose, pregelatinized starch, talc, titanium dioxide

## QUESTIONS OR COMMENTS
Call **1-800-755-4008** (English) or **1-888-466-8746** (Spanish)

---

## PEPCID COMPLETE (famotidine, calcium carbonate, and magnesium hydroxide) tablet, chewable
Johnson & Johnson

### DRUG FACTS

| Active ingredients (in each chewable tablet) | Purpose |
|---|---|
| Famotidine 10 mg | Acid reducer |
| Calcium carbonate 800 mg | Antacid |
| Magnesium hydroxide 165 mg | Antacid |

## USES
- relieves heartburn associated with acid indigestion and sour stomach

## WARNINGS
**Allergy alert**
Do not use if you are allergic to famotidine or other acid reducers.

## DO NOT USE
- if you have trouble or pain swallowing food
- vomiting with blood
- bloody or black stools. These may be signs of a serious condition. See your doctor
- with other acid reducers

## ASK A DOCTOR BEFORE USE IF YOU HAVE
- had heartburn over 3 months. This may be a sign of a more serious condition
- heartburn with lightheadedness, sweating or dizziness
- chest pain or shoulder pain with shortness of breath; sweating; pain spreading to arms, neck or shoulders; or lightheadedness
- frequent chest pain
- frequent wheezing, particularly with heartburn
- unexplained weight loss

- nausea or vomiting
- stomach pain

## ASK A DOCTOR OR PHARMACIST BEFORE USE IF YOU ARE
- presently taking a prescription drug. Antacids may interact with certain prescription drugs

## STOP USE AND ASK A DOCTOR IF
- your heartburn continues or worsens
- you need to take this product for more than 14 days

**If pregnant or breastfeeding,** ask a health professional before use.

**Keep out of reach of children.** In case of overdose, get medical help or contact a Poison Control Center right away.

## DIRECTIONS

| adults and children 12 years and over | do not swallow tablet whole: chew completely <br><br> to relieve symptoms, chew 1 tablet before swallowing <br><br> do not use more than 2 chewable tablets in 24 hours |
|---|---|
| children under 12 years | ask a doctor |

## OTHER INFORMATION
- each tablet contains: calcium 320 mg; magnesium 70 mg
- read the directions and warnings before use
- keep the carton. It contains important information
- store at 20-30°C (68-86°F)
- protect from moisture

## INACTIVE INGREDIENTS
**Tropical Fruit Flavor**
cellulose acetate, corn starch, corn syrup solids, crospovidone, dextrose, FD&C yellow no. 5 aluminum lake (tartrazine), FD&C yellow aluminum lake no. 6, flavors, gum arabic, hydroxypropyl cellulose, hypromellose, lactose, magnesium stearate, maltodextrin, mineral oil, sucralose, triacetin

## INACTIVE INGREDIENTS
**Berry Flavor**
cellulose acetate, corn starch, crospovidone, D&C red no. 7 calcium lake, dextrose, FD&C blue no. 1 aluminum lake, FD&C red no. 40 aluminum lake, flavors, gum arabic, hydroxypropyl cellulose, hypromellose, lactose, magnesium stearate, maltodextrin, mineral oil, sucralose

## INACTIVE INGREDIENTS
**Cool Mint Flavor**
cellulose acetate, corn starch, crospovidone, D&C yellow no. 10 aluminum lake, dextrose, FD&C blue no. 1 aluminum lake, flavors, gum arabic, hydroxypropyl cellulose, hypromellose, lactose, magnesium stearate, maltodextrin, mineral oil, sucralose

---

## PEPTIC RELIEF MAXIMUM STRENGTH
(bismuth subsalicylate) suspension
Aaron Industries, Inc.

### DRUG FACTS

| Active ingredients | Purpose |
|---|---|
| Bismuth subsalicylate 525 mg | Upset stomach reliever/ antidiarrheal |

## USES
- relieves:
  - upset stomach
  - heartburn
  - indigestion
  - diarrhea
  - nausea

## WARNINGS
### Reye's syndrome
Children and teenagers who have or are recovering from chicken pox or flu-like symptoms should not use this product. When using this product, if changes in behavior with nausea or vomiting occur, consult a doctor because these symptoms could be an early sign of Reye's syndrome, a rare but serious illness.

### Allergy alert
contains salicylate. Do not take if you are taking other salicylate products or are allergic to salicylates (including aspirin)

## DO NOT USE IF YOU HAVE
- an ulcer
- a bleeding problem
- bloody or black stool

## ASK A DOCTOR BEFORE USE IF YOU HAVE
- fever
- mucus in stool

## ASK A DOCTOR OR PHARMACIST BEFORE USE IF YOU ARE
- taking any drug for:
  - anticoagulation (thinning blood)
  - diabetes
  - gout
  - arthritis

## WHEN USING THIS PRODUCT
- a temporary, but harmless, darkening of the stool and/or tongue may occur

## STOP USE AND ASK A DOCTOR IF
- symptoms get worse
- ringing in the ears or loss of hearing occurs
- diarrhea lasts more than 2 days

**If pregnant or breastfeeding,** ask a health professional before use.

**Keep this and all drugs out of the reach of children.** In case of accidental overdose, seek professional assistance or contact a Poison Control Center immediately.

## DIRECTIONS
- shake well before use
- for accurate dosing, use dose cup
- drink plenty of clear fluids to help prevent dehydration caused by diarrhea

| adults and children 12 years and over | 1 dose (2 tablespoons or 30 ml) every hour as needed |
| | do not exceed 4 doses (8 tablespoons or 120 ml) in 24 hours |
| | use until diarrhea stops but not more than 2 days |
| children under 12 years | ask a doctor |

## OTHER INFORMATION
- each tablespoon contains: sodium 6 mg
- sugar free
- low sodium
- keep tightly closed
- avoid excessive heat (over 104°F or 40°C)
- protect from freezing

Total salicylate per tablespoon: 236 mg

## INACTIVE INGREDIENTS
benzoic acid, flavor, magnesium aluminum silicate, methyl cellulose, purified water, D&C red 22, D&C red 28, saccharin sodium, salicylic acid, sodium salicylate, sorbic acid

## QUESTIONS OR COMMENTS
Visit www.peptic-drug-facts.com

---

# PEPTIC RELIEF (bismuth subsalicylate) suspension
## Aaron Industries, Inc.

## DRUG FACTS

| Active ingredients | Purpose |
| --- | --- |
| Bismuth subsalicylate 262 mg | Upset stomach reliever/ antidiarrheal |

## USES
- relieves:
  - upset stomach
  - heartburn
  - indigestion
  - diarrhea
  - nausea

## WARNINGS
### Reye's syndrome
Children and teenagers who have or arerecovering from chicken pox or flu-like symptoms should not use this product. When using this product, if changes in behavior with nausea or vomiting occur, consult adoctor because these symptoms could be an early sign of Reye's syndrome, a rare but serious illness.

### Allergy alert
**Contains salicylate**

## DO NOT TAKE IF YOU ARE
- taking other salicylate products
- allergic to salicylates (including aspirin)

## DO NOT USE IF YOU HAVE
- an ulcer
- a bleeding problem
- bloody or black stool

## ASK A DOCTOR BEFORE USE IF YOU HAVE
- fever
- mucus in stool

## ASK A DOCTOR OR PHARMACIST BEFORE USE IF YOU ARE
- taking any drug for:
  - anticoagulation (thinning blood)
  - diabetes
  - gout
  - arthritis

## WHEN USING THIS PRODUCT
- a temporary, but harmless, darkening of the stool and/or tongue may occur

## STOP USE AND ASK A DOCTOR IF
- symptoms get worse
- ringing in the ears or loss of hearing occurs
- diarrhea lasts more than 2 days

**If pregnant or breastfeeding,** ask a health professional before use.

**Keep this and all drugs out of the reach of children.** In case of accidental overdose, seek professional assistance or contact a Poison Control Center immediately.

## DIRECTIONS
- shake well before use
- for accurate dosing, use dose cup
- drink plenty of clear fluids to help prevent dehydration caused by diarrhea

| adults and children 12 years and over | 1 dose (2 tablespoons or 30 ml) every ½ to 1 hour as needed |
| | do not exceed 8 doses (16 tablespoons or 240 ml) in 24 hours |
| | use until diarrhea stops but not more than 2 days |
| children under 12 years | ask a doctor |

## OTHER INFORMATION
- each tablespoon contains: sodium 6 mg
- sugar free
- low sodium
- keep tightly closed
- avoid excessive heat (over 104°F or 40°C)
- protect from freezing

Total salicylate per tablespoon: 130 mg

## INACTIVE INGREDIENTS
benzoic acid, flavor, magnesium aluminum silicate, methyl cellulose, purified water, D&C red 22, D&C red 28, saccharin sodium, salicylic acid, sodium salicylate, sorbic acid

## QUESTIONS OR COMMENTS
visit www.peptic-drug-facts.com

---

# PEPTO-BISMOL (bismuth subsalicylate) caplet
## Procter & Gamble Manufacturing Company

## DRUG FACTS

| Active ingredient (in each caplet) | Purpose |
| --- | --- |
| Bismuth subsalicylate 262 mg | Upset stomach reliever and antidiarrheal |

## USES
- relieves:
  - travelers' diarrhea
  - diarrhea
- upset stomach due to overindulgence in food and drink, including:
  - heartburn
  - indigestion
  - nausea
  - gas
  - belching
  - fullness

## WARNINGS
**Reye's syndrome**
Children and teenagers who have or are recovering from chicken pox or flu-like symptoms should not use this product. If changes in behavior with nausea and vomiting occur, consult a doctor because these symptoms could be an early sign of Reye's syndrome, a rare but serious illness

**Allergy alert**
Contains salicylate. Do not take if you are allergic to salicylates (including aspirin) or are taking other salicylate products.

## DO NOT USE IF YOU HAVE
- an ulcer
- a bleeding problem
- bloody or black stool

## ASK A DOCTOR BEFORE USE IF YOU HAVE
- fever
- mucus in the stool

## ASK A DOCTOR OR PHARMACIST BEFORE USE IF YOU ARE
- taking any drug for:
  - anticoagulation (thinning the blood)
  - diabetes
  - gout
  - arthritis

## WHEN USING THIS PRODUCT
- a temporary, but harmless, darkening of the stool and/or tongue may occur

## STOP USE AND ASK A DOCTOR IF
- symptoms get worse or last more than 2 days
- ringing in the ears or loss of hearing occurs
- diarrhea lasts more than 2 days

**If pregnant or breastfeeding,** ask a health professional before use.

**Keep out of reach of children.** In case of overdose, get medical help or contact a Poison Control Center right away.

## DIRECTIONS
- swallow with water, do not chew
- drink plenty of clear fluids to help prevent dehydration caused by diarrhea

| adults and children 12 years and over | 2 caplets every ½ to 1 hour as needed |
| | do not exceed 8 doses (16 caplets) in 24 hours |
| | use until diarrhea stops but not more than 2 days |
| children under 12 years | ask a doctor |

## OTHER INFORMATION
- each caplet contains: calcium 27 mg, sodium 3 mg, salicylate 99 mg
- low sodium
- sugar free
- avoid excessive heat (over 104°F or 40°C)

## INACTIVE INGREDIENTS
calcium carbonate, magnesium stearate, mannitol, microcrystalline cellulose, polysorbate 80, povidone, D&C red 27 aluminum lake, silicon dioxide, sodium starch glycolate

## QUESTIONS OR COMMENTS
Call **1-800-717-3786** or visit www.pepto-bismol.com

# PEPTO-BISMOL CHERRY CHEWABLE TABLETS (bismuth subsalicylate) tablet
Procter & Gamble Manufacturing Company

## DRUG FACTS

| Active ingredient (in each tablet) | Purpose |
|---|---|
| Bismuth subsalicylate 262 mg | Upset stomach reliever and antidiarrheal |

### USES
- relieves:
  - heartburn
  - indigestion
  - upset stomach
  - nausea
  - diarrhea
- traveler's diarrhea and gas, belching, and fullness due to overindulgence in food and drink

### WARNINGS
**Reye's syndrome**
Children and teenagers who have or are recovering from chicken pox or flulike symptoms should not use this product. When using this product, if changes in behavior with nausea or vomiting occur, consult a doctor because these symptoms could be an early sign of Reye's syndrome, a rare but serious illness.

**Allergy alert**
Contains salicylate. Do not take if you are allergic to salicylates (including aspirin) or are taking other salicylate products.

### DO NOT USE IF YOU HAVE
- an ulcer
- a bleeding problem
- bloody or black stool

### ASK A DOCTOR BEFORE USE IF YOU HAVE
- fever
- mucus in the stool

### ASK A DOCTOR OR PHARMACIST BEFORE USE IF YOU ARE
- taking any drug for:
  - anticoagulation (thinning the blood)
  - diabetes
  - gout
  - arthritis

### WHEN USING THIS PRODUCT
- a temporary, but harmless, darkening of the stool and/or tongue may occur

### STOP USE AND ASK A DOCTOR IF
- symptoms get worse
- ringing in the ears or loss of hearing occurs
- diarrhea lasts more than 2 days

**If pregnant or breastfeeding,** ask a health professional before use.

**Keep out of reach of children.** In case of overdose, get medical help or contact a Poison Control Center right away.

### DIRECTIONS
- chew or dissolve in mouth
- drink plenty of clear fluids to help prevent dehydration caused by diarrhea

| | |
|---|---|
| adults and children 12 years and over | 2 tablets every ½ to 1 hour as needed |
| | do not exceed 8 doses (16 tablets) in 24 hours |
| | use until diarrhea stops, but not more than 2 days |
| children under 12 years | ask a doctor |

### OTHER INFORMATION
- each tablet contains: sodium less than 1 mg, salicylate 99 mg
- very low sodium
- sugar free
- avoid excessive heat (more than 104°F or 40°C)

### INACTIVE INGREDIENTS
adipic acid, calcium carbonate, flavor, magnesium stearate, mannitol, povidone, D&C red no. 27 aluminum lake, FD&C red no. 40 aluminum lake, saccharin sodium, talc

### QUESTIONS OR COMMENTS
Call **1-800-717-3786**

# PEPTO-BISMOL CHERRY LIQUID (bismuth subsalicylate) liquid
Procter & Gamble Manufacturing Company

## DRUG FACTS

| Active ingredient (in each 15 ml tablespoon) | Purpose |
|---|---|
| Bismuth subsalicylate 262 mg | Upset stomach reliever and antidiarrheal |

### USES
- relieves:
  - heartburn
  - indigestion
  - upset stomach
  - nausea
  - diarrhea
- traveler's diarrhea and gas, belching, and fullness due to overindulgence in food and drink

### WARNINGS
**Reye's syndrome**
Children and teenagers who have or are recovering from chicken pox or flulike symptoms should not use this product. When using this product, if changes in behavior with nausea or vomiting occur, consult a doctor because these symptoms could be an early sign of Reye's syndrome, a rare but serious illness.

**Allergy alert**
Contains salicylate. Do not take if you are allergic to salicylates (including aspirin) or are taking other salicylate products.

### DO NOT USE IF YOU HAVE
- an ulcer
- a bleeding problem
- bloody or black stool

### ASK A DOCTOR BEFORE USE IF YOU HAVE
- fever
- mucus in the stool

**ASK A DOCTOR OR PHARMACIST BEFORE USE IF YOU ARE**
- taking any drug for:
  - anticoagulation (thinning the blood)
  - diabetes
  - gout
  - arthritis

**WHEN USING THIS PRODUCT**
- a temporary, but harmless, darkening of the stool and/or tongue may occur

**STOP USE AND ASK A DOCTOR IF**
- symptoms get worse
- ringing in the ears or loss of hearing occurs
- diarrhea lasts more than 2 days

**If pregnant or breastfeeding,** ask a health professional before use.

**Keep out of reach of children.** In case of overdose, get medical help or contact a Poison Control Center right away.

**DIRECTIONS**
- shake well before use
- for accurate dosing, use dose cup
- drink plenty of clear fluids to help prevent dehydration caused by diarrhea

| adults and children 12 years and over | 1 dose (2 tbsp or 30 ml) every ½ to 1 hour as needed<br><br>do not exceed 8 doses (16 tbsp or 240 ml) in 24 hours<br><br>use until diarrhea stops, but not more than 2 days |
|---|---|
| children under 12 years | ask a doctor |

**OTHER INFORMATION**
- each tbsp contains: sodium 6 mg
- low sodium
- sugar free
- protect from freezing
- avoid excessive heat (more than 104°F or 40°C)

**INACTIVE INGREDIENTS**
benzoic acid, flavor, magnesium aluminum silicate, methylcellulose, D&C red no. 22, D&C red no. 28, saccharin sodium, salicylic acid, sodium salicylate, sorbic acid, sucralose, water

**QUESTIONS OR COMMENTS**
Call 1-800-717-3786

---

# PEPTO-BISMOL INSTACOOL (bismuth subsalicylate) tablet, chewable
The Procter & Gamble Manufacturing Company

## DRUG FACTS

| Active ingredient (in each tablet) | Purpose |
|---|---|
| Bismuth subsalicylate 262 mg | Upset stomach reliever and antidiarrheal |

**USES**
- relieves:
  - travelers' diarrhea
  - diarrhea
- upset stomach due to overindulgence in food and drink, including:
  - heartburn
  - indigestion
  - nausea
  - gas
  - belching
  - fullness

**WARNINGS**
**Reye's syndrome**
Children and teenagers who have or are recovering from chicken pox or flu-like symptoms should not use this product. When using this product, if changes in behavior with nausea and vomiting occur, consult a doctor because these symptoms could be an early sign of Reye's syndrome, a rare but serious illness.

**Allergy alert**
Contains salicylate. Do not take if you are allergic to salicylates (including aspirin) or are taking other salicylate products.

**DO NOT USE IF YOU HAVE**
- an ulcer
- a bleeding problem
- bloody or black stool

**ASK A DOCTOR BEFORE USE IF YOU HAVE**
- fever
- mucus in the stool

**ASK A DOCTOR OR PHARMACIST BEFORE USE IF YOU ARE**
- taking any drug for:
  - anticoagulation (thinning the blood)
  - diabetes
  - gout
  - arthritis

**WHEN USING THIS PRODUCT**
- a temporary, but harmless, darkening of the stool and/or tongue may occur

**STOP USE AND ASK A DOCTOR IF**
- symptoms get worse or last more than 2 days
- ringing in the ears or loss of hearing occurs
- diarrhea lasts more than 2 days

**If pregnant or breastfeeding,** ask a health professional before use.

**Keep out of reach of children.** In case of overdose, get medical help or contact a Poison Control Center right away.

**DIRECTIONS**
- chew or dissolve in mouth
- drink plenty of clear fluids to help prevent dehydration caused by diarrhea

| adults and children 12 years and over | 2 tablets every ½ to 1 hour as needed<br><br>do not exceed 8 doses (16 tablets) in 24 hours<br><br>use until diarrhea stops but not more than 2 days |
|---|---|
| children under 12 years | ask a doctor |

## OTHER INFORMATION

- each tablet contains: calcium 85 mg, sodium less than 1 mg, salicylate 100 mg
- very low sodium
- sugar free
- avoid excessive heat (over 104°F or 40°C)

## INACTIVE INGREDIENTS

calcium carbonate, flavor, magnesium stearate, mannitol, povidone, D&C red no. 27 aluminum lake, saccharin sodium, talc

## QUESTIONS OR COMMENTS

Call **1-800-717-3786**

---

# PERCOGESIC ORIGINAL STRENGTH
(acetaminophen and diphenhydramine hydrochloride) tablet, coated

Medtech Products Inc.

## DRUG FACTS

| Active ingredients (in each tablet) | Purpose |
|---|---|
| Acetaminophen 325 mg | Pain reliever/fever reducer |
| Diphenhydramine hydrochloride 12.5 mg | Antihistamine |

## USES

- for temporary relief of minor aches and pains due to:
  - headache
  - backache
  - muscular aches
  - arthritis pain
  - colds
  - flu
  - fever
  - toothache
  - premenstrual and menstrual cramps

## WARNINGS
**Liver Warning**
This product contains acetaminophen. Severe liver damage may occur if:

- adult or child 12 years and older takes more than 8 tablets in 24 hours, which is the maximum daily amount
- taken with other drugs containing acetaminophen
- adult has 3 or more alcoholic drinks every day while using this product

## ASK A DOCTOR BEFORE USE

- if the user has liver disease

## DO NOT USE

- with any other drug containing acetaminophen (prescription or nonprescription). If you are not sure whether a drug contains acetaminophen, ask a doctor or pharmacist

## ASK A DOCTOR OR PHARMACIST BEFORE USE

- if the user is taking the blood thinning drug warfarin

## ASK A DOCTOR OR PHARMACIST BEFORE USE

- if you are taking sedatives or tranquilizers

## WHEN USING THIS PRODUCT

- marked drowsiness may occur
- avoid alcoholic beverages
- alcohol, sedatives, and tranquilizers may cause drowsiness
- may cause excitability, especially in children
- be careful driving a motor vehicle or operating machinery

## STOP USE AND ASK A DOCTOR IF

- pain persists for more than 10 days
- fever persists for more than 3 days (unless directed by a doctor)
- condition worsens or new symptoms occur
- redness or swelling is present. These may be signs of a serious condition

**If you are pregnant or nursing a baby**, seek the advice of a health care professional before using this product.

**Keep this and all drugs out of the reach of children.**

## OVERDOSE WARNING

Taking more than the recommended dose (overdose) could cause serious health problems, including liver damage. In case of overdose, get medical help or contact a Poison Control Center right away. Prompt medical attention is critical for adults as well as children even if you do not notice any signs or symptoms. Do not exceed the recommended dosage.

## DIRECTIONS

| adults and children 12 years and older | take 1 or 2 tablets every 4 hours. Maximum daily dose is 8 tablets. |
|---|---|
| children under 12 years of age | do not use |

## OTHER INFORMATION

- store at controlled room temperature 15-30°C (59-86°F)
- avoid excessive heat
- keep carton for complete product information

## INACTIVE INGREDIENTS

croscarmellose sodium, FD&C yellow no. 6 lake, hypromellose, magnesium silicate, magnesium stearate, microcrystalline cellulose, mineral oil, polyethylene glycol, polyvinylpyrrolidone, pregelatinized starch, silica, sodium starch glycolate and stearic acid

## QUESTIONS OR COMMENTS

Call **1-800-443-4908**

---

# PERI-COLACE TABLETS (docusate sodium and sennosides) tablet

Purdue Products LP

## DRUG FACTS

| Active ingredients | Purpose |
|---|---|
| Docusate sodium 50 mg | Stool softener |
| Sennosides 8.6 mg | Laxative |

## USES

- for overnight relief from occasional constipation (irregularity)
- generally produce bowel movement in 6 to 12 hours
- relieve occasional constipation (irregularity)

## WARNINGS

- use laxatives for no longer than seven (7) days, unless directed otherwise by a doctor
- do not use if you are presently taking mineral oil unless told to do so by a doctor

**ASK A DOCTOR BEFORE USE IF YOU HAVE**
- stomach pain
- nausea
- vomiting
- noticed a sudden change in bowel habits that lasts over two weeks

**STOP USE AND ASK A DOCTOR IF YOU HAVE**
- rectal bleeding
- fail to have a bowel movement after use of a laxative. These could be signs of a serious condition.

**If pregnant or breastfeeding,** ask a health professional before use.

**Keep out of reach of children.** In case of overdose, get medical help or contact a Poison Control Center right away.

**OTHER INFORMATION**
- each tablet contains: 50 mg docusate sodium and 8.6 mg sennosides
- tablets: 10s, 30s, 60s

**RECOMMENDED DOSES**
- take only by mouth
- doses may be taken as a single daily dose, preferable in the evening, or in divided doses

| adults and children 12 years of age and older | take 2-4 tablets daily |
| children 6 to under 12 years | take 1-2 tablets daily |
| children 2 to under 6 years of age | take up to 1 tablet daily |
| children under 2 | ask a doctor |

## PERSA-GEL 10 (benzoyl peroxide)
Johnson & Johnson Consumer Companies, Inc

### DRUG FACTS

| Active ingredients | Purpose |
| --- | --- |
| Benzoyl peroxide 10 % | Acne medication |

**USE**
- for the treatment of acne

**WARNING**
**For external use only.**

**DO NOT USE**
- if you have very sensitive skin
- if you are sensitive to benzoyl peroxide

**WHEN USING THIS PRODUCT**
- keep away from eyes, lips and mouth
- avoid unnecessary sun exposure and use a sunscreen
- avoid contact with hair or dyed fabric, including carpet and clothing which may be bleached by this product
- skin irritation may occur, characterized by redness, burning, itching, peeling, or possibly swelling. Mild irritation may be reduced by using the product less frequently or in a lower concentration. If irritation becomes severe, discontinue use; if irritation still continues, consult a doctor
- using other topical acne medications at the same time or immediately following the use of this product may increase dryness or irritation of the skin. If this occurs, only one medication should be used unless directed by a doctor

**Keep out of reach of children.** If swallowed, get medical help or contact a Poison Control Center right away.

**DIRECTIONS**
- cleanse the skin thoroughly before applying medication
- cover the entire affected area with a thin layer 1-3 times daily
- if bothersome dryness or peeling occurs, reduce application to once a day

**OTHER INFORMATION**
- keep tightly closed
- avoid storing at extreme temperatures (below 40°F-above 100°F)

**INACTIVE INGREDIENTS**
carbomer, disodium EDTA, hydroxypropyl methylcellulose, laureth-4, sodium hydroxide, water

## PHAZYME (simethicone) capsule, gelatin coated
GlaxoSmithKline Consumer Healthcare LP

### DRUG FACTS

| Active ingredient (in each softgel) | Purpose |
| --- | --- |
| Simethicone 180 mg | Anti-gas |

**USE**
- relieves bloating, pressure or fullness commonly referred to as gas

**WARNINGS**
**Keep out of reach of children.**

**STOP USE AND ASK A DOCTOR**
- if condition persists

**DIRECTIONS**
- swallow one or two softgels as needed after a meal
- do not exceed two softgels per day except under the advice and supervision of a physician

**OTHER INFORMATION**
- store at room temperature 59-86°F (15-30°C)

**INACTIVE INGREDIENTS**
FD&C yellow no. 6, gelatin, glycerin, white edible ink

**QUESTIONS OR COMMENTS**
Call toll-free **1-866-255-5204** (English/Spanish) weekdays

## PLAN B ONE-STEP (levonorgestrel) tablet
Duramed Pharmaceuticals, Inc.

**INDICATIONS AND USAGE**
- plan B One-Step is a progestin-only emergency contraceptive indicated for prevention of pregnancy following unprotected intercourse or a known or suspected contraceptive failure. To obtain optimal efficacy, the tablet should be taken as soon as possible within 72 hours of intercourse
- plan B One-Step is available only by prescription for women younger than age 17 years, and available over the counter for women 17 years and older
- plan B One-Step is not indicated for routine use as a contraceptive

- plan B One-Step is a progestin-only emergency contraceptive indicated for prevention of pregnancy following unprotected intercourse or a known or suspected contraceptive failure. Plan B One-Step is available only by prescription for women younger than age 17 years, and available over the counter for women 17 years and older. Plan B One-Step is not intended for routine use as a contraceptive. (1)

## DOSAGE AND ADMINISTRATION
- take Plan B One-Step orally as soon as possible within 72 hours after unprotected intercourse or a known or suspected contraceptive failure. Efficacy is better if the tablet is taken as soon as possible after unprotected intercourse. Plan B One-Step can be used at any time during the menstrual cycle
- if vomiting occurs within two hours of taking the tablet, consideration should be given to repeating the dose
- one tablet taken orally as soon as possible within 72 hours after unprotected intercourse. Efficacy is better if the tablet is taken as soon as possible after unprotected intercourse. (2)

## DOSAGE FORMS AND STRENGTHS
- the Plan B One-Step tablet is supplied as an almost white, round tablet containing 1.5 mg of levonorgestrel and is marked G00 on one side
- 1.5 mg tablet (3)

## CONTRAINDICATIONS
- plan B One-Step is contraindicated for use in the case of known or suspected pregnancy
- known or suspected pregnancy (4)

## WARNINGS AND PRECAUTIONS
- ectopic pregnancy: Women who become pregnant or complain of lower abdominal pain after taking Plan B One-Step should be evaluated for ectopic pregnancy. (5.1)
- plan B One-Step is not effective in terminating an existing pregnancy. (5.2)
- effect on menses: Plan B One-Step may alter the next expected menses. If menses is delayed beyond 1 week, pregnancy should be considered. (5.3)
- STI/HIV: Plan B One-Step does not protect against STI/HIV. (5.4)

### Ectopic pregnancy
- ectopic pregnancies account for approximately 2% of all reported pregnancies. Up to 10% of pregnancies reported in clinical studies of routine use of progestin-only contraceptives are ectopic
- a history of ectopic pregnancy is not a contraindication to use of this emergency contraceptive method. Healthcare providers, however, should consider the possibility of an ectopic pregnancy in women who become pregnant or complain of lower abdominal pain after taking Plan B One-Step. A follow-up physical or pelvic examination is recommended if there is any doubt concerning the general health or pregnancy status of any woman after taking Plan B One-Step

### Existing pregnancy
Plan B One-Step is not effective in terminating an existing pregnancy.

### Effects on menses
- some women may experience spotting a few days after taking Plan B One-Step. Menstrual bleeding patterns are often irregular among women using progestin-only oral contraceptives and women using levonorgestrel for postcoital and emergency contraception
- if there is a delay in the onset of expected menses beyond 1 week, consider the possibility of pregnancy

### STI/HIV
Plan B One-Step does not protect against HIV infection (AIDS) or other sexually transmitted infections (STIs).

### Physical examination and follow-up
A physical examination is not required prior to prescribing Plan B One-Step. A follow-up physical or pelvic examination is recommended if there is any doubt concerning the general health or pregnancy status of any woman after taking Plan B One-Step.

### Fertility following discontinuation
A rapid return of fertility is likely following treatment with Plan B One-Step for emergency contraception; therefore, routine contraception should be continued or initiated as soon as possible following use of Plan B One-Step to ensure ongoing prevention of pregnancy.

## ADVERSE REACTIONS
- the most common adverse reactions (≥10%) in clinical trials included heavier menstrual bleeding (31%), nausea (14%), lower abdominal pain (13%), fatigue (13%), headache (10%), and dizziness (10%). (6.1)
- to report SUSPECTED ADVERSE REACTIONS, contact Barr Laboratories at 1-800-330-1271 or FDA at 1-800-FDA-1088 or www.fda.gov/medwatch

### Clinical trials experience
- because clinical trials are conducted under widely varying conditions, adverse reaction rates observed in the clinical trials of a drug cannot be directly compared to rates in the clinical trials of another drug and may not reflect the rates observed in clinical practice
- plan B One-Step was studied in a randomized, double-blinded multicenter clinical trial. In this study, all women who had received at least one dose of study medication were included in the safety analysis: 1,379 women in the Plan B One-Step group, and 1,377 women in the Plan B group (2 doses of 0.75 mg levonorgestrel taken 12 hours apart). The mean age of women given Plan B One-Step was 27 years. The racial demographic of those enrolled was 54% Chinese, 12% Other Asian or Black, and 34% were Caucasian in each treatment group. 1.6% of women in the Plan B One-Step group and 1.4% in Plan B group were lost to follow-up
- The most common adverse events (>10%) in the clinical trial for women receiving Plan B One-Step included heavier menstrual bleeding (30.9%), nausea (13.7%), lower abdominal pain (13.3%), fatigue (13.3%), and headache (10.3%). Table 1 lists those adverse events that were reported in > 4% of Plan B One-Step users

**Table 1. Adverse Events in > 4% of Women, by % Frequency**

| Most Common Adverse Events (MedDRA) | Plan B One-Step N = 1359 (%) |
|---|---|
| Heavier menstrual bleeding | 30.9 |
| Nausea | 13.7 |
| Lower abdominal pain | 13.3 |
| Fatigue | 13.3 |
| Headache | 10.3 |
| Dizziness | 9.6 |
| Breast tenderness | 8.2 |
| Delay of menses (> 7 days) | 4.5 |

## Postmarketing experience

The following adverse reactions have been identified during post-approval use of Plan B (2 doses of 0.75 mg levonorgestrel taken 12 hours apart). Because these reactions are reported voluntarily from a population of uncertain size, it is not always possible to reliably estimate their frequency or establish a causal relationship to drug exposure.

### Gastrointestinal disorders
Abdominal Pain, Nausea, Vomiting

### General disorders and administration site conditions
Fatigue

### Nervous system disorders
Dizziness, Headache

### Reproductive system and breast disorders
Dysmenorrhea, Irregular Menstruation, Oligomenorrhea, Pelvic Pain

## DRUG INTERACTIONS

Drugs or herbal products that induce enzymes, including CYP3A4, that metabolize progestins may decrease the plasma concentrations of progestins, and may decrease the effectiveness of progestin-only pills. Some drugs or herbal products that may decrease the effectiveness of progestin-only pills include:

- barbiturates
- bosentan
- carbamazepine
- felbamate
- griseofulvin
- oxcarbazepine
- phenytoin
- rifampin
- St. John's wort
- topiramate

Significant changes (increase or decrease) in the plasma levels of the progestin have been noted in some cases of co-administration with HIV protease inhibitors or with non-nucleoside reverse transcriptase inhibitors.

Consult the labeling of all concurrently used drugs to obtain further information about interactions with progestin-only pills or the potential for enzyme alterations.

Drugs or herbal products that induce certain enzymes, such as CYP3A4, may decrease the effectiveness of progestin-only pills. (7)

## USE IN SPECIFIC POPULATIONS

- Nursing Mothers: Small amounts of progestin pass into the breast milk of nursing women taking progestin-only pills for long-term contraception, resulting in detectable steroid levels in infant plasma. (8.3)
- Plan B One-Step is not intended for use in premenarcheal (8.4) or postmenopausal females (8.5)

### Pregnancy
Many studies have found no harmful effects on fetal development associated with long-term use of contraceptive doses of oral progestins. The few studies of infant growth and development that have been conducted with progestin-only pills have not demonstrated significant adverse effects.

### Nursing mothers
In general, no adverse effects of progestin-only pills have been found on breastfeeding performance or on the health, growth, or development of the infant. However, isolated post-marketing cases of decreased milk production have been reported. Small amounts of progestins pass into the breast milk of nursing mothers taking progestin-only pills for long-term contraception, resulting in detectable steroid levels in infant plasma.

### Pediatric use
Safety and efficacy of progestin-only pills for long-term contraception have been established in women of reproductive age. Safety and efficacy are expected to be the same for postpubertal adolescents less than 17 years and for users 17 years and older. Use of Plan B One-Step emergency contraception before menarche is not indicated.

### Geriatric use
This product is not intended for use in postmenopausal women.

### Race
No formal studies have evaluated the effect of race. However, clinical trials demonstrated a higher pregnancy rate in Chinese women with both Plan B and the Yuzpe regimen (another form of emergency contraception). There was a non-statistically significant increased rate of pregnancy among Chinese women in the Plan B One-Step trial. The reason for this apparent increase in the pregnancy rate with emergency contraceptives in Chinese women is unknown.

### Hepatic impairment
No formal studies were conducted to evaluate the effect of hepatic disease on the disposition of Plan B One-Step.

### Renal impairment
No formal studies were conducted to evaluate the effect of renal disease on the disposition of Plan B One-Step.

## DRUG ABUSE AND DEPENDENCE

Levonorgestrel is not a controlled substance. There is no information about dependence associated with the use of Plan B One-Step.

## OVERDOSAGE

There are no data on overdosage of Plan B One-Step, although the common adverse event of nausea and associated vomiting may be anticipated.

## DESCRIPTION

The Plan B One-Step tablet contains 1.5 mg of a single active steroid ingredient, levonorgestrel [18,19-Dinorpregn-4-en-20-yn-3-one-13-ethyl-17-hydroxy-, (17 α)-(-)-], a totally synthetic progestogen. The inactive ingredients are colloidal silicon dioxide, corn starch, lactose monohydrate, magnesium stearate, potato starch, and talc.

Levonorgestrel has a molecular weight of 312.45, and the following structural and molecular formulas: $C_{21}H_{28}O_2$ Levonorgestrel Structural Formula

## CLINICAL PHARMACOLOGY

### Mechanism of action
Emergency contraceptive pills are not effective if a woman is already pregnant. Plan B One-Step is believed to act as an emergency contraceptive principally by preventing ovulation or fertilization (by altering tubal transport of sperm and/or ova). In addition, it may inhibit implantation (by altering the endometrium). It is not effective once the process of implantation has begun.

### Pharmacokinetics
### Absorption
Following a single dose administration of Plan B One-Step in 30 women under fasting conditions, maximum plasma concentrations of levonorgestrel of 19.1 ng/mL were reached at 1.7 hours. See Table 2.

Table 2. Pharmacokinetic Parameter Values Following Single Dose Administration of Plan B One-Step (levonorgestrel) tablet 1.5 mg to 30 Healthy Female Volunteers under Fasting Conditions

| | Mean (± SD) | | | | |
| | $C_{max}$ (ng/mL) | $AUC_t$ (ng·hr/mL)* | $AUC_{inf}$ (ng·hr/mL)* | $T_{max}$ (hr)† | $t_{1/2}$ (hr) |
|---|---|---|---|---|---|
| Levonorgestrel | 19.1 (9.7) | 294.8 (208.8) | 307.5 (218.5) | 1.7 (1.0-4.0) | 27.5 (5.6) |

$C_{max}$ = maximum concentration

$AUC_t$ = area under the drug concentration curve from time 0 to time of last determinable concentration

$AUC_{inf}$ = area under the drug concentration curve from time 0 to infinity

$T_{max}$ = time to maximum concentration
$t_{1/2}$ = elimination half life

*N=29

† median (range)

Effect of Food: The effect of food on the rate and the extent of levonorgestrel absorption following single oral administration of Plan B One-Step has not been evaluated.

### Distribution
The apparent volume of distribution of levonorgestrel is reported to be approximately 1.8 L/kg. It is about 97.5 to 99% protein-bound, principally to sex hormone binding globulin (SHBG) and, to a lesser extent, serum albumin.

### Metabolism
Following absorption, levonorgestrel is conjugated at the 17β-OH position to form sulfate conjugates and, to a lesser extent, glucuronide conjugates in plasma. Significant amounts of conjugated and unconjugated 3α, 5β-tetrahydrolevonorgestrel are also present in plasma, along with much smaller amounts of 3α, 5α-tetrahydrolevonorgestrel and 16βhydroxylevonorgestrel. Levonorgestrel and its phase I metabolites are excreted primarily as glucuronide conjugates. Metabolic clearance rates may differ among individuals by several-fold, and this may account in part for the wide variation observed in levonorgestrel concentrations among users.

### Excretion
About 45% of levonorgestrel and its metabolites are excreted in the urine and about 32% are excreted in feces, mostly as glucuronide conjugates.

### SPECIFIC POPULATIONS
#### Pediatric
This product is not intended for use in the premenarcheal population, and pharmacokinetic data are not available for this population.

#### Geriatric
This product is not intended for use in postmenopausal women, and pharmacokinetic data are not available for this population.

#### Race
No formal studies have evaluated the effect of race. However, clinical trials demonstrated a higher pregnancy rate in Chinese women with both Plan B and the Yuzpe regimen (another form of emergency contraception). There was a non-statistically significant increased rate of pregnancy among Chinese women in the Plan B One-Step trial. The reason for this apparent increase in the pregnancy rate with emergency contraceptives in Chinese women is unknown [see USE IN SPECIFIC POPULATIONS (8.6)].

### Hepatic impairment
No formal studies were conducted to evaluate the effect of hepatic disease on the disposition of Plan B One-Step.

### Renal impairment
No formal studies were conducted to evaluate the effect of renal disease on the disposition of Plan B One-Step.

### Drug-drug interactions
No formal drug-drug interaction studies were conducted with Plan B One-Step [see DRUG INTERACTIONS (7)].

## NONCLINICAL TOXICOLOGY
### Carcinogenesis, mutagenesis, impairment of fertility
Carcinogenicity: There is no evidence of increased risk of cancer with short-term use of progestins. There was no increase in tumorgenicity following administration of levonorgestrel to rats for 2 years at approximately 5 μg/day, to dogs for 7 years at up to 0.125 mg/kg/day, or to rhesus monkeys for 10 years at up to 250 μg/kg/day. In another 7 year dog study, administration of levonorgestrel at 0.5 mg/kg/day did increase the number of mammary adenomas in treated dogs compared to controls. There were no malignancies.

Genotoxicity: Levonorgestrel was not found to be mutagenic or genotoxic in the Ames Assay, in vitro mammalian culture assays utilizing mouse lymphoma cells and Chinese hamster ovary cells, and in an in vivo micronucleus assay in mice.

Fertility: There are no irreversible effects on fertility following cessation of exposures to levonorgestrel or progestins in general.

## CLINICAL STUDIES
A double-blind, randomized, multicenter, multinational study evaluated and compared the efficacy and safety of three different regimens for emergency contraception. Subjects were enrolled at 15 sites in 10 countries; the racial/ethnic characteristics of the study population overall were 54% Chinese, 34% Caucasian, and 12% Black or Asian (other than Chinese). 2,381 healthy women with a mean age of 27 years, who needed emergency contraception within 72 hours of unprotected intercourse were involved and randomly allocated into one of the two levonorgestrel groups. A single dose of 1.5 mg of levonorgestrel (Plan B One-Step) was administered to women allocated into group 1. Two doses of 0.75 mg levonorgestrel 12 hours apart (Plan B) were administered to women in group 2. In the Plan B One-Step group, 16 pregnancies occurred in 1,198 women and in the Plan B group, 20 pregnancies occurred in 1,183 women. The number of pregnancies expected in each group was calculated based on the timing of intercourse with regard to each woman's menstrual cycle. Among women receiving Plan B One-Step, 84% of expected pregnancies were prevented and among those women taking Plan B, 79% of expected pregnancies were prevented. The expected pregnancy rate of 8% (with no contraceptive use) was reduced to approximately 1% with Plan B One-Step.

Emergency contraceptives are not as effective as routine contraception since their failure rate, while low based on a single use, would accumulate over time with repeated use [see INDICATIONS AND USAGE (1)].

In the clinical study, bleeding disturbances were the most common adverse event reported after taking the levonorgestrel-containing regimens. More than half of the women had menses within two days of the expected time; however, 31% of women experienced change in their bleeding pattern during the study period; 4.5% of women had menses more than 7 days after the expected time.

## HOW SUPPLIED/STORAGE AND HANDLING
The Plan B One-Step (levonorgestrel) tablet 1.5 mg is available in a PVC/aluminum foil blister package. The tablet is almost white, round, and marked G00 on one side.

NDC 51285-942-88 (1 tablet unit of use package)

Store Plan B One-Step at 20° to 25°C (68° to 77°F) [see USP Controlled Room Temperature].

## PATIENT COUNSELING INFORMATION
**Information for patients**
- Take Plan B One-Step as soon as possible and not more than 72 hours after unprotected intercourse or a known or suspected contraceptive failure
- If you vomit within two hours of taking the tablet, immediately contact your healthcare provider to discuss whether to take another tablet
- Seek medical attention if you experience severe lower abdominal pain 3 to 5 weeks after taking Plan B One-Step, in order to be evaluated for an ectopic pregnancy
- After taking Plan B One-Step, consider the possibility of pregnancy if your period is delayed more than one week beyond the date you expected your period
- Do not use Plan B One-Step as routine contraception
- Plan B One-Step is not effective in terminating an existing pregnancy
- Plan B One-Step does not protect against HIV-infection (AIDS) and other sexually transmitted diseases/infections
- For women younger than age 17 years, Plan B One-Step is available only by prescription

## QUESTIONS OR COMMENTS
Call **1-800-330-1271** or visit www.PlanBOneStep.com

---

# POLYSPORIN (polymyxin B sulfate and bacitracin zinc) powder
Johnson & Johnson Consumer Products Company

## DRUG FACTS

| Active ingredients (in each gram) | Purpose |
| --- | --- |
| Bacitracin 500 units | First aid antibiotic |
| Polymyxin B 10,000 units | First aid antibiotic |

## USES
- first aid to help prevent infection in minor:
  - cuts
  - scrapes
  - burns

## WARNINGS
**For external use only.**

## DO NOT USE
- if you are allergic to any of the ingredients
- in the eyes
- over large areas of the body

## ASK A DOCTOR BEFORE USE IF YOU HAVE
- deep or puncture wounds
- animal bites
- serious burns

## STOP USE AND ASK A DOCTOR IF
- you need to use longer than 1 week
- condition persists or gets worse
- rash or other allergic reaction develops

---

**Keep out of reach of children.** If swallowed, get medical help or contact a Poison Control Center right away.

## DIRECTIONS
- clean the affected area
- apply a light dusting of the powder on the area 1 to 3 times daily
- may be covered with a sterile bandage

## OTHER INFORMATION
- store at 20°C-25°C (68°F-77°F)
- do not refrigerate

## INACTIVE INGREDIENT
lactose base

## QUESTIONS OR COMMENTS
Call **1-800-223-0182**

---

# PRECISE PAIN RELIEVING CREAM (menthol and methyl salicylate) cream
McNeil Consumer Healthcare, Division of McNeil-PPC, Inc.

## DRUG FACTS

| Active ingredients | Purpose |
| --- | --- |
| Menthol 10% | Topical analgesic |
| Methyl salicylate 30% | Topical analgesic |

## USES
- temporarily relieves minor aches and pains of muscles and joints associated with:
  - simple backache
  - arthritis
  - sprains
  - bruises
  - strains

## WARNINGS
**For external use only.**

## DO NOT USE
- on wounds or damaged skin
- with a heating pad
- on a child under 12 years of age with arthritis-like conditions

## ASK A DOCTOR BEFORE USE IF YOU HAVE
- redness over the affected area

## WHEN USING THIS PRODUCT
- avoid contact with eyes or mucous membranes
- do not bandage tightly

## STOP USE AND ASK A DOCTOR IF
- condition worsens or symptoms persist for more than 7 days
- symptoms clear up and occur again within a few days
- excessive skin irritation occurs

**Keep out of reach of children.** In case of accidental ingestion, get medical help or contact a Poison Control Center right away. **(1-800-222-1222)**

## DIRECTIONS
- use only as directed

| adults and children 12 years of age and older | apply to affected area not more than 3 to 4 times daily |
|---|---|
| children under 12 years of age | ask a doctor |

## OTHER INFORMATION
- store between 20-25°C (68-77°F). Protect from freezing
- see bottom panel for lot number and expiration date

## INACTIVE INGREDIENTS
C12-15 alkyl benzoate, carbomer, cocoglycerides, distearyl ether, edetate disodium, ethylparaben, fragrance, glyceryl laurate, glyceryl stearate, methylparaben, myristyl alcohol, phenoxyethanol, propylparaben, sodium hydroxide, steareth-2, steareth-21, stearyl alcohol, water

## QUESTIONS OR COMMENTS
Call **1-877-895-3665** (English) or **1-888-466-8746** (Spanish): weekdays 9:00 AM to 4:30 PM EST

---

# PREMSYN PMS PREMENSTRUAL SYNDROME RELIEF (acetaminophen, pamabrom and pyrilamine maleate) caplet
Chattem, Inc.

## DRUG FACTS

| Active ingredients (in each caplet) | Purposes |
|---|---|
| Acetaminophen 500 mg | Pain reliever |
| Pamabrom 25 mg | Diuretic |
| Pyrilamine maleate 15 mg | Antihistamine |

## USES
- for the temporary relief of these symptoms associated with menstrual periods:
  - cramps
  - headache
  - bloating
  - backache
  - water-weight gain
  - muscular aches
  - irritability

## WARNINGS
**Liver warning**
This product contains acetaminophen. Severe liver damage may occur if you take:
- more than 8 caplets in 24 hours, which is the maximum daily amount
- with other drugs containing acetaminophen
- 3 or more alcoholic drinks every day while using this product

## DO NOT USE
- with any other drug containing acetaminophen (prescription or nonprescription). If you are not sure whether a drug contains acetaminophen, ask a doctor or pharmacist

## ASK A DOCTOR BEFORE USE IF YOU HAVE
- liver disease
- glaucoma
- a breathing problem such as emphysema or chronic bronchitis
- difficulty in urination due to enlargement of the prostate gland

## ASK A DOCTOR OR PHARMACIST BEFORE USE IF YOU ARE
- taking the blood thinning drug warfarin
- taking sedatives or tranquilizers

## WHEN USING THIS PRODUCT
- you may get drowsy, avoid alcoholic beverages
- alcohol, sedatives and tranquilizers may increase drowsiness
- use caution when driving or operating machinery
- excitability may occur, especially in children

## STOP USE AND ASK A DOCTOR IF
- pain gets worse or lasts for more than 10 days
- fever gets worse or lasts for more than 3 days
- new symptoms occur
- redness or swelling is present

**If pregnant or breastfeeding,** ask a health professional before use.

**Keep out of reach of children.** In case of overdose, get medical help or contact a Poison Control Center right away. Quick medical attention is critical for adults as well as for children even if you do not notice any signs or symptoms.

## DIRECTIONS

| adults and children 12 years and over | take 2 caplets with water every 6 hours as needed |
|---|---|
| | do not exceed 8 caplets in a 24 hour period or as directed by a doctor |
| | do not use more than directed (see warnings) |
| children under 12 years | ask a doctor |

## INACTIVE INGREDIENTS
crospovidone, magnesium stearate, povidone, pregelatinized starch, sodium starch glycolate, stearic acid (224-186)

---

# PREPARATION H COOLING GEL (phenylephrine hydrochloride, witch hazel) gel
Wyeth Consumer Healthcare

## DRUG FACTS

| Active ingredients | Purpose |
|---|---|
| Phenylephrine hydrochloride 0.25% | Vasoconstrictor |
| Witch hazel 50.0% | Astringent |

## USES
- helps relieve the local itching and discomfort associated with hemorrhoids
- temporary relief of irritation and burning
- temporarily shrinks hemorrhoidal tissue
- aids in protecting irritated anorectal areas

**WARNINGS**
**For external use only.**

**ASK A DOCTOR BEFORE USE IF YOU HAVE**
- heart disease
- high blood pressure
- thyroid disease
- diabetes
- difficulty in urination due to enlargement of the prostate gland

**ASK A DOCTOR OR PHARMACIST BEFORE USE IF YOU ARE**
- presently taking a prescription drug for high blood pressure or depression

**WHEN USING THIS PRODUCT**
- do not exceed the recommended daily dosage unless directed by a doctor
- do not put this product into the rectum by using fingers or any mechanical device or applicator

**STOP USE AND ASK A DOCTOR IF**
- bleeding occurs
- condition worsens or does not improve within 7 days

**If pregnant or breastfeeding,** ask a health professional before use.

**Keep out of reach of children.** If swallowed, get medical help or contact a Poison Control Center right away.

**DIRECTIONS**

| adults | when practical, cleanse the affected area by patting or blotting with an appropriate cleansing wipe |
| | Gently dry by patting or blotting with a tissue or a soft cloth before applying gel |
| | when first opening the tube, puncture foil seal with top end of cap |
| | apply externally to the affected area up to 4 times daily, especially at night, in the morning or after each bowel movement |
| children under 12 years of age | ask a doctor |

**OTHER INFORMATION**
- store at 20-25°C (68-77°F)

**INACTIVE INGREDIENTS**
aloe barbadensis leaf juice, edetate disodium, hydroxyethyl cellulose, methylparaben, polysorbate 80, propylene glycol, propylparaben, purified water, sodium citrate, sulisobenzone, vitamin E acetate

**QUESTIONS OR COMMENTS**
Call weekdays 9 AM to 5 PM EST at **1-800-99 PrepH** or **1-800-997-7374.**

# PREPARATION H HEMORRHOIDAL OINTMENT (mineral oil, petrolatum, phenylephrine hydrochloride) ointment

Pfizer Consumer Healthcare

## DRUG FACTS

| Active ingredients | Purpose |
|---|---|
| Mineral oil 14% | Protectant |
| Petrolatum 71.9% | Protectant |
| Phenylephrine hydrochloride 0.25% | Vasoconstrictor |

**USES**
- helps relieve the local itching and discomfort associated with hemorrhoids
- temporarily shrinks hemorrhoidal tissue and relieves burning
- temporarily provides a coating for relief of anorectal discomforts
- temporarily protects the inflamed, irritated anorectal surface to help make bowel movements less painful

**WARNINGS**
**For external and/or intrarectal use only.**

**ASK A DOCTOR BEFORE USE IF YOU HAVE**
- heart disease
- high blood pressure
- thyroid disease
- diabetes
- difficulty in urination due to enlargement of the prostate gland

**ASK A DOCTOR OR PHARMACIST BEFORE USE IF YOU ARE**
- presently taking a prescription drug for high blood pressure or depression

**WHEN USING THIS PRODUCT**
- do not exceed the recommended daily dosage unless directed by a doctor

**STOP USE AND ASK A DOCTOR IF**
- bleeding occurs
- condition worsens or does not improve within 7 days
- introduction of applicator into the rectum causes additional pain

**If pregnant or breastfeeding,** ask a health professional before use.

**Keep out of reach of children.** If swallowed, get medical help or contact a Poison Control Center right away.

## DIRECTIONS

| adults | when practical, cleanse the affected area by patting or blotting with an appropriate cleansing wipe. Gently dry by patting or blotting with a tissue or a soft cloth before applying ointment |
| | when first opening the tube, puncture foil seal with top end of cap |
| | apply to the affected area up to 4 times daily, especially at night, in the morning or after each bowel movement |
| | intrarectal use: remove cover from applicator, attach applicator to tube, lubricate applicator well and gently insert applicator into the rectum |
| | thoroughly cleanse applicator after each use and replace cover |
| | also apply ointment to external area |
| | regular use provides continual therapy for relief of symptoms |
| children under 12 years of age | ask a doctor |

## OTHER INFORMATION
- store at 20-25°C (68-77°F)

## INACTIVE INGREDIENTS
benzoic acid, butylated hydroxyanisole, corn oil, glycerin, lanolin, lanolin alcohols, methylparaben, mineral oil, paraffin, propylparaben, purified water, shark liver oil, thymus vulgaris (thyme) flower/leaf oil, tocopherols excipient, white wax

## QUESTIONS OR COMMENTS
Call weekdays 9 AM to 5 PM EST at **1-800-99PrepH** or **1-800-997-7374.**

---

# PREPARATION H HYDROCORTISONE
(hydrocortisone) cream
Pfizer Consumer Healthcare

## DRUG FACTS

| Active ingredient | Purpose |
|---|---|
| Hydrocortisone 1% | Anti-itch |

## USES
- temporary relief of external anal itching
- temporary relief of itching associated with minor skin irritations and rashes
- other uses of this product should be only under the advice and supervision of a doctor

## WARNINGS
**For external use only.**

## DO NOT USE
- for the treatment of diaper rash. Consult a doctor

## WHEN USING THIS PRODUCT
- avoid contact with the eyes
- do not exceed the recommended daily dosage unless directed by a doctor
- do not put into the rectum by using fingers or any mechanical device or applicator

## STOP USE AND ASK A DOCTOR IF
- bleeding occurs
- condition worsens
- symptoms persist for more than 7 days or clear up and occur again within a few days. Do not begin use of any other hydrocortisone product unless you have consulted a doctor

**Keep out of reach of children.** If swallowed, get medical help or contact a Poison Control Center right away.

## DIRECTIONS

| adults | when practical, cleanse the affected area by patting or blotting with an appropriate cleansing wipe. Gently dry by patting or blotting with a tissue or soft cloth before application of this product |
| | when first opening the tube, puncture foil seal with top end of cap |
| adults and children 12 years of age and older | apply to the affected area not more than 3 to 4 times daily |
| children under 12 years of age | do not use, consult a doctor |

## OTHER INFORMATION
- store at 20-25°C (68-77°F)

## INACTIVE INGREDIENTS
anhydrous citric acid, butylated hydroxyanisole, carboxymethylcellulose sodium, cetyl alcohol, citric acid monohydrate, edetate disodium, glycerin, glyceryl oleate, glyceryl stearate, lanolin, methylparaben, propyl gallate, propylene glycol, propylparaben, purified water, simethicone emulsion, sodium benzoate, sodium lauryl sulfate, stearyl alcohol, white petrolatum, xanthan gum

## QUESTIONS OR COMMENTS
Call weekdays 9 AM to 5 PM EST at **1-800-99PrepH** or **1-800-997-7374.**

---

# PREPARATION H MAX STRENGTH CREAM
(glycerin, petrolatum, phenylephrine hydrochloride, pramoxine hydrochloride) cream
Pfizer Consumer Healthcare

## DRUG FACTS

| Active ingredients | Purpose |
|---|---|
| Glycerin 14.4% | Protectant |
| Phenylephrine hydrochloride 0.25% | Vasoconstrictor |
| Pramoxine hydrochloride 1% | Local anesthetic |
| White petrolatum 15% | Protectant |

## USES
- for temporary relief of pain, soreness and burning
- helps relieve the local itching and discomfort associated with hemorrhoids
- temporarily shrinks hemorrhoidal tissue
- temporarily provides a coating for relief of anorectal discomforts
- temporarily protects the inflamed, irritated anorectal surface to help make bowel movements less painful

## WARNINGS
**For external use only.**

## ASK A DOCTOR BEFORE USE IF YOU HAVE
- heart disease
- high blood pressure
- thyroid disease
- diabetes
- difficulty in urination due to enlargement of the prostate gland

## ASK A DOCTOR OR PHARMACIST BEFORE USE IF YOU ARE
- presently taking a prescription drug for high blood pressure or depression

## WHEN USING THIS PRODUCT
- do not exceed the recommended daily dosage unless directed by a doctor
- do not put into the rectum by using fingers or any mechanical device or applicator

## STOP USE AND ASK A DOCTOR IF
- bleeding occurs
- condition worsens or does not improve within 7 days
- an allergic reaction develops
- the symptom being treated does not subside or if redness, irritation, swelling, pain, or other symptoms develop or increase

**If pregnant or breastfeeding,** ask a health professional before use.

**Keep out of reach of children.** If swallowed, get medical help or contact a Poison Control Center right away.

## DIRECTIONS

| adults | when practical, cleanse the affected area by patting or blotting with an appropriate cleansing wipe. Gently dry by patting or blotting with a tissue or a soft cloth before applying cream |
| --- | --- |
| | when first opening the tube, puncture foil seal with top end of cap |
| | apply externally or in the lower portion of the anal canal only |
| | apply externally to the affected area up to 4 times daily, especially at night, in the morning or after each bowel movement |

| Intearectal use | for application in the lower anal canal: remove cover from dispensing cap. Attach dispensing cap to tube. Lubricate dispensing cap well, then gently insert dispensing cap partway into the anus |
| --- | --- |
| | thoroughly cleanse dispensing cap after each use and replace cover |
| children under 12 years of age | ask a doctor |

## OTHER INFORMATION
- store at 20-25°C (68-77°F)

## INACTIVE INGREDIENTS
aloe barbadensis leaf extract, anhydrous citric acid, butylated hydroxyanisole, carboxymethylcellulose sodium, cetyl alcohol, citric acid monohydrate, dexpanthenol, edetate disodium, glyceryl monostearate, methylparaben, mineral oil, polyoxyl lauryl ether, polyoxyl stearyl ether, propyl gallate, propylene glycol, propylparaben, purified water, sodium benzoate, stearyl alcohol, tocopherols excipient, vitamin E acetate, xanthan gum

## QUESTIONS OR COMMENTS
Call weekdays 9 AM to 5 PM EST at **1-800-99PrepH** or **1-800-997-7374**.

---

# PREPARATION H MEDICATED WIPES (witch hazel) cloth

Wyeth Consumer Healthcare

## DRUG FACTS

| Active ingredient | Purpose |
| --- | --- |
| Witch hazel 50.0% | Astringent |

## USES
- helps relieve the local itching and discomfort associated with hemorrhoids
- temporary relief of irritation and burning
- aids in protecting irritated anorectal areas

## WARNINGS
**For external use only.**

## WHEN USING THIS PRODUCT
- do not exceed the recommended daily dosage unless directed by a doctor
- do not put this product into the rectum by using fingers or any mechanical device or applicator

## STOP USE AND ASK A DOCTOR IF
- bleeding occurs
- condition worsens or does not improve within 7 days

**If pregnant or breastfeeding,** ask a health professional before use.

**Keep out of reach of children.** If swallowed, get medical help or contact a Poison Control Center right away.

## DIRECTIONS
- open the lid on the top of the wipes pouch
- peel back wipes seal, remove completely and discard
- grab the top wipe at the edge of the center fold and pull out of pouch
- close lid after each use to retain moisture

| adults | unfold wipe and cleanse the area by gently wiping, patting or blotting. If necessary, repeat until all matter is removed from the area |
| | use up to 6 times daily or after each bowel movement and before applying topical hemorrhoidal treatments, and then discard |
| children under 12 years of age | consult a doctor |

## OTHER INFORMATION
• store at 20-25°C (68-77°F)
• for best results, flush only one or two wipes at a time

## INACTIVE INGREDIENTS
aloe barbadensis leaf juice, anhydrous citric acid, capryl/capramidopropyl betaine, diazolidinyl urea, glycerin, methylparaben, propylene glycol, propylparaben, purified water, sodium citrate

## QUESTIONS OR COMMENTS
Call weekdays 9 AM to 5 PM EST at **1-800-99PrepH** or **1-800-997-7374**.

---

# PREPARATION H SUPPOSITORIES (cocoa butter, phenylephrine hydrochloride) suppository
Pfizer Consumer Healthcare

## DRUG FACTS

| Active ingredients | Purpose |
|---|---|
| Cocoa butter 85.39% | Protectant |
| Phenylephrine hydrochloride 0.25% | Vasoconstrictor |

## USES
• helps relieve the local itching and discomfort associated with hemorrhoids
• temporarily relieves burning and shrinks hemorrhoidal tissue
• temporarily provides a coating for relief of anorectal discomforts
• temporarily protects the inflamed, irritated anorectal surface to help make bowel movements less painful

## WARNINGS
**For rectal use only.**

## ASK A DOCTOR BEFORE USE IF YOU HAVE
• heart disease
• high blood pressure
• thyroid disease
• diabetes
• difficulty in urination due to enlargement of the prostate gland

## ASK A DOCTOR OR PHARMACIST BEFORE USE IF YOU ARE
• presently taking a prescription drug for high blood pressure or depression

## WHEN USING THIS PRODUCT
• do not exceed the recommended daily dosage unless directed by a doctor

## STOP USE AND ASK A DOCTOR IF
• bleeding occurs
• condition worsens or does not improve within 7 days

**If pregnant or breastfeeding,** ask a health professional before use.

**Keep out of reach of children.** If swallowed, get medical help or contact a Poison Control Center right away.

## DIRECTIONS

| adults | when practical, cleanse the affected area by patting or blotting with an appropriate cleansing wipe. Gently dry by patting or blotting with a tissue or a soft cloth before insertion of this product |
| | detach one suppository from the strip; remove the foil wrapper before inserting into the rectum as follows: |
| | hold suppository with rounded end up |
| | as shown, carefully separate foil tabs by inserting tip of fingernail at end marked "peel down" |
| | slowly and evenly peel apart (do not tear) foil by pulling tabs down both sides, to expose the suppository |
| | remove exposed suppository from wrapper |
| | insert one suppository into the rectum up to 4 times daily, especially at night, in the morning or after each bowel movement |
| children under 12 years of age | ask a doctor |

## OTHER INFORMATION
• store at 20-25°C (68-77°F)

## INACTIVE INGREDIENTS
corn starch, methylparaben, propylparaben, shark liver oil

## QUESTIONS OR COMMENTS
Call weekdays 9 AM to 5 PM EST at **1-800-99PrepH** or **1-800-997-7374**.

---

# PREVACID 24 HR (lansoprazole) capsule, delayed release
Novartis Consumer Health, Inc.

## DRUG FACTS

| Active ingredient | Purpose |
|---|---|
| Lansoprazole 15 mg | Acid reducer |

## USES
• treats frequent heartburn (occurs 2 or more days a week)
• not intended for immediate relief of heartburn; this drug may take 1 to 4 days for full effect

## WARNINGS
**Allergy alert**
Do not use if you are allergic to lansoprazole.

## DO NOT USE
• if you have trouble or pain swallowing food, vomiting with blood, or bloody or black stools. These may be signs of a serious condition. See your doctor

## ASK A DOCTOR OR PHARMACIST BEFORE USE IF YOU ARE TAKING
- warfarin (blood-thinning medicine)
- prescription antifungal or anti-yeast medicines
- digoxin (heart medicine)
- theophylline (asthma medicine)
- tacrolimus (immune system medicine)
- atazanavir (medicine for HIV infection)

## STOP USE AND ASK A DOCTOR IF
- your heartburn continues or worsens
- you need to take this product for more than 14 days
- you need to take more than 1 course of treatment every 4 months

**If pregnant or breastfeeding,** ask a health professional before use.

**Keep out of reach of children.** In case of overdose get medical help or contact a Poison Control Center right away.

## DIRECTIONS

| adults 18 years of age and older | this product is to be used once a day (every 24 hours), every day for 14 days |
| --- | --- |
| | it may take 1 to 4 days for full effect, although some people get complete relief of symptoms within 24 hours |
| 14-day course of treatment | swallow 1 capsule with a glass of water before eating in the morning |
| | take every day for 14 days |
| | do not take more than 1 capsule a day |
| | swallow whole; do not crush or chew capsules |
| | do not use for more than 14 days unless directed by your doctor |
| repeated 14-day course (if needed) | you may repeat a 14-day course every 4 months |
| | do not take for more than 14 days or more often than every 4 months unless directed by a doctor |
| children under 18 years of age | ask a doctor before use |
| | heartburn in children may sometimes be caused by a serious condition. |

## OTHER INFORMATION
- read the directions, warnings and package insert before use
- keep the carton and package insert. They contain important information
- store at 20-25°C (68-77° F)
- keep product out of high heat and humidity
- protect product from moisture

## INACTIVE INGREDIENTS
colloidal silicon dioxide, D&C red no. 28, FD&C blue no. 1, FD&C green no. 3, FD&C red no. 40, gelatin, hydroxypropyl cellulose, low substituted hydroxypropyl cellulose, magnesium carbonate, methacrylic acid copolymer, polyethylene glycol, polysorbate 80, starch, sucrose, sugar sphere, talc, titanium dioxide

## QUESTIONS OR COMMENTS
Call **1-800-452-0051**

## PRILOSEC OTC (omeprazole magnesium) tablet, delayed release
Procter & Gamble Manufacturing Company

## DRUG FACTS

| Active ingredient (in each tablet) | Purpose |
| --- | --- |
| Omeprazole magnesium delayed-release tablet 20.6 mg (equivalent to 20 mg omeprazole) | Acid reducer |

## USES
- treats frequent heartburn (occurs 2 or more days a week)
- not intended for immediate relief of heartburn; this drug may take 1 to 4 days for full effect

## WARNINGS
**Allergy alert**
Do not use if you are allergic to omeprazole

## DO NOT USE
- if you have trouble or pain swallowing food, vomiting with blood, or bloody or black stools. These may be signs of a serious condition. See your doctor

## ASK A DOCTOR BEFORE USE IF YOU HAVE
- had heartburn over 3 months. This may be a sign of a more serious condition
- heartburn with lightheadedness, sweating or dizziness
- chest pain or shoulder pain with shortness of breath; sweating; pain spreading to arms, neck or shoulders; or lightheadedness
- frequent chest pain
- frequent wheezing, particularly with heartburn
- unexplained weight loss
- nausea or vomiting
- stomach pain

## ASK A DOCTOR OR PHARMACIST BEFORE USE IF YOU ARE TAKING
- warfarin, clopidogrel, or cilostazol (blood-thinning medicines)
- prescription antifungal or anti-yeast medicines
- diazepam (anxiety medicine)
- digoxin (heart medicine)
- tacrolimus (immune system medicine)
- prescription antiretrovirals (medicines for HIV infection)

## STOP USE AND ASK A DOCTOR IF
- your heartburn continues or worsens
- you need to take this product for more than 14 days
- you need to take more than 1 course of treatment every 4 months

**If pregnant or breastfeeding,** ask a health professional before use.

**Keep out of reach of children.** In case of overdose, get medical help or contact a Poison Control Center right away.

## DIRECTIONS

| for adults 18 years of age and older | this product is to be used once a day (every 24 hours), every day for 14 days |
| | it may take 1 to 4 days for full effect; some people get complete relief of symptoms within 24 hours |
| 14-day course of treatment | swallow 1 tablet with a glass of water before eating in the morning take every day for 14 days |
| | do not take more than 1 tablet a day |
| | do not use for more than 14 days unless directed by your doctor |
| | swallow whole. Do not chew or crush tablets. |
| repeated 14-day course (if needed) | you may repeat a 14-day course every 4 months |
| | do not take for more than 14 days or more often than every 4 months unless directed by a doctor |
| children under 18 years of age | ask a doctor. |
| | heartburn in children may sometimes be caused by a serious condition |

## OTHER INFORMATION
- read the directions and warnings before use
- keep the carton. It contains important information
- store at 20-25°C (68-77°F) and protect from moisture

## INACTIVE INGREDIENTS
glyceryl monostearate, hydroxypropyl cellulose, hypromellose, iron oxide, magnesium stearate, methacrylic acid copolymer, microcrystalline cellulose, paraffin, polyethylene glycol 6000, polysorbate 80, polyvinylpyrrolidone, sodium stearyl fumarate, starch, sucrose, talc, titanium dioxide, triethyl citrate

## QUESTIONS OR COMMENTS
Call **1-800-289-9181**

---

## PRIMATENE (ephedrine hydrochloride, guaifenesin) tablet

Wyeth Consumer Healthcare

## DRUG FACTS

| Active ingredients (in each tablet) | Purpose |
| --- | --- |
| Ephedrine hydrochloride, USP 12.5 mg | Bronchodilator |
| Guaifenesin, USP 200 mg | Expectorant |

## USES
- for temporary relief of occasional symptoms of mild asthma:
  - wheezing
  - tightness of chest
  - shortness of breath

- helps loosen phlegm (mucus) and thin bronchial secretions to rid bronchial passageways of bothersome mucus, and to make coughs more productive

## WARNINGS
**Asthma alert**
Because asthma can be life threatening, see a doctor if you:
- are not better in 60 minutes
- get worse
- need 12 tablets in any day
- use more than 8 tablets a day for more than 3 days a week
- have more than 2 asthma attacks in a week

## DO NOT USE
- unless a doctor said you have asthma
- if you are now taking a prescription monoamine oxidase inhibitor (MAOI) (certain drugs taken for depression, psychiatric or emotional conditions, or Parkinson's disease), or for 2 weeks after stopping the MAOI drug. If you do not know if your prescription drug contains an MAOI, ask a doctor or pharmacist before taking this product

## ASK A DOCTOR BEFORE USE IF YOU HAVE
- ever been hospitalized for asthma
- heart disease
- high blood pressure
- diabetes
- thyroid disease
- seizures
- narrow angle glaucoma
- a psychiatric or emotional condition
- trouble urinating due to an enlarged prostate gland
- cough that occurs with too much phlegm (mucus)
- cough that lasts or is chronic such as occurs with smoking, asthma, chronic bronchitis, or emphysema

## ASK A DOCTOR OR PHARMACIST BEFORE USE IF YOU ARE
- taking prescription drugs for asthma, obesity, weight control, depression, or psychiatric or emotional conditions
- taking any drug that contains phenylephrine, pseudoephedrine, ephedrine, or caffeine (such as for allergy, cough-cold, or pain)

## STOP USE AND ASK A DOCTOR IF
- cough lasts more than 7 days, comes back, or is accompanied by fever, rash, or persistent headache. These could be signs of a serious condition

## WHEN USING THIS PRODUCT
- increased blood pressure or heart rate can occur, which could lead to more serious problems such as heart attack and stroke. Your risk may increase if you take more frequently or more than the recommended dose
- nervousness, sleeplessness, rapid heart beat, tremor, and seizure may occur. If these symptoms persist or get worse, consult a doctor right away
- avoid caffeine-containing foods or beverages
- avoid dietary supplements containing ingredients reported or claimed to have a stimulant effect

**If pregnant or breastfeeding,** ask a health professional before use.

**Keep out of reach of children.** In case of overdose, get medical help or contact a Poison Control Center right away.

## DIRECTIONS
- do not exceed dosage
- this adult product is not intended for use in children under 12 years of age

| adults and children 12 years of age and over | take 1-2 tablets every 4 hours, as needed, not to exceed 12 tablets in 24 hours |
|---|---|
| children under 12 years of age | do not use |

## OTHER INFORMATION
- store at 20-25°C (68-77°F)

## INACTIVE INGREDIENTS
colloidal silicon dioxide, crospovidone, D&C yellow no. 10 aluminum lake, FD&C yellow no. 6 aluminum lake, magnesium stearate, microcrystalline cellulose, povidone

## QUESTIONS OR COMMENTS
Call weekdays from 9 AM to 5 PM EST at **1-800-535-0026**

---

# RECLEAR AF (clotrimazole) solution
NDC Laboratories

## DRUG FACTS

| Active ingredient | Purpose |
|---|---|
| Clotrimazole 1 % | Antifungal |

## USES
- kills fungus on skin under the nail
- treat, soothes and conditions skin without irritation
- treatment of most tinea pedis (athlete's foot)
- effectively relieves itching, burning, cracking and scaling accompanying such conditions

**For external use only.**

## DO NOT USE
- on children under 2 years of age except under the advice and supervision of a physician. Avoid contact with the eyes. If accidental eye contact occurs, rinse thoroughly with water. If irritation occurs or if there is no improvement within 4 weeks, discontinue use and consult a physician

## DIRECTIONS
- clean the affected area and dry thoroughly
- apply a thin layer of the product over affected area twice daily (morning and night) or as directed by a physician. Supervise children in the use of this product
- for athlete's foot: pay special attention to the spaces between toes, wear well-fitting, ventilated shoes, and change shoes and socks at least once daily.
- for athlete's foot and ringworm, use daily for 4 weeks; for jock itch, use daily for 2 weeks. If condition persists longer, consult a physician
- this product is not effective on the scalp or nails
- apply to skin around and under entire nail and cuticle
- saturate and work into open front edge to soak back to skin under the nail

**If pregnant/breastfeeding,** consult a physician before using.

**Keep out of reach of children.** If swallowed, get medical help or contact a Poison Control Center immediately.

## INACTIVE INGREDIENTS
benzalkonium chloride, cocamidopropyl betaine, glycerin, hydroxypropylcellulose, PEG-8, propylene glycol, SDA-40 B, melaleuca alternifolia oil (tea tree)

---

# REFRESH CLASSIC (polyvinyl alcohol, povidone)
solution/drops

Allergan, Inc.

## DRUG FACTS

| Active ingredients | Purpose |
|---|---|
| Polyvinyl alcohol 1.4% | Eye lubricant |
| Povidone 0.6% | Eye lubricant |

## USES
- for the temporary relief of burning, irritation, and discomfort due to dryness of the eye or exposure to wind or sun
- may be used as a protectant against further irritation

## WARNINGS
**For external use only.**

## DO NOT USE
- if solution changes color or becomes cloudy

## STOP USE AND ASK A DOCTOR IF
- you experience eye pain, changes in vision, continued redness or irritation of the eye, or if the condition worsens or persists for more than 72 hours

**Keep out of reach of children.** If swallowed, get medical help or contact a Poison Control Center right away.

## DIRECTIONS
- to open, twist and pull tab to remove
- instill 1 or 2 drops in the affected eye(s) as needed and discard container
- to avoid contamination, do not touch tip of container to any surface
- do not reuse. Once opened, discard
- do not touch unit-dose tip to eye

## OTHER INFORMATION
- use only if single-use container is intact
- use before expiration date marked on container
- store at 59-86°F (15-30°C)
- retain carton for future reference

## INACTIVE INGREDIENTS
purified water and sodium chloride; may also contain hydrochloric acid and/or sodium hydroxide to adjust pH

## QUESTIONS OR COMMENTS
Call **1-800-433-8871**, M-F 6 AM-4:30 PM Pacific Time or visit www.refreshbrand.com

---

# REFRESH LIQUIGEL (carboxymethylcellulose sodium) solution/drops
Allergan, Inc.

## DRUG FACTS

| Active ingredient | Purpose |
|---|---|
| Carboxymethylcellulose sodium 1% | Eye lubricant |

## USES
- for the temporary relief of burning, irritation, and discomfort due to dryness of the eye or exposure to wind or sun
- may be used as a protectant against further irritation

## WARNINGS
**For external use only.**

## DO NOT USE
- if solution changes color or becomes cloudy, do not use

## STOP USE AND ASK A DOCTOR IF
- you experience:
  - eye pain
  - changes in vision
  - continued redness or irritation of the eye
  - the condition worsens or persists for more than 72 hours

**Keep out of reach of children.** If swallowed, get medical help or contact a Poison Control Center right away.

## DIRECTIONS
- instill 1 or 2 drops in the affected eye(s) as needed
- to avoid contamination, do not touch tip of container to any surface. Replace cap after using

## OTHER INFORMATION
- use only if imprinted tape seals on top and bottom flaps are intact and clearly legible
- use before expiration date marked on container
- store at 59-86°F (15-30°C)
- retain carton for future reference

## INACTIVE INGREDIENTS
boric acid, calcium chloride, magnesium chloride, potassium chloride, purified water, purite (stabilized oxychloro complex), sodium borate, sodium chloride

## QUESTIONS OR COMMENTS
Call **1-800-433-8871** M-F 6 AM-4:30 PM Pacific Time or visit refreshbrand.com

---

## REFRESH OPTIVE (carboxymethylcellulose sodium and glycerin) solution/drops
Allergan, Inc.

### DRUG FACTS

| Active ingredients | Purpose |
| --- | --- |
| Carboxymethylcellulose sodium 0.5% | Eye lubricant |
| Glycerin 0.9% | Eye lubricant |

## USES
- for the temporary relief of burning, irritation, and discomfort due to dryness of the eye or exposure to wind or sun
- may be used as a protectant against further irritation

## WARNINGS
**For external use only.**

## DO NOT USE
- if solution changes color

## STOP USE AND ASK A DOCTOR IF
- you experience:
  - eye pain
  - changes in vision
  - continued redness or irritation of the eye
  - the condition worsens or persists for more than 72 hours

**Keep out of reach of children.** If swallowed, get medical help or contact a Poison Control Center right away.

## DIRECTIONS
- instill 1 or 2 drops in the affected eye(s) as needed
- to avoid contamination, do not touch tip of container to any surface. Replace cap after using

## OTHER INFORMATION
- use only if imprinted tape seals on top and bottom flaps are intact and clearly legible
- use before expiration date marked on container
- store at 59-86°F (15-30°C)
- retain carton for future reference

## INACTIVE INGREDIENTS
boric acid, calcium chloride dihydrate, erythritol, levocarnitine, magnesium chloride hexahydrate, potassium chloride, purified water, purite (stabilized oxychloro complex), sodium borate decahydrate, sodium citrate dihydrate

## QUESTIONS OR COMMENTS
Call **1-800-433.8871** M-F 6 AM-4:30 PM Pacific Time or visit www.refreshbrand.com

---

## REFRESH OPTIVE SENSITIVE
(carboxymethylcellulose sodium and glycerin) solution/drops

Allergan, Inc.

### DRUG FACTS

| Active ingredients | Purpose |
| --- | --- |
| Carboxymethylcellulose sodium 0.5% | Eye lubricant |
| Glycerin 0.9% | Eye lubricant |

## USES
- for the temporary relief of burning, irritation, and discomfort due to dryness of the eye or exposure to wind or sun
- may be used as a protectant against further irritation

## WARNINGS
**For external use only.**

## DO NOT USE
- if solution changes color

## STOP USE AND ASK A DOCTOR IF
- you experience:
  - eye pain
  - changes in vision
  - continued redness or irritation of the eye
  - the condition worsens or persists for more than 72 hours

**Keep out of reach of children.** If swallowed, get medical help or contact a Poison Control Center right away.

## DIRECTIONS
- to open, twist and pull tab to remove
- instill 1 or 2 drops in the affected eye(s) as needed and discard container
- to avoid contamination, do not touch tip of container to any surface. Do not reuse. Once opened, discard
- do not touch unit-dose tip to eye

*If used for post-operative (e.g., LASIK) dryness and discomfort, follow your eye doctor's instructions.

## OTHER INFORMATION
- use only if single-use container is intact
- use before expiration date marked on container
- store at 59-86°F (15-30°C)
- retain carton for future reference

## INACTIVE INGREDIENTS
boric acid, calcium chloride dihydrate, erythritol, levocarnitine, magnesium chloride hexahydrate, potassium chloride, purified water, sodium borate decahydrate, and sodium citrate dihydrate

## QUESTIONS OR COMMENTS
Call **1-800-433-8871** M-F 6 AM-4:30 PM Pacific Time or visit www.refreshbrand.com

## REFRESH REDNESS RELIEF (phenylephrine hydrochloride and polyvinyl alcohol) solution/drops
Allergan, Inc.

### DRUG FACTS

| Active ingredients | Purpose |
| --- | --- |
| Phenylephrine hydrochloride 0.12% | Redness reliever |
| Polyvinyl alcohol 1.4% | Eye lubricant |

## USES
- relieves redness of the eye due to minor eye irritations
- for use as a lubricant to prevent further irritation or to relieve dryness of the eye

## WARNINGS
**For external use only.**
- overuse of this product may produce increased redness of the eye
- when using this product pupils may become enlarged temporarily

## DO NOT USE
- if solution changes color or becomes cloudy

## ASK A DOCTOR BEFORE USE IF YOU HAVE
- narrow angle glaucoma

## STOP USE AND ASK A DOCTOR IF
- you experience:
  - eye pain
  - changes in vision
  - continued redness or irritation of the eye
  - the condition worsens or persists for more than 72 hours

**Keep out of reach of children.** If swallowed, get medical help or contact a Poison Control Center right away

## DIRECTIONS
- instill 1 or 2 drops in the affected eye(s) up to four times daily
- to avoid contamination, do not touch tip of container to any surface. Replace cap after using

## OTHER INFORMATION
- use only if imprinted tape seals on top and bottom flaps are intact and clearly legible
- not for use while wearing soft contact lenses
- use before expiration date marked on container
- store at 59-86°F (15-30°C)
- retain this carton for future reference

## INACTIVE INGREDIENTS
benzalkonium chloride, edetate disodium; purified water, sodium acetate, sodium phosphate, dibasic; sodium phosphate, monobasic, sodium thiosulfate; may contain hydrochloric acid and/or sodium hydroxide to adjust pH

## QUESTIONS OR COMMENTS
Call **1-800-433-8871** M-F 6 AM-4:30 PM Pacific Time or visit refreshbrand.com

## REFRESH TEARS (carboxymethylcellulose sodium) drops
Allergan, Inc.

### DRUG FACTS

| Active ingredient | Purpose |
| --- | --- |
| Carboxymethylcellulose sodium 0.5% | Eye lubricant |

## USES
- for the temporary relief of burning, irritation, and discomfort due to dryness of the eye or exposure to wind or sun
- may be used as a protectant against further irritation

## WARNINGS
**For external use only.**

## DO NOT USE
- if solution changes color or becomes cloudy

## STOP USE AND ASK A DOCTOR IF
- you experience:
  - eye pain
  - changes in vision
  - continued redness or irritation of the eye
  - the condition worsens or persists for more than 72 hours

**Keep out of reach of children.** If swallowed, get medical help or contact a Poison Control Center right away.

## DIRECTIONS
- instill 1 or 2 drops in the affected eye(s) as needed
- to avoid contamination, do not touch tip of container to any surface. Replace cap after using

## OTHER INFORMATION
- use only if imprinted tape seals on top and bottom flaps are intact and clearly legible
- use before expiration date marked on container
- retain carton for future reference

## INACTIVE INGREDIENTS
boric acid, calcium chloride, magnesium chloride, potassium chloride, purified water, purite (stabilized oxychloro complex), sodium borate, sodium chloride; may also contain hydrochloric acid and/or sodium hydroxide to adjust pH.

## QUESTIONS OR COMMENTS
Call **1-800-433-8871** Mon-Fri 6 AM-4:30 PM Pacific Time or visit www.refreshbrand.com

## REVALESKIN (octinoxate and oxybenzone) cream
Stiefel Laboratories Inc

### DRUG FACTS

| Active ingredients | Purpose |
|---|---|
| Octinoxate 7.5%<br>Oxybenzone 4.0% | Sunscreen |

### USES
- helps prevent sunburn
- higher SPF gives more sunburn protection

### WARNINGS
**For external use only.**
UV exposure from the sun increases the risk of skin cancer, premature skin aging, and other skin damage. It is important to decrease UV exposure by limiting time in the sun, wearing protective clothing, and using a sunscreen.

### WHEN USING THIS PRODUCT
- keep out of eyes. Rinse with water to remove

### STOP USE AND ASK A DOCTOR IF
- rash or irritation develops and lasts

**Keep out of the reach of children.** If swallowed, get medical help or contact a Poison Control Center right away.

### DIRECTIONS
- in the morning, wash your face with REVALESKIN Facial Cleanser, pat dry, and apply REVALESKIN Day Cream evenly to your face and neck. When used as a sunscreen, apply before sun exposure and as needed
- children under 6 months of age: ask a doctor

### OTHER INFORMATION
- store at 20-25°C (68-77°F)

### INACTIVE INGREDIENTS
acrylates/C10-30 alkyl acrylate crosspolymer, caprylic/capric triglyceride, carbomer, citrus grandis (grapefruit) peel extract, coffea arabica fruit extract, cyclohexasiloxane, cyclopentasiloxane, dimethicone/vinyl dimethicone crosspolymer, disodium EDTA, ethylhexylglycerin, glycerin, glycine soja (soybean) protein, glycosphingolipids, FD&C green no. 3, hydrogenated polyisobutene, isononyl isononanoate, oleth-20, oxido reductases, pentylene glycol, phenoxyethanol, phospholipids, polybutene, polyquaternium-51, polysorbate 80, PPG-3 benzyl ether myristate, silica, sodium hyaluronate, sodium PCA, sodium polyacrylate, steareth-2, stearic acid, stearyl alcohol, tocopheryl acetate, trehalose, triacetin, triethanolamine, urea, water, FD&C yellow no. 5

## RID COMPLETE LICE ELIMINATION KIT
(piperonyl butoxide, pyrethrum extract, permethrin) shampoo, gel, spray
Bayer HealthCare

### DRUG FACTS

| Active ingredients | Purpose |
|---|---|
| Piperonyl butoxide (4%) | Lice treatment |
| Pyrethrum extract (equivalent to 0.33% pyrethrins) | Lice treatment |

### STEP 1
*LICE KILLING SHAMPOO*

### USES
- treats head, pubic (crab), and body lice

### WARNINGS
**For external use only.**

### DO NOT USE
- near the eyes
- inside the nose, mouth, or vagina
- on lice in eyebrows or eyelashes. See a doctor if lice are present in these areas

### ASK A DOCTOR BEFORE USE IF YOU ARE
- allergic to ragweed

May cause breathing difficulty or an asthmatic attack.

### WHEN USING THIS PRODUCT
- keep eyes tightly closed and protect eyes with a washcloth or towel
- if product gets into the eyes, flush with water right away
- scalp itching or redness may occur

### STOP USE AND ASK A DOCTOR IF
- breathing difficult occurs
- eye irritation occurs
- skin or scalp irritation continues or infection occurs

**Keep out of reach children.** If swallowed, get medical help or contact poison control center right away.

### DIRECTIONS
- important: read warnings before use
- adults and children 2 years and over:

**Inspect**
- check each household member with a magnifying glass in bright light for lice/nits (eggs)
- look for tiny nits near scalp, beginning at back of neck and behind ears
- examine small sections of hair at a time
- unlike dandruff which moves when touched, nits stick to the hair
- if either lice or nits are found, treat with this product

**Treat**
- apply thoroughly to DRY HAIR or other affected area. For head lice, first apply behind ears and to back of neck
- allow product to remain for 10 minutes, but no longer
- use warm water to form a lather, shampoo, then thoroughly rinse
- for head lice, towel dry hair and comb out tangles

**Remove lice and their eggs (nits)**
- use a fine-tooth or special lice/nit comb. Remove any remaining nits by hand (using a throw-away glove)
- hair should remain slightly damp while removing nits
- if hair dries during combing, dampen slightly with water
- for head lice, part hair into sections. Do one section at a time starting on top of head. Longer hair may take 1 to 2 hours
- lift a 1-to 2-inch wide strand of hair. Place comb as close to scalp as possible and comb with a firm, even motion away from scalp
- pin back each strand of hair after combing
- clean comb often. Wipe nits away with tissue and discard in a plastic bag. Seal bag and discard to prevent lice from coming back
- after combing, thoroughly recheck for lice/nits. Repeat combing if necessary
- check daily for any lice/nits that you missed

- a second treatment must be done in 7 to 10 days to kill any newly hatched lice
- if infestation continues, see a doctor for other treatments
- children under 2 years: ask a doctor

## OTHER INFORMATION
- keep carton for important product information
- see consumer information insert for additional information
- avoid excessive heat

## INACTIVE INGREDIENTS
ammonium laureth sulfate, dehydrated alcohol, fragrance, isopropyl alcohol, PEG-25 hydrogenated castor oil, polyquaternium-10, purified water

## QUESTIONS OR COMMENTS
Call **(1-800-RID-LICE) (1-800-743-5423)** (Mon-Fri 9 AM-5 PM EST) or visit www.ridlice.com

## STEP 2

### *LICE & EGG COMB-OUT GEL*

### DRUG FACTS

| INGREDIENTS | PURPOSE |
|---|---|
| Purified water | Facilitate egg and nit removal |
| Glycerin | |
| Hydroxyethylcellulose | |
| PG-hydroxyethycellulose cocodimonium chloride | |
| Polysorbate 20 | |
| DMDM hydantoin | |
| Fragrance | |
| iodopropynyl butylcarbamate | |

## USE
- to make egg and nit removal from the hair faster and easier

## WARNINGS
**For external use only.**

**Keep out of reach of children.**

## DIRECTIONS FOR USE
- before using, read Consumer Information Insert for complete directions
- use AFTER shampooing with RID Lice Killing Shampoo or other similar product to kill lice and eggs
- towel dry hair and comb out tangles with regular comb
- apply RID Lice & Egg Comb-Out Gel to one section of damp hair at a time
- massage well to ensure that the product covers the entire section
- pay special attention to the areas behind the ears and at the nape of the neck where nits and eggs are more likely to be found
- comb out the dead lice, eggs, and nits with the enclosed RID Comb. (See insert for additional combing instructions). This step is very important
- if hair dries during combing, dampen slightly with water and re-apply gel as needed
- rinse thoroughly with warm water, after you have combed entire head. Disinfect combs with hot water (130°F)

## OTHER INFORMATION
- protect from freezing and excessive heat
- it is important to wash in hot water (130°F) all clothing, bedding, towels, and hair products (combs, brushes) used by infested persons

- dry clean non-washable fabrics
- to eliminate infestation of furniture and bedding that cannot be washed or dry cleaned, a multi-use lice spray may be used
- this product does not kill lice or their eggs. Use this product only after treating with RID Lice Killing Shampoo or other similar product

## INACTIVE INGREDIENTS
purified water, glycerin, hydroxyethylcellulose, PG-hydroxyethylcellulose cocodimonium chloride, polysorbate 20, DMDM hydantoin, fragrance, iodopropynyl butylcarbamate.

## QUESTIONS OR COMMENTS
Call **(1-800-743-5423)** (Mon-Fri 9 AM-5 PM EST) or visit www.ridlice.com **1-800-RID-LICE**

## STEP 3

### *HOME LICE, BEDBUG & DUST MITE SPRAY*

**Not For Use On Humans**

### DRUG FACTS

| Active ingredient | Purpose |
|---|---|
| Permethrin* | 0.50% |
| Other ingredients** | 99.50% |
| Total. | 100.00% |

\*Cis/trans ratio: Max 55% (+/-) cis and Min 45% (+/-) trans.

\*\*Contains petroleum distillate

## FIRST AID
Call poison control center or doctor immediately for treatment advice. Have the product container or label with you when calling a poison control center or doctor, or going for treatment. For MEDICAL Emergencies or other information Call 1-800-RID-LICE (1-800-743-5423).

For TRANSPORT Emergencies ONLY Call 1-877-315-9819.

| If Swallowed | Immediately call a poison control center or doctor |
|---|---|
| | Do not induce vomiting unless told to do so by a poison control center or doctor |
| | Do not give any liquid to the person |
| | Do not give anything by mouth to an unconscious person. |
| If in Eyes | Hold eye open and rinse slowly and gently with water for 15-20 minutes |
| | Remove contact lenses, if present, after the first 5 minutes, then continue rinsing eye |
| If Inhaled | Move person to fresh air |
| | If person is not breathing, call 911 or an ambulance, then give artificial respiration, preferably by mouth-to-mouth, if possible |
| If on Skin or Clothing | Take off contaminated clothing |
| | Rinse skin immediately with plenty of water for 15-20 minutes |

## NOTE TO PHYSICIAN
Contains petroleum distillate - vomiting may cause aspiration pneumonia.

## PRECAUTIONARY STATEMENTS HAZARDS TO HUMANS & DOMESTIC ANIMALS

### CAUTION

Harmful if swallowed or absorbed through skin. Avoid inhalation of spray mist. Causes eye irritation. Avoid contact with skin, eyes or clothing. Wash thoroughly with soap and water after handling. Avoid contamination of feed and foodstuffs. Remove pets and birds and cover fish aquaria before space spraying or surface applications. This product is not for use on humans. Vacate room after treatment and ventilate before reoccupying. Do not allow children or pets to contact treated areas until surfaces are dry.

### PHYSICAL OR CHEMICAL HAZARDS

Contents under pressure. Do not use or store near heat or open flame. Do not puncture or incinerate container. Exposure to temperatures above 130°F (54°C) may cause bursting.

### DIRECTIONS FOR USE

It is a violation of Federal law to use this product in a manner inconsistent with its labeling.

In the home, cover all food processing surfaces and utensils during treatment or thoroughly wash before use. Cover or remove exposed food. We recommend that those with asthma or severe allergies consult their doctor before using this product and have someone else apply this product

### COMPLETELY ELIMINATE LICE FROM YOUR FAMILY AND HOME.

#### STEP 1: TREAT

- Apply RID Lice Killing Shampoo according to label directions
- Repeat this step 7 to 10 days later to help prevent reinfestation

#### STEP 2: REMOVE

- After Step 1, comb out the eggs and nits in the hair with a fine-toothed comb or with the RID comb (included)
- You can use RID Lice & Egg Comb-Out Gel on damp hair to make removal faster and easier

#### STEP 3: CONTROL

- Use RID Home Lice, Bedbug & Dust Mite Spray to kill lice and their eggs on mattresses, furniture, car interiors, and other non-washable items
- Wash bed linens, clothing, and other items in hot water and dry in high heat

### IMPORTANT: READ DETAILED DIRECTIONS INSIDE BEFORE USING.

**This kit contains 3 products** (Lice Killing Shampoo, Lice & Egg Comb-Out Gel, Home Lice Control Spray) **to completely eliminate lice from your family and home. The 4 ounce bottle of shampoo and 2 ounce tube of gel should be enough product to treat one person. However, amount of product needed will vary by hair length. See below for guidelines.**

### LICE KILLING SHAMPOO

| Hair Length | Approximate Amount For 1 Adult/Child | |
|---|---|---|
| Short (ear length or shorter) | First Application: | 1 ounces - 2 ounces |
| | Second Application: | 1 ounces - 2 ounces |
| | **Total: 4 ounces** | **2 ounces** |
| Medium (shoulder length) | First Application: | 1 ounces - 3 ounces |
| | Second Application: | 2 ounces - 3 ounces |
| | **Total: 6 ounces** | **4 ounces** |
| Long (past shoulder length) | First Application: | 3 ounces - 4 ounces |
| | Second Application: | 3 ounces - 4 ounces |
| | **Total: 8 ounces** | **6 ounces** |

### LICE & EGG COMB-OUT GEL

| Hair Length | Approximate Amount For 1 Adult/Child | |
|---|---|---|
| Short (ear length or shorter) | First Application: | ½ tube |
| | Second Application: | ½ tube |
| | **Total:** | **1 Tube (2 ounces )** |
| Medium/Long (shoulder length or longer) | First Application: | 1 tube (2 ounces ) |
| | Second Application: | 1 tube (2 ounces ) |
| | **Total:** | **2 Tubes (4 ounces )** |

### SHAKE WELL BEFORE USING

Remove protective cap, hold container upright with nozzle away from you. Depress valve and spray from a distance of 8-10 inches (12-15 inches for baseboards, moldings and floors). Test product on an inconspicuous area before applying to check for possible staining or discoloration. Inspect again after drying. Spray to the point of dampness but not run-off. Over application may cause damage. Will not stain surfaces or fabrics where water alone causes no damage.

This product is Step 3 in the Bayer Corporation's Lice Control System. Step 1: Kill lice with RID Lice Killing Shampoo. Re-apply in 10 days. Step 2: Comb out eggs & nits with RID Lice & Egg Comb-Out Gel. Step 3: Clean home. Use RID Home Lice, Bedbug & Dust Mite Spray for non-washable items. Washables should be washed in hot water and dried in high heat.

**To kill Lice and Louse Eggs:** Spray the entire area to be treated. Spray each square foot for three seconds. Allow all sprayed articles to dry thoroughly before use. If lice infestation should occur on humans, use a product labeled for use on humans. Spray only those garments and parts of bedding, including mattresses and furniture that cannot be either laundered or dry cleaned. Do not use on sheets or pillowcases.

**Bedbugs:** Spray mattress, particularly around tufts and seams. Take beds apart and spray into all joints. Treat baseboards, moldings and floors. After mattress is dry, cover with mattress cover and sheet. Do not use mattress without a cover. Retreat if infestation occurs, but not more than once every two weeks.

**To Kill House Dust Mites (*Dermaplophagoides* spp.):** RID Home Lice, Bedbug & Dust Mite Spray controls house dust mites that may cause asthma, hay fever, rhinitis, watery eyes and sneezing. One treatment lasts for up to 8 weeks. **On Upholstered Furniture** - test fabric in an inconspicuous area to insure dyes will not bleed. Spray all fabric surfaces until damp. Do not use on delicate fabrics. Allow furniture to dry thoroughly before using. **On Carpets** - spray over entire carpet until damp. Hold the nozzle approximately 12 to 18 inches from the carpet surface and spray in a sweeping motion. Use an overlapping pattern to insure total coverage. After application, brush the surface of the carpet with a broom or brush to insure deep penetration. Allow carpet to dry thoroughly before reentering the treated area. Drying time can be accelerated by using a fan. **On Mattresses** - spray the top, bottom and sides of mattresses until damp, paying particular attention to tufts and seams. Allow to dry thoroughly before using. After mattress is dry, cover with mattress cover and sheet. Do not use mattress without a cover. Vacuum entire area once dry. Since vacuuming stirs dust up in the air those with allergies should have another person vacuum or should wear a dust mask and use vacuum with a high efficiency particulate (HEPA) filter.

---

# ROBITUSSIN CHEST CONGESTION
(guaifenesin) liquid

Wyeth Consumer Healthcare

## DRUG FACTS

| Active ingredient (in each 5 ml tsp) | Purpose |
|---|---|
| Guaifenesin, USP 100 mg | Expectorant |

## USE
- helps loosen phlegm (mucus) and thin bronchial secretions to make coughs more productive

## WARNINGS

### ASK A DOCTOR BEFORE USE IF YOU HAVE
- cough that occurs with too much phlegm (mucus)
- cough that lasts or is chronic such as occurs with smoking, asthma, chronic bronchitis, or emphysema

### STOP USE AND ASK A DOCTOR IF
- cough lasts more than 7 days, comes back, or is accompanied by fever, rash, or persistent headache. These could be signs of a serious condition

**If pregnant or breastfeeding,** ask a health professional before use.

**Keep out of reach of children.** In case of overdose, get medical help or contact a Poison Control Center right away.

## DIRECTIONS
- do not take more than 6 doses in any 24-hour period
- this adult product is not intended for use in children under 12 years of age

| Age | Dose |
|---|---|
| adults and children 12 years and over | 2-4 teaspoons every 4 hours |
| children under 12 years | do not use |

## OTHER INFORMATION
- each teaspoon contains: sodium 2 mg
- store at 20-25°C (68-77°F)
- alcohol-free
- dosage cup provided

## INACTIVE INGREDIENTS
anhydrous citric acid, artificial flavor, caramel, FD&C red no. 40, glycerin, high fructose corn syrup, liquid glucose, menthol, propylene glycol, purified water, saccharin sodium, sodium benzoate

**QUESTIONS OR COMMENTS**
Call weekdays from 9 AM to 5 PM EST at **1-800-762-4675**

# ROBITUSSIN COUGH & CHEST CONGESTION DM MAX (dextromethorphan hydrobromide and guaifenesin) liquid

Wyeth Consumer Healthcare

## DRUG FACTS

| Active ingredients (in each 5 ml tsp) | Purpose |
|---|---|
| Dextromethorphan hydrobromide, USP 10 mg | Cough suppressant |
| Guaifenesin, USP 200 mg | Expectorant |

## USES
- temporarily relieves cough due to minor throat and bronchial irritation as may occur with a cold
- helps loosen phlegm (mucus) and thin bronchial secretions to drain bronchial tubes

## WARNINGS

### DO NOT USE
- if you are now taking a prescription monoamine oxidase inhibitor (MAOI) (certain drugs for depression, psychiatric, or emotional conditions, or Parkinson's disease), or for 2 weeks after stopping the MAOI drug. If you do not know if your prescription drug contains an MAOI, ask a doctor or pharmacist before taking this product

### ASK A DOCTOR BEFORE USE IF YOU HAVE
- cough that occurs with too much phlegm (mucus)
- cough that lasts or is chronic such as occurs with smoking, asthma, chronic bronchitis, or emphysema

### STOP USE AND ASK A DOCTOR IF
- cough lasts more than 7 days, comes back, or is accompanied by fever, rash, or persistent headache. These could be signs of a serious condition

**If pregnant or breastfeeding,** ask a health professional before use.

**Keep out of reach of children.** In case of overdose, get medical help or contact a Poison Control Center right away.

## DIRECTIONS
- shake well before using
- do not take more than 6 doses in any 24-hour period
- this adult product is not intended for use in children under 12 years of age

| Age | Dose |
|---|---|
| adults and children 12 years and over | 2 teaspoons every 4 hours |
| children under 12 years | do not use |

## OTHER INFORMATION
- each teaspoon contains: sodium 5 mg
- store at 20-25°C (68-77°F)
- alcohol-free
- dosage cup provided

## INACTIVE INGREDIENTS

anhydrous citric acid, artificial & natural flavors, carboxymethylcellulose sodium, D&C red no. 33, FD&C red no. 40, glycerin, high fructose corn syrup, menthol, microcrystalline cellulose, polyethylene glycol, povidone, propylene glycol, purified water, saccharin sodium, sodium benzoate, sorbitol solution, xanthan gum

## QUESTIONS OR COMMENTS

Call weekdays from 9 AM to 5 PM EST at **1-800-762-4675**

# ROBITUSSIN COUGH AND CHEST CONGESTION DM/ SUGAR-FREE
(dextromethorphan hydrobromide and guaifenesin) liquid
Wyeth Consumer Healthcare

## DRUG FACTS

| Active ingredients (in each 5 ml tsp) | Purpose |
|---|---|
| Dextromethorphan hydrobromide, USP 10 mg | Cough suppressant |
| Guaifenesin, USP 100 mg | Expectorant |

## USES
- temporarily relieves cough due to minor throat and bronchial irritation as may occur with a cold
- helps loosen phlegm (mucus) and thin bronchial secretions to drain bronchial tubes

## WARNINGS

### DO NOT USE
- if you are now taking a prescription monoamine oxidase inhibitor (MAOI) (certain drugs for depression, psychiatric, or emotional conditions, or Parkinson's disease), or for 2 weeks after stopping the MAOI drug. If you do not know if your prescription drug contains an MAOI, ask a doctor or pharmacist before taking this product

### ASK A DOCTOR BEFORE USE IF YOU HAVE
- cough that occurs with too much phlegm (mucus)
- cough that lasts or is chronic such as occurs with smoking, asthma, chronic bronchitis, or emphysema

### STOP USE AND ASK A DOCTOR IF
- cough lasts more than 7 days, comes back, or is accompanied by fever, rash, or persistent headache. These could be signs of a serious condition

**If pregnant or breastfeeding,** ask a health professional before use.

**Keep out of reach of children.** In case of overdose, get medical help or contact a Poison Control Center right away.

## DIRECTIONS
- do not take more than 6 doses in any 24-hour period
- this adult product is not intended for use in children under 12 years of age

| adults and children 12 years and over | 2 teaspoons every 4 hours |
|---|---|
| children under 12 years | do not use |

## OTHER INFORMATION
**Robitussin Cough & Chest Congestion DM**
- each teaspoon contains: sodium 7 mg
- store at 20-25°C (68-77°F)
- dosage cup provided

**Robitussin Cough & Chest Congestion Sugar Free DM**
- each teaspoon contains: sodium 4 mg
- store at 20-25°C (68-77°F)
- alcohol-free
- dosage cup provided

## INACTIVE INGREDIENTS
**Robitussin Cough & Chest Congestion DM**
anhydrous citric acid, FD&C red no. 40, glycerin, high fructose corn syrup, menthol, natural flavor, propylene glycol, purified water, sodium benzoate, sodium citrate, sucralose

**Robitussin Cough & Chest Congestion Sugar Free DM**
acesulfame potassium, artificial & natural flavor, citric acid monohydrate, glycerin, methylparaben, polyethylene glycol, povidone, propylene glycol, purified water, saccharin sodium, sodium benzoate

## QUESTIONS OR COMMENTS
Call weekdays from 9 AM to 5 PM EST at **1-800-762-4675**

# ROBITUSSIN COUGH AND COLD CF
(dextromethorphan hydrobromide, guaifenesin and phenylephrine hydrochloride) liquid
Wyeth Consumer Healthcare

## DRUG FACTS

| Active ingredients (in each 5 ml tsp) | Purpose |
|---|---|
| Dextromethorphan hydrobromide, USP 10 mg | Cough suppressant |
| Guaifenesin, USP 100 mg | Expectorant |
| Phenylephrine hydrochloride, USP 5 mg | Nasal decongestant |

## USES
- helps loosen phlegm (mucus) and thin bronchial secretions to drain bronchial tubes
- temporarily relieves these symptoms occurring with a cold:
  - nasal congestion
  - cough due to minor throat and bronchial irritation

## WARNINGS

### DO NOT USE
- if you are now taking a prescription monoamine oxidase inhibitor (MAOI) (certain drugs for depression, psychiatric, or emotional conditions, or Parkinson's disease), or for 2 weeks after stopping the MAOI drug. If you do not know if your prescription drug contains an MAOI, ask a doctor or pharmacist before taking this product

### ASK A DOCTOR BEFORE USE IF YOU HAVE
- heart disease
- high blood pressure
- thyroid disease
- diabetes
- trouble urinating due to an enlarged prostate gland
- cough that occurs with too much phlegm (mucus)
- cough that lasts or is chronic such as occurs with smoking, asthma, chronic bronchitis, or emphysema

**WHEN USING THIS PRODUCT**
• do not use more than directed

**STOP USE AND ASK A DOCTOR IF**
• you get nervous, dizzy, or sleepless
• symptoms do not get better within 7 days or are accompanied by fever
• cough lasts more than 7 days, comes back, or is accompanied by fever, rash, or persistent headache. These could be signs of a serious condition

**If pregnant or breastfeeding,** ask a health professional before use.

**Keep out of reach of children.** In case of overdose, get medical help or contact a Poison Control Center right away.

**DIRECTIONS**
• do not take more than 6 doses in any 24-hour period
• this adult product is not intended for use in children under 12 years of age

| adults and children 12 years and over | 2 teaspoons every 4 hours |
|---|---|
| children under 12 years | do not use |

**OTHER INFORMATION**
• each teaspoon contains: **sodium 3 mg**
• store at 20-25°C (68-77°F)
• dosage cup provided

**INACTIVE INGREDIENTS**
anhydrous citric acid, FD&C red no. 40, glycerin, menthol, natural & artificial flavor, propylene glycol, purified water, sodium benzoate, sodium citrate, sorbitol solution, sucralose

**QUESTIONS OR COMMENTS**
Call weekdays from 9 AM to 5 PM EST at **1-800-762-4675**

---

# CHILDREN'S ROBITUSSIN COUGH AND COLD CF (dextromethorphan hydrobromide, guaifenesin and phenylephrine hydrochloride) liquid
Wyeth Consumer Healthcare

## DRUG FACTS

| Active ingredients (in each 5 ml tsp) | Purpose |
|---|---|
| Dextromethorphan hydrobromide, USP 5 mg | Cough suppressant |
| Guaifenesin, USP 50 mg | Expectorant |
| Phenylephrine hydrochloride, USP 2.5 mg | Nasal decongestant |

**USES**
• helps loosen phlegm (mucus) and thin bronchial secretions to drain bronchial tubes
• temporarily relieves these symptoms occurring with a cold:
  • nasal congestion
  • cough due to minor throat and bronchial irritation

**WARNINGS**
**DO NOT USE**
• if you are now taking a prescription monoamine oxidase inhibitor (MAOI) (certain drugs for depression, psychiatric, or emotional conditions, or Parkinson's disease), or for 2 weeks after stopping the MAOI drug. If you do not know if your prescription drug contains an MAOI, ask a doctor or pharmacist before taking this product

**ASK A DOCTOR BEFORE USE IF YOU HAVE**
• heart disease
• high blood pressure
• thyroid disease
• diabetes
• trouble urinating due to an enlarged prostate gland
• cough that occurs with too much phlegm (mucus)
• cough that lasts or is chronic such as occurs with smoking, asthma, chronic bronchitis or emphysema

**WHEN USING THIS PRODUCT**
• do not use more than directed

**STOP USE AND ASK A DOCTOR IF**
• you get nervous, dizzy, or sleepless
• symptoms do not get better within 7 days or are accompanied by a fever
• cough lasts more than 7 days, comes back, or is accompanied by fever, rash, or persistent headache. These could be signs of a serious condition

**If pregnant or breastfeeding,** ask a health professional before use.

**Keep out of the reach of children.** In case of overdose, get medical help or contact a Poison Control Center right away.

**DIRECTIONS**
• do not take more than 6 doses in any 24-hour period

| children under 4 years | do not use |
|---|---|
| children 4 to under 6 years | 1 teaspoon every 4 hours |
| children 6 to under 12 years | 2 teaspoons every 4 hours |
| adults and children 12 years and over | 4 teaspoons every 4 hours |

**OTHER INFORMATION**
• each teaspoon contains: sodium 3 mg
• store at 20-25°C (68-77°F)
• dosage cup provided

**INACTIVE INGREDIENTS**
anhydrous citric acid, artificial flavor, FD&C red no. 40, glycerin, propylene glycol, purified water, sodium benzoate, sodium citrate, sorbitol solution, sucralose

**QUESTIONS OR COMMENTS**
Call weekdays from 9 AM to 5 PM EST at **1-800-762-4675**

# ROBITUSSIN COUGH AND COLD CF MAX
(dextromethorphan hydrobromide and guaifenesin, phenylephrine hydrochloride) liquid

Wyeth Consumer Healthcare

## DRUG FACTS

| Active ingredients (in each 5 ml tsp) | Purpose |
|---|---|
| Dextromethorphan hydrobromide, USP 10 mg | Cough suppressant |
| Guaifenesin, USP 200 mg | Expectorant |
| Phenylephrine hydrochloride, USP 5 mg | Nasal decongestant |

## USES
- helps loosen phlegm (mucus) and thin bronchial secretions to drain bronchial tubes
- temporarily relieves these symptoms occurring with a cold:
  - nasal congestion
  - cough due to minor throat and bronchial irritation

## WARNINGS

### DO NOT USE
- if you are now taking a prescription monoamine oxidase inhibitor (MAOI) (certain drugs for depression, psychiatric, or emotional conditions, or Parkinson's disease), or for 2 weeks after stopping the MAOI drug. If you do not know if your prescription drug contains an MAOI, ask a doctor or pharmacist before taking this product

### ASK A DOCTOR BEFORE USE IF YOU HAVE
- heart disease
- high blood pressure
- thyroid disease
- diabetes
- trouble urinating due to an enlarged prostate gland
- cough that occurs with too much phlegm (mucus)
- cough that lasts or is chronic such as occurs with smoking, asthma, chronic bronchitis or emphysema

### ASK A DOCTOR OR PHARMACIST BEFORE USE IF YOU ARE
- taking any other oral nasal decongestant or stimulant

### WHEN USING THIS PRODUCT
- do not use more than directed

### STOP USE AND ASK A DOCTOR IF
- you get nervous, dizzy, or sleepless
- symptoms do not get better within 7 days or are accompanied by fever
- cough lasts more than 7 days, comes back, or is accompanied by fever, rash, or persistent headache. These could be signs of a serious condition

**If pregnant or breastfeeding,** ask a health professional before use.

**Keep out of reach of children.** In case of overdose, get medical help or contact a Poison Control Center right away.

### DIRECTIONS
- do not take more than 6 doses in any 24-hour period
- this adult product is not intended for use in children under 12 years of age

| adults and children 12 years and over | 2 teaspoons every 4 hours |
|---|---|
| children under 12 years | do not use |

## OTHER INFORMATION
- each teaspoon contains: sodium 3 mg
- store at 20-25°C (68-77°F)
- do not refrigerate
- dosage cup provided

## INACTIVE INGREDIENTS
anhydrous citric acid, FD&C red no. 40, glycerin, menthol, natural flavor, polyethylene glycol, propylene glycol, purified water, sodium benzoate, sodium citrate, sorbitol solution, sucralose, xanthan gum

## QUESTIONS OR COMMENTS
Call weekdays from 9 AM to 5 PM EST at **1-800-762-4675**

# ROBITUSSIN COUGH AND COLD D
(dextromethorphan hydrobromide, guaifenesin, pseudoephedrine hydrochloride) liquid

Wyeth Consumer Healthcare

## DRUG FACTS

| Active ingredients (in each 5 ml tsp) | Purpose |
|---|---|
| Dextromethorphan hydrobromide, USP 15 mg | Cough suppressant |
| Guaifenesin, USP 200 mg | Expectorant |
| Pseudoephedrine hydrochloride, USP 30 mg | Nasal decongestant |

## USES
- helps loosen phlegm (mucus) and thin bronchial secretions to drain bronchial tubes
- temporarily relieves these symptoms occurring with a cold:
  - nasal congestion
  - cough due to minor throat and bronchial irritation

## WARNINGS

### DO NOT USE
- if you are now taking a prescription monoamine oxidase inhibitor (MAOI) (certain drugs for depression, psychiatric, or emotional conditions, or Parkinson's disease), or for 2 weeks after stopping the MAOI drug. If you do not know if your prescription drug contains an MAOI, ask a doctor or pharmacist before taking this product

### ASK A DOCTOR BEFORE USE IF YOU HAVE
- heart disease
- high blood pressure
- thyroid disease
- diabetes
- trouble urinating due to an enlarged prostate gland
- cough that occurs with too much phlegm (mucus)
- cough that lasts or is chronic such as occurs with smoking, asthma, chronic bronchitis or emphysema

### WHEN USING THIS PRODUCT
- do not use more than directed

**STOP USE AND ASK A DOCTOR IF**
- you get nervous, dizzy, or sleepless
- symptoms do not get better within 7 days or are accompanied by fever
- cough lasts more than 7 days, comes back, or is accompanied by fever, rash, or persistent headache. These could be signs of a serious condition

**If pregnant or breastfeeding,** ask a health professional before use.

**Keep out of reach of children.** In case of overdose, get medical help or contact a Poison Control Center right away.

**DIRECTIONS**
- do not take more than 4 doses in any 24-hour period
- this adult product is not intended for use in children under 12 years of age

| adults and children 12 years and over | 2 teaspoons every 4 hours |
|---|---|
| children under 12 years | do not use |

**OTHER INFORMATION**
- each teaspoon contains: sodium 4 mg
- store at 20-25°C (68-77°F)
- dosage cup provided

**INACTIVE INGREDIENTS**
anhydrous citric acid, artificial flavor, FD&C red no. 40, glycerin, menthol, polyethylene glycol, propylene glycol, purified water, sodium benzoate, sodium citrate, sorbitol solution, sucralose

**QUESTIONS OR COMMENTS**
Call weekdays from 9 AM to 5 PM EST at **1-800-762-4675**

# ROBITUSSIN COUGH AND CHEST CONGESTION DM MAX (dextromethorphan hydrobromide and guaifenesin) liquid
Wyeth Consumer Healthcare

## DRUG FACTS

| Active ingredients (in each 5 ml tsp) | Purpose |
|---|---|
| Dextromethorphan hydrobromide, USP 10 mg | Cough suppressant |
| Guaifenesin, USP 200 mg | Expectorant |

**USES**
- temporarily relieves cough due to minor throat and bronchial irritation as may occur with a cold
- helps loosen phlegm (mucus) and thin bronchial secretions to drain bronchial tubes

**WARNINGS**

**DO NOT USE**
- if you are now taking a prescription monoamine oxidase inhibitor (MAOI) (certain drugs for depression, psychiatric, or emotional conditions, or Parkinson's disease), or for 2 weeks after stopping the MAOI drug. If you do not know if your prescription drug contains an MAOI, ask a doctor or pharmacist before taking this product

**ASK A DOCTOR BEFORE USE IF YOU HAVE**
- cough that occurs with too much phlegm (mucus)
- cough that lasts or is chronic such as occurs with smoking, asthma, chronic bronchitis, or emphysema

**STOP USE AND ASK A DOCTOR IF**
- cough lasts more than 7 days, comes back, or is accompanied by fever, rash, or persistent headache. These could be signs of a serious condition

**If pregnant or breastfeeding,** ask a health professional before use.

**Keep out of reach of children.** In case of overdose, get medical help or contact a Poison Control Center right away.

**DIRECTIONS**
- shake well before using
- do not take more than 6 doses in any 24-hour period
- this adult product is not intended for use in children under 12 years of age

| adults and children 12 years and over | 2 teaspoons every 4 hours |
|---|---|
| children under 12 years | do not use |

**OTHER INFORMATION**
- each teaspoon contains: sodium 5 mg
- store at 20-25°C (68-77°F)
- alcohol-free
- dosage cup provided

**INACTIVE INGREDIENTS**
anhydrous citric acid, artificial & natural flavors, carboxymethylcellulose sodium, D&C red no. 33, FD&C red no. 40, glycerin, high fructose corn syrup, menthol, microcrystalline cellulose, polyethylene glycol, povidone, propylene glycol, purified water, saccharin sodium, sodium benzoate, sorbitol solution, xanthan gum

**QUESTIONS OR COMMENTS**
Call weekdays from 9 AM to 5 PM EST at **1-800-762-4675**

# ROBITUSSIN COUGH AND COLD LONG-ACTING (chlorpheniramine maleate and dextromethorphan hydrobromide) liquid
Richmond Division of Wyeth

## DRUG FACTS

| Active ingredients (in each 5 ml tsp) | Purpose |
|---|---|
| Chlorpheniramine maleate, USP 2 mg | Antihistamine |
| Dextromethorphan hydrobromide, USP 15 mg | Cough suppressant |

**USES**
- temporarily relieves cough due to minor throat and bronchial irritation as may occur with a cold
- temporarily relieves these symptoms due to hay fever or other upper respiratory allergies:
  - runny nose
  - sneezing
  - itchy, watery eyes
  - itching of the nose or throat

**WARNINGS**

**DO NOT USE**
- to sedate a child or to make a child sleepy
- if you are now taking a prescription monoamine oxidase inhibitor (MAOI) (certain drugs for depression, psychiatric, or emotional conditions, or Parkinson's disease), or for 2 weeks after stopping the MAOI drug. If you do not know if

your prescription drug contains an MAOI, ask a doctor or pharmacist before taking this product

**ASK A DOCTOR BEFORE USE IF YOU HAVE**
- trouble urinating due to an enlarged prostate gland
- glaucoma
- a cough that occurs with too much phlegm (mucus)
- a breathing problem or chronic cough that lasts or as occurs with smoking, asthma, chronic bronchitis or emphysema

**ASK A DOCTOR OR PHARMACIST BEFORE USE IF YOU ARE**
- taking sedatives or tranquilizers

**WHEN USING THIS PRODUCT**
- do not use more than directed
- marked drowsiness may occur
- avoid alcoholic drinks
- alcohol, sedatives, and tranquilizers may increase drowsiness
- be careful when driving a motor vehicle or operating machinery
- excitability may occur, especially in children

**STOP USE AND ASK A DOCTOR IF**
- cough lasts more than 7 days, comes back, or is accompanied by fever, rash, or persistent headache. These could be signs of a serious condition

**If pregnant or breastfeeding,** ask a health professional before use.

**Keep out of reach of children.** In case of overdose, get medical help or contact a Poison Control Center right away.

**DIRECTIONS**
- do not take more than 4 doses in any 24-hour period
- this adult product is not intended for use in children under 12 years of age

| children under 12 years | do not use |
|---|---|
| adults and children 12 years and over | 2 teaspoons every 6 hours |

**OTHER INFORMATION**
- store at 20-25°C (68-77°F)
- dosage cup provided

**INACTIVE INGREDIENTS**
anhydrous citric acid, artificial & natural flavors, FD&C red no. 40, glycerin, lactic acid, menthol, propylene glycol, purified water, sodium benzoate, sodium citrate, sorbitol solution, sucralose

**QUESTIONS OR COMMENTS**
Call weekdays from 9 AM to 5 PM EST at **1-800-762-4675**

---

# CHILDREN'S ROBITUSSIN COUGH AND COLD LONG-ACTING (chlorpheniramine maleate and dextrometrorphan hydrobromide) liquid
Wyeth Consumer Healthcare

## DRUG FACTS

| Active ingredients (in each 5 ml tsp) | Purpose |
|---|---|
| Chlorpheniramine maleate, USP 1 mg | Antihistamine |
| Dextromethorphan hydrobromide, USP 7.5 mg | Cough suppressant |

**USES**
- temporarily relieves cough due to minor throat and bronchial irritation as may occur with a cold
- temporarily relieves these symptoms due to hay fever or other upper respiratory allergies:
  - runny nose
  - sneezing
  - itchy, watery eyes
  - itching of the nose or throat

**WARNINGS**

**DO NOT USE**
- to sedate a child or to make a child sleepy
- if you are now taking a prescription monoamine oxidase inhibitor (MAOI) (certain drugs for depression, psychiatric, or emotional conditions, or Parkinson's disease), or for 2 weeks after stopping the MAOI drug. If you do not know if your prescription drug contains an MAOI, ask a doctor or pharmacist before taking this product

**ASK A DOCTOR BEFORE USE IF YOU HAVE**
- trouble urinating due to an enlarged prostate gland
- glaucoma
- a cough that occurs with too much phlegm (mucus)
- a breathing problem or chronic cough that lasts or as occurs with smoking, asthma, chronic bronchitis or emphysema

**ASK A DOCTOR OR PHARMACIST BEFORE USE IF YOU ARE**
- taking sedatives or tranquilizers

**WHEN USING THIS PRODUCT**
- do not use more than directed
- marked drowsiness may occur
- avoid alcoholic drinks
- alcohol, sedatives, and tranquilizers may increase drowsiness
- be careful when driving a motor vehicle or operating machinery
- excitability may occur, especially in children

**STOP USE AND ASK A DOCTOR IF**
- cough lasts more than 7 days, comes back, or is accompanied by fever, rash, or persistent headache. These could be signs of a serious condition

**If pregnant or breastfeeding,** ask a health professional before use.

**Keep out of reach of children.** In case of overdose, get medical help or contact a Poison Control Center right away.

**DIRECTIONS**
- do not take more than 4 doses in any 24-hour period

| under 6 years | do not use |
|---|---|
| 6 to under 12 years | 2 teaspoons every 6 hours |
| 12 years and older | 4 teaspoons every 6 hours |

**OTHER INFORMATION**
- each teaspoon contains: sodium 3 mg
- store at 20-25°C (68-77°F)
- dosage cup provided

**INACTIVE INGREDIENTS**
anhydrous citric acid, artificial & natural flavors, FD&C red no. 40, glycerin, lactic acid, propylene glycol, purified water, sodium benzoate, sodium citrate, sorbitol solution, sucralose

**QUESTIONS OR COMMENTS**
Call weekdays from 9 AM to 5 PM EST at **1-800-762-4675**

# ROBITUSSIN COUGH GELS LONG-ACTING
(dextromethorphan hydrobromide) capsule, liquid filled

Wyeth Consumer Healthcare

## DRUG FACTS

| Active ingredient | Purpose |
|---|---|
| Dextromethorphan hydrobromide, USP 15 mg | Cough suppressant |

### USE
- temporarily relieves cough due to minor throat and bronchial irritation as may occur with a cold

### WARNINGS

### DO NOT USE
- if you are now taking a prescription monoamine oxidase inhibitor (MAOI) (certain drugs for depression, psychiatric, or emotional conditions, or Parkinson's disease), or for 2 weeks after stopping the MAOI drug. If you do not know if your prescription drug contains an MAOI, ask a doctor or pharmacist before taking this product

### ASK A DOCTOR BEFORE USE IF YOU HAVE
- a cough that occurs with too much phlegm (mucus)
- a cough that lasts or is chronic as occurs with smoking, asthma, or emphysema

### STOP USE AND ASK A DOCTOR IF
- cough lasts more than 7 days, comes back, or is accompanied by fever, rash, or persistent headache. These could be signs of a serious condition

**If pregnant or breastfeeding,** ask a health professional before use.

**Keep out of reach of children.** In case of overdose, get medical help or contact a Poison Control Center right away.

### DIRECTIONS
- do not take more than 8 capsules in any 24-hour period
- this adult product is not intended for use in children under 12 years of age

| adults and children 12 years and over | take 2 capsules every 6 to 8 hours, as needed |
|---|---|
| children under 12 years | do not use |

### OTHER INFORMATION
- store at 20-25°C (68-77°F)
- avoid excessive heat above 40°C (104°F)
- protect from light

### INACTIVE INGREDIENTS
FD&C blue no. 1, FD&C red no. 40, gelatin, glycerin, mannitol, medium chain triglycerides, pharmaceutical ink, polyethylene glycol, povidone, propyl gallate, propylene glycol, purified water, sorbitol, sorbitol anhydrides

### QUESTIONS OR COMMENTS
Call weekdays from 9 AM to 5 PM EST at **1-800-762-4675**

# CHILDREN'S ROBITUSSIN COUGH LONG-ACTING (dextromethorphan hydrobromide) liquid

Wyeth Consumer Healthcare

## DRUG FACTS

| Active ingredient (in each 5 ml tsp) | Purpose |
|---|---|
| Dextromethorphan hydrobromide, USP 7.5 mg | Cough suppressant |

### USE
- temporarily relieves cough due to minor throat and bronchial irritation as may occur with a cold

### WARNINGS

### DO NOT USE
- if you are now taking a prescription monoamine oxidase inhibitor (MAOI) (certain drugs for depression, psychiatric, or emotional conditions, or Parkinson's disease), or for 2 weeks after stopping the MAOI drug. If you do not know if your prescription drug contains an MAOI, ask a doctor or pharmacist before taking this product

### ASK A DOCTOR BEFORE USE IF YOU HAVE
- cough that occurs with too much phlegm (mucus)
- cough that lasts or is chronic such as occurs with smoking, asthma, or emphysema

### STOP USE AND ASK A DOCTOR IF
- cough lasts more than 7 days, comes back, or is accompanied by fever, rash, or persistent headache. These could be signs of a serious condition

**If pregnant or breastfeeding,** ask a health professional before use.

**Keep out of reach of children.** In case of overdose, get medical help or contact a Poison Control Center right away.

### DIRECTIONS
- do not take more than 4 doses in any 24-hour period

| children under 4 years | do not use |
|---|---|
| children 4 to under 6 years | 1 teaspoon every 6 to 8 hours |
| children 6 to under 12 years | 2 teaspoons every 6 to 8 hours |
| adults and children 12 years and older | 4 teaspoons every 6 to 8 hours |

### OTHER INFORMATION
- each teaspoon contains: sodium 5 mg
- store at 20-25°C (68-77°F)
- dosage cup provided

### INACTIVE INGREDIENTS
anhydrous citric acid, artificial flavor, FD&C red no. 40, glycerin, high fructose corn syrup, propylene glycol, purified water, saccharin sodium, sodium benzoate, sodium chloride, sodium citrate

### QUESTIONS OR COMMENTS
Call weekdays from 9 AM to 5 PM EST at **1-800-762-4675**

## ROBITUSSIN LINGERING COLD LONG-ACTING COUGHGELS (dextromethorphan hydrobromide) capsule, liquid filled
Pfizer

### DRUG FACTS

| Active ingredient | Purpose |
|---|---|
| Dextromethorphan hydrobromide, USP 15 mg | Cough suppressant |

### USE
- temporarily relieves cough due to minor throat and bronchial irritation as may occur with a cold

### WARNINGS

**DO NOT USE**
- if you are now taking a prescription monoamine oxidase inhibitor (MAOI) (certain drugs for depression, psychiatric, or emotional conditions, or Parkinson's disease), or for 2 weeks after stopping the MAOI drug. If you do not know if your prescription drug contains an MAOI, ask a doctor or pharmacist before taking this product

**ASK A DOCTOR BEFORE USE IF YOU HAVE**
- a cough that occurs with too much phlegm (mucus)
- a cough that lasts or is chronic as occurs with smoking, asthma, or emphysema

**STOP USE AND ASK A DOCTOR IF**
- cough lasts more than 7 days, comes back, or is accompanied by fever, rash, or persistent headache. These could be signs of a serious condition

**If pregnant or breastfeeding,** ask a health professional before use.

**Keep out of reach of children.** In case of overdose, get medical help or contact a Poison Control Center right away.

### DIRECTIONS
- do not take more than 8 capsules in any 24-hour period
- this adult product is not intended for use in children under 12 years of age

| adults and children 12 years and over | take 2 capsules every 6 to 8 hours, as needed |
|---|---|
| children under 12 years | do not use |

### OTHER INFORMATION
- store at 20-25°C (68-77°F)
- avoid excessive heat above 40°C (104°F)
- protect from light

### INACTIVE INGREDIENTS
FD&C blue no. 1, FD&C red no. 40, fractionated coconut oil, gelatin, glycerin, mannitol, pharmaceutical ink, polyethylene glycol, povidone, propyl gallate, propylene glycol, purified water, sorbitol, sorbitol anhydrides

### QUESTIONS OR COMMENTS
Call weekdays from 9 AM-5 PM EST at **1-800-762-4675**

## ROBITUSSIN LINGERING COLD LONG-ACTING COUGH (dextromethorphan hydrobromide) liquid
Pfizer

### DRUG FACTS

| Active ingredient (in each 5 ml tsp) | Purpose |
|---|---|
| Dextromethorphan hydrobromide, USP 15 mg | Cough suppressant |

### USE
- temporarily relieves cough due to minor throat and bronchial irritation as may occur with a cold

### WARNINGS

**DO NOT USE**
- if you are now taking a prescription monoamine oxidase inhibitor (MAOI) (certain drugs for depression, psychiatric, or emotional conditions, or Parkinson's disease), or for 2 weeks after stopping the MAOI drug. If you do not know if your prescription drug contains an MAOI, ask a doctor or pharmacist before taking this product

**ASK A DOCTOR BEFORE USE IF YOU HAVE**
- a cough that occurs with too much phlegm (mucus)
- a cough that lasts or is chronic such as occurs with smoking, asthma, or emphysema

**STOP USE AND ASK A DOCTOR IF**
- cough lasts more than 7 days, comes back, or is accompanied by fever, rash, or persistent headache. These could be signs of a serious condition

**If pregnant or breastfeeding,** ask a health professional before use.

**Keep out of reach of children.** In case of overdose, get medical help or contact a Poison Control Center right away.

### DIRECTIONS
- do not take more than 4 doses in any 24-hour period
- this adult product is not intended for use in children under 12 years of age

| children under 12 years | do not use |
|---|---|
| adults and children 12 years and over | 2 teaspoons every 6 to 8 hours |

### OTHER INFORMATION
- store at 20-25°C (68-77°F)
- dosage cup provided

### INACTIVE INGREDIENTS
alcohol, anhydrous citric acid, artificial & natural flavors, FD&C red no. 40, glycerin, high fructose corn syrup, liquid glucose, menthol, purified water, saccharin sodium, sodium benzoate

### QUESTIONS OR COMMENTS
Call weekdays from 9 AM-5 PM EST at **1-800-762-4675**

## ROBITUSSIN NIGHT TIME COUGH AND COLD (diphenhydramine hydrochloride and phenylephrine hydrochloride) liquid

Wyeth Consumer Healthcare

### DRUG FACTS

| Active ingredients (in each 5 ml tsp) | Purpose |
|---|---|
| Diphenhydramine hydrochloride, USP 6.25 mg | Antihistamine/cough suppressant |
| Phenylephrine hydrochloride, USP 2.5 mg | Nasal Decongestant |

### USES
- temporarily relieves these symptoms occurring with a cold, hay fever, or other upper respiratory allergies:
  - nasal congestion
  - cough
  - runny nose
  - sneezing
  - itchy, watery eyes
  - itching of the nose or throat

### WARNINGS

### DO NOT USE
- to sedate a child or to make a child sleepy
- if you are now taking a prescription monoamine oxidase inhibitor (MAOI) (certain drugs for depression, psychiatric, or emotional conditions, or Parkinson's disease), or for 2 weeks after stopping the MAOI drug. If you do not know if your prescription drug contains an MAOI, ask a doctor or pharmacist before taking this product
- with any other product containing diphenhydramine, even one used on skin

### ASK A DOCTOR BEFORE USE IF YOU HAVE
- heart disease
- high blood pressure
- thyroid disease
- diabetes
- trouble urinating due to an enlarged prostate gland
- glaucoma
- cough that occurs with too much phlegm (mucus)
- a breathing problem or a chronic cough that lasts or as occurs with smoking, asthma, chronic bronchitis, or emphysema

### ASK A DOCTOR OR PHARMACIST BEFORE USE IF YOU ARE
- taking sedatives or tranquilizers

### WHEN USING THIS PRODUCT
- do not use more than directed
- marked drowsiness may occur
- avoid alcoholic drinks
- alcohol, sedatives, and tranquilizers may increase drowsiness
- be careful when driving a motor vehicle or operating machinery
- excitability may occur, especially in children

### STOP USE AND ASK A DOCTOR IF
- you get nervous, dizzy, or sleepless
- symptoms do not get better within 7 days or are accompanied by fever
- cough lasts more than 7 days, comes back, or is accompanied by fever, rash, or persistent headache. These could be signs of a serious condition

**If pregnant or breastfeeding,** ask a health professional before use.

**Keep out of reach of children.** In case of overdose, get medical help or contact a Poison Control Center right away.

### DIRECTIONS
- do not take more than 6 doses in any 24-hour period
- do not exceed recommended dosage
- this adult product is not intended for use in children under 12 years of age

| adults and children 12 years and over | 4 teaspoons every 4 hours |
|---|---|
| children under 12 years | do not use |

### OTHER INFORMATION
- each teaspoon contains: sodium 3 mg
- store at 20-25°C (68-77°F)
- dosage cup provided

### INACTIVE INGREDIENTS
anhydrous citric acid, artificial flavors, FD&C red no. 40, glycerin, menthol, polyethylene glycol, propyl gallate, propylene glycol, purified water, sodium benzoate, sodium citrate, sorbitol solution, sucralose

### QUESTIONS OR COMMENTS
Call weekdays from 9 AM to 5 PM EST at **1-800-762-4675**

## ROBITUSSIN NIGHT TIME COUGH, COLD & FLU (acetaminophen, chlorpheniramine maleate, dextromethorphan hydrobromide and phenylephrine hydrochloride) liquid

Wyeth Consumer Healthcare

### DRUG FACTS

| Active ingredients (in each 5 ml tsp) | Purpose |
|---|---|
| Acetaminophen, USP 160 mg | Pain reliever/Fever reducer |
| Chlorpheniramine maleate, USP 1 mg | Antihistamine |
| Dextromethorphan hydrobromide, USP 5 mg | Cough suppressant |
| Phenylephrine hydrochloride, USP 2.5 mg | Nasal decongestant |

### USES
- temporarily relieves these symptoms occurring with a cold or flu, hay fever, or other upper respiratory allergies:
  - headache
  - nasal congestion
  - sore throat
  - fever
  - cough
  - minor aches and pains
  - runny nose
  - sneezing
  - itchy, watery eyes
  - itching of the nose or throat

## WARNINGS

**Liver warning:**
This product contains acetaminophen. Severe liver damage may occur if user takes:

- more than 5 doses in 24 hours
- with other drugs containing acetaminophen
- 3 or more alcoholic drinks every day while using this product

**Sore throat warning**
If sore throat is severe, persists for more than 2 days, is accompanied or followed by fever, headache, rash, nausea, or vomiting, consult a doctor promptly.

## DO NOT USE

- to sedate a child or to make a child sleepy
- if user is now taking a prescription monoamine oxidase inhibitor (MAOI) (certain drugs for depression, psychiatric, or emotional conditions, or Parkinson's disease), or for 2 weeks after stopping the MAOI drug. If you do not know if your prescription drug contains an MAOI, ask a doctor or pharmacist before taking this product
- with any other drug containing acetaminophen (prescription or nonprescription). Ask a doctor or pharmacist before using with other drugs if you are not sure

## ASK A DOCTOR BEFORE USE IF USER HAS

- liver disease
- heart disease
- high blood pressure
- thyroid disease
- diabetes
- trouble urinating due to an enlarged prostate gland
- glaucoma
- cough that occurs with too much phlegm (mucus)
- a breathing problem or chronic cough that lasts or as occurs with smoking, asthma, chronic bronchitis, or emphysema

## ASK A DOCTOR OR PHARMACIST BEFORE USE IF USER IS

- taking any other pain reliever/fever reducer
- taking sedatives or tranquilizers

## WHEN USING THIS PRODUCT

- do not use more than directed
- marked drowsiness may occur
- avoid alcoholic drinks
- alcohol, sedatives, and tranquilizers may increase drowsiness
- be careful when driving a motor vehicle or operating machinery
- excitability may occur, especially in children

## STOP USE AND ASK A DOCTOR IF

- user gets nervous, dizzy, or sleepless
- pain, cough, or nasal congestion gets worse or lasts more than 5 days (children) or 7 days (adults)
- fever gets worse or lasts more than 3 days
- redness or swelling is present
- cough comes back or occurs with rash or headache that lasts. These could be signs of a serious condition
- new symptoms occur

**If pregnant or breastfeeding,** ask a health professional before use.

**Keep out of reach of children.** In case of overdose, get medical help or contact a Poison Control Center right away. Prompt medical attention is critical for adults as well as for children, even if you do not notice any signs or symptoms.

## DIRECTIONS

- do not take more than 5 doses in any 24-hour period
- do not exceed recommended dosage. Taking more than the recommended dose (overdose) may cause serious liver damage

- this adult product is not intended for use in children under 12 years of age

| Age | Dose |
|---|---|
| adults and children 12 years and over | 4 teaspoons every 4 hours |
| children under 12 years | do not use |

## OTHER INFORMATION

- each teaspoon contains: sodium 2 mg
- store at 20-25°C (68-77°F)
- dosage cup provided

## INACTIVE INGREDIENTS

anhydrous citric acid, artificial & natural flavors, FD&C red no. 40, glycerin, lactic acid, menthol, polyethylene glycol, propyl gallate, propylene glycol, purified water, sodium benzoate, sodium citrate, sorbitol solution, sucralose

## QUESTIONS OR COMMENTS

Call weekdays from 9 AM to 5 PM EST at **1-800-762-4675**

---

# ROBITUSSIN PEAK COLD COUGH PLUS CHEST CONGESTION DM/SUGAR-FREE COUGH PLUS CHEST CONGESTION DM
(dextromethorphan hydrobromide, guaifenesin) liquid
Pfizer

## DRUG FACTS

| Active ingredients (in each 5 ml tsp) | Purpose |
|---|---|
| Dextromethorphan hydrobromide, USP 10 mg | Cough suppressant |
| Guaifenesin, USP 100 mg | Expectorant |

## USES

- temporarily relieves cough due to minor throat and bronchial irritation as may occur with a cold
- helps loosen phlegm (mucus) and thin bronchial secretions to drain bronchial tubes

## WARNINGS

### DO NOT USE

- if you are now taking a prescription monoamine oxidase inhibitor (MAOI) (certain drugs for depression, psychiatric, or emotional conditions, or Parkinson's disease), or for 2 weeks after stopping the MAOI drug. If you do not know if your prescription drug contains an MAOI, ask a doctor or pharmacist before taking this product

### ASK A DOCTOR BEFORE USE IF YOU HAVE

- cough that occurs with too much phlegm (mucus)
- cough that lasts or is chronic such as occurs with smoking, asthma, chronic bronchitis or emphysema

### STOP USE AND ASK A DOCTOR IF

- cough lasts more than 7 days, comes back, or is accompanied by fever, rash, or persistent headache. These could be signs of a serious condition.

**If pregnant or breastfeeding,** ask a health professional before use.

**Keep out of reach of children.** In case of overdose, get medical help or contact a Poison Control Center right away.

### DIRECTIONS
- do not take more than 6 doses in any 24-hour period
- this adult product is not intended for use in children under 12 years of age

| adults and children 12 years and over | 2 teaspoons every 4 hours |
|---|---|
| children under 12 years | do not use |

### OTHER INFORMATION
**Robitussin Peak Cold Cough+Chest Congestion DM**
- each teaspoon contains: sodium 7 mg
- store at 20-25°C (68-77°F). Do not refrigerate
- dosage cup provided

**Robitussin Peak Cold Sugar-Free Cough+Chest Congestion DM**
- each teaspoon contains: sodium 3 mg
- store at 20-25°C (68-77°F). Do not refrigerate
- alcohol-free
- dosage cup provided

### INACTIVE INGREDIENTS
**Robitussin Peak Cold Cough+Chest Congestion DM**
anhydrous citric acid, FD&C red no. 40, glycerin, high fructose corn syrup, menthol, natural flavor, propylene glycol, purified water, sodium benzoate, sodium citrate, sucralose

**Robitussin Peak Cold Sugar-Free Cough+Chest Congestion DM**
acesulfame potassium, artificial & natural flavor, citric acid monohydrate, glycerin, methylparaben, polyethylene glycol, povidone, propylene glycol, purified water, saccharin sodium, sodium benzoate

### QUESTIONS OR COMMENTS
Call weekdays from 9 AM to 5 PM EST at **1-800-762-4675**

---

# ROBITUSSIN PEAK COLD MAXIMUM STRENGTH MULTI-SYMPTOM COLD
(dextromethorphan hydrobromide, guaifenesin, phenylephrine hydrochloride) liquid
Pfizer

## DRUG FACTS

| Active ingredients (in each 5 ml tsp) | Purpose |
|---|---|
| Dextromethorphan hydrobromide, USP 10 mg | Cough suppressant |
| Guaifenesin, USP 200 mg | Expectorant |
| Phenylephrine hydrochloride, USP 5 mg | Nasal decongestant |

### USES
- helps loosen phlegm (mucus) and thin bronchial secretions to drain bronchial tubes
- temporarily relieves these symptoms occurring with a cold:
  - nasal congestion
  - cough due to minor throat and bronchial irritation

### WARNINGS

**DO NOT USE**
- if you are now taking a prescription monoamine oxidase inhibitor (MAOI) (certain drugs for depression, psychiatric, or emotional conditions, or Parkinson's disease), or for 2 weeks after stopping the MAOI drug. If you do not know if your prescription drug contains an MAOI, ask a doctor or pharmacist before taking this product

**ASK A DOCTOR BEFORE USE IF YOU HAVE**
- heart disease
- high blood pressure
- thyroid disease
- diabetes
- trouble urinating due to an enlarged prostate gland
- cough that occurs with too much phlegm (mucus)
- cough that lasts or is chronic such as occurs with smoking, asthma, chronic bronchitis or emphysema

**ASK A DOCTOR OR PHARMACIST BEFORE USE IF YOU ARE**
- taking any other oral nasal decongestant or stimulant

**WHEN USING THIS PRODUCT**
- do not use more than directed

**STOP USE AND ASK A DOCTOR IF**
- you get nervous, dizzy, or sleepless
- symptoms do not get better within 7 days or are accompanied by fever
- cough lasts more than 7 days, comes back, or is accompanied by fever, rash, or persistent headache. These could be signs of a serious condition

**If pregnant or breastfeeding,** ask a health professional before use.

**Keep out of reach of children.** In case of overdose, get medical help or contact a Poison Control Center right away.

### DIRECTIONS
- shake well before using
- do not take more than 6 doses in any 24-hour period
- this adult product is not intended for use in children under 12 years of age

| adults and children 12 years and over | 2 teaspoons every 4 hours |
|---|---|
| children under 12 years | do not use |

### OTHER INFORMATION
- each teaspoon contains: sodium 3 mg
- store at 20-25°C (68-77°F)
- do not refrigerate
- dosage cup provided

### INACTIVE INGREDIENTS
anhydrous citric acid, FD&C red no. 40, glycerin, menthol, natural flavor, polyethylene glycol, propylene glycol, purified water, sodium benzoate, sodium citrate, sorbitol solution, sucralose, xanthan gum

### QUESTIONS OR COMMENTS
Call weekdays from 9 AM to 5 PM EST at **1-800-762-4675**

# ROBITUSSIN PEAK COLD MAXIMUM STRENGTH COUGH PLUS CHEST CONGESTION DM (dextromethorphan hydrobromide, guaifenesin) liquid

Pfizer

## DRUG FACTS

| Active ingredients (in each 5 ml tsp) | Purpose |
|---|---|
| Dextromethorphan hydrobromide, USP 10 mg | Cough suppressant |
| Guaifenesin, USP 200 mg | Expectorant |

### USES
- temporarily relieves cough due to minor throat and bronchial irritation as may occur with a cold
- helps loosen phlegm (mucus) and thin bronchial secretions to drain bronchial tubes

### WARNINGS

#### DO NOT USE
- if you are now taking a prescription monoamine oxidase inhibitor (MAOI) (certain drugs for depression, psychiatric, or emotional conditions, or Parkinson's disease), or for 2 weeks after stopping the MAOI drug. If you do not know if your prescription drug contains an MAOI, ask a doctor or pharmacist before taking this product

#### ASK A DOCTOR BEFORE USE IF YOU HAVE
- cough that occurs with too much phlegm (mucus)
- cough that lasts or is chronic such as occurs with smoking, asthma, chronic bronchitis, or emphysema

#### STOP USE AND ASK A DOCTOR IF
- cough lasts more than 7 days, comes back, or is accompanied by fever, rash, or persistent headache. These could be signs of a serious condition

**If pregnant or breastfeeding,** ask a health professional before use.

**Keep out of reach of children.** In case of overdose, get medical help or contact a Poison Control Center right away.

### DIRECTIONS
- shake well before using
- do not take more than 6 doses in any 24-hour period
- this adult product is not intended for use in children under 12 years of age

| adults and children 12 years and over | 2 teaspoons every 4 hours |
|---|---|
| children under 12 years | do not use |

### OTHER INFORMATION
- each teaspoon contains: sodium 5 mg
- store at 20-25°C (68-77°F)
- do not refrigerate
- dosage cup provided

### INACTIVE INGREDIENTS
anhydrous citric acid, carboxymethylcellulose sodium, D&C red no. 33, FD&C red no. 40, glycerin, high fructose corn syrup, menthol, microcrystalline cellulose, natural and artificial flavor, polyethylene glycol, povidone, propylene glycol, purified water, saccharin sodium, sodium benzoate, sorbitol solution, xanthan gum

### QUESTIONS OR COMMENTS
Call weekdays from 9 AM to 5 PM EST at **1-800-762-4675**

---

# ROBITUSSIN PEAK COLD MULTI-SYMPTOM COLD (dextromethorphan hydrobromide, guaifenesin and phenylephrine hydrochloride) liquid

Pfizer

## DRUG FACTS

| Active ingredients (in each 5 ml tsp) | Purpose |
|---|---|
| Dextromethorphan hydrobromide, USP 10 mg | Cough suppressant |
| Guaifenesin, USP 100 mg | Expectorant |
| Phenylephrine hydrochloride, USP 5 mg | Nasal decongestant |

### USES
- helps loosen phlegm (mucus) and thin bronchial secretions to drain bronchial tubes
- temporarily relieves these symptoms occurring with a cold:
  - nasal congestion
  - cough due to minor throat and bronchial irritation

### WARNINGS

#### DO NOT USE
- if you are now taking a prescription monoamine oxidase inhibitor (MAOI) (certain drugs for depression, psychiatric, or emotional conditions, or Parkinson's disease), or for 2 weeks after stopping the MAOI drug. If you do not know if your prescription drug contains an MAOI, ask a doctor or pharmacist before taking this product

#### ASK A DOCTOR BEFORE USE IF YOU HAVE
- heart disease
- high blood pressure
- thyroid disease
- diabetes
- trouble urinating due to an enlarged prostate gland
- cough that occurs with too much phlegm (mucus)
- cough that lasts or is chronic such as occurs with smoking, asthma, chronic bronchitis, or emphysema

#### ASK A DOCTOR OR PHARMACIST BEFORE USE IF YOU ARE
- taking any other oral nasal decongestant or stimulant

#### WHEN USING THIS PRODUCT
- do not use more than directed

#### STOP USE AND ASK A DOCTOR IF
- you get nervous, dizzy, or sleepless
- symptoms do not get better within 7 days or are accompanied by fever
- cough lasts more than 7 days, comes back, or is accompanied by fever, rash, or persistent headache. These could be signs of a serious condition

**If pregnant or breastfeeding,** ask a health professional before use.

**Keep out of reach of children.** In case of overdose, get medical help or contact a Poison Control Center right away.

## DIRECTIONS
- do not take more than 6 doses in any 24-hour period
- this adult product is not intended for use in children under 12 years of age

| adults and children 12 years and over | 2 teaspoons every 4 hours |
|---|---|
| children under 12 years | do not use |

## OTHER INFORMATION
- each teaspoon contains: sodium 3 mg
- store at 20-25°C (68-77°F). Do not refrigerate
- dosage cup provided

## INACTIVE INGREDIENTS
anhydrous citric acid, FD&C red no. 40, glycerin, menthol, natural & artificial flavor, propylene glycol, purified water, sodium benzoate, sodium citrate, sorbitol solution, sucralose

## QUESTIONS OR COMMENTS
Call weekdays from 9 AM to 5 PM EST at **1-800-762-4675**

---

# ROBITUSSIN PEAK COLD NASAL RELIEF
(acetaminophen, and phenylephrine hydrochloride) tablet
Pfizer

## DRUG FACTS

| Active ingredients (in each tablet) | Purpose |
|---|---|
| Acetaminophen, USP 325 mg | Pain reliever/fever reducer |
| Phenylephrine hydrochloride, USP 5 mg | Nasal decongestant |

## USES
- temporarily relieves these symptoms associated with a cold or flu, hay fever or other upper respiratory allergies:
  - nasal congestion
  - sinus congestion and pressure
  - reduces swelling of nasal passages
  - restores freer breathing through the nose
  - headache
  - sore throat
  - minor aches and pains
- temporarily reduces fever

## WARNINGS
**Liver warning**
This product contains acetaminophen. Severe liver damage may occur if you take:
- more than 12 tablets in any 24-hour period, which is the maximum daily amount
- with other drugs containing acetaminophen
- 3 or more alcoholic drinks every day while using this product

**Sore throat warning**
If sore throat is severe, persists for more than 2 days, is accompanied or followed by fever, headache, rash, nausea, or vomiting, consult a doctor promptly.

**DO NOT USE**
- if you are now taking a prescription monoamine oxidase inhibitor (MAOI) (certain drugs for depression, psychiatric, or emotional conditions, or Parkinson's disease), or for 2 weeks after stopping the MAOI drug. If you do not know if your prescription drug contains an MAOI, ask a doctor or pharmacist before taking this product
- with any other drug containing acetaminophen (prescription or nonprescription). If you are not sure whether a drug contains acetaminophen ask a doctor or pharmacist

**ASK A DOCTOR BEFORE USE IF YOU HAVE**
- liver disease
- heart disease
- high blood pressure
- thyroid disease
- diabetes
- trouble urinating due to an enlarged prostate gland

**ASK A DOCTOR OR PHARMACIST BEFORE USE IF YOU ARE**
- taking the blood thinning drug warfarin
- taking any other oral nasal decongestant or stimulant
- taking any other pain reliever/fever reducer

**WHEN USING THIS PRODUCT**
- do not use more than directed

**STOP USE AND ASK A DOCTOR IF**
- you get nervous, dizzy, or sleepless
- pain or nasal congestion gets worse or lasts more than 7 days
- fever gets worse or lasts more than 3 days
- redness or swelling is present
- new symptoms occur

**If pregnant or breastfeeding,** ask a health professional before use.

**Keep out of reach of children.** In case of overdose, get medical help or contact a Poison Control Center right away. Prompt medical attention is critical for adults as well as for children, even if you do not notice any signs or symptoms.

## DIRECTIONS
- do not use more than 12 tablets in any 24-hour period
- do not exceed recommended dosage. Taking more than the recommended dose (overdose) may cause serious liver damage
- this adult product is not intended for use in children under 12 years of age

| adults and children 12 years and over | 2 tablets every 4 hours |
|---|---|
| children under 12 years | do not use |

## OTHER INFORMATION
- store at 20-25°C (68-77°F)
- tamper-evident individual blisters

## INACTIVE INGREDIENTS
calcium stearate, croscarmellose sodium, crospovidone, hypromellose, microcrystalline cellulose, polyethylene glycol, povidone, pregelatinized starch, stearic acid

## QUESTIONS OR COMMENTS
Call weekdays from 9 AM to 5 PM EST at **1-800-762-4675**

# ROBITUSSIN PEAK COLD NIGHTTIME MULTI-SYMPTOM COLD (acetaminophen, diphenhydramine hydrochloride, and phenylephrine hydrochloride) liquid

Richmond Division of Wyeth

## DRUG FACTS

| Active ingredients (in each 5 ml tsp) | Purpose |
|---|---|
| Acetaminophen, USP 160 mg | Pain reliever/fever reducer |
| Diphenhydramine hydrochloride, USP 6.25 mg | Antihistamine/cough suppressant |
| Phenylephrine hydrochloride, USP 2.5 mg | Nasal decongestant |

## USES
- temporarily relieves these symptoms occurring with a cold or flu, hay fever, or other upper respiratory allergies:
  - headache
  - nasal congestion
  - sore throat
  - cough
  - minor aches and pains
  - runny nose
  - sneezing
  - itchy, watery eyes
  - itching of the nose or throat
- temporarily reduces fever

## WARNINGS
**Liver warning**
This product contains acetaminophen. Severe liver damage may occur if user takes:

- more than 24 teaspoons in any 24-hour period, which is the maximum daily amount
- with other drugs containing acetaminophen
- 3 or more alcoholic drinks every day while using this product

**Sore throat warning**
If sore throat is severe, persists for more than 2 days, is accompanied or followed by fever, headache, rash, nausea, or vomiting, consult a doctor promptly.

## DO NOT USE
- to sedate a child or to make a child sleepy
- if you are now taking a prescription monoamine oxidase inhibitor (MAOI) (certain drugs for depression, psychiatric, or emotional conditions, or Parkinson's disease), or for 2 weeks after stopping the MAOI drug. If you do not know if your prescription drug contains an MAOI, ask a doctor or pharmacist before taking this product
- with any other drug containing acetaminophen (prescription or nonprescription). If you are not sure whether a drug contains acetaminophen ask a doctor or pharmacist
- with any other product containing diphenhydramine, even one used on skin

## ASK A DOCTOR BEFORE USE IF USER HAS
- liver disease
- heart disease
- high blood pressure
- thyroid disease
- diabetes
- trouble urinating due to an enlarged prostate gland
- glaucoma
- cough that occurs with too much phlegm (mucus)
- a breathing problem or chronic cough that lasts or as occurs with smoking, asthma, chronic bronchitis, or emphysema

## ASK A DOCTOR OR PHARMACIST BEFORE USE IF USER IS
- taking the blood thinning drug warfarin
- taking any other oral nasal decongestant or stimulant
- taking any other pain reliever/fever reducer
- taking sedatives or tranquilizers

## WHEN USING THIS PRODUCT
- do not use more than directed
- marked drowsiness may occur
- avoid alcoholic drinks
- alcohol, sedatives, and tranquilizers may increase drowsiness
- be careful when driving a motor vehicle or operating machinery
- excitability may occur, especially in children

## STOP USE AND ASK A DOCTOR IF
- user gets nervous, dizzy, or sleepless
- pain, cough, or nasal congestion gets worse or lasts more than 5 days (children) or 7 days (adults)
- fever gets worse or lasts more than 3 days
- redness or swelling is present
- cough comes back or occurs with rash or headache that lasts. These could be signs of a serious condition
- new symptoms occur

**If pregnant or breastfeeding,** ask a health professional before use.

**Keep out of reach of children.** In case of overdose, get medical help or contact a Poison Control Center right away. Prompt medical attention is critical for adults as well as for children, even if you do not notice any signs or symptoms.

## DIRECTIONS
- do not take more than 6 doses in any 24-hour period
- do not exceed recommended dosage. Taking more than the recommended dose (overdose) may cause serious liver damage
- this adult product is not intended for use in children under 12 years of age

| adults and children 12 years and over | 4 teaspoons every 4 hours |
|---|---|
| children under 12 years | do not use |

## OTHER INFORMATION
- each teaspoon contains: sodium 4 mg
- store at 20-25°C (68-77°F)

## INACTIVE INGREDIENTS
anhydrous citric acid, artificial flavor, edetate disodium, FD&C red no. 40, glycerin, menthol, polyethylene glycol, propyl gallate, propylene glycol, purified water, sodium benzoate, sodium citrate, sorbitol solution, sucralose

## QUESTIONS OR COMMENTS
Call weekdays from 9 AM to 5 PM EST at **1-800-762-4675**

## ROBITUSSIN PEAK COLD NIGHTTIME NASAL RELIEF (acetaminophen, chlorpheniramine maleate, and phenylephrine hydrochloride) tablet

Richmond Division of Wyeth

### DRUG FACTS

| Active ingredients (in each tablet) | Purpose |
|---|---|
| Acetaminophen, USP 325 mg | Pain reliever/Fever reducer |
| Chlorpheniramine maleate, USP 2 mg | Antihistamine |
| Phenylephrine hydrochloride, USP 5 mg | Nasal decongestant |

### USES
- temporarily relieves these symptoms associated with a cold, or flu:
  - headache
  - nasal congestion
  - sore throat
  - fever
  - minor aches and pains
- temporarily relieves minor aches, pains and headache as well as these symptoms of hay fever or other upper respiratory allergies:
  - runny nose
  - sneezing
  - nasal congestion
  - itching of the nose or throat
  - itchy, watery eyes
- temporarily relieves minor aches, pains, headache and nasal congestion as well as sinus congestion and pressure, and reduces swelling of nasal passages

### WARNINGS
**Liver warning**
This product contains acetaminophen. Severe liver damage may occur if you take:
- more than 12 tablets in any 24-hour period, which is the maximum daily amount
- with other drugs containing acetaminophen
- 3 or more alcoholic drinks every day while using this product

**Sore throat warning**
If sore throat is severe, persists for more than 2 days, is accompanied or followed by fever, headache, rash, nausea, or vomiting, consult a doctor promptly.

### DO NOT USE
- to sedate a child or to make a child sleepy
- if you are now taking a prescription monoamine oxidase inhibitor (MAOI) (certain drugs for depression, psychiatric, or emotional conditions, or Parkinson's disease), or for 2 weeks after stopping the MAOI drug. If you do not know if your prescription drug contains an MAOI, ask a doctor or pharmacist before taking this product
- with any other drug containing acetaminophen (prescription or nonprescription). If you are not sure whether a drug contains acetaminophen ask a doctor or pharmacist

### ASK A DOCTOR BEFORE USE IF YOU HAVE
- liver disease
- heart disease
- high blood pressure
- thyroid disease
- diabetes
- trouble urinating due to an enlarged prostate gland
- glaucoma
- a breathing problem such as emphysema, asthma, or chronic bronchitis

### ASK A DOCTOR OR PHARMACIST BEFORE USE IF YOU ARE
- taking the blood thinning drug warfarin
- taking any other oral nasal decongestant or stimulant
- taking any other pain reliever/fever reducer
- taking sedatives or tranquilizers

### WHEN USING THIS PRODUCT
- do not use more than directed
- drowsiness may occur
- avoid alcoholic drinks
- alcohol, sedatives, and tranquilizers may increase drowsiness
- be careful when driving a motor vehicle or operating machinery
- excitability may occur, especially in children

### STOP USE AND ASK A DOCTOR IF
- you get nervous, dizzy, or sleepless
- pain or nasal congestion gets worse or lasts more than 7 days
- fever gets worse or lasts more than 3 days
- redness or swelling is present
- new symptoms occur

**If pregnant or breastfeeding,** ask a health professional before use.

**Keep out of reach of children.** In case of overdose, get medical help or contact a Poison Control Center right away. Prompt medical attention is critical for adults as well as for children, even if you do not notice any signs or symptoms.

### DIRECTIONS
- do not use more than 12 tablets in any 24-hour period
- do not exceed recommended dosage. Taking more than the recommended dose (overdose) may cause serious liver damage
- this adult product is not intended for use in children under 12 years of age

| adults and children 12 years and over | 2 tablets every 4 hours |
|---|---|
| children under 12 years | do not use |

### OTHER INFORMATION
- store at 20-25°C (68-77°F)
- tamper-evident individual blisters

### INACTIVE INGREDIENTS
calcium stearate, croscarmellose sodium, crospovidone, D&C yellow no. 10 aluminum lake, FD&C yellow no. 6 aluminum lake, hypromellose, microcrystalline cellulose, polyethylene glycol, povidone, pregelatinized starch, stearic acid

### QUESTIONS OR COMMENTS
Call weekdays from 9 AM to 5 PM EST at **1-800-762-4675**

# ROBITUSSIN TO GO COUGH & CHEST CONGESTION DM (dextromethorphan hydrobromide, and guaifenesin) liquid

Richmond Division of Wyeth

## DRUG FACTS

| Active ingredients (in each 10 ml pre-filled spoon) | Purpose |
|---|---|
| Dextromethorphan hydrobromide, USP 20 mg | Cough suppressant |
| Guaifenesin, USP 200 mg | Expectorant |

### USES
- temporarily relieves cough due to minor throat and bronchial irritation as may occur with a cold
- helps loosen phlegm (mucus) and thin bronchial secretions to drain bronchial tubes

### WARNINGS

### DO NOT USE
- If you are now taking a prescription monoamine oxidase inhibitor (MAOI) (certain drugs for depression, psychiatric, or emotional conditions, or Parkinson's disease), or for 2 weeks after stopping the MAOI drug. If you do not know if your prescription drug contains an MAOI, ask a doctor or pharmacist before taking this product

### ASK A DOCTOR BEFORE USE IF YOU HAVE
- cough that occurs with too much phlegm (mucus)
- cough that lasts or is chronic such as occurs with smoking, asthma, chronic bronchitis, or emphysema

### STOP USE AND ASK A DOCTOR IF
- cough lasts more than 7 days, comes back, or is accompanied by fever, rash, or persistent headache. These could be signs of a serious condition

**If pregnant or breastfeeding,** ask a health professional before use.

**Keep out of reach of children.** In case of overdose, get medical help or contact a Poison Control Center right away.

### DIRECTIONS
- do not take more than 6 doses in any 24-hour period
- this adult product is not intended for use in children under 12 years of age

| adults and children 12 years and over | 1 pre-filled spoon every 4 hours |
|---|---|
| children under 12 years | do not use |

### OTHER INFORMATION
- each pre-filled spoon contains: sodium 14 mg
- store at 20-25°C (68-77°F)

### INACTIVE INGREDIENTS
anhydrous citric acid, FD&C red no. 40, glycerin, high fructose corn syrup, menthol, natural flavor, propylene glycol, purified water, sodium benzoate, sodium citrate, sucralose

### QUESTIONS OR COMMENTS
Call weekdays from 9 AM to 5 PM EST at **1-800-762-4675**

# ROBITUSSIN TO GO COUGH & COLD CF (dextromethorphan hydrobromide, guaifenesin, and phenylephrine hydrochloride) liquid

Richmond Division of Wyeth

## DRUG FACTS

| Active ingredients (in each 10 ml pre-filled spoon) | Purpose |
|---|---|
| Dextromethorphan hydrobromide, USP 20 mg | Cough suppressant |
| Guaifenesin, USP 200 mg | Expectorant |
| Phenylephrine hydrochloride, USP 10 mg | Nasal decongestant |

### USES
- helps loosen phlegm (mucus) and thin bronchial secretions to drain bronchial tubes
- temporarily relieves these symptoms occurring with a cold:
  - nasal congestion
  - cough due to minor throat and bronchial irritation

### WARNINGS

### DO NOT USE
- if you are now taking a prescription monoamine oxidase inhibitor (MAOI) (certain drugs for depression, psychiatric, or emotional conditions, or Parkinson's disease), or for 2 weeks after stopping the MAOI drug. If you do not know if your prescription drug contains an MAOI, ask a doctor or pharmacist before taking this product

### ASK A DOCTOR BEFORE USE IF YOU HAVE
- heart disease
- high blood pressure
- thyroid disease
- diabetes
- trouble urinating due to an enlarged prostate gland
- cough that occurs with too much phlegm (mucus)
- cough that lasts or is chronic such as occurs with smoking, asthma, chronic bronchitis or emphysema

### WHEN USING THIS PRODUCT
- do not use more than directed

### STOP USE AND ASK A DOCTOR IF
- you get nervous, dizzy, or sleepless
- symptoms do not get better within 7 days or are accompanied by fever
- cough lasts more than 7 days, comes back, or is accompanied by fever, rash, or persistent headache. These could be signs of a serious condition

**If pregnant or breastfeeding,** ask a health professional before use.

**Keep out of reach of children.** In case of overdose, get medical help or contact a Poison Control Center right away.

### DIRECTIONS
- do not take more than 6 doses in any 24-hour period
- this adult product is not intended for use in children under 12 years of age

| adults and children 12 years and over | 1 pre-filled spoon every 4 hours |
|---|---|
| children under 12 years | do not use |

**OTHER INFORMATION**
- each pre-filled spoon contains: sodium 6 mg
- store at 20-25°C (68-77°F)

**INACTIVE INGREDIENTS**
anhydrous citric acid, FD&C red no. 40, glycerin, menthol, natural & artificial flavor, propylene glycol, purified water, sodium benzoate, sodium citrate, sorbitol solution, sucralose

**QUESTIONS OR COMMENTS**
Call weekdays from 9 AM to 5 PM EST at **1-800-762-4675**

---

# WOMEN'S ROGAINE EXTRA STRENGTH
(minoxidil) solution

Johnson & Johnson Healthcare Products, Division of McNeil-PPC, Inc.

## DRUG FACTS

| Active ingredient | Purpose |
|---|---|
| Minoxidil 2% w/v | Hair regrowth treatment |

**USE**
- to regrow hair on the scalp

**WARNINGS**
**For external use only.**

**Flammable:** Keep away from fire or flame.

**DO NOT USE IF**
- your degree of hair loss is different than that shown on the side of this carton, because this product may not work for you
- you have no family history of hair loss
- your hair loss is sudden and/or patchy
- your hair loss is associated with childbirth
- you do not know the reason for your hair loss
- you are under 18 years of age. Do not use on babies and children
- your scalp is red, inflamed, infected, irritated, or painful
- you use other medicines on the scalp

**ASK A DOCTOR BEFORE USE IF YOU HAVE**
- heart disease

**WHEN USING THIS PRODUCT**
- do not apply on other parts of the body
- avoid contact with the eyes. In case of accidental contact, rinse eyes with large amounts of cool tap water
- some people have experienced changes in hair color and/or texture
- it takes time to regrow hair. You may need to use this product 2 times a day for at least 4 months before you see results
- the amount of hair regrowth is different for each person. This product will not work for everyone

**STOP USE AND ASK A DOCTOR IF**
- chest pain, rapid heartbeat, faintness, or dizziness occurs
- sudden, unexplained weight gain occurs
- your hands or feet swell
- scalp irritation or redness occurs
- unwanted facial hair growth occurs
- you do not see hair regrowth in 4 months

**May be harmful if used when pregnant or breastfeeding.**

**Keep out of reach of children**. If swallowed, get medical help or contact a Poison Control Center right away.

**DIRECTIONS**
- apply one mL with dropper 2 times a day directly onto the scalp in the hair loss area
- using more or more often will not improve results
- continued use is necessary to increase and keep your hair regrowth, or hair loss will begin again

**OTHER INFORMATION**
- see hair loss pictures on side of carton
- before use, read all information on carton and enclosed booklet
- keep carton. It contains important information
- store at controlled room temperature 20°C-25°C (68°F-77°F)

**INACTIVE INGREDIENTS**
alcohol, propylene glycol, purified water

**QUESTIONS OR COMMENTS**
Call us at **1-800-ROGAINE (1-800-764-2463)**
visit rogaine.com
for more information about hair thinning, visit womenhairinstitute.com

---

# ROLAIDS MULTI-SYMPTOM (calcium carbonate and simethicone) bar, chewable

McNeil Consumer Healthcare, Division of McNeil-PPC, Inc.

## DRUG FACTS

| Active ingredients (in each chew) | Purpose |
|---|---|
| Calcium carbonate 1177 mg | Antacid |
| Simethicone 80 mg | Antigas |

**USES**
- relieves:
  - heartburn
  - sour stomach
  - acid indigestion
  - upset stomach due to these symptoms
  - bloating, pressure, and discomfort commonly referred to as gas

**WARNINGS**

**ASK A DOCTOR OR PHARMACIST BEFORE USE IF YOU ARE**
- now taking a prescription drug. Antacids may interact with certain prescription drugs

Do not take more than 6 chews in a 24-hour period, or use the maximum dosage for more than 2 weeks, except under the advice and supervision of a physician.

**Keep out of reach of children.**

**DIRECTIONS**
- chew and swallow 2 to 3 chews, hourly if needed

**OTHER INFORMATION**
- each chew contains: calcium 510 mg, magnesium 5 mg, sodium 2 mg
- contains soy
- store between 20-25°C (68-77°F) in a dry place
- do not use if pouch is torn or open
- see back panel of the pouch for lot number and expiration date

**INACTIVE INGREDIENTS**
confectioner's sugar, corn syrup, corn syrup solids, FD&C red no. 40, flavors, glycerin, gum acacia, hydrogenated coconut oil, maltodextrin, sorbitol, soy lecithin, soy protein isolate, titanium dioxide

**QUESTIONS OR COMMENTS**
Call 1-800-223-0182

---

# ROLAIDS REGULAR STRENGTH TABLETS
(calcium carbonate, and magnesium hydroxide) tablets
McNeil Consumer Healthcare

## DRUG FACTS

| Active ingredients (in each tablet) | Purpose |
|---|---|
| Calcium carbonate 550 mg | Antacid |
| Magnesium hydroxide 110 mg | Antacid |

## USES
• Relieves:
  • heartburn
  • acid indigestion
  • sour stomach
  • upset stomach due to these symptoms

## WARNINGS

### ASK A DOCTOR OR PHARMACIST BEFORE USE IF YOU ARE
• now taking a prescription drug. Antacids may interact with certain prescription drugs

Do not take more than 12 tablets in a 24 hour period, or use the maximum dosage for more than 2 weeks, except under the active and supervision of a physician. **Keep out of reach of children**

## DIRECTIONS
• chew 2 to 4 tablets, hourly if needed

## OTHER INFORMATION
• each tablet contains: calcium 220 mg, magnesium 45 mg
• store between 20°C to 25°C (68°F to 77°F) in a dry place

## INACTIVE INGREDIENTS
**Cherry**
acesulfame potassium, D&C red no. 27 aluminum lake, dextrose excipient, flavor, magnesium stearate, malodextrin, pregelatinized starch, soy protein isolate
**Peppermint**
acesulfame potassium, dextrose excipient, flavor, magnesium stearate, maltodextrin, pregelatinized starch

---

# SAFETUSSIN DM (dextromethorpan hydrobromide, and guaifenesin) liquid
Kramer Laboratories

## DRUG FACTS

| Active ingredients | Purpose |
|---|---|
| Dextromethorphan hydrobromide, USP 30 mg | Cough suppressant |
| Guaifenesin, USP 200 mg | Expectorant |

## USES
• temporarily relieves cough due to minor throat and bronchial irritation, loosens phlegm (mucus)
• helps rid bronchial passage of phlegm (mucus)

## WARNINGS
In case of overdose, get medical help or contact a Poison Control Center right away.

## DO NOT USE
• if you are now taking a prescription monoamine oxidase inhibitor (MAOI) (certain drugs for depression, psychiatric or emotional conditions, or Parkinson's disease), or for 2 weeks after stopping the MAOI drug. If you do not know if your child's prescription drug contains an MAOI, ask a doctor or pharmacist before giving this product

## DIRECTIONS
• take every 6 hours, not more than 4 doses in 24 hours

| 12 years and over | 2 teaspoons |
|---|---|
| 6 to 12 years | 1 teaspoon |
| 2 to 6 | ½ teaspoon/ask a doctor |
| under 2 years | do not use |

## INACTIVE INGREDIENTS
aspartame, benzoic acid, citric acid, glycerin, menthol, methylparaban, natural orange flavor, propylene glycol, propylparaben, purified water

---

# SALONPAS PAIN RELIEF (menthol, and methyl salicylate) patch
Hisamitsu Pharmaceutical Co., Inc.

## DRUG FACTS

| Active ingredients (in each patch) | Purpose |
|---|---|
| Menthol 3% | Topical analgesic |
| Methyl salicylate 10% (NSAID*) | |

*nonsteroidal anti-inflammatory drug

## USES
• temporarily relieves mild to moderate aches and pains of muscles and joints associated with:
  • strains
  • sprains
  • simple backache
  • arthritis
  • bruises

## WARNINGS
**For external use only.**

**Stomach bleeding warning**
This product contains an NSAID, which may cause stomach bleeding. The chance is small but higher if you:
• are age 60 or older
• have had stomach ulcers or bleeding problems
• take a blood thinning (anticoagulant) or steroid drug
• take other drugs containing an NSAID [aspirin, ibuprofen, naproxen, or others]
• have 3 or more alcoholic drinks every day while using this product
• take more or for a longer time than directed

## DO NOT USE
• on the face or rashes
• on wounds or damaged skin
• if allergic to aspirin or other NSAIDs
• with a heating pad

- when sweating (such as from exercise or heat)
- any patch from a pouch that has been open for 14 or more days
- right before or after heart surgery

## ASK A DOCTOR BEFORE USE IF

- you are allergic to topical products
- the stomach bleeding warning applies to you
- you have high blood pressure, heart disease, or kidney disease
- you are taking a diuretic

## WHEN USING THIS PRODUCT

- wash hands after applying or removing patch. Avoid contact with eyes. If eye contact occurs, rinse thoroughly with water
- the risk of heart attack or stroke may increase if you use more than directed or for longer than directed

## STOP USE AND ASK A DOCTOR IF

- you feel faint, vomit blood, or have bloody or black stools. These are signs of stomach bleeding
- rash, itching or skin irritation develops
- condition worsens
- symptoms last for more than 3 days
- symptoms clear up and occur again within a few days
- stomach pain or upset gets worse or lasts

**If pregnant or breastfeeding,** ask a doctor before use while breastfeeding and during the first 6 months of pregnancy.

Do not use during the last 3 months of pregnancy because it may cause problems in the unborn child or complications during delivery.

**Keep out of reach of children.** If put in mouth, get medical help or contact a Poison Control Center right away. Package not child resistant.

## DIRECTIONS

| adults 18 years and older | clean and dry affected area |
| --- | --- |
| | remove patch from backing film and apply to skin (see illustration) |
| | apply one patch to the affected area and leave in place for up to 8 to 12 hours |
| | if pain lasts after using the first patch, a second patch may be applied for up to another 8 to 12 hours |
| | only use one patch at a time |
| | do not use more than 2 patches per day |
| | do not use for more than 3 days in a row |
| children under 18 years of age | do not use |

## OTHER INFORMATION

- some individuals may not experience pain relief until several hours after applying the patch
- avoid storing product in direct sunlight
- protect product from excessive moisture
- store at 20-25°C (68-77°F)

## INACTIVE INGREDIENTS

alicyclic saturated hydrocarbon resin, backing cloth, film, mineral oil, polyisobutylene, polyisobutylene 1,200,000, styrene-isoprene-styrene block copolymer, synthetic aluminum silicate

# SALONPAS PAIN RELIEVING GEL-PATCH
## HOT-L (capsaicin and menthol) ointment
Hisamitsu Pharmaceutical Co., Inc.

## DRUG FACTS

| Active ingredients | Purpose |
| --- | --- |
| Capsicum extract 0.025% as Capsaicin Menthol 1.25% | Topical analgesic |

## USES

- for temporary relief of minor aches and muscles and joints associated with:
  - simple backache
  - arthritis
  - strains
  - bruises
  - sprains

## WARNINGS
**For external use only.**

## DO NOT USE

- on wounds or damaged skin
- with a heating pad
- if you are allergic to any ingredients of this product

## WHEN USING THIS PRODUCT

- do not use otherwise than as directed
- avoid contact with the eyes, mucous membranes or rashes
- do not bandage tightly
- discontinue use at least 1 hour before a bath or shower
- do not use immediately after a bath or shower

## STOP USE AND ASK A DOCTOR IF

- rash, itching or excessive skin irritation develops
- conditions worsen
- symptoms persist for more than 7 days
- symptoms clear up and occur within a few days

**If pregnant or breastfeeding,** ask a health professional before use.

**Keep out of reach of children.** If swallowed, get medical help or contact a Poison Control Center right away.

## DIRECTIONS

| adults and children 12 years of age and over | clean and dry affected area |
| --- | --- |
| | remove film from patch and apply to the skin. (see illustration.) |
| | apply to affected area not more than 3 to 4 times daily |
| | remove patch from the skin after at most 8 hours application |
| children under 12 years of age | consult a doctor |

## OTHER INFORMATION

- avoid storing product in direct sunlight and heat
- store at cool and dry place

## INACTIVE INGREDIENTS

aluminum silicate, edetate disodium, gelatin, glycerin, magnesium aluminometasilicate, oleyl alcohol, polyacrylic acid, polyethylene glycol, polyvinyl alcohol, sodium polyacrylate, sorbitan monooleate, tartaric acid, titanium dioxide, water

**QUESTIONS OR COMMENTS**
Call toll free **1-800-826-8861**, weekdays, 9 AM to 5 PM (PST) or visit www.salonpas.us

---

## SALONPAS PAIN RELIEVING JET (menthol, and methyl salicylate) aerosol, spray

Hisamitsu Pharmaceutical Co., Inc.

### DRUG FACTS

| Active ingredients | Purpose |
|---|---|
| Menthol 3%<br>Methyl salicylate 10% | Topical analgesic |

### USES
- for temporary relief of minor aches and pains of muscles and joints associated with:
  - strains
  - sprains
  - bruises
  - simple backache
  - arthritis

### WARNINGS
**For external use only.**

**Allergy alert**
If prone to allergic reaction from aspirin or salicylates, consult a doctor before use.

**Flammable**
- keep away from fire or flame
- do not use where sparks come out
- do not use in a confined space
- do not puncture or incinerate container. Contents under pressure
- do not expose to temperature exceeding 120° F (48° C)

### DO NOT USE
- on wounds or damaged skin
- with a heating pad
- if you are allergic to any ingredients of this product

### WHEN USING THIS PRODUCT
- do not use otherwise than as directed
- avoid contact with the eyes, mucous membranes or rashes
- do not bandage tightly
- avoid inhalation

### STOP USE AND ASK A DOCTOR IF
- rash, itching or excessive skin irritation develops
- conditions worsen
- symptoms persist for more than 7 days
- symptoms clear up and occur again within a few days

**If pregnant or breastfeeding,** ask a health professional before use.

**Keep out of reach of children.** If swallowed, get medical help or contact a Poison Control Center right away.

### DIRECTIONS

| adults and children 12 years of age and over | shake the can very well before use |
|---|---|
| | to avoid frostbite, hold the can 4 inches (10 cm) away from the skin, and spray each affected area for no longer than 1 second |
| | apply to affected area not more than 3 to 4 times daily |
| children under 12 years of age | consult a doctor |

### OTHER INFORMATION
- avoid storing product in direct sunlight and heat

### INACTIVE INGREDIENTS
alcohol

### QUESTIONS OR COMMENTS
Call toll free **1-800-826-8861**, weekdays, 9AM to 5PM (PST) or visit www.salonpas.us

---

## SALONPAS PAIN RELIEVING MASSAGE
(menthol, and methyl salicylate) aerosol, foam
Hisamitsu Pharmaceutical Co., Inc.

### DRUG FACTS

| Active ingredients | Purpose |
|---|---|
| Menthol 3%<br>Methyl salicylate 10% | Topical analgesic |

### USES
- for temporary relief of minor aches and pains of muscles and joints associated with:
  - strains
  - sprains
  - bruises
  - simple backache
  - arthritis

### WARNINGS
**For external use only.**

**Allergy alert**
If prone to allergic reaction from aspirin or salicylates, consult a doctor before use.

**Flammable**
- keep away from the fire or flame
- do not use where sparks come out
- do not use in a confined space
- do not puncture or incinerate container. Contents under pressure
- do not expose to temperature exceeding 120°F (48°C)

### DO NOT USE
- on wounds or damaged skin
- with a heating pad
- if you are allergic to any ingredients of this product

### WHEN USING THIS PRODUCT
- do not use otherwise than as directed
- avoid contact with the eyes, mucous membranes or rashes
- do not bandage tightly
- avoid inhalation

**STOP USE AND ASK A DOCTOR IF**
- rash, itching or excessive skin irritation develops
- conditions worsen
- symptoms persist for more than 7 days
- symptoms clear up and occur again within a few days

**If pregnant or breastfeeding,** ask a health professional before use.

**Keep out of reach of children.** If swallowed, get medical help or contact a Poison Control Center right away.

## DIRECTIONS

| adults and children 12 years of age and over | shake the can very well before use |
| --- | --- |
| | spray and dispense foam onto fingertips or palm no longer than 3 seconds, and massage well on the affected area until the crackling sound stops |
| | do not use upside down |
| | apply to affected area not more than 3 to 4 times daily |
| children under 12 years of age | consult a doctor |

## OTHER INFORMATION
- avoid storing product in direct sunlight and heat

## INACTIVE INGREDIENTS
alcohol, ceteth-20, hydroxyethylcellulose, laureth-2, PEG-40 hydrogenated castor oil, polysorbate 20, talc, water

## QUESTIONS OR COMMENTS
Call toll free **1-800-820-8861**, weekdays, 9 AM to 5 PM (PST) or visit www.salonpas.us

---

# SALONPAS PAIN RELIEVING PATCH-L
(menthol, and methyl salicylate) ointment
Hisamitsu Pharmaceutical Co., Inc.

## DRUG FACTS

| Active ingredients | Purpose |
| --- | --- |
| Menthol 1.5%<br>Methyl salicylate 10% | Topical analgesic |

## USES
- for temporary relief of minor aches and pains of muscles and joints associated with:
  - simple backache
  - arthritis
  - strains
  - bruises
  - sprains

## WARNINGS
**For external use only.**

### Allergy alert
If prone to allergic reaction from aspirin or salicylates, consult a doctor before use.

## DO NOT USE
- on wounds or damaged skin
- with a heating pad
- if you are allergic to any ingredients of this product

**WHEN USING THIS PRODUCT**
- do not use otherwise than as directed
- avoid contact with the eyes, mucous membranes or rashes
- do not bandage tightly

**STOP USE AND ASK A DOCTOR IF**
- rash, itching or excessive skin irritation develops
- conditions worsen
- symptoms persist for more than 7 days
- symptoms clear up and occur again within a few days

**If pregnant or breastfeeding,** ask a health professional before use.

**Keep out of reach of children.** If swallowed, get medical help or contact a Poison Control Center right away.

## DIRECTIONS

| adults and children 12 years of age and over | clean and dry affected area |
| --- | --- |
| | peel film from patch and apply to the skin. (see illustration) |
| | apply to affected area not more than 3 to 4 times daily |
| | remove patch from the skin after at most 8 hours application |
| children under 12 years of age | consult a doctor |

## OTHER INFORMATION
- avoid storing product in direct sunlight and heat
- store at cool and dry place

## INACTIVE INGREDIENTS
alicyclic saturated hydrocarbon resin, aluminum silicate, mineral oil, polyisobutylene, polyisobutylene 1,200,000, styrene-isoprene-styrene block copolymer

## QUESTIONS OR COMMENTS
Call toll free **1-800-826-8861**, weekdays, 9AM to 5PM (PST)
www.salonpas.us

---

# SARNA (camphor and menthol) lotion
Stiefel Laboratories, Inc

## DRUG FACTS

| Active ingredient | Purpose |
| --- | --- |
| Camphor 0.5%<br>Menthol 0.5% | external analgesic |

## USES
- for the temporary relief of pain and itching associated with minor skin irritations such as:
  - poison ivy
  - oak
  - sumac
  - sunburn
  - insect bites
  - minor cuts and scrapes

## WARNINGS
**For external use only.**

## WHEN USING THIS PRODUCT
- avoid contact with the eyes

**STOP USE AND ASK A DOCTOR IF**
- condition worsens
- symptoms persist for more than 7 days or clear up and occur again within a few days

**Keep out of reach of children.** If swallowed, get medical help or contact a Poison Control Center right away.

**DIRECTIONS**
- To open, squeeze cap tightly and turn pump counter-clockwise

| adults and children 2 years of age and older | apply to affected area not more than 3 to 4 times daily |
|---|---|
| children under 2 years of age | consult a doctor |

**INACTIVE INGREDIENTS**
carbomer 940, cetyl alcohol, DMDM hydantoin, fragrance, glyceryl stearate, isopropyl myristate, PEG-8 stearate, PEG-100 stearate, petrolatum, purified water, sodium hydroxide, stearic acid

**QUESTIONS OR COMMENTS**
Visit www.stiefelchc.com
Side effects may be reported to 1-888-438-7426.

---

## SCARGUARD MD (hydrocortisone silicone) liquid
Scarguard Labs, LLC

### DRUG FACTS

| Active ingredients | Purpose |
|---|---|
| Silicone 12.0% | Scar management |
| Hydrocortisone 0.5% | Anti-pruritic |

**USES**
- scar management
- for the temporary relief of itching associated with minor skin irritations, inflammation and rashes

**WARNINGS**
**For external use only.**

**DO NOT USE**
- on children under 2 years of age. Consult a doctor
- on mucous membranes

**WHEN USING THIS PRODUCT**
- avoid contact with the eyes
- use in a well ventilated area
- flammable until dry

**STOP USE AND ASK A DOCTOR IF**
- condition worsens
- symptoms persist for more than 7 days

**Keep out of reach of children.** If swallowed, get medical help or contact a Poison Control Center right away.

**DIRECTIONS**
- clean affected area with mild soap and water, dry thoroughly
- brush on twice daily
- allow to dry for 1 minute before coming into contact with clothing
- reapply if peeling
- children from 2-12 years of age, ask a doctor

**OTHER INFORMATION**
- store at 15°C to 30°C (59°F to 86°F)
- Keep bottle tightly closed or product will evaporate

**INACTIVE INGREDIENTS**
vitamin E, specially-formulated flexible collodion

**QUESTIONS OR COMMENTS**
Call **1-877-566-5935**

---

## SCARGUARD MD PHYSICIANS FORMULA
(hydrocortisone silicone) liquid
Scarguard Labs, LLC

### DRUG FACTS

| Active ingredients | Purpose |
|---|---|
| Silicone 12.75% | Scar management |
| Hydrocortisone 0.55% | Anti-pruritic |

**USES**
- scar management
- for the temporary relief of itching associated with minor skin irritations, inflammation and rashes

**WARNINGS**
**For external use only.**

**DO NOT USE**
- on children under 2 years of age. Consult a doctor
- on mucous membranes

**WHEN USING THIS PRODUCT**
- avoid contact with the eyes
- use in a well ventilated area
- flammable until dry

**STOP USE AND ASK A DOCTOR IF**
- condition worsens
- symptoms persist for more than 7 days

**Keep out of reach of children.** If swallowed, get medical help or contact a Poison Control Center right away.

**DIRECTIONS**
- clean affected area with mild soap and water, dry thoroughly
- brush on twice daily
- allow to dry for 1 minute before coming into contact with clothing
- reapply if peeling
- children from 2-12 years of age, ask a doctor

**OTHER INFORMATION**
- store at 15°C to 30°C (59°F to 86°F)
- keep bottle tightly closed or product will evaporate

**INACTIVE INGREDIENTS**
vitamin E, specially-formulated flexible collodion

**QUESTIONS OR COMMENTS**
Call **1-877-566-5935**

---

## SCAR ZONE ACNE (salicylic acid) cream
CCA Industries, Inc.

### DRUG FACTS

| Active ingredient | Purpose |
|---|---|
| Salicylic acid 2.0% | Acne treatment |

## USES
- Use for treatment of acne

## WARNINGS
**For external use only.**
- Avoid contact with eyes
- If product gets into eyes, rinse thoroughly with water
- Using this product and other topical acne treatments at the same time or immediately following use of this product may increase dryness or irritation of the skin
- If this occurs, only one treatment should be used unless directed by a physician

**Keep out of reach of children.** If swallowed, get medical attention or contact a Poison Control Center immediately.

## DIRECTIONS
- Cleanse thoroughly before applying treatment
- Cover the entire affected area twice daily

## INACTIVE INGREDIENTS
allantoin, BHT, butylene glycol, C13-14 isoparaffin, camellia sinensis (green tea) leaf extract, caprylic/capric triglyceride, caprylyl glycol, dimethicone, glycerin, glyceryl stearate, hexylene glycol, isohexadecane, laureth-7, PEG-100 stearate, phenoxyethanol, polyacrylamide, polyethylene, polysorbate 60, potassium hydroxide, potassium sorbate, squalane, trisodium edta, water (aqua)

## QUESTIONS OR COMMENTS
Call **1-800-595-6230** or visit www.scarzone.com. Report any issues associated with this product to the telephone number or address listed on this package.

# SCAR ZONE BURN PAIN RELIEF DOUBLE ACTION (lidocaine, and benzalkonium chloride) gel
CCA Industries, Inc.

## DRUG FACTS

| Active ingredients | Purpose |
|---|---|
| Lidocaine 2.00% | Topical analgesic/anesthetic |
| Benzalkonium chloride 0.13% | First aid antiseptic |

## USE
- for temporary relief of pain or discomfort, for first degree burns or superficial second degree burns and to help prevent infection in:
  - minor burns
  - cuts
  - scrapes

## WARNINGS
- seek medical attention immediately if burn is severe
- for external use only

**Keep out of reach of children.** In case of accidental ingestion, seek professional assistance or contact a Poison Control Center immediately.

## DO NOT USE
- in the eyes or over an area larger than the palm of your hand
- do not use longer than 1 week unless directed by a doctor

## ASK A DOCTOR BEFORE USE IF YOU HAVE
- a history of heart disease or serious burns

## STOP USE AND ASK A DOCTOR IF
- increased redness or weeping or pain persist or clears up and occurs again within a few days

## DIRECTIONS
- adults and children 2 years and over
  - clean the affected area
  - lightly apply to the affected area 1 to 3 times daily
  - may be covered with a sterile bandage
- children under 2 years, consult a doctor

## INACTIVE INGREDIENTS
allantoin, allium cepa (onion) bulb extract, aloe barbadensis leaf juice, benzyl alcohol, butylene glycol, calophyllum tacamahaca (tamanu) seed oil, camellia sinensis (green tea) leaf extract, centella asiatica extract, citric acid, glycerin, melaleuca alternifolia (tea tree) leaf oil, methylisothiazolinone, phenoxyethanol, phytonadione, polysorbate 60, propylene glycol, sodium polyacrylate, water (aqua)

## QUESTIONS OR COMMENTS
Call **1-800-595-6230** or visit www.scarzone.com. Report any issues associated with this product to the telephone number or address listed on this package.

# SCAR ZONE SCAR DIMINISHING (dimethicone (silicone), zinc oxide, and octinoxate) cream
CCA Industries, Inc.

## DRUG FACTS

| Active ingredients | Purpose |
|---|---|
| Dimethicone (silicone) 4.00% | Skin protectant |
| Zinc oxide 4.00% | Sunscreen |
| Octinoxate 7.50% | Sunscreen |

## USE
- helps prevent sunburn
- temporarily protects chapped or cracked skin

## WARNINGS
- for external use only
- avoid contact with eyes
- not intended for open wounds
- if still under treatment for wound or other skin conditions, consult your physician before using
- discontinue use if irritation occurs
- for children under six months of age, consult a doctor

**Keep out of reach of children.**

## DIRECTIONS
- gently massage into scar twice a day for 2-3 minutes

## INACTIVE INGREDIENTS
allium cepa (onion) bulb extract, butylene glycol, camellia sinensis (green tea) leaf extract, caprylic/capric triglyceride, cetyl dimethicone, cyclopentasiloxane, DMDM hydantoin, hydrogenated castor oil, hydrogenated polydecene, lauryl glucoside, PEG-8, PEG-22/dodecyl glycol copolymer, PEG-30 dipolyhydroxystearate, PEG/PPG-20/15 dimethicone, phythonadione, silica, sodium chloride, tocopheryl acetate, triethoxycaprylylsilane, water (aqua)

QUESTIONS OR COMMENTS
Call **1-800-595-6230** or visit www.scarzone.com. Report any
issues associated with this product to the telephone number or
address listed on this package.

## SCARLIGHT MD (hydroquinone) liquid
Scarguard Labs, LLC

### DRUG FACTS

| Active ingredients | Purpose |
|---|---|
| Hydroquinone 2% | Skin lightener |

### USE
- lightens dark (brownish) discoloration in the skin such as age
  and liver spots

### WARNINGS
**For external use only.**

### DO NOT USE
- on children under 12 years of age. Consult a doctor
- on mucous membranes

### WHEN USING THIS PRODUCT
- mild irritation may occur
- avoid contact with eyes. If contact occurs, rinse with water

### STOP USE AND ASK A DOCTOR IF
- irritation becomes severe
- condition worsens

**Keep out of reach of children.** If swallowed, get medical help
or contact a Poison Control Center right away.

### DIRECTIONS

| adults | brush a small amount twice daily. Rub in. |
|---|---|
| | limit sun exposure and use a sunscreen, a sun blocking agent or protective clothing to cover bleached skin when using and after using this product in order to prevent darkening from reoccurring |
| | discontinue if symptoms persist for more than 3 months |
| children under 12 years of age | consult a doctor before use |

### OTHER INFORMATION
- store at 15°C-30°C (59°F-86°F)
- keep bottle tightly closed or product will evaporate

### INACTIVE INGREDIENTS
retinoic acid, melatonin, MSM, BHT, na metabisulfite, arbutin,
cystamine, licorice root, dandelion root, hydroxyanisole, ascorbic
acid, hydroxypropylcellulose, kojic acid, azelaic acid, acetone,
propylene glycol, ethyl alcohol (SDA), distilled water q.s

### QUESTIONS OR COMMENTS
Call **1-877-566-5935**

## SCOT-TUSSIN DIABETES COUGH FORMULA
**WITH DM** (dextromethorphan hydrobromide) liquid
SCOT-TUSSIN Pharmacal Co., Inc.

### DRUG FACTS

| Active ingredient (each teaspoonful (5 ml) contains) | Purpose |
|---|---|
| Dextromethorphan hydrobromide 10 mg | Cough suppressant |

### USE
- temporarily quiets and calms a dry cough

### WARNINGS
### DO NOT USE
- more than the recommended dosage. If drowsiness occurs, do
  not drive or operate machinery
- if you are now taking a prescription monoamine oxidase
  inhibitor (MAOI) (certain drugs for depression, psychiatric,
  or emotional conditions, or Parkinson's disease) or for two
  weeks after stopping the MAOI drug. If you do not know if
  your prescription drug contains an MAOI, ask a doctor or
  pharmacist before taking this product

### ASK A DOCTOR BEFORE USE IF YOU HAVE
- a chronic cough such as occurs with smoking, asthma, chronic
  bronchitis or emphysema
- difficulty in urination due to enlargement of the prostate gland
- glaucoma
- a cough that occurs with too much phlegm (mucus)

### STOP USE AND ASK A DOCTOR IF
- Chough lasts more than seven days, returns or is accompanied
  by fever, rash or persistent headache

These could be signs of a serious condition.

**If pregnant or breastfeeding,** do not use.

**Keep out of reach of children.** In case of accidental overdose
get medical help or contact a poison control center right away.

### DIRECTIONS
- follow dosage chart
- do not exceed four doses in a 24 hour period

| adults | 2 teaspoonfuls (10 ml) every 6 to 8 hours |
|---|---|
| children 12 years and older | consult a doctor |
| children under 12 years old | do not use |

### OTHER INFORMATION
- store at 20°C-25°C (68°F-77°F)

### INACTIVE INGREDIENTS
citric acid, clear cherry-strawberry flavor, glycerin,
hydroxyethylcellulose, magnasweet, menthol, methyl-paraben,
potassium benzoate, propyl-paraben, propylene glycol, purified
water

## SCOT-TUSSIN DM SF MAXIMUM STRENGTH COUGH COLD (dextromethorphan hydrobromide, and chlorpheniramine maleate) liquid
SCOT-TUSSIN Pharmacal Co., Inc.

### DRUG FACTS

| Active ingredients (each teaspoonful (5 ml) contains) | Purpose |
|---|---|
| Dextromethorphan hydrobromide 15 mg | cough suppressant |
| Chlorpheniramine maleate 2 mg | antihistamine |

### USES
- temporarily relieves cough due to minor throat and bronchial irritation as may occur with a cold. Quiets and calms a dry cough
- temporarily relieves runny nose and sneezing, itching of the nose and throat, and itchy watery eyes due to upper respiratory symptoms

### WARNINGS
- do not use this product to sedate children

### DO NOT USE
- more than the recommended dosage
- if you are now taking a prescription monoamine oxidase inhibitor (MAOI); (certain drugs for depression, psychiatric, or emotional conditions, or Parkinson's disease) or for 2 weeks after stopping the MAOI drug. If you do not know if your prescription drug contains an MAOI, ask a doctor or pharmacist before taking this product

### WHEN USING THIS PRODUCT
- may cause drowsiness. Alcohol, sedatives and tranquilizers may increase the drowsiness effect. Avoid alcoholic beverages while taking this product if you are taking sedatives or tranquilizers, without first consulting your doctor. Use caution when driving a motor vehicle or operating machinery

### ASK A DOCTOR BEFORE USE IS YOU HAVE
- persistent or a chronic cough such as occurs with smoking, asthma, chronic bronchitis or emphysema, or if cough is accompanied by excessive phlegm
- difficulty in urination due to enlargement of the prostate gland
- glaucoma

### STOP USE AND ASK A DOCTOR IF
- cough lasts more than seven days, returns or is accompanied by fever, rash or persistent headache

These could be signs of a serious condition.

**If pregnant or breastfeeding,** do not use.

**Keep out of reach of children.** In case of overdose get medical help or contact a Poison Control Center right away.

### DIRECTIONS
- follow dosage chart
- do not exceed four doses in a 24 hour period

| adults | 2 teaspoonfuls (10 ml) every 6-8 hours |
|---|---|
| children 12 years old and older | consult a doctor |
| children under 12 years old | do not use |

### OTHER INFORMATION
- store at 20°C-25°C (68°F-77°F)

### INACTIVE INGREDIENTS
citric acid, clear cherry-strawberry flavor, glycerin, hydroxyethylcellulose, magnasweet, menthol, methyl-paraben, potassium benzoate, propyl-paraben, propylene glycol, purified water

## SCOT-TUSSIN EXPECTORANT SF COUGH (guaifenesin) liquid
SCOT-TUSSIN Pharmacal Co., Inc.

### DRUG FACTS

| Active ingredient (each teaspoonful (5 ml) contains) | Purpose |
|---|---|
| Guaifenesin 100 mg | Expectorant |

### USES
- helps loosen phlegm (mucus) to make coughs more productive thereby relieving chest congestion

### WARNINGS
- do not exceed recommended dosage
- *Phenylketonurics: contains phenylalanine

### WHEN USING THIS PRODUCT
- do not exceed recommended dosage

### ASK A DOCTOR BEFORE USE IF YOU HAVE
- a cough that occurs with too much phlegm (mucus)
- a chronic cough such as occurs with smoking, asthma, chronic bronchitis or emphysema

### STOP USE AND ASK A DOCTOR IF
- cough lasts more than seven days, returns or is accompanied by fever, rash, or persistent headache

These could be signs of a serious condition.

**If pregnant or breastfeeding,** do not use.

**Keep out of reach of children.** In case of overdose get medical help or contact a Poison Control Center right away.

### DIRECTIONS
- follow Dosage Chart
- do not exceed six doses in any 24 hour period

| adults | 2-4 teaspoonfuls (10-20 ml) every 4 hours |
|---|---|
| Children 12 years and older | Consult a Doctor |
| Children Under 12 years old | DO NOT USE |

### OTHER INFORMATION
- store at 20°C-25°C (68°F-77°F)

### INACTIVE INGREDIENTS
aspartame* (see warning) benzoic acid, citric acid, clear grape flavor, glycerin, hydroxypropylmethylcellulose, menthol, methyl-paraben, propyl-paraben, propylene glycol, purified water, *Phenylketonurics: contains phenylalanine

## SCOT-TUSSIN SENIOR SF DM EXP
(dextromethorphan hydrobromide, guaifenesin) liquid
SCOT-TUSSIN Pharmacal Co., Inc.

### DRUG FACTS

| Active ingredients (each teaspoonful (5 ml) contains) | Purpose |
|---|---|
| Dextromethorphan hydrobromide 15 mg | Cough suppressant |
| Guaifenesin 200 mg | Expectorant |

### USES
- temporarily relieves cough due to minor throat and bronchial irritation as may occur with a cold. Quiets and calms a dry cough
- helps loosen phlegm (mucus) and thin bronchial secretions to make coughs more productive thereby relieving chest congestion

### WARNINGS

**DO NOT USE**
- more than the recommended dosage
- do not use if you are now taking a prescription monoamine oxidase inhibitor (MAOI) (certain drugs for depression, psychiatric, or emotional conditions, or Parkinson's disease) or for 2 weeks after stopping the MAOI drug. If you do not know if your prescription drug contains an MAOI, ask a doctor or pharmacist before taking this product

**ASK A DOCTOR BEFORE USE IS YOU HAVE**
- a chronic cough such as occurs with smoking, asthma, chronic bronchitis or emphysema
- difficulty in urination due to enlargement of the prostate gland
- glaucoma
- a cough that occurs with too much phlegm (mucus)

**STOP USE AND ASK A DOCTOR IF**
- cough lasts more than seven days, returns or is accompanied by fever, rash or persistent headache

These could be signs of a serious condition.

**If pregnant or breastfeeding,** do not use.

**Keep out of reach of children.** In case of accidental overdose get medical help or contact a Poison Control Center right away.

### DIRECTIONS
- follow dosage chart
- do not exceed four doses in any 24 hour period

| adults | 1 teaspoonful (5 ml) every 4 to 6 hours |
|---|---|
| children 12 years old and older | consult a doctor |
| children under 12 years old | do not use |

### OTHER INFORMATION
- store at 20°C-25°C (68°F-77°F)

### INACTIVE INGREDIENTS
*aspartame, benzoic acid, citric acid, glycerin, hydroxypropylmethylcellulose, menthol, methyl-paraben, peppermint stick flavor, propyl-paraben, propylene glycol, purified water, *Phenylketonurics: contains phenylalanine

## SENOKOT (sennosides) tablet
Purdue Products LP

### DRUG FACTS

| Active ingredient (in each tablet) | Purpose |
|---|---|
| Sennosides 8.6 mg | Laxative |

### USES
- relieves occasional constipation (irregularity)
- generally produces a bowel movement in 6-12 hours

### WARNINGS

**DO NOT USE**
- laxative products for longer than 1 week unless directed by a doctor

**ASK A DOCTOR BEFORE USE IF YOU HAVE**
- stomach pain
- nausea
- vomiting
- noticed a sudden change in bowel habits that continues over a period of 2 weeks

**STOP USE AND ASK A DOCTOR IF**
- you have rectal bleeding or fail to have a bowel movement after use of a laxative

These may indicate a serious condition.

**If pregnant or breastfeeding,** ask a health professional before use.

**Keep out of reach of children.** In case of overdose, get medical help or contact a Poison Control Center right away.

### DIRECTIONS
- take preferably at bedtime or as directed by a doctor

| Age | Starting dosage | Maximum dosage |
|---|---|---|
| adults and children 12 years of age and over | 2 tablets once a day | 4 tablets twice a day |
| children 6 to under 12 years | 1 tablet once a day | 2 tablets twice a day |
| children 2 to under 6 years | ½ tablet once a day | 1 tablet twice a day |
| children under 2 years | ask a doctor | ask a doctor |

### OTHER INFORMATION
- each tablet contains: calcium 25 mg
- store at 25°C (77°F); excursions permitted between 15-30°C (59-86°F)

### INACTIVE INGREDIENTS
croscarmellose sodium, dicalcium phosphate, hypromellose, lactose anhydrous, magnesium stearate, microcrystalline cellulose, mineral oil, tartaric acid

## SENOKOT-S (sennosides and docusate sodium) tablet
Purdue Products LP

### DRUG FACTS

| Active ingredients (in each tablet) | Purpose |
|---|---|
| Docusate sodium 50 mg | Stool softener |
| Sennosides 8.6 mg | Laxative |

### USES
- relieves occasional constipation (irregularity)
- generally produces a bowel movement in 6-12 hours

### WARNINGS

### DO NOT USE
- if you are now taking mineral oil, unless directed by a doctor
- laxative products for longer than 1 week unless directed by a doctor

### ASK A DOCTOR BEFORE USE IF YOU HAVE
- stomach pain
- nausea
- vomiting
- noticed a sudden change in bowel habits that continues over a period of 2 weeks

### STOP USE AND ASK A DOCTOR IF
- you have rectal bleeding or fail to have a bowel movement after use of a laxative. These may indicate a serious condition.

**If pregnant or breastfeeding,** ask a health professional before use.

**Keep out of reach of children.** In case of overdose, get medical help or contact a Poison Control Center right away.

### DIRECTIONS
- take preferably at bedtime or as directed by a doctor

| Age | Starting dosage | Maximum dosage |
|---|---|---|
| adults and children 12 years of age and over | 2 tablets once a day | 4 tablets twice a day |
| children 6 to under 12 years | 1 tablet once a day | 2 tablets twice a day |
| children 2 to under 6 years | ½ tablet once a day | 1 tablet twice a day |
| children under 2 years | ask a doctor | ask a doctor |

### OTHER INFORMATION
- each tablet contains: calcium 20 mg, sodium 6 mg LOW SODIUM
- store at 25°C (77°F); excursions permitted between 15-30°C (59-86°F)

### INACTIVE INGREDIENTS
carnauba wax, colloidal silicon dioxide, croscarmellose sodium, dicalcium phosphate, D&C yellow no. 10 aluminum lake, FD&C yellow no. 6 aluminum lake, hypromellose, lactose anhydrous, magnesium stearate, microcrystalline cellulose, PEG 8000, sodium benzoate, stearic acid, tartaric acid, titanium dioxide

## SENOKOT XTRA (sennosides) tablet
Purdue Products LP

### DRUG FACTS

| Active ingredient (in each tablet) | Purpose |
|---|---|
| Sennosides 17.2 mg | Laxative |

### USES
- relieves occasional constipation (irregularity)
- generally produces a bowel movement in 6-12 hours

### WARNINGS

### DO NOT USE
- laxative products for longer than 1 week unless directed by a doctor

### ASK A DOCTOR BEFORE USE IF YOU HAVE
- stomach pain
- nausea
- vomiting
- noticed a sudden change in bowel movements that continues over a period of 2 weeks

### STOP USE AND ASK A DOCTOR IF
- you have rectal bleeding or fail to have a bowel movement after use of a laxative. These may indicate a serious condition.

**If pregnant or breastfeeding,** ask a health professional before use.

**Keep out of reach of children.** In case of overdose, get medical help or contact a Poison Control Center right away.

### DIRECTIONS
- take preferably at bedtime or as directed by a doctor

| Age | Starting dosage | Maximum dosage |
|---|---|---|
| adults and children 12 years of age and over | 1 tablets once a day | 2 tablets twice a day |
| children 6 to under 12 years | ½ tablet once a day | 1 tablet twice a day |
| children under 6 | ask a doctor | ask a doctor |

### OTHER INFORMATION
- each tablet contains: calcium 25 mg
- store at 25°C (77°F); excursions permitted between 15-30°C (59°F-86°F)

### INACTIVE INGREDIENTS
croscarmellose sodium, dicalcium phosphate, hypromellose, lactose anhydrous, magnesium stearate, microcrystalline cellulose, mineral oil, stearic acid, tartaric acid

## SIMPLY SALINE STERILE SALINE NASAL MIST (sodium chloride) spray
Church & Dwight Co., Inc.

### DRUG FACTS

| Active ingredient | Purpose |
|---|---|
| Sodium chloride, 0.9% | Nasal spray |
| Purified water | |

## USE
- relieves symptoms of dry irritated nose
- flushes dust, dirt, pollen and congestion from nasal and sinus passages

## WARNINGS
- the use of this dispenser by more than one person may spread infection
- keep out of reach of children
- contents under pressure
- do not puncture or incinerate

## DIRECTIONS
**To flush and irrigate**
- tilt head to the side over sink or use in shower. Insert nozzle into one nostril depressing as a gentle mist fills sinus passages and flows out nostrils

**To moisturize**
- insert nozzle into each nostril and press as moisture is restored to dry nasal passages. Use as often as needed (non-habit forming, non-addicting)

## OTHER INFORMATION
- store between 59°F-86°F (15°C-30°C)

---

# SINE OFF SINUS/COLD MEDICINE
(acetaminophen, chlorpheniramine maleate, and phenylephrine hydrochloride) caplet, film coated
Gemini Pharmaceuticals, Inc.

## DRUG FACTS

| Active ingredients (in each caplet) | Purpose |
| --- | --- |
| Acetaminophen 500 mg | Pain reliever |
| Chlorpheniramine maleate 2 mg | Antihistamine |
| Phenylephrine hydrochloride 5 mg | Nasal decongestant |

## USES
- temporarily relieves these symptoms of hay fever or other upper respiratory allergies:
  - headache
  - sinus congestion and pressure
  - nasal congestion
  - runny nose and sneezing
  - minor aches and pains
- temporarily relieves these additional symptoms of hay fever:
  - itching of the nose and throat
  - itchy, watery eyes
  - helps clear nasal passages
  - helps decongest sinus openings and passages

## WARNINGS
**Liver Warning**
This product contains acetaminophen. Severe liver damage may occur if you take:
- more than 8 caplets in 24 hours, which is maximum daily amount for this product
- with other drugs containing acetaminophen
- 3 or more alcoholic drinks every day while using this product

## DO NOT USE
- with any other drug containing acetaminophen (prescription or nonprescription). If you are not sure whether a drug contains acetaminophen, ask a doctor or pharmacist
- if you are allergic to acetaminophen or any of the inactive ingredients in this products

- if you are now taking prescription monoamine oxidase inhibitor (MAOI) (certain drugs for depression, psychiatric, or emotional conditions, or Parkinson's disease), or 2 weeks after stopping the MAOI Drug. If you do not know if your prescription drug contains an MAOI, ask a doctor or pharmacist before taking this product

## ASK A DOCTOR BEFORE USE IF YOU HAVE
- liver disease
- heart disease
- high blood pressure
- thyroid disease
- diabetes
- difficulty in urination due to enlargement of the prostrate gland
- a breathing problem such as emphysema or chronic bronchitis
- glaucoma

## ASK A DOCTOR OR PHARMACIST BEFORE USE IF YOU ARE
- taking the blood thinning drug warfarin
- taking sedatives or tranquilizers

## WHEN USING THIS PRODUCT
- do not exceed recommended dosage
- excitability may occur, especially in children
- drowsiness may occur
- alcohol, sedatives and tranquilizers may increase drowsiness
- avoid alcoholic drinks
- be careful when driving motor vehicle or operating machinery

## STOP USE AND ASK A DOCTOR IF
- nervousness, dizziness, or sleeplessness occurs
- pain or nasal congestion gets worse or lasts more than 7 days
- fever gets worse or lasts more than 3 days
- redness swelling is present
- new symptoms occur

These could be signs of a serious condition.

**If pregnant or breastfeeding,** ask a health professional before use.

**Keep out of reach of children.**

## OVERDOSE WARNING
Taking more than recommended dose (overdose) may cause liver damage. In case of overdose, get medical help or contact a Poison Control Center Right away. (1-800-222-1222). Quick medical attention is critical for adults as well as for children even if you do not notice any signs or symptoms.

## DIRECTIONS
- do not take more than directed (see overdose warning)

| adults and children 12 years and older | take 2 caplets every 4 to 6 hours as needed |
| --- | --- |
| | swallow whole - do not crush, chew or dissolve |
| | do not take more than 8 caplets in 24 hours |
| children under 12 years | do not use. This will provide more than the recommended dose (overdose) and may cause the liver damage |

## OTHER INFORMATION
- store at room temperature
- avoid excessive heat and humidity
- retain carton for complete product information

## INACTIVE INGREDIENTS
croscarmellose sodium, crospovidone, D&C yellow no. 10, FD&C yellow no. 6, hypromellose, magnesium stearate, microcrystalline cellulose, povidone, pregelatinized starch, propylene glycol, silicone dioxide, stearic acid, titanium dioxide, triacetin

## QUESTIONS OR COMMENTS
If you have any questions or comments, or to report an adverse event, please contact **1-888-876-6898**

# SINUCLEANSE NASAL WASH (sodium bicarbonate and sodium chloride)
Med-Systems, Inc.

## DRUG FACTS

| Active ingredients (in each packet) | Purpose |
|---|---|
| Sodium bicarbonate (USP 700 mg) | Nasal wash |
| Sodium chloride (USP 2300 mg) | |

## USES
- temporarily relieves symptoms associated with sinusitis, cold, flu or allergies:
  - sneezing
  - runny nose
  - nasal stuffiness
  - post nasal drip
- removes inhaled irritants (dust, pollen)
- promotes nasal and sinus drainage
- helps reduce swelling of nasal membranes

## WARNINGS
**STOP USE AND ASK A DOCTOR IF**
washing is uncomfortable or symptoms are not relieved.

**WHEN USING THIS PRODUCT**
- use by only one person
- wash with soap and water after each use
- top rack of dishwasher safe
- do not heat in microwave

**Keep out of reach from children.**

## DIRECTIONS
- consult instructions for use for proper use

| adults and children 4 years and over | use 1-2 packets up to every 2 hours as needed |
|---|---|
| children under 4 years | consult a physician |

## OTHER INFORMATION
- inspect saline solution packets for integrity
- do not use if open or torn
- protect saline solution packet from excessive heat and moisture

## INACTIVE INGREDIENTS
None

## QUESTIONS OR COMMENTS
Call **1-888-547-5492** or visit www.sinucleanse.com

# SINUTAB SINUS MAXIMUM STRENGTH
(acetaminophen and phenylephrine hydrochloride) caplet, film coated

McNeil Consumer Healthcare, Division of McNeil-PPC, Inc.

## DRUG FACTS

| Active ingredients (in each caplet) | Purpose |
|---|---|
| Acetaminophen 325 mg | Pain reliever |
| Phenylephrine hydrochloride 5 mg | Nasal decongestant |

## USES
- for the temporary relief of:
  - sinus congestion and pressure
  - headache
  - minor aches and pains
  - nasal congestion

## WARNINGS
**Alcohol warning**
If you consume 3 or more alcoholic drinks every day, ask your doctor whether you should take acetaminophen or other pain relievers or fever reducers. Acetaminophen may cause liver damage.

**DO NOT USE**
- with another product containing acetaminophen
- if you are now taking a prescription monoamine oxidase inhibitor (MAOI) (certain drugs for depression, psychiatric or emotional conditions, or Parkinson's disease), or for 2 weeks after stopping the MAOI drug. If you do not know if your prescription drug contains an MAOI, ask a doctor or pharmacist before taking this product

**ASK A DOCTOR BEFORE USE IF YOU HAVE**
- heart disease
- high blood pressure
- thyroid disease
- diabetes
- trouble urinating due to an enlarged prostate gland

**WHEN USING THIS PRODUCT**
- do not exceed recommended dose

**STOP USE AND ASK A DOCTOR IF**
- nervousness, dizziness, or sleeplessness occur
- pain or nasal congestion gets worse or lasts more than 7 days
- fever gets worse or lasts more than 3 days
- redness or swelling is present
- new symptoms occur

These could be signs of a serious condition.

**If pregnant or breastfeeding,** ask a health professional before use.

**Keep out of reach of children.**

**OVERDOSE WARNING**
Taking more than the recommended dose (overdose) may cause liver damage. In case of overdose, get medical help or contact a Poison Control Center right away. (1-800-222-1222) Quick medical attention is critical for adults as well as for children even if you do not notice any signs or symptoms.

## DIRECTIONS
• do not take more than directed (see overdose warning)

| adults and children 12 years and over | take 2 caplets every 4 hours<br>do not exceed 12 caplets in 24 hours |
|---|---|
| children under 12 years | do not use. This will provide more than the recommended dose (overdose) and may cause liver damage |

## OTHER INFORMATION
• store between 20°C-25°C (68°F-77°F)
• do not use if carton is opened or if blister unit is broken
• see side panel for lot number and expiration date

## INACTIVE INGREDIENTS
carnauba wax, corn starch, FD&C yellow no. 6 aluminum lake, hypromellose, magnesium stearate, microcrystalline cellulose, polyethylene glycol, polysorbate 80, powdered cellulose, pregelatinized starch, sodium starch glycolate, titanium dioxide

## QUESTIONS OR COMMENTS
Call 1-800-223-0182

## SOLARCAINE (lidocaine) spray
Schering-Plough Healthcare Products Inc.

## DRUG FACTS

| Active ingredient | Purpose |
|---|---|
| Lidocaine 0.5 % | External analgesic |

## USES
• temporarily relieves pain and itching due to:
  • sunburn
  • minor burns
  • minor cuts
  • scrapes
  • insect bites
  • minor skin irritations

## WARNINGS

**For external use only.**

**Flammable:** Do not use while smoking or near heat or flame

## DO NOT USE
• in large quantities, particularly over raw surfaces or blistered areas

## WHEN USING THIS PRODUCT
• keep out of eyes
• use only as directed. Intentional misuse by deliberately concentrating and inhaling the contents can be harmful or fatal
• do not puncture or incinerate. Contents under pressure. Do not store at temperatures above 120°F

## STOP USE AND ASK A DOCTOR IF
• condition gets worse
• symptoms last more than 7 days
• symptoms clear up and occur again in a few days

**Keep out of reach of children.** If swallowed, get medical help or contact a Poison Control Center right away.

## DIRECTIONS
• shake well

| adults and children 2 years of age and older | apply to affected area not more than 3 to 4 times daily |
|---|---|
| children under 2 years of age | ask a doctor |

• To apply to face, spray in palm of hand and gently apply

## INACTIVE INGREDIENTS
aloe barbadensis leaf juice, isobutane, propane, propylene glycol, glycerin, simethicone, tocopheryl acetate (vitamin E acetate), triethanolamine, carbomer, diazolidinyl urea, methylparaben, propylparaben, disodium cocoamphodipropionate, disodium EDTA

## SOMINEX (diphenhydramine hydrochloride) tablet or caplet
GlaxoSmithKline Consumer Healthcare LP

## DRUG FACTS

| Active ingredient | Purpose |
|---|---|
| Diphenhydramine hydrochloride 25 mg/tablet | Nighttime sleep-aid |
| Diphenhydramine hydrochloride 50 mg/caplet | |

## USE
• helps reduce difficulty falling asleep

## WARNINGS

## DO NOT USE
• in children under 12 years of age
• with any other product containing diphenhydramine, even one used on skin

## ASK A DOCTOR BEFORE USE IF YOU HAVE
• glaucoma
• a breathing problem such as emphysema or chronic bronchitis
• trouble urinating due to an enlarged prostate gland

## ASK A DOCTOR OR PHARMACIST BEFORE USE IF YOU ARE
• taking sedatives or tranquilizers

## WHEN USING THIS PRODUCT
• avoid alcoholic beverages

## STOP USE AND ASK A DOCTOR IF
• sleeplessness persists continuously for more than 2 weeks

Insomnia may be a symptom of serious underlying medical illness.

**If pregnant or breastfeeding,** ask a health professional before use.

**Keep out of reach of children.** In case of accidental overdose get medical help or contact a Poison Control Center right away.

## DIRECTIONS (Original formula)

| adults and children 12 years and older | take 2 tablets at bedtime if needed or as directed by your doctor |
|---|---|

## DIRECTIONS (Maximum strength)

| adults and children 12 years and older | take 1 caplet at bedtime if needed or as directed by your doctor |
|---|---|

## OTHER INFORMATION (Original formula)
- each tablet contains: calcium 70 mg
- store at room temperature
- avoid excessive heat (greater than 100°F) or humidity

## OTHER INFORMATION (Maximum strength)
- each caplet contains: calcium 50 mg
- store at room temperature
- avoid excessive heat (greater than 100°F) or humidity

## INACTIVE INGREDIENTS (Original formula)
dibasic calcium phosphate, FD&C blue no. 1 aluminum lake, magnesium stearate, microcrystalline cellulose, silicon dioxide, starch

## INACTIVE INGREDIENTS (Maximum strength)
carnauba wax, crospovidone, dibasic calcium phosphate, FD&C blue no. 1 aluminum lake, hypromellose, magnesium stearate, microcrystalline cellulose, polyethylene glycol, polysorbate 80, silicon dioxide, starch, titanium dioxide

## QUESTIONS OR COMMENTS
Call **1-800-245-1040** (English/Spanish) weekdays or visit www.sominex.com

---

# SOOTHE (glycerin and propylene glycol) solution/drops
Bausch & Lomb Incorporated

## DRUG FACTS

| Active Ingredients | Purpose |
|---|---|
| Glycerin (0.55%) | Lubricant |
| Propylene glycol (0.55%) | |

## USES
- relieves dryness of the eye
- prevents further irritation

## WARNINGS

## DO NOT USE
- if solution changes color or becomes cloudy

## WHEN USING THIS PRODUCT
- do not touch tip of container to any surface to avoid contamination
- replace cap after using

## STOP USE AND ASK A DOCTOR IF
- you experience eye pain, changes in vision, continued redness or irritation of the eye, or if condition worsens or persists for more than 72 hours

**Keep out of reach of children.** If swallowed, get medical help or contact a Poison Control Center right away.

## DIRECTIONS
- instill 1 to 2 drop(s) in the affected eye(s) as needed or directed by your doctor

## OTHER INFORMATION
- store at 15-25°C (59-77°F)

---

## INACTIVE INGREDIENTS
butylated hydroxyanisole (BHA), boric acid, carbamide peroxide, hydroxyalkyl-phosphonate 30%, sodium alginate, sodium borate

## QUESTIONS OR COMMENTS
Toll-free product information or to report a serious side effect associated with use of the product Call **1-800-553-5340**

---

# SOOTHE XP (light mineral oil and mineral oil) solution/drops
Bausch & Lomb Incorporated

## DRUG FACTS

| Active ingredients | Purpose |
|---|---|
| Light mineral oil (1.0%) | Emollient |
| Mineral oil (4.5%) | |

## USES
- temporary relief of burning and irritation due to dryness of the eye
- temporary relief of discomfort due to minor irritations of the eye or to exposure to wind or sun
- as a protectant to prevent further irritation or to relieve dryness of the eye

## WARNINGS
**For external use only.**

## DO NOT USE
- if solution changes color

## WHEN USING THIS PRODUCT
- do not touch the tip of container to any surface
- replace cap after using

## STOP USE AND ASK A DOCTOR IF
- you experience eye pain, changes in vision, continued redness or irritation of the eye, or if condition worsens or persists for more than 72 hours

**Keep out of reach of children.** If swallowed, get medical help or contact a Poison Control Center right away.

## DIRECTIONS
- remove contact lenses before use
- shake well before using
- instill 1 or 2 drop(s) in the affected eye(s) as needed or as directed by your doctor

## OTHER INFORMATION
- temporarily blurred vision is typical upon application
- drops appear as a milky white solution
- store at 15-25°C (59-77°F)

## INACTIVE INGREDIENTS
edetate disodium, octoxynol-40, polyhexamethylene biguanide (preservative), polysorbate-80, purified water, sodium chloride, sodium hydroxide and/or hydrochloric acid (to adjust pH), sodium phosphate dibasic, sodium phosphate monobasic

## QUESTIONS OR COMMENTS
Toll-free product Call **1-800-553-5340**

# SPORTSCREME (trolamine salicylate) cream
Chattem

## DRUG FACTS

| Active ingredient | Purpose |
|---|---|
| Trolamine salicylate 10% | Topical analgesic |

### USES
- temporarily relieves minor pain associated with:
  - arthritis
  - simple backache
  - bursitis
  - tendonitis
  - muscle strains
  - muscle sprains
  - bruises
  - cramps

### WARNINGS
**For external use only.**

**Allergy alert**
Do not use if you are allergic to salicylates (including aspirin) unless directed by a doctor.

### WHEN USING THIS PRODUCT
- use only as directed
- do not bandage tightly or use with a heating pad
- avoid contact with eyes or mucous membranes
- do not apply to wounds or damaged skin

### STOP USE AND ASK A DOCTOR IF
- condition worsens
- symptoms persist for more than 7 days or clear up and occur again within a few days
- redness is present
- irritation develops

**If pregnant or breastfeeding,** ask a health professional before use.

**Keep out of reach of children.** If swallowed, get medical help or contact a Poison Control Center right away.

### DIRECTIONS

| adults and children over 10 years | apply generously to affected area |
|---|---|
| | massage into painful area until thoroughly absorbed into skin |
| | repeat as necessary no more than 4 times daily for temporary relief |
| children 10 years or younger | ask a doctor |

### INACTIVE INGREDIENTS
cetyl alcohol, FD&C blue no. 1, FD&C yellow no. 5, fragrance, glycerin, methylparaben, mineral oil, potassium phosphate, propylparaben, stearic acid, triethanolamine, water (229-121)

# ST. JOSEPH CHEWABLE (aspirin) tablet
St. Josephs Health Products, LLC

## DRUG FACTS

| Active ingredient (in each tablet) | Purpose |
|---|---|
| Aspirin 81 mg (NSAID)* | Pain reliever |

*nonsteroidal anti-inflammatory drug

### USE
- temporarily relieves minor aches and pains

### WARNINGS
**Reye's Syndrome**
Children and teenagers who have or are recovering from chicken pox or flu-like symptoms should not use this product. When using this product, if changes in behavior with nausea and vomiting occur, consult a doctor because these symptoms could be an early sign of Reye's Syndrome, a rare but serious illness.

**Allergy alert**
Aspirin may cause a severe allergic reaction which may include:
- hives
- facial swelling
- asthma (wheezing)
- shock

**Stomach bleeding warning**
This product contains an NSAID, which may cause severe stomach bleeding. The chance is higher if you:
- are age 60 or older
- have had stomach ulcers or bleeding problems
- take other drugs containing prescription or nonprescription NSAIDs (aspirin, ibuprofen, naproxen, or others)
- have 3 or more alcoholic drinks every day while using this product
- take more or for a longer time than directed

### DO NOT USE
- if you have ever had an allergic reaction to any pain reliever or fever reducer

### ASK A DOCTOR BEFORE USE IF
- the stomach bleeding warning applies to you
- you have history of stomach problems such as heartburn
- you have high blood pressure, heart disease, liver cirrhosis, or kidney disease
- you have asthma
- you are taking a diuretic

### ASK A DOCTOR OR PHARMACIST BEFORE USE IF YOU ARE
- taking a prescription drug for:
  - gout
  - diabetes
  - arthritis

### STOP USE AND ASK A DOCTOR IF
- you experience any of the following signs of stomach bleeding:
  - feel faint
  - vomit blood
  - have bloody or black stools
  - have stomach pain that does not get better
- allergic reaction occurs
- ringing in the ears or loss of hearing occurs
- pain gets worse or lasts more than 10 days
- new symptoms occur
- redness or swelling is present

These could be signs of a serious condition.

**If pregnant or breastfeeding,** ask a health professional before use.

**It is especially important not to use aspirin during the last three months of pregnancy unless definitely directed to do so by a doctor because it may cause problems in the unborn child or complications during a delivery.**

**Keep out of reach of children.** In case of overdose, get medical help or contact a Poison Control Center right away. (1-800-222-1222)

## DIRECTIONS

| adults and children 12 years and over | • for temporary relief of minor aches and pains, take 4 to 8 tablets every 4 hours while symptoms persist<br>• do not exceed 48 tablets in 24 hours unless directed by a doctor |
|---|---|
| children under 12 years of age | do not use unless directed by a doctor |

## INACTIVE INGREDIENTS
butylated hydroytolene BHT, dextrates, FD&C yellow no. 6 aluminum lake, microcrystalline cellulose, modified corn starch, orange flavor, pregelatinized starch, sodium saccharin, stearic acid

## OTHER INFORMATION
• store between 20-25°C (68-77°F). Avoid high humidity
• do not use if "safety seal" is broken

# ST JOSEPH SAFETY-COATED (aspirin) tablet
St. Josephs Health Products, LLC

## DRUG FACTS

| Active ingredient (in each tablet) | Purpose: |
|---|---|
| Aspirin 81 mg (NSAID)* | Pain reliever |

*nonsteroidal anti-inflammatory drug

## USE
• temporarily relieves minor aches and pains

## WARNINGS
### Reye's Syndrome
Children and teenagers who have or are recovering from chicken pox or flu-like symptoms should not use this product. When using this product, if changes in behavior with nausea and vomiting occur, consult a doctor because these symptoms could be an early sign of Reye's Syndrome, a rare but serious illness.

### Allergy alert
Aspirin may cause a severe allergic reaction which may include:
• hives
• facial swelling
• asthma (wheezing)
• shock

### Stomach bleeding warning
This product contains an NSAID, which may cause severe stomach bleeding. The chance is higher if you:
• are age 60 or older
• have had stomach ulcers or bleeding problems
• take other drugs containing prescription or nonprescription NSAIDs (aspirin, ibuprofen, naproxen, or others)
• have 3 or more alcoholic drinks every day while using this product
• take more or for a longer time than directed

## DO NOT USE
• if you have ever had a allergic reaction to any pain reliever or fever reducer

## ASK A DOCTOR BEFORE USE IF
• the stomach bleeding warning applies to you
• you have history of stomach problems such as heartburn
• you have high blood pressure, heart disease, liver cirrhosis, or kidney disease
• you have asthma
• you are taking a diuretic

## ASK A DOCTOR OR PHARMACIST BEFORE USE IF YOU ARE
• taking a prescription drug for:
  • gout
  • diabetes
  • arthritis

## STOP USE AND ASK A DOCTOR IF
• you experience any of the following signs of stomach bleeding:
  • feel faint
  • vomit blood
  • have bloody or black stools
  • have stomach pain that does not get better
• allergic reaction occurs
• ringing in the ears or loss of hearing occurs
• pain gets worse or lasts more than 10 days
• new symptoms occur
• redness or swelling is present

These could be signs of a serious condition.

**If pregnant or breastfeeding,** ask a health professional before use.

**It is especially important not to use aspirin during the last three months of pregnancy unless definitely directed to do so by a doctor because it may cause problems in the unborn child or complications during a delivery.**

**Keep out of reach of children.** In case of overdose, get medical help or contact a Poison Control Center right away. (1-800-222-1222)

## DIRECTIONS

| adults and children 12 years and over | for temporary relief of minor aches and pains, take 4 to 8 tablets every 4 hours while symptoms persist<br><br>do not exceed 48 tablets in 24 hours unless directed by a doctor |
|---|---|
| children under 12 years of age | do not use unless directed by a doctor |

## INACTIVE INGREDIENTS
FD&C red no. 40, FD&C yellow no. 6, hypromellose, methacrylic acid copolymer, microcrystalline cellulose, pregelatinized starch, silica, silicon dioxide, sodium bicarbonate, sodium lauryl sulfate, stearic scid, talc, and triethyl citrate

## OTHER INFORMATION
• Store between 20-25°C (68-77°F). Avoid high humidity
• do not use if "safety seal" is broken
•

## STANBACK (aspirin and caffeine) powder
GlaxoSmithKline Consumer Healthcare LP

### DRUG FACTS

| Active ingredients | Purpose |
| --- | --- |
| Aspirin (NSAID*) 845 mg | Pain reliever/fever reducer |
| Caffeine 65 mg | Pain reliever aid |

*nonsteroidal anti-inflammatory drug

### USES
- temporarily relieves minor aches and pains due to:
  - headache
  - muscular aches
  - minor arthritis pain
  - colds
- temporarily reduces fever

### WARNINGS
**Reye's syndrome**
Children and teenagers who have or are recovering from chicken pox or flu-like symptoms should not use this product. When using this product, if changes in behavior with nausea and vomiting occur, consult a doctor because these symptoms could be an early sign of Reye's syndrome, a rare but serious illness.

**Allergy alert**
Aspirin may cause a severe allergic reaction which may include:
- hives
- facial swelling
- shock
- asthma (wheezing)

**Stomach bleeding warning**
This product contains an NSAID, which may cause severe stomach bleeding. The chance is higher if you:
- are age 60 or older
- have had stomach ulcers or bleeding problems
- take a blood thinning (anticoagulant) or steroid drug
- take other drugs containing prescription or nonprescription NSAIDs (aspirin, ibuprofen, naproxen, or others)
- have 3 or more alcoholic drinks every day while using this product
- take more or for a longer time than directed

### DO NOT USE
- if you have ever had an allergic reaction to aspirin or any other pain reliever/fever reducer

### ASK A DOCTOR BEFORE USE IF
- stomach bleeding warning applies to you
- you have a history of stomach problems, such as heartburn
- you have high blood pressure, heart disease, liver cirrhosis, or kidney disease
- you are taking a diuretic
- you have asthma

### ASK A DOCTOR OR PHARMACIST BEFORE USE IF YOU ARE
- taking a prescription drug for diabetes, gout, or arthritis

### WHEN USING THIS PRODUCT
- limit the use of caffeine-containing drugs, foods, or drinks because too much caffeine may cause nervousness, irritability, sleeplessness, and, occasionally, rapid heart beat. The recommended dose of this product contains about as much caffeine as a cup of coffee

### STOP USE AND ASK A DOCTOR IF
- an allergic reaction occurs. Seek medical help right away

- you experience any of the following signs of stomach bleeding:
  - feel faint
  - have stomach pain that does not get better
  - vomit blood
  - have bloody or black stools
- pain gets worse or lasts more than 10 days
- fever gets worse or lasts more than 3 days
- redness or swelling is present
- any new symptoms appear
- ringing in the ears or a loss of hearing occurs

These could be signs of a serious condition.

**If pregnant or breastfeeding,** ask a health professional before use.

It is especially important not to use aspirin during the last 3 months of pregnancy unless definitely directed to do so by a doctor because it may cause problems in the unborn child or complications during delivery.

**Keep out of reach of children.** In case of overdose, get medical help or contact a Poison Control Center right away.

### DIRECTIONS

| adults and children 12 years of age and over | place 1 powder packet on tongue every 6 hours, while symptoms persist. Drink a full glass of water with each dose, or may stir powder into a glass of water or other liquid |
| --- | --- |
| | do not take more than 4 powder packets in 24 hours unless directed by a doctor |
| children under 12 years of age | ask a doctor |

### OTHER INFORMATION
- each powder contains: potassium 55 mg
- store below 25°C (77°F)

### INACTIVE INGREDIENTS
docusate sodium, fumaric acid, lactose monohydrate, potassium chloride

### QUESTIONS OR COMMENTS
Call **1-866-255-5197** (English/Spanish) weekdays

- do not use if carton is opened or neck wrap or foil inner seal imprinted with "Safety Seal" is broken
- see end panel for lot and expiration date

## STAPHASEPTIC (benzethonium chloride, lidocaine hydrochloride) gel
Tec Laboratories, Inc.

### DRUG FACTS

| Active ingredients | Purpose |
| --- | --- |
| Benzethonium chloride 0.2% | First aid antiseptic |
| Lidocaine hydrochloride 2.5% | Topical pain reliever |

### USES
- first aid to help protect against skin infection in minor:
  - cuts
  - scrapes
  - burns
- temporarily relieves pain and itching associated with minor:
  - burns
  - cuts

- scrapes
- insect bites
- skin irritations

## WARNINGS
**For external use only.**

### ASK A DOCTOR BEFORE USE IF YOU HAVE
- deep or puncture wounds
- animal bites
- serious burns

### WHEN USING THIS PRODUCT
- do not use in or near the eyes
- do not apply to large areas of raw or blistered skin in large quantities

### STOP USE AND ASK A DOCTOR IF
- symptoms last more than 7 days or clear up and occur again within a few days
- condition worsens

**Keep out of reach of children.** If swallowed, get medical help or contact a Poison Control Center right away.

## DIRECTIONS

| adults and children 2 years of age and older | clean the affected area whenever possible |
| | apply to affected area not more that 3 to 4 times daily |
| | may be covered with a sterile bandage; if bandaged, let dry first |
| children under 2 years of age | do not use, consult a doctor |

## OTHER INFORMATION
Store at 59°F-86°F (15°C-30°C)

## INACTIVE INGREDIENTS
aminomethyl propanol, allantoin, carbomer, cocamide DEA, disodium EDTA, glycerine, polyolyl 35 castor oil, purified water, tea tree oil, white thyme oil

## QUESTIONS OR COMMENTS
Call **1-800-482-4464** or visit us at www.staphaseptic.com
Serious side effects may be reported to this number

---

# STRIDEX NATURALLY CLEAR (salicylic acid)
liquid patch

Blistex Inc.

## DRUG FACTS

| Active ingredient | Purpose |
| --- | --- |
| Salicylic acid 1% | acne medication |

## USES
- for the treatment and management of acne
- reduces the number of acne pimples and blackheads and allows the skin to heal
- helps to prevent new acne pimples from forming

## WARNINGS
**For external use only.**

### Allergy alert
Do not use this product it you have a known allergy to salicylic acid.

**Keep out of reach of children.** If swallowed get medical help or contact a posion control center right away.

## DIRECTIONS
- cleanse the skin thoroughly before applying medication
- use the pad to wipe the entire affected area
- repeat with a clean pad as necessary to remove remaining traces of
- dirt, because excessive drying of the skin may occur, start with one application daily, then gradually increase to two to three times daily as needed or as directed by a doctor
- if bothersome dryness or peeling occurs, reduce application to once a day or every other day
- do not leave pad on skin for an extended period of time
- keep away from eyes, lips and other mucous membrane

## OTHER INFORMATION
- using other topical acne medications at the same time or immediately following use of this product may increase dryness or irritation of the skin. If this occurs, only one medication should be used unless directed by doctor

---

# SUCRETS WILD CHERRY (dyclonine hydrochloride)
lozenge

Insight Pharmaceuticals

## DRUG FACTS

| Active ingredient (per lozenge) | Purpose |
| --- | --- |
| Dyclonine hydrochloride 2.0 mg | Sore throat/oral anesthetic |

## USES
- for the temporary relief of the following occasional mouth and throat symptoms:
  - pain
  - minor irritation
  - sore mouth
  - sore throat

## WARNINGS

### STOP USE AND ASK A DOCTOR IF
- sore throat is severe, lasts for more than 2 days, occurs with or is followed by fever, headache, rash, nausea, or vomiting
- sore mouth symptoms last more than 7 days, or irritation, pain, or redness continues or worsens

**If pregnant or breastfeeding,** ask a health professional before use.

**Keep out of reach of children.** In case of overdose, get medical help or contact a Poison Control Center right away.

## DIRECTIONS

| adults and children 6 years of age and older | allow lozenge to dissolve slowly in mouth. May be repeated every 2 hours as needed or as directed by a dentist or doctor |
| | do not take more than 10 lozenges per day |
| children under 6 years of age | ask a dentist or doctor |

## INACTIVE INGREDIENTS
corn syrup, FD&C blue 1, FD&C red 40, flavor, menthol, propylene glycol, purified water, sucrose, tartaric acid, titanium dioxide

QUESTIONS OR COMMENTS
Call **1-800-344-7239** or write to Consumer Affairs.
www.insightpharma.com

# SUCRETS CHILDREN'S FORMULA (dyclonine hydrochloride) lozenge

Insight Pharmaceuticals

## DRUG FACTS

| Active ingredient (per lozenge) | Purpose |
|---|---|
| Dyclonine hydrochloride (1.2 mg) | Sore throat/oral anesthetic |

### STOP USE AND ASK A DOCTOR IF

- sore throat is severe, lasts for more than 2 days, occurs with or is followed by fever, headache, rash, nausea, or vomiting
- sore mouth symptoms last more than 7 days, or irritation, pain, or redness continues or worsens

**If pregnant or breastfeeding,** ask a health professional before use.

**Keep out of reach of children.** In case of overdose, get medical help or contact a Poison Control Center right away.

### DIRECTIONS

| adults and children 6 years of age and older | allow lozenge to dissolve slowly in mouth. May be repeated every 2 hours as needed or as directed by a dentist or doctor. |
| | do not take more than 10 lozenges per day |
| children under 6 years of age | ask a dentist or doctor. |

### OTHER INFORMATION

- avoid storing at high temperature (greater than 100°F)
- use only if lozenge blister seals are unbroken

### INACTIVE INGREDIENTS:

citric acid, corn syrup, FD&C red no. 40, flavor, menthol, propylene glycol, purified water, sucrose.

### QUESTIONS OR COMMENTS

Call your Poison Control Center at: **1-800-222-1222**

# SUCRETS COMPLETE COOL CITRUS (dyclonine hydrochloride and menthol) lozenge

Insight Pharmaceuticals

## DRUG FACTS

| Active ingredients (per lozenge) | Purpose |
|---|---|
| Dyclonine hydrochloride 3.0 mg | Oral anesthetic/analgesic |
| Menthol 6.0 mg | Cough suppressant |

### USES

- temporarily relieves:
  - occasional minor irritation, pain, sore throat and sore mouth
  - cough associated with a cold or inhaled irritants

### WARNINGS

**Sore throat warning**
Severe or persistent sore throat or sore throat that occurs with or is followed by high fever, headache, rash, swelling and nausea may be serious. Ask doctor right away. Do not use more than 2 days or give to children under 2 years of age unless directed by a doctor.

### ASK A DOCTOR BEFORE USE IF YOU HAVE

- cough that lasts or is chronic such as occurs with smoking, asthma, or emphysema
- cough that occurs with too much phlegm (mucus)

### STOP USE AND ASK A DOCTOR IF

- sore mouth symptoms do not improve in 7 days
- irritation, pain or redness persists or worsens
- swelling, rash or fever develops
- cough lasts more than 7 days, comes back, or occurs with fever, or persistent headache.

These could be signs of a serious condition

**If pregnant or breastfeeding,** ask a health professional before use.

**Keep out of reach of children.** In case of overdose, get medical help or contact a Poison Control Center right away.

### DIRECTIONS

| adults and children 2 years of age and older | dissolve 1 lozenge slowly in the mouth. May be repeated every 2 hours as needed or as directed by a doctor or dentist |
| children under 2 years of age | consult a doctor or dentist |

### OTHER INFORMATION

- Avoid storing at high temperature (greater than 100°F)
- Use only if lozenge blister seals are unbroken

### INACTIVE INGREDIENTS

corn syrup, sucrose, water, propylene glycol, citric acid, zinc gluconate, tartaric acid, sodium ascorbate, acesulfame potassium, ascorbic acid, citrus flavor, D&C yellow no. 10.

### QUESTIONS OR COMMENTS

Call **1-800-344-7239** or visit www.insightpharma.com

# SUCRETS COUGH HONEY LEMON (dextromethorphan hydrobromide) lozenge

Insight Pharmaceuticals

## DRUG FACTS

| Active ingredient (per lozenge) | Purpose |
|---|---|
| Dextromethorphan hydrobromide 10 mg | Cough Suppressant |

### USES

- temporarily suppresses coughs due to minor throat and bronchial irritation associated with a cold or inhaled irritants

### WARNINGS

### DO NOT USE

- if taking a prescription monoamine oxidase inhibitor (MAOI) (certain drugs for depression, psychiatric, or emotional conditions, or Parkinson's disease), or for 2 weeks after stopping the MAOI drug. If you do not know if your prescription drug contains an MAOI, ask a doctor or pharmacist before taking this product

**ASK A DOCTOR BEFORE USE IF YOU HAVE**
- chronic cough that lasts or occurs with smoking, asthma, chronic bronchitis or emphysema
- cough that occurs with too much phlegm (mucus)

**STOP USE AND ASK A DOCTOR IF**
- cough lasts more than 7 days, comes back, or occurs with fever, rash or headache that lasts

These could be signs of a serious condition.

**If pregnant or breastfeeding,** ask a health professional before use.

**Keep out of reach of children.** In case of overdose, get medical help or contact a Poison Control Center right away.

## DIRECTIONS

| adults | take 3 lozenges every 6-8 hours |
| | do not take more than 12 lozenges per day |
| children under 12 years of age | ask a doctor. |

## INACTIVE INGREDIENTS
corn syrup, D&C yellow no. 10, hydrogenated palm oil, menthol, N&A honey lemon flavor, sugar

## QUESTIONS OR COMMENTS
Call **1-800-344-7239** or write to Consumer Affairs. www.insightpharma.com

## SUCRETS HERBAL HONEY LEMON GINSENG
(menthol and pectin) lozenge
Insight Pharmaceuticals

## DRUG FACTS

| Active ingredient (per lozenge) | Purpose |
| --- | --- |
| Menthol 5.0 mg | Cough suppressant |
| Pectin 6.0 mg | Demulcent |

## USES
- temporarily relieves:
  - occasional minor irritation, pain, sore throat and sore mouth
  - cough associated with a cold or inhaled irritants
  - for protection of irritated areas in sore mouth and throat

## WARNINGS
**Sore throat warning**
Severe or persistent sore throat or sore throat that occurs with or is followed by high fever, headache, rash, nausea or vomiting may be serious. Ask doctor right away. Do not use more than 2 days or give to children under 2 years of age unless directed by a doctor.

**ASK A DOCTOR BEFORE USE IF YOU HAVE**
- cough that lasts or is chronic such as occurs with smoking, asthma, or emphysema
- cough that occurs with too much phlegm (mucus)

**STOP USE AND ASK A DOCTOR IF**
- sore mouth symptoms do not improve in 7 days
- cough lasts more than 7 days, comes back, or occurs with fever, rash or persistent headache

These could be signs of a serious condition.

**If pregnant or breastfeeding,** ask a health professional before use.

**Keep out of reach of children.** In case of overdose, get medical help or contact a Poison Control Center right away.

## DIRECTIONS

| adults and children 3 years of age and older | dissolve 1 lozenge slowly in the mouth. May be repeated every 1 hour as needed or as directed by a doctor or dentist |
| children under 3 years of age | consult a doctor or dentist |

## OTHER INFORMATION
- avoid storing at high temperature (greater than 100°F)
- use only if lozenge blister seals are unbroken

## INACTIVE INGREDIENTS
acesulfame potassium, asorbic acid, corn syrup, D&C yellow no. 10, green tea extract, natural and artificial honey and lemon flavors, propylene glycol, siberian ginseng powder, sodium ascorbate, sucrose

## QUESTIONS OR COMMENTS
Call **1-800-344-7239** or visit www.insightpharma.com

## SUDAFED 12 HOUR (pseudoephedrine hydrochloride) tablet, film coated, extended release
McNeil Consumer Healthcare, Division of McNeil-PPC, Inc.

## DRUG FACTS

| Active ingredient (in each tablet) | Purpose |
| --- | --- |
| Pseudoephedrine hydrochloride 120 mg | Nasal decongestant |

## USES
- temporarily relieves nasal congestion due to the common cold, hay fever or other upper respiratory allergies
- temporarily relieves sinus congestion and pressure

## WARNINGS
**DO NOT USE**
- if you are now taking a prescription monoamine oxidase inhibitor (MAOI) (certain drugs for depression, psychiatric or emotional conditions, or Parkinson's disease), or for 2 weeks after stopping the MAOI drug. If you do not know if your prescription drug contains an MAOI, ask a doctor or pharmacist before taking this product

**ASK A DOCTOR BEFORE USE IF YOU HAVE**
- heart disease
- high blood pressure
- thyroid disease
- diabetes
- trouble urinating due to an enlarged prostate gland

**WHEN USING THIS PRODUCT**
- do not exceed recommended dosage

**STOP USE AND ASK A DOCTOR IF**
- nervousness, dizziness, or sleeplessness occur
- symptoms do not improve within 7 days or occur with a fever

**If pregnant or breastfeeding,** ask a health professional before use.

**Keep out of reach of children.** In case of overdose, get medical help or contact a Poison Control Center right away. (1-800-222-1222)

## DIRECTIONS

| adults and children 12 years and over | take 1 tablet every 12 hours |
| | do not take more than 2 tablets in 24 hours |
| children under 12 years | do not use this product in children under 12 years of age |

## OTHER INFORMATION
- store at 59°F-77°F in a dry place. Protect from light
- do not use if carton is opened or if blister unit is broken
- see side panel for lot number and expiration date

## INACTIVE INGREDIENTS
candelilla wax, hypromellose, magnesium stearate, microcrystalline cellulose, polyethylene glycol, povidone, and titanium dioxide; printed with edible blue ink

## QUESTIONS OR COMMENTS
Call **1-888-217-2117**

---

# SUDAFED 24 HOUR (pseudoephedrine hydrochloride) tablet, extended release
McNeil Consumer Healthcare, Division of McNeil-PPC, Inc.

## DRUG FACTS

| Active ingredient (in each tablet) | Purpose |
|---|---|
| Pseudoephedrine hydrochloride 240 mg | Nasal decongestant |

## USES
- temporarily relieves nasal congestion due to the common cold, hay fever or other upper respiratory allergies
- reduces swelling of nasal passages
- relieves sinus pressure

## WARNINGS

### DO NOT USE
- if you are now taking a prescription monoamine oxidase inhibitor (MAOI) (certain drugs for depression, psychiatric or emotional conditions, or Parkinson's disease), or for 2 weeks after stopping the MAOI drug. If you do not know if your prescription drug contains an MAOI, ask a doctor or pharmacist before taking this product

### ASK A DOCTOR BEFORE USE IF YOU HAVE
- heart disease
- high blood pressure
- thyroid disease
- diabetes
- trouble urinating due to an enlarged prostate gland
- had obstruction or narrowing of the bowel. Rarely, tablets of this kind may cause bowel obstruction (blockage), usually in people with severe narrowing of the bowel (esophagus, stomach or intestine)

### WHEN USING THIS PRODUCT
- do not exceed recommended dosage

## STOP USE AND ASK A DOCTOR IF
- nervousness, dizziness, or sleeplessness occur
- symptoms do not improve within 7 days or occur with a fever
- you experience persistent abdominal pain or vomiting

**If pregnant or breastfeeding,** ask a health professional before use.

**Keep out of reach of children.** In case of overdose, get medical help or contact a Poison Control Center right away. (1-800-222-1222)

## DIRECTIONS

| adults and children 12 years and over | swallow one whole tablet with water every 24 hours |
| | do not exceed one tablet in 24 hours |
| | do not divide, crush, chew or dissolve the tablet |
| | the tablet does not completely dissolve and may be seen in the stool (this is normal) |
| children under 12 years | do not use |

## OTHER INFORMATION
- each tablet contains: sodium 10 mg
- store at 15°C-25°C (59°F-77°F) in a dry place
- do not use if carton is opened or if individual blister seals are broken or opened
- see side panel for lot number and expiration date

## INACTIVE INGREDIENTS
cellulose, cellulose acetate, hydroxypropyl cellulose, hypromellose, magnesium stearate, polyethylene glycol, polysorbate 80, povidone, sodium chloride, and titanium dioxide

## QUESTIONS OR COMMENTS
Call **1-888-217-2117**

---

# SUDAFED OM (oxymetazoline hydrochloride) spray
McNeil Consumer Healthcare, Division of McNeil-PPC, Inc.

## DRUG FACTS

| Active ingredient (in each spray) | Purpose |
|---|---|
| Oxymetazoline hydrochloride 0.05% | Nasal decongestant |

## USES
- temporarily relieves nasal congestion due to:
  - the common cold
  - hay fever
  - upper respiratory allergies
- helps clear nasal passages; shrinks swollen membranes
- temporarily restores freer breathing through the nose
- helps decongest sinus openings and passages
- temporarily relieves sinus congestion and pressure

## WARNINGS

### ASK A DOCTOR BEFORE USE IF YOU HAVE
- heart disease
- thyroid disease
- diabetes
- high blood pressure
- trouble urinating due to an enlarged prostate gland

**WHEN USING THIS PRODUCT**
- do not exceed recommended dose
- use of this container by more than one person may cause infection
- temporary discomfort such as burning, stinging, sneezing, or increased nasal discharge may occur
- frequent or prolonged use may cause nasal congestion to recur or worsen

**STOP USE AND ASK A DOCTOR IF**
- symptoms persist for more than 3 days

**If pregnant or breastfeeding,** ask a health professional before use.

**Keep out of reach of children.** In case of overdose, get medical help or contact a Poison Control Center right away. (1-800-222-1222)

**DIRECTIONS**

| adults and children 6 years to under 12 years of age (with adult supervision) | 2 or 3 sprays in each nostril, not more often than every 10 to 12 hours |
| | do not exceed 2 doses in any 24 hour period |
| children under 6 years | do not use |

**OTHER INFORMATION**
- store between 20-25°C (68-77°F)
- do not use if bottle wrap imprinted with "SUDAFED OM" is broken or missing
- see bottom panel for lot number and expiration date

**INACTIVE INGREDIENTS**
benzalkonium chloride solution, benzyl alcohol, dibasic sodium phosphate, edetate disodium, glycerin, hypromellose, monobasic sodium phosphate, polyethylene glycol, propylene glycol, purified water

**QUESTIONS OR COMMENTS**
Call 1-888-217-2117

## SUDAFED PE CONGESTION (phenylephrine hydrochloride) tablet
McNeil Consumer Healthcare

**DRUG FACTS**

| Active ingredient (in each tablet) | Purpose |
|---|---|
| Phenylephrine hydrochloride 10 mg | Nasal decongestant |

**USES**
- temporarily relieves sinus congestion and pressure
- temporarily relieves nasal congestion due to:
  - the common cold
  - hay fever
  - other upper-respiratory allergies

**WARNINGS**

**DO NOT USE**
- if you are now taking a prescription monoamine oxidase inhibitor (MAOI) (certain drugs for depression, psychiatric or emotional conditions or Parkinson's disease), or for 2 weeks after stopping the MAOI drug if your prescription drug contains an MAOI, ask a doctor or pharmacist before taking this product.

**ASK A DOCTOR BEFORE USE IF YOU HAVE**
- heart disease
- high blood pressure
- thyroid disease
- diabetes
- trouble urinating due to an enlarged prostate gland

**WHEN USING THIS PRODUCT**
- do not exceed recommended dose

**STOP USE AND ASK A DOCTOR IF**
- nervousness, dizziness, or sleeplessness occurs
- symptoms do not improve within 7 days or occur with a fever

**If pregnant or breastfeeding,** ask a health professional before use.

**Keep out of reach of children.** In case of overdose, get medical help or contact a Poison Control Center right away (1-800-222-1222).

**DIRECTIONS**

| adults and children 12 years and over | take 1 tablet every 4 hours |
| | do not take more than 6 tablets in 24 hours |
| children under 12 years | do not use |

**INACTIVE INGREDIENTS**
carnauba wax, corn starch, D&C yellow no. 10 aluminum lake, FD&C red no. 40 aluminum lake, FD&C yellow no. 6 aluminum lake, magnesium stearate, microcrystalline cellulose, polyethylene glycol, polyvinyl alcohol, powdered cellulose, pregelatinized starch, sodium starch glycolate, talc, titanium dioxide

**OTHER INFORMATION**
- store between 20-25°C (68-77°F)

**QUESTIONS OR COMMENTS**
Call 1-888-217-2117

## SUDAFED PE COUGH AND COLD
(acetaminophen, dextromethorphan hydrobromide, guaitenesin, and phenylephrine hydrochloride) caplet
McNeil Consumer Healthcare

**DRUG FACTS**

| Active ingredients (in each caplet) | Purpose |
|---|---|
| Acetaminophen 325 mg | Pain reliever/fever reducer |
| Dextromethorphan hydrobromide 10 mg | Cough suppressant |
| Guaitenesin 100 mg | Expectorant |
| Phenylephrine hydrochloride 5 mg | Nasal decongestant |

**USES**
- temporarily relieves these symptoms due to the common cold:
  - nasal congestion
  - headache
  - minor aches and pains
  - cough
  - sore throat
- helps loosen phlegm (mucus) and thin bronchial secretions to drain bronchial tubes and make coughs more productive
- temporarily reduces fever

## WARNINGS

### Liver warning

This product contains acetaminophen. Severe liver damage may occur if you take:

- more than 12 caplets in 24 hours, which is the maximum daily amount
- with other drugs containing acetaminophen
- 3 or more alcoholic drinks every day while using this product

### Sore throat warning

If sore throat is severe, persists for more than 2 days, is accompanied or followed by fever, headache, rash, nausea, or vomiting, consult a doctor promptly.

### DO NOT USE

- with any other drug containing acetaminophen (prescription or nonprescription). If you are not sure whether a drug contains acetaminophen, ask a doctor or pharmacist
- if you are now taking a prescription monoamine oxidase inhibitor (MAOI) (certain drugs for depression, psychiatric or emotional conditions or Parkinson's disease), or for 2 weeks after stopping the MAOI drug, if you do not know if your prescription drug contains an MAOI, ask a doctor or pharmacist before taking this product
- if you have ever had an allergic reaction to this product or any of its ingredients

### ASK A DOCTOR BEFORE USE IF YOU HAVE

- liver disease
- heart disease
- high blood pressure
- thyroid disease
- diabetes
- trouble urinating due to an enlarged prostate gland
- persistent or chronic cough such as occurs with smoking, asthma, chronic bronchitis or emphysema
- cough that occurs with too much phlegm (mucus)

### ASK A DOCTOR OR PHARMACIST BEFORE USE IF

- you are taking the blood-thinning drug warfarin

### WHEN USING THIS PRODUCT

- do not exceed recommended dose

### STOP USE AND ASK A DOCTOR IF

- nervousness, dizziness, or sleeplessness occur
- pain, cough, or nasal congestion gets worse or lasts more than 7 days
- fever gets worse or lasts more than 3 days
- redness or swelling is present
- new symptoms occur
- cough comes back or occurs with rash or headache that lasts

These could be signs of a serious condition.

**If pregnant or breastfeeding,** ask a health professional before use.

Keep out of reach of children.

### OVERDOSE WARNING

Taking more than the recommended dose (overdose) may cause liver damage. In case of overdose, get medical help or contact a Poison Control Center right away (1-800-222-1222). Quick medical attention Is critical for adults as well as for children even if you do not notice any signs or symptoms.

### DIRECTIONS

- do not use more than directed (see overdose warning)

| adults and children 12 years and over | take 2 caplets every 4 hours |
| | do not take more than 12 tablets in 24 hours |
| children under 12 years | do not use this adult product for children under 12 years of age; this will provide more than the recommended dose (overdose) and may cause liver damage |

### INACTIVE INGREDIENTS

carnauba wax, croscarmellose sodium, FD&C yellow no. 5 aluminum lake (tartrazine), FD&C yellow no. 6 aluminum lake, hydroxypropyl cellulose, hypromellose, magnesium stearate, microcrystalline cellulose, polyethylene gtycol, polysorbate 80, pregelatinized starch, titanium dioxide

### OTHER INFORMATION

- contains FD&C yellow no. 5 aluminum lake (tartrazine) as a color additive
- each caplet contains: sodium 3 mg
- store between 20-25°C (58-77°F)

### QUESTIONS OR COMMENTS

Call **1-888-217-2117**

---

# CHILDREN'S SUDAFED PE COLD & COUGH

(dextromethorphan hydrobromide and phenylephrine hydrochloride) liquid

McNeil

## DRUG FACTS

| Active ingredients (in each 5 mL) | Purpose |
|---|---|
| Dextromethorphan hydrobromide 5 mg | Cough suppressant |
| Phenylephrine hydrochloride 2.5 mg | Nasal decongestant |

* 5 mL = one teaspoonful

### USES

- temporarily relieves nasal congestion due to the common cold, hay fever, or other upper-respiratory allergies:
  - cough
  - nasal congestion

### WARNINGS

### DO NOT USE

- for a child who is taking a prescription monoamine oxidase inhibitor (MAOI) (certain drugs for depression, psychiatric or emotional conditions or Parkinson's disease), or for 2 weeks after stopping the MAOI drug. If you do not know if your child's prescription drug contains an MAOI, ask a doctor or pharmacist before giving this product

### ASK A DOCTOR BEFORE USE IF THE CHILD HAS

- heart disease
- high blood pressure
- thyroid disease
- diabetes
- persistent or chronic cough such as occurs with asthma
- cough that occurs with too much phlegm (mucus)
- a sodium-restricted diet

### WHEN USING THIS PRODUCT

- do not exceed recommended dose

**STOP USE AND ASK A DOCTOR IF**
- nervousness, dizziness, or sleeplessness occur
- symptoms do not improve within 7 days or occur with a fever
- cough gets worse or lasts for more than 7 days
- cough tends to come back or occurs with fever, rash or headache that lasts
- these could be signs of a serious condition

**Keep out of reach of children.** In case of overdose, get medical help or contact a Poison Control Center right away (1-800-222-1222).

**DIRECTIONS**
- find right dose below
- use only enclosed dosing cup designed for use with this product. Do not use any other dosing device
- if needed, repeat dose every 4 hours
- do not use more than 6 times in 24 hours

| under 4 years | do not use |
|---|---|
| 4 to 5 years | 1 teaspoonful (5 mL) |
| 6 to 11 years | 2 teaspoonfuls (10 mL) |

**INACTIVE INGREDIENTS**
anhydrous citric acid, carboxymethylcellulose sodium, edetate disodium, FD&C blue no. 1, FD&C red no. 40, flavors, glycerin, purified water, sodium benzoate, sodium citrate, sorbitol solution, sucralose

**OTHER INFORMATION**
- each teaspoonful contains: sodium 15 mg
- store between 20-25°C (68-77°F). Protect from light
- store in outer carton until contents are used

**QUESTIONS OR COMMENTS**
Call **1-888-217-2117**

## CHILDREN'S SUDAFED NASAL DECONGESTANT GRAPE LIQUID

(Pseudoephedrine hydrochloride) liquid

McNeil-PPC Inc.

### DRUG FACTS

| Active ingredient (in each 5 mL*) | Purpose |
|---|---|
| Pseudoephedrine hydrochloride 15 mg | Nasal decongestant |

\* 5 mL = one teaspoonful

**USES**
- temporarily relieves nasal congestion due to the common cold, hay fever, or other upper-respiratory allergies
- temporarily relieves sinus congestion and pressure
- promotes nasal and/or sinus drainage

**WARNINGS**

**DO NOT USE**
- for a child who is taking a prescription monoamine oxidase inhibitor (MAOI) (certain drugs for depression, psychiatric or emotional conditions or Parkinson's disease), or for 2 weeks after stopping the MAOI drug. If you do not know if your child's prescription drug contains an MAOI, ask a doctor or pharmacist before giving this product

**ASK A DOCTOR BEFORE USE IF THE CHILD HAS**
- heart disease
- high blood pressure
- thyroid disease
- diabetes

**WHEN USING THIS PRODUCT**
- do not exceed recommended dose

**STOP USE AND ASK A DOCTOR IF**
- nervousness, dizziness, or sleeplessness occur
- symptoms do not improve within 7 days or occur with a fever

**Keep out of reach of children.** In case of overdose, get medical help or contact a Poison Control Center right away (1-800-222-1222).

**DIRECTIONS**
- find right dose below
- use only enclosed dosing cup designed for use with this product. Do not use any other dosing device
- if needed, repeat dose every 4 hours
- do not use more than 4 times in 24 hours

| under 4 years | do not use |
|---|---|
| 4 to 5 years | 1 teaspoonful (5 mL) |
| 6 to 11 years | 2 teaspoonfuls (10 mL) |

**INACTIVE INGREDIENTS**
anhydrous citric acid, edetate disodium, FD&C blue no. 1, FD&C red no. 40, flavor, glycerin, menthol, poloxamer 407, polyethylene glycol, povidone K-90, purified water, saccharin sodium, sodium benzoate, sodium citrate, sorbitol solution

**OTHER INFORMATION**
- each teaspoonful contains: sodium 5 mg
- store between 20-25°C (68-77°F). Protect from light
- store in outer carton until contents are used

**QUESTIONS OR COMMENTS**
Call **1-888-217-2117**

## SUDAFED PE NON-DROWSY SINUS HEADACHE MAXIMUM STRENGTH

(acetaminophen and phenylephrine hydrochloride) caplet, film coated

McNeil Consumer Healthcare, Division of McNeil-PPC, Inc.

Covidien Ltd.

### DRUG FACTS

| Active ingredients (in each caplet) | Purpose |
|---|---|
| Acetaminophen 325 mg | Pain reliever |
| Phenylephrine hydrochloride 5 mg | Nasal decongestant |

**USES**
- temporarily relieves headache, minor aches, and pains
- temporarily relieves nasal congestion

## WARNINGS

### Alcohol warning

If you consume 3 or more alcoholic drinks every day, ask your doctor whether you should take acetaminophen or other pain relievers or fever reducers. Acetaminophen may cause liver damage.

### DO NOT USE

- with another product containing acetaminophen
- if you are now taking a prescription monoamine oxidase inhibitor (MAOI) (certain drugs for depression, psychiatric or emotional conditions, or Parkinson's disease), or for 2 weeks after stopping the MAOI drug. If you do not know if your prescription drug contains an MAOI, ask a doctor or pharmacist before taking this product

### ASK A DOCTOR BEFORE USE IF YOU HAVE

- heart disease
- high blood pressure
- thyroid disease
- diabetes
- trouble urinating due to an enlarged prostate gland

### WHEN USING THIS PRODUCT

- do not exceed recommended dose

### STOP USE AND ASK A DOCTOR IF

- nervousness, dizziness, or sleeplessness occur
- pain or nasal congestion gets worse or lasts more than 7 days
- fever gets worse or lasts more than 3 days
- redness or swelling is present
- new symptoms occur

These could be signs of a serious condition.

**If pregnant or breastfeeding,** ask a health professional before use.

**Keep out of reach of children.**

### OVERDOSE WARNING

Taking more than the recommended dose (overdose) may cause liver damage. In case of overdose, get medical help or contact a Poison Control Center right away. (1-800-222-1222) Quick medical attention is critical for adults as well as for children even if you do not notice any signs or symptoms.

### DIRECTIONS

- do not use more than directed (see overdose warning)

| adults and children 12 years and over | take 2 caplets every 4 hours |
| | do not take more than 12 caplets in 24 hours |
| children under 12 years | do not use; this will provide more than the recommended dose (overdose) and may cause liver damage |

### OTHER INFORMATION

- store between 20-25°C (68-77°F)
- do not use if carton is opened or if blister unit is broken
- see side panel for lot number and expiration date

### INACTIVE INGREDIENTS

carnauba wax, corn starch, FD&C yellow no. 6 aluminum lake, hypromellose, magnesium stearate, microcrystalline cellulose, polyethylene glycol, polysorbate 80, powdered cellulose, pregelatinized starch, sodium starch glycolate, titanium dioxide

### QUESTIONS OR COMMENTS

Call **1-888-217-2117**

# SUDAFED PE SINUS AND ALLERGY
(chlorpheniramine maleate and phenylephrine hydrochloride) tablet

McNeil Consumer Healthcare

## DRUG FACTS

| Active ingredient (in each tablet) | Purpose |
|---|---|
| Chlorpheniramine maleate 4 mg | Antihistamine |
| Phenylephrine hydrochloride 10 mg | Nasal decongestant |

### USES

- temporarily relieves these symptoms due to hay fever (allergic rhinitis) or other upper-respiratory allergies:
  - runny nose
  - sneezing
  - itchy, watery eyes
  - nasal congestion
  - itching of the nose or throat
  - sinus congestion and pressure

## WARNINGS

### DO NOT USE

- if you are now taking a prescription monoamine oxidase inhibitor (MAOI) (certain drugs for depression, psychiatric or emotional conditions or Parkinson's disease), or for 2 weeks after stopping the MAOI drug. If you do not know if your prescription drug contains an MAOI, ask a doctor or pharmacist before taking this product

### ASK A DOCTOR BEFORE USE IF YOU HAVE

- heart disease
- high blood pressure
- thyroid disease
- diabetes
- trouble urinating due to an enlarged prostate gland
- a breathing problem such as emphysema or chronic bronchitis
- glaucoma

### ASK A DOCTOR OR PHARMACIST BEFORE YOU USE IF YOU ARE

- taking sedatives or tranquilizers

### WHEN USING THIS PRODUCT

- do not exceed recommended dose
- excitability may occur, especially in children
- drowsiness may occur
- alcohol, sedatives, and tranquilizers may increase drowsiness
- avoid alcoholic drinks
- be careful when driving a motor vehicle or operating machinery

### STOP USE AND ASK A DOCTOR IF

- nervousness, dizziness, or sleeplessness occurs
- symptoms do not improve within 7 days or occur with a fever

**If pregnant or breastfeeding,** ask a health professional before use.

**Keep out of reach of children.** In case of overdose, get medical help or contact a Poison Control Center right away (1-800-222-1222).

### DIRECTIONS

| adults and children 12 years and over | take 1 tablet every 4 hours |
| | do not take more than 6 tablets in 24 hours |

| children under 12 years | do not use |
|---|---|

## INACTIVE INGREDIENTS
carnauba wax, corn starch, magnesium stearate, microcrystalline cellulose, polyethylene glycol, polyvinyl alcohol, powdered cellulose, pregelatinized starch, sodium starch glycolate, talc, titanium dioxide

## OTHER INFORMATION
• store between 20-25°C (68-77°F)

## QUESTIONS OR COMMENTS
Call **1-888-217-2117**

# SUDAFED SINUS CONGESTION MOISTURIZING NASAL SPRAY (oxymetazoline hydrochloride) spray

McNeil Consumer Healthcare, Division of McNeil-PPC, Inc.

## DRUG FACTS

| Active ingredient (in each spray) | Purpose |
|---|---|
| Oxymetazoline hydrochloride 0.05% | Nasal decongestant |

## USES
• temporarily relieves nasal congestion due to:
  • the common cold
  • hay fever
  • upper respiratory allergies
• helps clear nasal passages; shrinks swollen membranes
• temporarily restores freer breathing through the nose
• helps decongest sinus openings and passages; temporarily relieves sinus congestion and pressure

## WARNINGS

### ASK A DOCTOR BEFORE USE IF YOU HAVE
• heart disease
• thyroid disease
• diabetes
• high blood pressure
• trouble urinating due to an enlarged prostate gland

### WHEN USING THIS PRODUCT
• do not exceed recommended dose
• use of this container by more than one person may cause infection
• temporary discomfort such as burning, stinging, sneezing, or increased nasal discharge may occur
• frequent or prolonged use may cause nasal congestion to recur or worsen

### STOP USE AND ASK A DOCTOR
• if symptoms persist for more than 3 days

**If pregnant or breastfeeding,** ask a health professional before use.

**Keep out of reach of children.** In case of overdose, get medical help or contact a Poison Control Center right away. (1-800-222-1222)

## DIRECTIONS

| adults and children 6 years to under 12 years of age (with adult supervision) | 2 or 3 sprays in each nostril, not more often than every 10 to 12 hours |
|---|---|
| | do not exceed 2 doses in any 24 hour period |
| children under 6 years | do not use |

## OTHER INFORMATION
• store between 20-25°C (68-77°F)
• do not use if bottle wrap imprinted with "SUDAFED OM" is broken or missing
• see bottom panel for lot number and expiration date

## INACTIVE INGREDIENTS
benzalkonium chloride solution, benzyl alcohol, dibasic sodium phosphate, edetate disodium, glycerin, hypromellose, monobasic sodium phosphate, polyethylene glycol, propylene glycol, purified water

## QUESTIONS OR COMMENTS
Call **1-888-217-2117**

# SUDAFED 12 HOUR PRESSURE AND PAIN
(naproxen sodium and pseudoephedrine hydrochloride) caplet, film coated, extended release

McNeil Consumer Healthcare, Division of McNeil-PPC, Inc.

## DRUG FACTS

| Active ingredients (in each caplet) | Purpose |
|---|---|
| Naproxen sodium 220 mg (naproxen 200 mg) (NSAID)* | Pain reliever/fever reducer |
| Pseudoephedrine hydrochloride 120 mg, extended-release | Nasal decongestant |

* nonsteroidal anti-inflammatory drug

## USES
• temporarily relieves these cold, sinus, and flu symptoms:
  • sinus pressure
  • minor body aches and pains
  • headache
  • nasal and sinus congestion (promotes sinus drainage and restores freer breathing through the nose)
  • fever

## WARNINGS
**Allergy alert**
Naproxen sodium may cause a severe allergic reaction, especially in people allergic to aspirin. Symptoms may include:

• hives
• facial swelling
• asthma (wheezing)
• shock
• skin reddening
• rash
• blisters

If an allergic reaction occurs, stop use and seek medical help right away.

**Stomach bleeding warning**
This product contains an NSAID, which may cause severe stomach bleeding. The chance is higher if you:
- arc age 60 or older
- have had stomach ulcers or bleeding problems
- take a blood thinning (anticoagulant) or steroid drug
- take other drugs containing prescription or nonprescription NSAIDs (aspirin, ibuprofen, naproxen, or others)
- have 3 or more alcoholic drinks every day while using this product
- take more or for a longer time than directed

**DO NOT USE**
- if you have ever had an allergic reaction to any other pain reliever/fever reducer right before or after heart surgery
- if you are now taking a prescription monoamine oxidase inhibitor (MAOI) (certain drugs for depression, psychiatric, or emotional conditions, or Parkinson's disease), or for 2 weeks after stopping the MAOI drug. If you do not know if your prescription drug contains an MAOI, ask a doctor or pharmacist before taking this product
- in children under 12 years of age

**ASK A DOCTOR BEFORE USE IF**
- the stomach bleeding warning applies to you
- you have a history of stomach problems, such as heartburn
- you have high blood pressure, heart disease, liver cirrhosis, or kidney disease
- you are taking a diuretic
- you have problems or serious side effects from taking pain relievers or fever reducers
- you have:
  - asthma
  - diabetes
  - thyroid disease
  - trouble urinating due to an enlarged prostate gland

**ASK A DOCTOR OR PHARMACIST BEFORE USE IF YOU ARE**
- under a doctor's care for any serious condition
- taking any other drug

**WHEN USING THIS PRODUCT**
- take with food or milk if stomach upset occurs
- the risk of heart attack or stroke may increase if you use more than directed or for longer than directed

**STOP USE AND ASK A DOCTOR IF**
- you experience any of the following signs of stomach bleeding:
  - feel faint
  - vomit blood
  - have bloody or black stools
  - have stomach pain that does not get better
- redness or swelling is present in the painful area
- any new symptoms appear
- fever gets worse or lasts more than 3 days
- you have difficulty swallowing or the caplet feels stuck in your throat
- you get nervous, dizzy, or sleepless
- nasal congestion lasts more than 7 days

**If pregnant or breastfeeding,** ask a health professional before use.

It is especially important not to use naproxen sodium during the last 3 months of pregnancy unless definitely directed to do so by a doctor because it may cause problems in the unborn child or complications during delivery.

**Keep out of reach of children.** In case of overdose, get medical help or contact a Poison Control Center right away. (1-800-222-1222)

**DIRECTIONS**
- do not take more than directed
- the smallest effective dose should be used
- swallow whole; do not crush or chew
- drink a full glass of water with each dose

| adults and children 12 years and older | 1 caplet every 12 hours<br><br>do not take more than 2 caplets in 24 hours |
|---|---|
| children under 12 years | do not use |

**OTHER INFORMATION**
- each caplet contains: **sodium 20 mg**
- do not use if carton is opened or if blister unit is broken
- store at 20-25°C (68-77°F)
- store in a dry place

**INACTIVE INGREDIENTS**
colloidal silicon dioxide, hypromellose, lactose monohydrate, magnesium stearate, microcrystalline cellulose, polyethylene glycol, polysorbate 80, povidone, talc, titanium dioxide

**QUESTIONS OR COMMENTS**
Call **1-888-217-2117**

---

**SYSTANE** (polyethylene glycol, and propylene glycol) solution/drops
Alcon Research Ltd

**DRUG FACTS**

| Active ingredients | Purpose |
|---|---|
| Polyethylene Glycol 400 0.4% | Lubricant |
| Propylene Glycol 0.3% | Lubricant |

**USE**
- for the temporary relief of burning and irritation due to dryness of the eye

**WARNINGS**
**For external use only.**

**DO NOT USE**
- if this product changes color or becomes cloudy
- if you are sensitive to any ingredient in this product

**WHEN USING THIS PRODUCT**
- do not touch tip of container to any surface to avoid contamination
- do not reuse
- once opened, discard

**STOP USE AND ASK A DOCTOR IF**
- you feel eye pain
- changes in vision occur
- redness or irritation of the eye(s) gets worse, persists or lasts more than 72 hours

**Keep out of reach of children.** If swallowed, get medical help or contact a Poison Control Center right away.

**DIRECTIONS**
- Instill 1 or 2 drops in the affected eye(s) as needed

## OTHER INFORMATION
- Store at room temperature
- Protect from light

## INACTIVE INGREDIENTS
boric acid, calcium chloride, hydroxypropyl guar, magnesium chloride, potassium chloride, purified water, sodium chloride, zinc chloride; may contain hydrochloric acid and/or sodium hydroxide to adjust pH

## QUESTIONS AND COMMENTS
In the U.S. call **1-800-757-9195** or visit www.systane.com
MedInfo@AlconLabs.com

---

# SYSTANE ULTRA (polyethylene glycol, and propylene glycol) solution/drops
Alcon Research Ltd

## DRUG FACTS

| Active ingredients | Purpose |
|---|---|
| Polyethylene glycol 400 0.4% | Lubricant |
| Propylene glycol 0.3% | Lubricant |

## USES
- for the temporary relief of burning and irritation due to dryness of the eye

## WARNINGS
**For external use only.**

## DO NOT USE
- if this product changes color or becomes cloudy
- if you are sensitive to any ingredient in this product

## WHEN USING THIS PRODUCT
- do not touch tip of container to any surface to avoid contamination
- do not reuse
- once opened, discard

## STOP USE AND ASK A DOCTOR IF
- you feel eye pain
- changes in vision occur
- redness or irritation of the eye(s) gets worse, persists or lasts more than 72 hours

**Keep out of reach of children.** If swallowed, get medical help or contact a Poison Control Center right away.

## DIRECTIONS
- Instill 1 or 2 drops in the affected eye(s) as needed

## OTHER INFORMATION
- Store at room temperature

## INACTIVE INGREDIENTS
aminomethylpropanol, boric acid, hydroxypropyl guar, potassium chloride, purified water, sodium chloride, sorbitol; may contain hydrochloric acid and/or sodium hydroxide to adjust pH

## QUESTIONS AND COMMENTS
In the U.S. Call **1-800-757-9195** or visit www.systane.com

---

# TAGAMET HB (cimetidine) tablet
GlaxoSmithKline Consumer Healthcare LP

## DRUG FACTS

| Active ingredient (in each tablet) | Purpose |
|---|---|
| Cimetidine 200 mg | Acid reducer |

## USES
- relieves heartburn associated with acid indigestion and sour stomach
- prevents heartburn associated with acid indigestion and sour stomach brought on by eating or drinking certain food and beverages

## WARNINGS
**Allergy alert**
Do not use if you are allergic to cimetidine or other acid reducers

## DO NOT USE
- if you have trouble or pain swallowing food, vomiting with blood, or bloody or black stools. These may be signs of a serious condition. See your doctor
- with other acid reducers

## ASK A DOCTOR BEFORE USE IF YOU HAVE
- frequent chest pain
- frequent wheezing, particularly with heartburn
- unexplained weight loss
- nausea or vomiting
- stomach pain
- had heartburn over 3 months. This may be a sign of a more serious condition
- heartburn with lightheadedness, sweating or dizziness
- chest pain or shoulder pain with:
  - shortness of breath
  - sweating
  - pain spreading to arms, neck or shoulders
  - lightheadedness

## ASK A DOCTOR OR PHARMACIST BEFORE USE IF YOU ARE TAKING
- theophylline (oral asthma medicine)
- warfarin (blood thinning medicine)
- phenytoin (seizure medicine)

If you are not sure you are taking one of these medicines, talk to your doctor or pharmacist.

**Drug Interaction Warnings**
Tagamet HB 200 may interfere with the action of drugs prescribed by your doctor. Check with your doctor before taking Tagamet HB 200 if you are taking blood thinning medication (e.g. warfarin) or drugs prescribed for asthma (e.g. theophylline) or epilepsy (e.g. phenytoin).

## STOP USE AND ASK A DOCTOR IF
- your heartburn continues or worsens
- stomach pain continues
- you need to take this product for more than 14 days

**If pregnant or breastfeeding,** ask a health professional before use.

**Keep out of reach of children.** In case of overdose, get medical help or contact a Poison Control Center right away.

## DIRECTIONS

| adults and children 12 years and over | to relieve symptoms, swallow 1 tablet with a glass of water |
| | to prevent symptoms, swallow 1 tablet with a glass of water right before or any time up to 30 minutes before eating food or drinking beverages that cause heartburn |
| | do not take more than 2 tablets in 24 hours |
| children under 12 years | ask a doctor |

## OTHER INFORMATION
- store at 15-30°C (59-86°F)
- each tablet individually sealed in blister pack; do not use if blister or foil is open or torn

## INACTIVE INGREDIENTS
cellulose, corn starch, hypromellose, magnesium stearate, polyethylene glycol, polysorbate 80, povidone, sodium lauryl sulfate, sodium starch glycolate, titanium dioxide

## QUESTIONS AND COMMENTS
Call toll-free **1-800-482-4394** (English/Spanish) weekdays

---

## TANAC (benzocaine) liquid
Insight Pharmaceuticals LLC

### DRUG FACTS

| Active ingredient | Purpose |
|---|---|
| Benzocaine 10% | Oral pain reliever |

## USES
- temporarily relieves pain due to:
  - canker sores
  - cold sores
  - fever blisters
  - minor irritations or injury of the mouth and gums

## WARNINGS
**Allergy alert**
Do not use this product if you have a history of allergy to local anesthetics such as procaine, butacaine, benzocaine, or other "caine" anesthetics.

## WHEN USING THIS PRODUCT
- avoid contact with the eyes
- do not use more than directed
- do not use for more than 7 days unless directed by a dentist or doctor

## STOP USE AND ASK A DENTIST OR DOCTOR IF
- sore mouth symptoms do not improve in 7 days
- symptoms clear up and occur again within a few days
- irritation, pain or redness persists or worsens
- swelling, rash, or fever develops

**Keep out of reach of children.** In case of accidental overdose, get medical help or contact a Poison Control Center right away.

## DIRECTIONS
- remove imprinted safety seal from bottle cap

| adults and children 2 years of age and older | apply product with cotton swab or clean fingertip to the affected area. |
| | Use up to 4 times daily or as directed by a dentist or doctor |
| children under 12 years of age | should be supervised in the use of this product |
| children under 2 years of age | ask a dentist or doctor |

## OTHER INFORMATION
- do not use if imprinted bottle seal is broken or missing prior to opening
- keep carton for full drug facts

## INACTIVE INGREDIENTS
benzalkonium chloride, peppermint oil, polyethylene glycol 400, propylene glycol, sodium saccharin, tannic acid

## QUESTIONS OR COMMENTS
Call **1-800-344-7239**

---

## TAVIST ALLERGY (clemastine fumarate) tablet
Novartis Consumer Health, Inc.

### DRUG FACTS

| Active ingredient | Purpose |
|---|---|
| Clemastine fumarate, USP 1.34 mg (equivalent to 1 mg clemastine) | Antihistamine |

## USES
- temporarily reduces these symptoms of the common cold, hay fever and other respiratory allergies:
  - runny nose
  - itchy, watery eyes
  - sneezing
  - itching of the nose or throat

## WARNINGS

**ASK DOCTOR BEFORE USE IF YOU HAVE**
- a breathing problem such as emphysema or chronic bronchitis
- glaucoma
- trouble urinating due to enlargement of the prostate gland

**ASK A DOCTOR OR PHARMACIST BEFORE USE IF YOU ARE**
- taking sedative or tranquillizers

**WHEN USING THIS PRODUCT**
- avoid alcoholic drinks
- drowsiness may occur
- alcohol, sedative, and tranquillizers may increase drowsiness
- be careful when driving a motor vehicle or operating machinery
- excitability may occur, especially in children

**If pregnant or breastfeeding,** ask a health professional before use.

**Keep out of reach of children** In case of overdose, get medical help or contact a Poison Control Center right away.

## DIRECTIONS

| adults and children 12 years of age and over | take 1 tablet every 12 hours<br><br>do not take more than 2 tablets in 24 hours unless directed by a doctor |
|---|---|
| children under 12 years of age | consult a doctor |

## OTHER INFORMATION
- sodium free
- store at controlled room temperature 20-25°C (68-77°F)

## INACTIVE INGREDIENTS
lactose, povidone, starch, stearic acid, talc

## QUESTIONS OR COMMENTS
Call 1-800-452-0051

## TEARS NATURALE FORTE (dextran, glycerin, and hypromellose) solution/drops
Alcon Inc.

## DRUG FACTS

| Active ingredients | Purpose |
|---|---|
| Dextran 70 0.1% | Lubricant |
| Glycerin 0.2% | Lubricant |
| Hypromellose 0.3% | Lubricant |

## USES
- for the temporary relief of burning and irritation due to dryness of the eye and for use as a protectant against further irritation. For the temporary relief of discomfort due to minor irritations of the eye or to exposure to wind or sun

## WARNINGS
**For external use only.**

## DO NOT USE
- if this solution changes color or becomes cloudy
- if you are sensitive to any ingredient in this product

## WHEN USING THIS PRODUCT
- remove contact lenses before using
- do not touch tip of container to any surface to avoid contamination
- replace cap after each use

## STOP USE AND ASK A DOCTOR IF
- you feel eye pain
- changes in vision occur
- redness or irritation of the eye(s) gets worse or lasts more than 72 hours

**Keep out of reach of children.** If swallowed, get medical help or contact a Poison Control Center right away.

## DIRECTIONS
- Instill 1 or 2 drops in the affected eye(s) as needed

## OTHER INFORMATION
- store at room temperature

## INACTIVE INGREDIENTS
boric acid, calcium chloride, glycine, hydrochloric acid and/or sodium hydroxide (to adjust pH), magnesium chloride, polyquad (polyquaternlum-1) 0.001% preservative, polysorbate 80, potassium chloride, purified water, sodium chloride, zinc chloride

## QUESTIONS OR COMMENTS
In the U.S. Call **1-800-757-9195** or visit www.tearsnaturale.com

## TECNU RASH RELIEF (grindelia robusta, plantago major, and calendula officinalis) spray
Tec Laboratories, Inc.

## DRUG FACTS

| Active ingredient | Purpose |
|---|---|
| Grindelia robusta 3x | Anti-itch/skin protection |
| Plantago major 4x | Anti-itch/pain relieving/wound healing |
| Calendula officinalis 3x | Wound healing/scar prevention |

## USES
- temporarily relieves the pain and violent itching of hot, burning, irritated or inflamed skin and rashes due to:
  - poison oak
  - poison ivy
  - poison sumac
  - prickly heat rash
  - hives
  - insect bites
  - minor cuts, scrapes and burns
- temporarily protects, cools, and soothes:
  - rashes
  - minor skin irritations
  - promotes healing to help prevent scar tissue formation

## WARNINGS
**For external use only.**

## DO NOT USE
- on severe draining rashes
- if pregnant or nursing, ask a health professional before use

## WHEN USING THIS PRODUCT
- Keep out of reach of children
- if swallowed, get medical help or contact a poison control center right away
- keep out of eyes

## STOP USE AND ASK A DOCTOR IF
- condition worsens, or if symptoms persist for more than 7 days, or clear up and occur again within a few days

## DIRECTIONS

| adults and children 2 years of age and older | when practical, wash affected area with soap and water or Tecnu Extreme Poison Ivy Scrub before the first application to remove poison oil<br><br>spray onto affected area as needed |
|---|---|
| children under 2 years of age | consult a doctor before use |

## OTHER INFORMATION
- store at room temperature (59-86°F/15-30°C)

## INACTIVE INGREDIENTS
disodium EDTA, glycerine, green tea extract, menthol, polyoxyl 35 castor oil, purified water, SD alcohol 40B (14% by weight), tea tree oil, white thyme oil

**QUESTIONS OR COMMENTS**
Call **1-800-ITCHING** or visit www.1800ITCHING.COM
Serious side effects may also be reported to this number

## THERA-GESIC (menthol and methyl salicylate) cream
Mission Pharmcal Company

### DRUG FACTS

| Active ingredients | Purpose |
|---|---|
| Menthol 1% | Analgesic |
| Methyl Salicylate 15% | Counterirritant |

### USES
- temporary relief of minor aches and pains of muscles and joints associated with:
  - arthritis
  - simple backaches
  - strains
  - bruises
  - sprains

### WARNINGS
**For external use only.**
- use only as directed
- avoid contact with eyes or mucous membranes
- do not bandage tightly
- do not bandage, wrap, or cover until after washing the areas where Thera-Gesic has been applied

### DO NOT USE
- immediately after shower or bath
- if skin is sensitive to oil of wintergreen (methyl salicylate)
- on wounds or damaged skin

### ASK A DOCTOR BEFORE USE
- for children under 2 and through 12 years of age
- if prone or sensitive to allergic reaction from aspirin or salicylate

### WHEN USING THIS PRODUCT
- discontinue use if skin irritation develops, or redness is present
- do not swallow
- do not use a heating pad after application of Thera-Gesic
- do not recline on or cover treated area

### STOP USE AND ASK A DOCTOR IF
- condition worsens
- if symptoms persist for more than 7 days or clear up and occur again within a few days

**Keep out of reach of children to avoid accidental poisoning.** If swallowed, get medical help or contact a Poison Control Center right away.

### DIRECTIONS

| adults and children 12 or more years of age | apply thin layers of creme into and around the sore or painful area, not more than 3 to 4 times daily. The number of thin layers controls the intensity. One thin layer provides a mild effect, two thin layers provide a strong effect and three thin layers provide a very strong effect |
|---|---|

### OTHER INFORMATION
- once Thera-Gesic has penetrated the skin, the area may be washed, leaving it dry, clean, and fragrance-free without decreasing the effectiveness of the product
- store at 20-25°C (68-77°F)

### INACTIVE INGREDIENTS
carbomer 934, dimethicone, glycerine, methylparaben, propylparaben, sodium lauryl sulfate, trolamine, water

### QUESTIONS OR COMMENT
Call **1-800-452-0051**

## THERAFLU COLD AND COUGH
(dextromethorphan hydrobromide, pheniramine maleate, and phenylephrine hydrochloride) powder for solution
Novartis Consumer Healthcare, Inc.

### DRUG FACTS

| Active ingredients (in each packet) | Purpose |
|---|---|
| Dextromethorphan hydrobromide 20 mg | Cough suppressant |
| Pheniramine maleate 20 mg | Antihistamine |
| Phenylephrine hydrochloride 10 mg | Nasal decongestant |

### USES
- temporarily relieves these symptoms due to a cold:
  - nasal and sinus congestion
  - cough due to minor throat and bronchial irritation
- temporarily relieves these symptoms due to hay fever or other upper respiratory allergies:
  - runny nose
  - sneezing
  - itchy nose and throat
  - itchy, watery eyes

### WARNINGS

### DO NOT USE
- if you are now taking a prescription monoamine oxidase inhibitor (MAOI) (certain drugs for depression, psychiatric, or emotional conditions, or Parkinson's disease), or for 2 weeks after stopping the MAOI drug. If you do not know if your prescription drug contains an MAOI, ask a doctor or pharmacist before taking this product

### ASK A DOCTOR BEFORE USE IF YOU HAVE
- heart disease
- high blood pressure
- thyroid disease
- diabetes
- glaucoma
- a breathing problem such as emphysema, asthma, or chronic bronchitis
- trouble urinating due to an enlarged prostate gland
- cough that occurs with smoking, too much phlegm (mucus) or chronic cough that lasts
- a sodium-restricted diet

### ASK A DOCTOR OR PHARMACIST BEFORE USE IF YOU ARE
- taking sedatives or tranquilizers

**WHEN USING THIS PRODUCT**
- do not exceed recommended dosage
- avoid alcoholic drinks
- may cause marked drowsiness
- alcohol, sedatives, and tranquilizers may increase drowsiness
- be careful when driving a motor vehicle or operating machinery
- excitability may occur, especially in children

**STOP USE AND ASK A DOCTOR IF**
- nervousness, dizziness, or sleeplessness occur
- symptoms do not improve within 7 days or occur with a fever
- cough persists for more than 7 days
- comes back or occurs with a fever, rash, or persistent headache

These could be signs of a serious condition.

**If pregnant or breastfeeding,** ask a health care professional before use.

**Keep out of reach of children.** In case of overdose, get medical help or contact a poison control center right away.

**DIRECTIONS**
- take one packet every 4 hours
- do not exceed 6 packets in 24 hours, or as directed by a doctor

| adults and children 12 years of age and over | dissolve contents of one packet in 8 ounces hot water, sip while hot consume entire drink within 10-15 minutes |
|---|---|
| children under 12 years of age | consult a doctor |

- If using a microwave, add contents of one packet to 8 ounces of cool water; stir briskly before and after heating. Do not overheat

**OTHER INFORMATION**
- each packet contains: sodium 46 mg
- store at controlled room temperature 20-25°C (68-77°F)

**INACTIVE INGREDIENTS**
acesulfame K. citric acid, D&C yellow no. 10, FD&C yellow no. 6, lecithin, magnesium stearate, maltodextrin, natural flavors, silicon dioxide, sodium citrate, sucrose, tribasic calcium phosphate

**QUESTIONS OR COMMENTS**
Call 1-800-452-0051

# THERAFLU MAX-D (acetaminophen, dextromethorphan hydrobromide, guaifenesin, pseudoephedrine hydrochloride) powder, for solution
Novartis Consumer Health, Inc.

## DRUG FACTS

| Active ingredient (in each packet) | Purpose |
|---|---|
| Acetaminophen 1000 mg | Pain reliever/fever reducer |
| Dextromethorphan hydrobromide 30 mg | Cough suppressant |
| Guaifenesin 400 mg | Expectorant |
| Pseudoephedrine hydrochloride 60 mg | Nasal decongestant |

**USES**
- temporarily relieves these symptoms due to a cold:
  - minor aches and pains
  - headache
  - minor sore throat pain
  - cough
  - nasal congestion
  - helps decongest sinus openings and passages
- temporarily reduces fever
- helps loosen phlegm (mucus) and thin bronchial secretions to drain bronchial tubes and make coughs more productive

**WARNINGS**
**Liver warning**
This product contains acetaminophen. Severe liver damage may occur if you take:
- more than 4 packets in 24 hours, which is the maximum daily amount
- with other drugs containing acetaminophen
- 3 or more alcoholic drinks every day while using this product

**Sore throat warning**
If sore throat is severe, persists for more than 2 days, is accompanied or followed by fever, headache, rash, nausea, or vomiting consult a doctor promptly.

**DO NOT USE**
- in a child under 4 years of age
- if you are allergic to acetaminophen
- with any other drug containing acetaminophen (prescription or nonprescription). If you are not sure whether a drug contains acetaminophen, ask a doctor or pharmacist
- if you are now taking a prescription monoamine oxidase inhibitor (MAOI) (certain drugs for depression, psychiatric or emotional conditions, or Parkinson's disease) or for 2 weeks after stopping the MAOI drug. If you do not know if your prescription drug contains an MAOI, ask a doctor or pharmacist before taking this product

**ASK A DOCTOR BEFORE USE IF YOU HAVE**
- liver disease
- heart disease
- diabetes
- thyroid disease
- high blood pressure
- trouble urinating due to an enlarged prostate gland
- cough that occurs with too much phlegm (mucus)
- cough that lasts or is chronic such as occurs with smoking, asthma, chronic bronchitis, or emphysema

**ASK A DOCTOR OR A PHARMACIST BEFORE USING IF**
- taking the blood thinning drug warfarin

**WHEN USING THIS PRODUCT**
- do not exceed recommended dosage

**STOP USE AND ASK A DOCTOR IF**
- nervousness, dizziness or sleeplessness occur
- pain, nasal congestion or cough gets worse or lasts more than 7 days
- fever gets worse or lasts more than 3 days
- redness or swelling is present
- new symptoms occur
- cough comes back or occurs with fever, rash or headache that lasts

These could be signs of a serious condition.

**If pregnant or breastfeeding,** ask a health care professional before use.

**Keep out of reach of children.** In case of overdose, get medical help or contact a Poison Control Center right away. Prompt medical attention is critical for adults as well as for children even if you do not notice any signs or symptoms.

## DIRECTIONS
- do not use more than directed

| children under 4 years of age | do not use |
|---|---|
| children 4 to under 12 years of age | do not use unless directed by a doctor |
| adults and children 12 years of age and over | take one packet every 6 hours; do not take more than 4 packets in 24 hours unless directed by a doctor |

- dissolve contents of one packet into 8 ounces hot water: sip while hot. Consume entire drink within 10-15 minutes
- if using a microwave, add contents of one packet to 8 ounces of cool water; stir briskly before and after heating. Do not overheat

## OTHER INFORMATION
- each packet contains: calcium 10 mg, potassium 10 mg, sodium 15 mg
- **Phenylketonurics:** contains phenylalanine 23.6 mg per packet
- store at controlled room temperature 20-25°C (68-77°F)

## INACTIVE INGREDIENTS
acesulfame K, aspartame, citric acid, D&C yellow no. 10, FD&C red no. 40, flavors, maltodextrin, silicon dioxide, sodium citrate, sucrose, tribasic calcium phosphate

## QUESTIONS OR COMMENTS
Call **1-800-452-0051**

---

# THERAFLU SUGAR FREE NIGHTTIME SEVERE COLD AND COUGH (acetaminophen, diphenhydramine hydrochloride, phenylephrine hydrochloride) powder, for solution
Novartis Consumer Health, Inc.

## DRUG FACTS

| Active ingredient | Purpose |
|---|---|
| Acetaminophen 650 mg | Pain reliever/fever reducer |
| Diphenhydramine hydrochloride 25 mg | Antihistamine/cough suppressant |
| phenylephrine hydrochloride 10 mg | Nasal decongestant |

## USES
- temporarily relieves these symptoms due to a cold:
  - minor aches and pains
  - minor sore throat pain
  - headache
  - nasal and sinus congestion
  - runny nose or throat
  - itchy, watery eyes due to hay fever
  - cough due to minor throat and bronchial irritation
- temporarily reduces fever

## WARNINGS
### Liver warning
This product contains acetaminophen. Severe liver damage may occur if you take:
- more than 6 packets in 24 hours, which is the maximum daily amount
- with other drugs containing acetaminophen
- 3 or more alcoholic drinks every day while using this product

### Sore throat warning
If sore throat is severe, persists for more than 2 days, is accompanied or followed by fever, headache, rash, nausea, or vomiting consult a doctor promptly.

### DO NOT USE
- in a child under 4 years of age
- if you are allergic to acetaminophen
- with any other drug containing acetaminophen (prescription or nonprescription). If you are not sure whether a drug contains acetaminophen, as a doctor or a pharmacist
- with any other product containing diphenhydramine, even one used on the skin
- if you are now taking a prescription monoamine oxidase inhibitor (MAOI) (certain drugs for depression, psychiatric, or emotional conditions, or Parkinson's disease), or for 2 weeks after stopping the MAOI drug. If you do not know if your prescription drug contains an MAOI, ask a doctor or pharmacist before taking this product

### ASK DOCTOR BEFORE USE IF YOU HAVE
- liver disease
- heart disease
- high blood pressure
- thyroid disease
- diabetes
- glaucoma
- a sodium restricted diet
- trouble urinating due to an enlarged prostrate gland
- a breathing problem such as emphysema, asthma or chronic bronchitis
- cough that occurs with too much phlegm (mucus)
- cough that lasts or is chronic such as occurs with smoking, asthma or emphysema

### ASK A DOCTOR OR PHARMACIST BEFORE USE IF YOU ARE
- taking sedatives or tranquilizers
- the blood thinning drug warfarin

### WHEN USING THIS PRODUCT
- do not exceed recommended dosage
- avoid alcoholic drinks
- marked drowsiness may occur
- alcoholic, sedatives and tranquilizers may increase drowsiness
- be careful when driving a motor vehicle or operating machinery
- excitability may occur, especially in children

### STOP USE AND ASK A DOCTOR IF
- nervousness, dizziness, or sleeplessness occurs
- fever gets worse or lasts more than 3 days
- redness or swelling is present
- new symptoms occur
- symptoms do not get better or worsen
- pain, cough or nasal congestion gets worse or lasts more than 7 days
- cough comes back or occurs with fever, rash or headache that lasts

These could be signs of a serious condition.

**If pregnant or breast feeding**, ask a health care professional before use.

**Keep out of reach of children.** In case of overdose, get medical help or contact a Poison Control Center right away. Prompt medical attention is critical for adults as well as for children even if you do not notice any signs or symptoms.

## DIRECTIONS
- do not use more than directed

| children under 4 years of age | do not use |
|---|---|
| children 4 to under 12 years of age | do not use unless directed by a doctor |
| adults and children 12 years of age and over | one packet every 4 hours; do not take more than 6 packets in 24 hours unless directed by a doctor |

- dissolve contents of one packet into 8 ounces hot water: sip while hot. Consume entire drink with 10 - 15 minutes
- if using a microwave, add contents of one packet to 8 ounces of cool water; stir briskly before and after heating, do not overheat

## OTHER INFORMATION
- each packet contains: potassium 10 mg, sodium 23 mg
- **Phenylketonurics:** contains phenylalanine 13 mg per packet
- store at controlled room temperature 20 -25°C (68-77°F).
- protect from excessive heat and moisture

## INACTIVE INGREDIENTS
acesulfame K, aspartame, citric acid, D&C yellow no. 10, FD&C blue no. 1, FD&C red no. 40, flavors, maltodextrin, silicon dioxide, sodium citrate, tribasic calcium phosphate

## QUESTIONS OR COMMENTS
Call **1-800-452-0051**

## TIGER BALM (oil of wintergreen and menthol) liniment
Haw Par Healthcare Ltd.
Tiger Balm (Malaysia) Sdn. Bhd.

## DRUG FACTS

| Active ingredients | Purpose |
|---|---|
| Oil of Wintergreen 28% | Topical analgesic |
| Menthol 16% | Topical analgesic |

## USES
- for temporary relief of minor aches and pains of muscles and joints associated with:
  - simple backache
  - arthritis
  - bruises
  - sprains and strains

## WARNINGS
**For external use only.**

## WHEN USING THIS PRODUCT
- use only as directed
- avoid contact with eyes and mucous membranes
- do not apply to wounds, damaged or irritated skin
- do not bandage or cover with wrap or use heating pad
- do not use 1 hour prior to bathing or 30 minutes after bathing

## STOP USE AND ASK A DOCTOR IF
- condition worsens
- severe skin irritation occurs
- pain persists for more than 7 days
- pain clears up and then recurs a few days later

**If pregnant or breastfeeding, or if you have sensitive skin,** ask a healthcare professional before use.

**Keep out of reach of children.** If swallowed, get medical help or contact a Poison Control Center immediately.

## DIRECTIONS

| for adults and children over 12 | rub well on the affected area repeat 3-4 times daily |
|---|---|
| for children 12 years of age or younger | consult a doctor before use |

## OTHER INFORMATION
- this product may cause allergic reaction in some individuals. Test on small area before use

## INACTIVE INGREDIENTS
eucalyptus oil, spike lavender oil, light mineral oil

## QUESTIONS OR COMMENTS
Call **510-887-1899**

## TIGER BALM WHITE REGULAR STRENGTH
(camphor and menthol) ointment
Tiger Balm (Malaysia) Sdn. Bhd.

## DRUG FACTS

| Active ingredients | Purpose |
|---|---|
| Camphor 11% | Topical analgesic |
| Menthol 8% | Topical analgesic |

## USES
- for temporary relief of minor aches and pains of muscles and joints associated with:
  - simple backache
  - arthritis
  - bruises
  - strains and sprains

## WARNINGS
**For external use only.**

## WHEN USING THIS PRODUCT
- use only as directed
- avoid contact with eyes and mucous membranes
- do not apply to wounds, damaged or irritated skin
- do not bandage or cover with wrap or use heating pad
- do not use 1 hour prior to bathing or 30 minutes after bathing

## STOP USE AND ASK A DOCTOR IF
- condition worsens
- severe skin irritation occurs
- pain persists for more than 7 days
- pain clears up and then recurs a few days later

**If pregnant or breastfeeding,** or if you have sensitive skin, ask a healthcare professional before use.

**Keep out of reach of children.** If swallowed, get medical help or contact a Poison Control Center immediately.

## DIRECTIONS

| | |
|---|---|
| for adults and children over 12 | rub well on the affected area repeat 3 to 4 times daily |
| for children 12 years of age or younger | consult a doctor before use |

## OTHER INFORMATION
- this product may cause allergic reaction in some individuals. Test on small area before use

## INACTIVE INGREDIENTS
cajuput oil, clove oil, dementholised mint oil and paraffin petrolatum

## QUESTIONS OR COMMENTS
Call **510-887-1899**

---

## TIGER BALM ARTHRITIS RUB (camphor and menthol) cream
Prince of Peace Enterprises, Inc.

## DRUG FACTS

| Active ingredients | Purpose |
|---|---|
| Camphor 11% | Topical analgesic |
| Menthol 11% | Topical analgesic |

## USES
- for the temporary relief of minor aches and pains associated with:
  - arthritis
  - backache
  - stiffness
  - muscle strains and sprains

## WARNINGS
**For external use only.**

## WHEN USING THIS PRODUCT
- use only as directed
- avoid contact with eyes and mucous membranes
- do not apply to wounds, damaged or irritated skin
- do not bandage or cover with wrap or use heating pad
- do not use 1 hour prior to bathing or 30 minutes after bathing

## STOP USE AND ASK A DOCTOR IF
- condition worsens
- severe skin irritation occurs
- pain persists for more than 7 days
- pain clears up and then recurs a few days later

**If pregnant or breastfeeding,** or if you have sensitive skin, ask a healthcare professional before use.

**Keep out of reach of children.** If swallowed, get medical help or contact a Poison Control Center immediately.

## DIRECTIONS
- shake well before using
- apply generously to affected areas and massage gently until cream is absorbed into the skin

| | |
|---|---|
| for adults and children over 12 | rub well on the affected area repeat 3-4 times daily |
| for children 12 years of age or younger | consult a doctor before use |

## OTHER INFORMATION
- this product may cause allergic reaction in some individuals. Test on small area before use
- as part of its warming action, temporary redness may occur

## INACTIVE INGREDIENTS
cajuput oil, chondroitin sulfate, cinnamon oil, clove oil, deionized water, dementholised mint oil, diazolidinyl urea, glucosamine sulfate, methyl paraben, methylsulfonylmethane (MSM), PEG-120 methyl glucose dioleate, propyl paraben, propylene glycol

## QUESTIONS OR COMMENTS
Call **510-887-1899**

---

## TIGER BALM RED EXTRA STRENGTH
(camphor and menthol) ointment
Tiger Balm (Malaysia) Sdn. Bhd.

## DRUG FACTS

| Active ingredients | Purpose |
|---|---|
| Camphor 11% | Topical analgesic |
| Menthol 10% | Topical analgesic |

## USES
- for temporary relief of minor aches and pains of muscles and joints associated with:
  - simple backache
  - arthritis
  - bruises
  - strains and sprains

## WARNINGS
**For external use only.**

## WHEN USING THIS PRODUCT
- use only as directed
- avoid contact with eyes and mucous membranes
- do not apply to wounds, damaged or irritated skin
- do not bandage or cover with wrap or use heating pad
- do not use 1 hour prior to bathing or 30 minutes after bathing

## STOP USE AND ASK A DOCTOR IF
- condition worsens
- severe skin irritation occurs
- pain persists for more than 7 days
- pain clears up and then recurs a few days later

**If pregnant or breastfeeding,** or if you have sensitive skin, ask a healthcare professional before use.

**Keep out of reach of children.** If swallowed, get medical help or contact a Poison Control Center immediately.

## DIRECTIONS

| | |
|---|---|
| for adults and children over 12 | rub well on the affected area repeat 3 to 4 times daily |
| for children 12 years of age or younger | consult a doctor before use |

## OTHER INFORMATION
- this product may cause allergic reaction in some individuals. Test on small area before use
- Tiger Balm Red Extra Strength may stain cloth items. To avoid possibility of stains, use Tiger Balm White Regular Strength or Tiger Balm Ultra Strength

**INACTIVE INGREDIENTS**
cajuput oil, cassia oil, clove oil, dementholised mint oil and paraffin petrolatum

**QUESTIONS OR COMMENTS**
Call **510-887-1899**

# TIGER BALM ULTRA STRENGTH (camphor and menthol) ointment
Tiger Balm (Malaysia) Sdn. Bhd.

## DRUG FACTS

| Active ingredients | Purpose |
|---|---|
| Camphor 11% | Topical analgesic |
| Menthol 11% | Topical analgesic |

### USES
- for temporary relief of minor aches and pains of muscles and joints associated with:
  - simple backache
  - arthritis
  - bruises
  - strains and sprains

### WARNINGS
**For external use only.**

### WHEN USING THIS PRODUCT
- use only as directed
- avoid contact with eyes and mucous membranes
- do not apply to wounds, damaged or irritated skin
- do not bandage or cover with wrap or use heating pad
- do not use 1 hour prior to bathing or 30 minutes after bathing

### STOP USE AND ASK A DOCTOR IF
- condition worsens
- severe skin irritation occurs
- pain persists for more than 7 days
- pain clears up and then recurs a few days later

**If pregnant or breastfeeding,** or if you have sensitive skin, ask a healthcare professional before use.

**Keep out of reach of children.** If swallowed, get medical help or contact a Poison Control Center immediately.

### DIRECTIONS

| for adults and children over 12 | rub well on the affected area. Repeat 3 to 4 times daily |
|---|---|
| for children 12 years of age or younger | consult a doctor before use |

### OTHER INFORMATION
- this product may cause allergic reaction in some individuals. Test on small area before use

### INACTIVE INGREDIENTS
cajuput oil, cassia oil, clove oil, dementholised mint oil and paraffin petrolatum

### QUESTIONS OR COMMENTS
Call **510-887-1899**

# TINEACIDE SOLUTION (tolnaftate) liquid
Blaine Labs Inc.

## DRUG FACTS

| Active ingredient | Purpose |
|---|---|
| Tolnaftate 1% | Antifungal treatment |

### USES
- cures most *dermatophytosis* (athlete's foot), *tinea cruris* (jock itch) and *tinea corporis* (ringworm)

**Keep out of reach of children.** In case of accidental ingestion contact a poison control center immediately.

### WARNINGS
**DO NOT USE**
- on children under 2 years of age unless directed by a physician

**For external use only.**
- avoid contact with eyes

### STOP USE AND ASK A DOCTOR IF
- irritation occurs
  - if there is no improvement within 4 weeks (for athlete's foot or ringworm) or within 2 weeks (for jock itch).

### DIRECTIONS
- Wash the affected area and dry thoroughly. apply a thin layer over affected area twice daily (morning and night) or as directed by a physician. supervise children in the use of the product.
- For athlete's foot: pay special attention to spaces between the toes; wear well-fitting, ventilated shoes, and change socks and shoes at least once daily. for athlete's foot and ring worm: use daily for 4 weeks. For jock itch: use daily for 2 weeks. if condition persists longer, consult a physician.

### INACTIVE INGREDIENTS
safflower oil, mineral oil, jojoba oil, BHT, BHA, colloidal silver, tocopheryl acetate, methyl paraben, propyl paraben

# TRIAMINIC CHEST & NASAL CONGESTION
(guaifenesin and phenylephrine hydrochloride)
Novartis

## DRUG FACTS

| Active ingredients (in each 5 mL, 1 teaspoonful) | Purpose |
|---|---|
| guaifenesin 50 mg | Expectorant |
| phenylephrine hydrochloride 2.5 mg | Nasal decongestant |

### USES
- helps loosen phlegm (mucus) and thins bronchial secretions to make coughs more productive
- temporarily relieves nasal aid sinus congestion as may occur with a cold

### WARNINGS
**DO NOT USE**
- in a child under 4 years of age
- in a child who is taking a prescription monoamine oxidase inhibitor (MAOI) (certain drugs for depression, psychiatric or emotional conditions, or Parkinson's disease), or for 2 weeks

after stopping the MAOI drug. If you do not know if the child's prescription drug contains an MAOI, ask a doctor or pharmacist before giving this product

### ASK A DOCTOR BEFORE USE IF THE CHILD HAS
- heart disease
- high blood pressure
- thyroid disease
- diabetes
- cough that occurs with too much phlegm (mucus)
- chronic cough that lasts or as occurs with asthma

### WHEN USING THIS PRODUCT
- do not exceed recommended dosage

### STOP USE AND ASK A DOCTOR IF
- nervousness, dizziness or sleeplessness occurs
- symptoms do not improve within 7 days or occur with a fever
- cough persists for more than 7 days, comes back or occurs with a fever, rash or persistent headache. These could be signs of a serious condition

**Keep out of reach of children.** In case of overdose, get medical help or contact a Poison Control Center right away.

### DIRECTIONS
- may be given every 4 hours
- do not give more than 6 doses in 24 hours unless directed by a doctor

| Children under 4 years of age | do not use |
|---|---|
| Children 4 to under 6 years of age | 1 teaspoonful (5 mL) |
| Children 6 to under 12 years of age | 2 teaspoonful (10 mL) |

### OTHER INFORMATION
- each teaspoonful contains: sodium 3 mg
- store at controlled room temperature 20-25°C (68-77°F)

### INACTIVE INGREDIENTS
acesultame K, benzoic acid, citric acid, D&C yellow no. 10, edetate disodium, FD&C yellow no. 6, flavors, maltitol solution, propylene glycol, purified water, sodium citrate

### QUESTIONS OR COMMENTS
Call **1-800-452-0051**

---

# TRIAMINIC CHILDREN'S COLD AND ALLERGY (chlorpheniramine maleate, phenylephrine hydrochloride) syrup
Novartis Consumer Health, Inc.

## DRUG FACTS

| Active ingredient | Purpose |
|---|---|
| Chlorpheniramine maleate 1 mg | Antihistamine |
| Phenylephrine hydrochloride 2.5 mg | Nasal decongestant |

### USES
- temporarily relieves:
  - itchy, watery eyes
  - runny nose
  - itchy nose or throat
  - sneezing
  - nasal and sinus congestion as may occur with a cold

### WARNINGS
### DO NOT USE
- in a child under 4 years of age
- in a child who is taking a prescription monoamine oxidase inhibitor (MAOI) (certain drugs for depression, psychiatric or emotional conditions, or Parkinson's disease), or for 2 weeks after stopping the MAOI drug. If you do not know if the child's prescription drug contains an MAOI, ask a doctor or pharmacist before giving this product
- for the purpose of making your child sleepy

### ASK A DOCTOR BEFORE USE IF THE CHILD HAS
- heart disease
- high blood pressure
- thyroid disease
- diabetes
- glaucoma
- a breathing problem such as asthma or chronic bronchitis

### ASK A DOCTOR OR PHARMACIST BEFORE USE IF
- the child is taking sedatives or tranquilizers

### WHEN USING THIS PRODUCT
- do not exceed recommended dosage
- marked drowsiness may occur
- sedatives and tranquilizers may increase drowsiness
- excitability may occur, especially in children

### STOP USING THIS PRODUCT IF
- nervousness, dizziness or sleeplessness occurs
- symptoms do not improve within 7 days or occur with a fever. These could be signs of a serious condition

**Keep out of reach of children** In case of overdose, get medical help or contact a Poison Control Center right away.

### DIRECTIONS
- may be given every 4 hours
- do not give more than 6 doses in 24 hours unless directed by a doctor

| children under 4 years of age | do not use |
|---|---|
| children 4 to under 6 years of age | do not use unless directed by a doctor |
| children 6 to under 12 years of age | 2 teaspoonfuls (10 mL) |

### OTHER INFORMATION
- each teaspoonful contains: sodium 3 mg
- store at controlled room temperature 20-25°C (68-77°F)
- child-resistant safety cap tamper evident feature: do not use if safety seal imprinted with "Triaminic" around the bottle cap is broken or missing

### INACTIVE INGREDIENTS
acesulfame K, benzoic acid, citric acid, edetate disodium, FD&C yellow no. 6, flavors, maltitol solution, purified water, sodium citrate

### QUESTIONS OR COMMENTS
Call **1-800-452-0051** 24 hours a day, 7 days a week or visit www.triaminic.com

# TRIAMINIC CHILDREN'S NIGHTTIME COLD AND COUGH (diphenhydramine hydrochloride, phenylephrine hydrochloride) syrup

Novartis Consumer Health, Inc.

## DRUG FACTS

| Active ingredient | Purpose |
|---|---|
| Diphenhydramine hydrochloride 6.25 mg | Antihistamine/cough suppressant |
| Phenylephrine hydrochloride 2.5 | Nasal decongestant |

## USES
- temporarily relieves:
  - sneezing
  - itchy nose or throat
  - runny nose
  - itchy, watery eyes due to hay fever
  - nasal and sinus congestion
  - cough due to minor throat and bronchial irritation as may occur with a cold

## WARNINGS
### DO NOT USE
- in a child under 4 years of age
- in a child who is taking a prescription monoamine oxidase inhibitor (MAOI) (certain drugs for depression, psychiatric or emotional conditions, or Parkinson's disease), or for 2 weeks after stopping the MAOI drug. If you do not know if the child's prescription drug contains an MAOI, ask a doctor or pharmacist before giving this product
- with any other product containing diphenhydramine, even one used on skin
- for the purpose of making your child sleepy

### ASK A DOCTOR BEFORE USE IF THE CHILD HAS
- heart disease
- high blood pressure
- thyroid disease
- diabetes
- glaucoma
- cough that occurs with too much phlegm (mucus)
- chronic cough that lasts, or as occurs with asthma
- a breathing problem such as chronic bronchitis

### ASK A DOCTOR OR PHARMACIST BEFORE USE IF
- the child is taking sedatives or tranquilizers

### WHEN USING THIS PRODUCT
- do not exceed recommended dosage
- marked drowsiness may occur
- sedatives and tranquilizers may increase drowsiness
- excitability may occur, especially in children

### STOP USE AND ASK A DOCTOR IF
- nervousness, dizziness or sleeplessness occurs
- symptoms do not improve within 7 days or occur with a fever
- cough persists for more than 7 days, comes back or occurs with a fever, rash or persistent headache. These could be signs of a serious condition

**Keep out of reach of children.** In case of overdose, get medical help or contact a Poison Control Center right away.

## DIRECTIONS
- may be given every 4 hours
- do not give more than 6 doses in 24 hours unless directed by a doctor
- find the right dose on chart below
- use enclosed dosing cup only. Keep for use with this product only. Do not use any other dosing device

| children under 4 years of age | do not use |
|---|---|
| children 4 to under 6 years of age | do not use unless directed by a doctor |
| children 6 to under 12 years of age | 2 teaspoonfuls (10 mL) |

## OTHER INFORMATON
- each teaspoonful contains: sodium 6 mg
- store at controlled room temperature 20-25°C (68-77°F)

## INACTIVE INGREDIENTS
acesulfame K, benzoic acid, citric acid, edetate disodium, FD&C blue no. 1, FD&C red no. 40, flavors, maltitol solution, propylene glycol, purified water, sodium citrate

## QUESTIONS OR COMMENTS
Call **1-800-452-0051** 24 hours a day, 7 days a week

# TRIAMINIC CHILDREN'S SYRUP FEVER REDUCER PAIN RELIEVER (acetaminophen) syrup

Novartis Consumer Health, Inc.

## DRUG FACTS

| Active ingredient (in each 5 mL, 1 teaspoonful) | Purpose |
|---|---|
| Acetaminophen 160 mg | Pain reliever/fever reducer |

## USES
- temporarily relieves minor aches and pains due to:
  - the common cold
  - flu
  - headache
  - minor sore throat pain
  - toothache
- temporarily reduces fever

## WARNINGS
**Liver warning**
This product contains acetaminophen. Severe liver damage may occur if your child takes:

- more than 5 doses in 24 hours, which is the maximum daily amount
- with other drugs containing acetaminophen

**Sore throat warning**
If sore throat is severe, persists for more than 2 days, is accompanied or followed by fever, headache, rash, nausea, or vomiting consult a doctor promptly.

### DO NOT USE
- if your child is allergic to acetaminophen
- with any other drug containing acetaminophen (prescription or nonprescription). If you are not sure whether a drug contains acetaminophen, ask a doctor or pharmacist

### ASK DOCTOR BEFORE USE IF YOUR
- child has liver disease

### ASK A DOCTOR OR PHARMACIST BEFORE USE IF YOUR
- child is taking the blood thinning drug warfarin

## WHEN USING THIS PRODUCT
- do not exceed recommended dosage

## STOP USE AND ASK A DOCTOR IF
- pain gets worse or lasts more than 5 days
- fever gets worse or lasts more than 3 days
- redness or swelling is present
- new symptoms occur

**Keep out of reach of children.** In case of overdose, get medical help or contact a Poison Control Center right away. Prompt medical attention is critical for adults as well as for children even if you do not notice any signs or symptoms.

## DIRECTIONS
- this product does not contain directions or complete warnings for adult use
- do not give more than directed
- may be given every 4 hours
- do not give more than 5 doses in 24 hours unless directed by a doctor

| Age | Weight | Dose |
|---|---|---|
| under 2 years of age | under 24 lbs | ask a doctor |
| 2 to 3 years of age | 24-35 lbs | 1 teaspoon (5 mL) |
| 4 to 5 years of age | 36-47 lbs | 1 ½ teaspoons (7.5 mL) |
| 6 to 8 years of age | 48-59 lbs | 2 teaspoons (10 mL) |
| 9 to 10 years of age | 60-71 lbs | 2 ½ teaspoons (12.5 mL) |
| 11 years of age | 72-95 lbs | 3 teaspoons (15 mL) |

## OTHER INFORMATION
- each teaspoonful contains: **sodium 5 mg** for grape flavor, **sodium 6 mg** for bubblegum flavor
- contains no aspirin
- store at controlled room temperature 20-25°C (68-77°F)

## INACTIVE INGREDIENTS
**for grape flavor**
citric acid, edetate disodium, FD&C blue no. 1, FD&C red no. 40, flavor, glycerin, polyethylene glycol, purified water, sodium benzoate, sodium citrate, sorbitol, sucrose

**for bubblegum flavor**
benzoic acid, citric acid, dibasic sodium phosphate, edetate disodium, FD&C red no. 40, flavor, glycerin, polyethylene glycol, purified water, sorbitol, sucrose

## QUESTIONS OR COMMENTS
Call **1-800-452-0051**. For more information plus helpful tips visit www.triaminic.com

---

## TUCKS HEMORRHOIDAL OINTMENT (mineral oil, pramoxine hydrochloride, and zinc oxide)
McNeil-PPC, Inc.

## DRUG FACTS

| Active ingredients | Purpose |
|---|---|
| Mineral oil 46.6% | Protectant |
| Pramoxine hydrochloride 1% | Pain reliever |
| Zinc oxide 12.5% | Protectant |

## USES
- temporarily relieves these local symptoms associated with hemorrhoids and other anorectal disorders:
  - pain
  - soreness
  - burning
  - itching
- temporarily forms a protective coating over inflamed tissues to help prevent drying of tissues

## WARNINGS
**For external use only.**

## WHEN USING THIS PRODUCT
- do not use more than directed unless told to do so by a doctor
- do not put into the rectum by using fingers or any mechanical device or applicator

## STOP USE AND ASK A DOCTOR IF
- allergic reaction occurs
- rectal bleeding occurs
- redness, irritation, swelling, pain, or other symptoms begin or increase
- condition worsens or does not improve within 7 days

**Keep out of reach of children.** If swallowed, get medical help or contact a Poison Control Center right away.

## DIRECTIONS

| adults | apply externally to the affected area up to 5 times daily |
|---|---|
| | when practical, clean the affected area with mild soap and warm water and rinse thoroughly |
| | gently dry by patting or blotting with toilet tissue or a soft cloth before applying |
| | to use dispensing cap |
| | attach it to tube, lubricate well, then gently insert part way into anus |
| | squeeze tube to deliver medication |
| | thoroughly cleanse dispensing cap after use |
| children under 12 years of age | ask a doctor |

## OTHER INFORMATION
- store at 20°C-25°C (58°F-77°F)

## INACTIVE INGREDIENTS
benzyl benzoate, calcium phosphate dibasic, cocoa butter, glyceryl monooleate, glyceryl monostearate, kaolin, Peruvian balsam, polyethylene wax

## QUESTIONS OR COMMENTS
Call **1-800-223-0182** Monday to Friday, 8 AM to 8 PM EST

# TUMS (calcium carbonate) tablet, chewable
GlaxoSmithKline Consumer Healthcare LP

## DRUG FACTS

| Active ingredient (per tablet) | Purpose |
|---|---|
| Calcium carbonate USP 500 mg | Antacid |

### USES
- relieves:
  - heartburn
  - sour stomach
  - acid indigestion
  - upset stomach associated with these symptoms

### WARNINGS

**ASK A DOCTOR OR PHARMACIST BEFORE USE IF YOU ARE**
- taking a prescription drug. Antacids may interact with certain prescription drugs

**WHEN USING THIS PRODUCT**
- do not take more than 15 tablets in 24 hours
- do not use the maximum dosage for more than 2 weeks

**Keep out of reach of children.**

### DIRECTIONS
- chew 2-4 tablets as symptoms occur, or as directed by a doctor
- chew 2 tablets twice daily with a meal

### OTHER INFORMATION
- store below 30°C (86°F)

### INACTIVE INGREDIENTS (Assorted fruit)
sucrose, calcium carbonate, corn starch, talc, mineral oil, natural and artificial flavors, adipic acid, sodium polyphosphate, red 40 lake, blue no. 1 lake

### INACTIVE INGREDIENT (Peppermint)
sucrose, calcium carbonate, corn starch, talc, mineral oil, natural flavor, sodium polyphosphate

### QUESTIONS OR COMMENTS
Call **1-800-897-7535** weekdays or visit www.tums.com

# TUMS DUAL ACTION (famotidine, calcium carbonate, magnesium hydroxide) tablet, chewable
GlaxoSmithKline LLC

## DRUG FACTS

| Active ingredients (in each chewable tablet) | Purpose |
|---|---|
| Famotidine 10 mg | Acid reducer |
| Calcium carbonate 800 mg | Antacid |
| Magnesium hydroxide 165 mg | Antacid |

### USE
- relieves heartburn associated with acid indigestion and sour stomach

### WARNINGS
**Allergy alert**
Do not use if you are allergic to famotidine or other acid reducers

**DO NOT USE**
- if you have trouble or pain swallowing food, vomiting with blood, or bloody or black stools. These may be signs of a serious condition. See you doctor
- with other acid reducers

**ASK A DOCTOR BEFORE USE IF YOU HAVE**
- had heartburn over 3 months. This may be a sign of a more serious condition
- heartburn with lightheadedness, sweating, or dizziness
- chest pain or shoulder pain with shortness of breath
  - sweating
  - pain spreading to arms, neck or shoulders
  - lightheadedness
- frequent chest pain
- frequent wheezing, particularly with heartburn
- unexplained weight loss
- nausea or vomiting
- stomach pain

**ASK A DOCTOR OR PHARMACIST BEFORE USE IF YOU ARE**
- presently taking a prescription drug. Antacids may interact with certain prescription drugs

**STOP USE AND ASK A DOCTOR IF**
- your heartburn continues or worsens
- you need to take this product for more than 14 days

**If pregnant or breastfeeding**, ask a health professional before use.

**Keep out of reach of children.** In case of overdose, get medical help or contact a Poison Control Center right away.

### DIRECTIONS

| adults and children 12 years and over | do not swallow tablet whole; chew completely |
|---|---|
| | to relieve symptoms, chew 1 tablet before swallowing |
| | do not use more than 2 chewable tablets in 24 hours |
| children under 12 years | ask a doctor |

### OTHER INFORMATION
- each tablet contains: calcium 320 mg; magnesium 65 mg
- **Phenylketonurics:** contains phenylalanine 2.2 mg per tablet
- read the directions and warnings before use
- read the bottle label. It contains important information
- store at 20-25°C (68-77°F)
- protect from moisture

### INACTIVE INGREDIENTS
aspartame, D&C red no. 7 calcium, dextrates, FD&C blue no. 1 lake, FD&C red no. 40 lake, flavor, glyceryl monostearate, lactose anhydrous, lactose monohydrate, magnesium stearate, microcrystalline cellulose, polyacrylate dispersion, polysorbate 80, povidone, pregelatinized starch, sodium starch glycolate, talc

### QUESTIONS OR COMMENTS
Call toll-free **1-800-897-7535** (English/Spanish) weekdays or visit www.tums.com

## TUMS EXTRA (calcium carbonate) tablet, chewable
GlaxoSmithKline Consumer Healthcare LP

### DRUG FACTS

| Active ingredient (per tablet) | Purpose |
|---|---|
| Calcium carbonate USP 750 mg | Antacid |

### USES
- relieves
  - heartburn
  - sour stomach
  - acid indigestion
  - upset stomach associated with these symptoms
  - daily source of extra calcium

### WARNINGS

**ASK A DOCTOR OR PHARMACIST BEFORE USE IF YOU ARE**
- taking a prescription drug. Antacids may interact with certain prescription drugs

**WHEN USING THIS PRODUCT**
- do not take more than 10 tablets in 24 hours
- do not use the maximum dosage for more than 2 weeks

**Keep out of reach of children.**

### DIRECTIONS
- chew 2-4 tablets as symptoms occur, or as directed by a doctor
- chew 2 tablets twice daily with a meal for use as calcium supplement

### INACTIVE INGREDIENTS (Assorted fruit)
sucrose, calcium carbonate, corn starch, talc, mineral oil, natural and artificial flavors, adipic acid, sodium polyphosphate, red 40 lake, yellow 6 lake, yellow 5 (tartrazine) lake, blue 1 lake

### INACTIVE INGREDIENTS (Assorted berries)
sucrose, calcium carbonate, corn starch, talc, mineral oil, adipic acid, artificial flavors, sodium polyphosphate, red 40 lake, blue 1 lake

### INACTIVE INGREDIENTS (Sugar free orange cream)
calcium carbonate, sorbitol, acacia, natural and artificial flavors, calcium stearate, adipic acid, yellow 6 lake, aspartame

### INACTIVE INGREDIENT (Assorted tropical fruit)
sucrose, calcium carbonate, corn starch, talc, mineral oil, natural and artificial flavors, sodium polyphosphate, red 40 lake, yellow 6 lake, yellow 5 (tartrazine) lake

### INACTIVE INGREDIENTS (Wintergreen)
sucrose, calcium carbonate, corn starch, talc, mineral oil, artificial flavor, sodium polyphosphate, yellow 5 (tartrazine) lake, blue 1 lake

### INACTIVE INGREDIENTS (Cherry)
adipic acid, corn starch, FD&C red no. 40 aluminum lake, flavor, mineral oil, sodium polyphosphate, sucrose, talc

### OTHER INFORMATION
- for calcium and sodium content see Supplement Facts
- store below 30°C (86°F)

### OTHER INFORMATION (Sugar free orange cream)
- **Phenylketonurics:** Contains phenylalanine, less than 1 mg per tablet

### OTHER INFORMATION (Cherry)
- each tablet contains: **elemental calcium 300 mg, sodium 2 mg**
- store below 30°C (86°F)

### QUESTIONS OR COMMENTS
Call **1-800-897-7535** weekdays or visit www.tums.com

## TUMS KIDS (calcium carbonate) tablet, chewable
GlaxoSmithKline Consumer Healthcare LP

### DRUG FACTS

| Active ingredient (per tablet) | Purpose |
|---|---|
| Calcium carbonate USP 750 mg | Antacid |

### USES
- relieves
  - sour stomach
  - acid indigestion
  - upset stomach associated with these symptoms or overindulgence in food and drink
  - calcium supplement

### WARNINGS

**ASK A DOCTOR OR PHARMACIST BEFORE USE IF**
- the child is presently taking a prescription drug. Antacids may interact with certain prescription drugs

**WHEN USING THIS PRODUCT**
- do not take more than 2 tablets (2-4 year olds) or 4 tablets (5-11 year olds) in 24 hours or use the maximum dosage for more than 2 weeks except under the advice and supervision of a doctor

**Keep out of reach of children.**

### DIRECTIONS
- find the right dose on chart below based on weight (preferred), otherwise use age
- chew ½ to 1 tablet as symptoms occur or as directed by a doctor

| Weight | Age | Dose |
|---|---|---|
| under 24 lbs | under 2 yrs | ask a doctor |
| 24-47 lbs | 2-4 yrs | ½ tablet |
| over 48 lbs | over 4 yrs | 1 tablet |

- as a calcium supplement: 2-4-year-olds: chew 1 tablet per day with a meal; adults and children over 4 years old: chew 1 tablet three times a day with meal

### OTHER INFORMATION
- for calcium/magnesium/sodium content see Supplement Facts
- store below 25°C (77°F). Keep the container tightly closed

### INACTIVE INGREDIENTS
calcium carbonate, sorbitol, dextrose, sucrose, microcrystalline cellulose, magnesium stearate, adipic acid, natural and artificial flavors, maltodextrin, guar gum, red 40 lake, blue 1 lake
contains: gluten (wheat)

### QUESTIONS OR COMMENTS
Call **1-800-897-7535** weekdays or visit www.tums.com

# TUMS SMOOTHIES (calcium carbonate) chewable, tablet
GlaxoSmithKline Consumer Healthcare LP

## DRUG FACTS

| Active ingredient (per tablet) | Purpose |
| --- | --- |
| Calcium carbonate USP 750 mg | Antacid/calcium supplement |

### USES
- relieves
  - heartburn
  - sour stomach
  - acid indigestion
  - upset stomach associated with these symptoms
  - calcium supplement

### WARNINGS

**ASK A DOCTOR OR PHARMACIST BEFORE USE IF YOU ARE**
- taking a prescription drug. Antacids may interact with certain prescription drugs

**WHEN USING THIS PRODUCT**
- do not take more than 10 tablets in 24 hours
- do not use the maximum dosage for more than 2 weeks

**Keep out of reach of children.**

### DIRECTIONS
- chew 2-4 tablets as symptoms occur, or as directed by a doctor
- chew 2 tablets twice a day with a meal as calcium supplement

### INACTIVE INGREDIENTS (Assorted fruit)
calcium carbonate, sorbitol, dextrose, sucrose, microcrystalline cellulose, magnesium stearate, adipic acid, corn starch, maltodextrin, guar gum, natural and artificial flavors, red 40 lake, yellow 6 lake, yellow 5 (tartrazine) lake, blue 1 lake; contains: milk, gluten (wheat)

### INACTIVE INGREDIENTS (Berry fusion)
calcium carbonate, sorbitol, dextrose, sucrose, microcrystalline cellulose, magnesium stearate, natural and artificial flavors, adipic acid, corn starch, guar gum, maltodextrin, red 40 lake, blue 1 lake; contains: gluten (wheat), soy

### INACTIVE INGREDIENT (Assorted tropical fruit)
calcium carbonate, sorbitol, dextrose, sucrose, microcrystalline cellulose, magnesium stearate, natural and artificial flavors, corn starch, guar gum, maltodextrin, adipic acid, yellow 6 lake, red 40 lake, blue 1 lake. Contains: soy

### INACTIVE INGREDIENTS (Peppermint)
calcium carbonate, sorbitol, dextrose, sucrose, microcrystalline cellulose, magnesium stearate, corn starch, guar gum, maltodextrin, natural and artificial flavors

### INACTIVE INGREDIENTS (Cocoa and creme)
calcium carbonate, sorbitol, dextrose, sucrose, cocoa powder, microcrystalline cellulose, natural and artificial flavors, magnesium stearate, corn starch, maltodextrin, guar gum, silicon dioxide; contains: milk, soy

### OTHER INFORMATION
- for calcium/magnesium/sodium content see Supplement Facts
- store below 25°C (77°F). Keep the container tightly closed

### QUESTIONS OR COMMENTS
Call **1-800-897-7535** weekdays or visit www.tums.com

# TUMS ULTRA (calcium carbonate) tablet
GlaxoSmithKline Consumer Healthcare LP

## DRUG FACTS

| Active ingredient (per tablet) | Purpose |
| --- | --- |
| Calcium carbonate USP 1,000 mg | Antacid |

### USES
- relieves:
  - heartburn
  - sour stomach
  - acid indigestion
  - upset stomach associated with these symptoms
- source of extra calcium

### WARNINGS

**ASK A DOCTOR OR PHARMACIST BEFORE USE IF YOU ARE**
- taking a prescription drug. Antacids may interact with certain prescription drugs

**WHEN USING THIS PRODUCT**
- do not take more than 7 tablets in 24 hours
- do not use the maximum dosage for more than 2 weeks

**Keep out of reach of children.**

### DIRECTIONS
- chew 2-3 tablets as symptoms occur, or as directed by a doctor
- chew 2 tablets twice a day with a meal as calcium supplement

### OTHER INFORMATION
- for calcium and sodium content see Supplement Facts
- store below 30°C (86°F)

### INACTIVE INGREDIENTS (Assorted fruit)
sucrose, calcium carbonate, corn starch, talc, mineral oil, natural and artificial flavors, adipic acid, sodium polyphosphate, red 40 lake, yellow 6 lake, yellow 5 (tartrazine) lake, blue 1 lake

### INACTIVE INGREDIENTS (Assorted tropical fruit)
sucrose, calcium carbonate, corn starch, talc, mineral oil, natural and artificial flavors, sodium polyphosphate, red 40 lake, yellow 6 lake, yellow 5 (tartrazine) lake

### INACTIVE INGREDIENTS (Assorted berry)
sucrose, calcium carbonate, corn starch, talc, mineral oil, adipic acid, artificial flavors, sodium polyphosphate, red 40 lake, blue 1 lake

### INACTIVE INGREDIENT (Peppermint)
sucrose, calcium carbonate, corn starch, talc, mineral oil, natural flavor, sodium polyphosphate

### INACTIVE INGREDIENT (Spearmint)
sucrose, calcium carbonate, corn starch, natural and artificial flavors, talc, mineral oil, sodium polyphosphate, blue 1 lake

### QUESTIONS OR COMMENTS
Call **1-800-897-7535** weekdays or visit www.tums.com

# DIABETIC TUSSIN COUGH DROPS (menthol)
lozenge

Health Care Products

## DRUG FACTS

| Active ingredient (in each cough drop) | Purpose |
|---|---|
| Menthol 5.8 mg | Cough suppressant/oral anesthetic |

## USES
- temporarily relieves:
  - coughs as may occur with a cold or inhaled irritants
  - occasional minor irritation and sore throat

## WARNINGS
**Sore throat warning**
If sore throat is severe, persists for more than 2 days, is accompanied or followed by fever, headache, rash, swelling, nausea or vomiting, consult a doctor promptly. These symptoms may be serious.

## ASK A DOCTOR BEFORE USE IF YOU HAVE
- persistent or chronic cough such as occurs with smoking, asthma, or emphysema
- cough accompanied by excessive phlegm (mucus)

## WHEN USING THIS PRODUCT
- do not exceed recommended dosage

## STOP USE AND CONSULT A DOCTOR IF
- cough persists for more than 7 days, tends to recur, or is accompanied by fever, rash, or persistent headache. These could be signs of a serious condition
- sore throat is severe, or irritation, pain or redness lasts or worsens
- sore mouth does not improve in 7 days

**If pregnant or breastfeeding,** ask a health professional before use.

**Keep this and all drugs out of the reach of children.**

## DIRECTIONS

| adults & children 3 years & over | allow 1 drop to dissolve slowly in mouth. May be repeated every two hours as necessary or as directed by a doctor |
|---|---|
| children under 3 years | ask a doctor |

## OTHER INFORMATION
- 6 calories per drop
- **Phenylketonurics:** contains **phenylalanine 2 mg** per drop product may be useful for diabetics on the advice of a doctor.

| Dietary Exchange* information | 1 Drop = FREE Exchange 10 Drops = 1 Fruit |
|---|---|

\* The dietary exchanges are based on the Exchange List for Meal Planning.

## INACTIVE INGREDIENTS
acesulfame potassium eucalyptus oil, flavoring hydrogenated starch hydrolysate, isomalt, sucralose and water, soybean oil used as a processing aid

## QUESTIONS OR COMMENTS
Call: **1-800-899-3116**, Mon-Thurs. 9:00 AM-5:00 PM EST, Fri. 9:00 AM-2:30 PM EST.
Serious side effects associated with use of this product may be reported to this number.

# DIABETIC TUSSIN DM (dextromethorphan hydrobromide and guaifenesin) liquid

Health Care Products

## DRUG FACTS

| Active ingredients (in each 5 mL) | Purpose |
|---|---|
| Dextromethorphan hydrobromide 10 mg | Cough suppressant |
| Guaifenesin 100 mg | Expectorant |

## USES
- temporarily relieves cough
- helps loosen phlegm (mucus) and thin bronchial secretions to rid bronchial passageways of bothersome mucus

## WARNINGS
**DO NOT USE**
- if you are now taking a prescription monoamine oxidase inhibitor (MAOI) (certain drugs for depression, psychiatric or emotional conditions, or Parkinson's disease), or for two weeks after stopping the MAOI drug
- If you do not know if your prescription drug contains an MAOI, ask a doctor or pharmacist before taking this product

## ASK A DOCTOR BEFORE USE IF YOU HAVE
- a cough that occurs with too much phlegm (mucus)
- a chronic cough that lasts or as occurs with smoking, asthma, chronic bronchitis, or emphysema

## STOP USE AND ASK A DOCTOR IF
- cough lasts more than 7 days, comes back, or occurs with fever, rash, or headache that lasts. These could be signs of a serious condition

**If pregnant or breastfeeding,** ask a health professional before use.

**Keep out of reach of children.** In case of overdose, get medical help or contact a Poison Control Center right away.

## DIRECTIONS
- take every 4 hours
- do not exceed 6 doses in 24 hours

| adults & children 12 years & over | 10 mL (2 teaspoonfuls) |
|---|---|
| children 6 years to under 12 years | 5 mL (1 teaspoonful) |
| children 2 years to under 6 years | 2.5 mL (½ teaspoonful) |
| children under 2 years | ask a doctor |

## OTHER INFORMATION
- **Phenylketonurics:** contains **phenylalanine 8.4 mg** per teaspoonful (5 mL)

**Storage**
- store at room temperature 20-25°C (68-77°F)
- keep tightly closed

## INACTIVE INGREDIENTS

acesulfame potassium, artificial cherry flavor, artificial vanilla flavor, aspartame, hypromellose, menthol, methylparaben, potassium sorbate, purified water, citric acid may be used to adjust pH

## QUESTIONS OR COMMENTS

Call **1-800-899-3116**, Mon-Thurs 9:00 AM-5:00 PM EST, Fri 9:00 AM-2:30 PM EST.
Serious side effects associated with use of this product may be reported to this number.

# DIABETIC TUSSIN DM MAXIMUM STRENGTH (dextromethorphan hydrobromide and guaifenesin) liquid

Health Care Products

## DRUG FACTS

| Active ingredients (in each 5 mL) | Purpose |
|---|---|
| Dextromethorphan hydrobromide 10 mg | Cough suppressant |
| Guaifenesin 200 mg | Expectorant |

## USES

- temporarily relieves cough
- helps loosen phlegm (mucus) and thin bronchial secretions to rid bronchial passageways of bothersome mucus

## WARNINGS

### DO NOT USE

- if you are now taking a prescription monoamine oxidase inhibitor (MAOI) (certain drugs for depression, psychiatric or emotional conditions, or Parkinson's disease), or for two weeks after stopping the MAOI drug
- if you do not know if your prescription drug contains an MAOI, ask a doctor or pharmacist before taking this product

### ASK A DOCTOR BEFORE USE IF YOU HAVE

- a cough that occurs with too much phlegm (mucus)
- a chronic cough that lasts or as occurs with smoking, asthma, chronic bronchitis, or emphysema

### STOP USE AND ASK A DOCTOR IF

- cough lasts more than 7 days, comes back, or occurs with fever, rash, or headache that lasts. These could be signs of a serious condition.

**If pregnant or breastfeeding,** ask a health professional before use.

**Keep out of reach of children.** In case of overdose, get medical help or contact a Poison Control Center right away.

### DIRECTIONS

- take every 4 hours
- do not exceed 6 doses in 24 hours

| adults & children 12 years & over | 10 mL (2 teaspoonfuls) |
|---|---|
| children under 12 years of age | ask a doctor |

## OTHER INFORMATION

**Phenylketonurics:** contains **phenylalanine 8.4 mg** per teaspoonful (5 mL)

## Storage

- store at room temperature 20-25°C (68-77°F)
- keep tightly closed

## INACTIVE INGREDIENTS

acesulfame K, artificial cherry & vanilla flavors, aspartame, hypromellose, menthol, methylparaben, polyethylene glycol, potassium sorbate, and purified water, citric acid may be used to adjust pH.

## QUESTIONS OR COMMENTS

Call **1-800-899-3116,** Mon-Thurs 9:00 AM-5:00 PM EST, Fri 9:00 AM-2:30 PM EST.
Serious side effects associated with use of this product may be reported to this number.

# DIABETIC TUSSIN EXPECTORANT
(guaifenesin) liquid

Health Care Products

## DRUG FACTS

| Active ingredient (in each 5 mL) | Purpose |
|---|---|
| Guaifenesin 100 mg | Expectorant |

## USES

- helps loosen phlegm (mucus) and thin bronchial secretions to rid bronchial passageways of bothersome mucus

## WARNINGS

### ASK A DOCTOR BEFORE USE IF YOU HAVE

- a cough that occurs with too much phlegm (mucus)
- a persistent or chronic cough such as occurs with smoking, asthma, chronic bronchitis, or emphysema

### STOP USE AND ASK A DOCTOR IF

- cough lasts more than 7 days, comes back, or occurs with fever, rash, or headache that lasts. These could be signs of a serious condition

**If pregnant or breastfeeding,** ask a health professional before use.

**Keep out of reach of children.** In case of overdose, get medical help or contact a Poison Control Center right away.

### DIRECTIONS

- take every 4 hours
- do not exceed 6 doses in 24 hours

| adults & children 12 years and over | 10 mL-20 mL (2 - 4 teaspoonfuls) |
|---|---|
| children 6 years to under 12 years | 5 mL-10 mL (1 - 2 teaspoonfuls) |
| children 2 years to under 6 years | 2.5 mL-5 mL (½ - 1 teaspoonful) |
| children under 2 years | ask a doctor |

## OTHER INFORMATION

- **Phenylketonurics:** contains **phenylalanine 8.4 mg** per teaspoonful (5 mL)

## Storage

- store at room temperature 20-25°C (68-77°F)
- keep tightly closed

## INACTIVE INGREDIENTS
acesulfame K, artificial cherry flavor, artificial vanilla flavor, aspartame, hypromellose, menthol, methylparaben, potassium sorbate, purified water, citric acid may be used to adjust pH.

## QUESTIONS OR COMMENTS
Call **1-800-899-3116**, Mon-Thurs 9:00 AM-5:00 PM EST, Fri 9:00 AM-2:30 PM EST.

Serious side effects associated with use of this product may be reported to this number.

---

# DIABETIC TUSSIN NIGHTTIME COLD AND FLU (acetaminophen, dextromethorphan hydrobromide, and diphenhydramine hydrochloride) liquid
Health Care Products

## DRUG FACTS

| Active ingredients (in each 5 mL) | Purpose |
| --- | --- |
| Acetaminophen 325 mg | Pain relief |
| Dextromethorphan hydrobromide 10 mg | Cough suppressant |
| Diphenhydramine hydrochloride 12.5 mg | Antihistamine |

## USES
- temporarily relieves common cold/flu symptoms including:
  - cough due to minor throat and bronchial irritation
  - sore throat
  - headache
  - minor aches and pains
  - muscular aches
  - fever
  - runny nose and sneezing

## WARNINGS
**Liver warning**
This product contains acetaminophen. Severe liver damage may occur if:

- adults take more than 6 doses in 24 hours, which is the maximum daily amount
- child takes more than 5 doses in 24 hours, which is the maximum daily amount
- taken with other drugs containing acetaminophen
- adult has 3 or more alcoholic drinks everyday while using this product

**Sore throat warning**
If sore throat is severe, persists for more than two days, is accompanied or followed by fever, headache, rash, nausea, or vomiting, consult a doctor promptly.

## DO NOT USE
- with any other drug containing acetaminophen (prescription or nonprescription). If you are not sure whether a drug contains acetaminophen, ask a doctor or pharmacist
- if you are now taking a prescription monoamine oxidase inhibitor (MAOI) (certain drugs for depression, psychiatric or emotional conditions, or Parkinson's disease), or for 2 weeks after stopping the MAOI drug. If you do not know if your prescription drug contains an MAOI, ask a doctor or pharmacist before taking this product
- with any other product containing diphenhydramine, even one used on the skin

## ASK A DOCTOR BEFORE USE IF YOU HAVE
- liver disease
- glaucoma
- a breathing problem such as emphysema or chronic bronchitis
- trouble urinating due to enlargement of the prostate gland
- cough that occurs with too much phlegm (mucus)
- a chronic cough that lasts or as occurs with smoking, asthma, chronic bronchitis, or emphysema

## ASK A DOCTOR OR PHARMACIST BEFORE USE
- if the user is taking the blood thinning drug warfarin, tranquilizers or sedatives

## WHEN USING THIS PRODUCT
- you may get very drowsy
- avoid alcoholic drinks
- alcohol, sedatives and tranquilizers may increase drowsiness
- be careful when driving a motor vehicle or operating machinery
- excitability may occur, especially in small children

## STOP USE AND ASK A DOCTOR IF
- redness or swelling is present
- fever gets worse or lasts more than 3 days
- new symptoms occur
- cough lasts more than 7 days, comes back, or occurs with fever, rash, or headache that lasts. These could be signs of a serious condition

**If pregnant or breastfeeding,** ask a health professional before use.

**Keep out of reach of children.** In case of overdose, get medical help or contact a Poison Control Center right away. Prompt medical attention is critical even if you do not notice any signs or symptoms.

## DIRECTIONS
- take every 4 to 6 hours
- do not exceed more than 5 doses in 24 hours for children under 12 years of age
- do not exceed more than 6 doses in 24 hours for adults and children over 12 years of age

| adults & children 12 years & over | 10 mL (2 teaspoonfuls) |
| --- | --- |
| children 6 years to under 12 years | 5 mL (1 teaspoonful) |
| children under 6 years | ask a doctor |

## OTHER INFORMATION
- **Phenylketonurics:** contains **phenylalanine 8.4 mg** per teaspoonful (5 mL)
- store at room temperature 20-25°C (68-77°F)

## INACTIVE INGREDIENTS
acesulfame potassium, aspartame, citric acid, hypromellose, menthol, methylparaben, natural & artificial orange flavor, polyethylene glycol, potassium sorbate, propylene glycol, purified water, sodium citrate may be used to adjust pH.

## QUESTIONS OR COMMENTS
Call: **1-800-899-3116**, Mon-Thurs 9:00 AM-5:00 PM EST, Fri 9:00 AM-2:30 PM EST.
Serious side effects associated with use of this product may be reported to this number.

# TYLENOL REGULAR STRENGTH
(acetaminophen) tablet
McNeil Consumer Healthcare

## DRUG FACTS

| Active ingredient (in each tablet) | Purpose |
|---|---|
| Acetaminophen 325 mg | Pain reliever/fever reducer |

## USES
- to reduce fever and for the temporary relief of minor aches and pains due to:
  - headache.
  - muscular aches.
  - backache.
  - minor pain of arthritis.
  - the common cold.
  - toothache.
  - premenstrual and menstrual cramps.
- temporarily reduces fever

## WARNINGS
### Liver warning
This product contains acetaminophen. Severe liver damage may occur if:
- adult takes more than 12 tablets in 24 hours, which is the maximum daily amount
- child take more than 5 doses in 24 hours
- taken with other drugs containing acetaminophen
- adult has 3 or more alcoholic drinks every day while using this product

## DO NOT USE
- with any other drug containing acetaminophen (prescription or nonprescription). If you are not sure whether a drug contains acetaminophen, ask a doctor or pharmacist
- if you are allergic to acetaminophen or any of the inactive ingredients in this product

## ASK A DOCTOR BEFORE USE IF
- the user has liver disease

## ASK A DOCTOR OR PHARMACIST BEFORE USE
- if the user is taking the blood thinning drug warfarin

## STOP USE AND ASK A DOCTOR IF:
- pain gets worse or lasts more than 10 days in adults and children
- pain gets worse or lasts more than 5 days in children under 12 years
- fever gets worse or lasts more than 3 days
- new symptoms occur
- redness or swelling is present

These could be signs of a serious condition.

**If pregnant or breastfeeding,** ask a health professional before use.

**Keep out of reach of children.**

## OVERDOSE WARNING
Taking more than the recommended dose (overdose) may cause liver damage. In case of overdose, get medical help or contact a Poison Control Center right away. (1-800-222-1222). Quick medical attention is critical for adults as well as for children even if you do not notice any signs or symptoms.

## DIRECTIONS
- do not take more than directed

| adults & children 12 years and over | take 2 tablets every 4 to 6 hours while symptoms last |
| --- | --- |
| | do not take more than 12 tablets in 24 hours |
| children 6-11 years | take 1 tablet every 4 to 6 hours while symptoms last |
| | do not take more than 5 tablets in 24 hours |
| children under 6 years | do not use adult regular strength products in children under 6 years of age; this will provide more than the recommended dose (overdose) of tylenol and may cause liver damage |

## OTHER INFORMATION
- Temper evident packaging
- carton: do not use if carton is opened or red neck wrap or foil inner seal imprinted with "Safety Seal" is broken
- Dispensit: do not use if pouch is opened
- label: do not use if red neck wrap or foil inner seal imprinted with "Safety Seal" is broken

## INACTIVE INGREDIENTS
corn starch, magnesium stearate, powdered cellulose, pregelatinized starch, sodium starch glycolate

## QUESTIONS OR COMMENTS
Call 1-877-TYLENOL (English) or **1-888-466-8746**

# CHILDREN'S TYLENOL (acetaminophen)
suspension
McNeil Consumer Healthcare, Division of McNeil-PPC, Inc.

## DRUG FACTS

| Active ingredient (in each 5 mL = 1 teaspoon) | Purpose |
|---|---|
| Acetaminophen 160 mg | Pain reliever/fever reducer |

## USES
- temporarily:
  - reduces fever
- relieves minor aches and pains due to:
  - the common cold
  - flu
  - headache
  - sore throat
  - toothache

## WARNINGS
### Liver warning
This product contains acetaminophen. Severe liver damage may occur if your child takes

- more than 5 doses in 24 hours, which is the maximum daily amount
- with other drugs containing acetaminophen

### Sore throat warning
If sore throat is severe, persists for more than 2 days, is accompanied or followed by fever, headache, rash, nausea, or vomiting, consult a doctor promptly.

**DO NOT USE**

- with any other drug containing acetaminophen (prescription or nonprescription). If you are not sure whether a drug contains acetaminophen, ask a doctor or pharmacist
- if your child is allergic to acetaminophen or any of the inactive ingredients in this product

**ASK A DOCTOR BEFORE USE IF YOUR CHILD HAS**

- liver disease

**ASK A DOCTOR OR PHARMACIST BEFORE USE IF YOUR CHILD IS**

- taking the blood thinning drug warfarin

**WHEN USING THIS PRODUCT**

- do not exceed recommended dose (see overdose warning)

**STOP USE AND ASK A DOCTOR IF**

- pain gets worse or lasts more than 5 days
- fever gets worse or lasts more than 3 days
- new symptoms occur
- redness or swelling is present

These could be signs of a serious condition.

**Keep out of reach of children.**

**OVERDOSE WARNING**

Taking more than the recommended dose (overdose) may cause liver damage. In case of overdose, get medical help or contact a Poison Control Center right away (1-800-222-1222). Quick medical attention is critical for adults as well as for children even if you do not notice any signs or symptoms.

**DIRECTIONS**

- this product does not contain directions or complete warnings for adult use
- do not give more than directed (see overdose warning)
- shake well before using
- find right dose on chart below. If possible, use weight to dose; otherwise, use age
- use only enclosed dosing cup designed for use with this product. Do not use any other dosing device
- if needed, repeat dose every 4 hours while symptoms last
- do not give more than 5 times in 24 hours
- do not give for more than 5 days unless directed by a doctor

| Weight (lb) | Age (yr) | Dose (tsp or mL) |
|---|---|---|
| under 24 | under 2 years | ask a doctor |
| 24-35 | 2-3 years | 1 tsp or 5 mL |
| 36-47 | 4-5 years | 1 ½ tsp or 7.5 mL |
| 48-59 | 6-8 years | 2 tsp or 10 mL |
| 60-71 | 9-10 years | 2 ½ tsp or 12.5 mL |
| 72-95 | 11 years | 3 tsp or 15 mL |

**OTHER INFORMATION**

- each teaspoon contains: sodium 2 mg
- store between 20-25°C (68-77°F)
- do not use if bottle wrap, or foil inner seal imprinted with "Safety Seal" is broken or missing
- see bottom panel for lot number and expiration date

**INACTIVE INGREDIENTS**

anhydrous citric acid, butylparaben, D&C red no. 33, FD&C blue no. 1, flavors, glycerin, high fructose corn syrup, microcrystalline cellulose and carboxymethylcellulose sodium, propylene glycol, purified water, sodium benzoate, sorbitol solution, sucralose, xanthan gum

**QUESTIONS OR COMMENTS**
Call **1-877-895-3665**

# TYLENOL ALLERGY MULTI-SYMPTOM
(acetaminophen, chlorpheniramine maleate, and phenylephrine hydrochloride) gelcaps & caplets
McNeil-PPC, Inc.

## DRUG FACTS

| Active ingredient (in each gelcap and caplet) | Purpose |
|---|---|
| Acetaminophen 325 mg | Pain reliever |
| Chlorpheniramine maleate 2 mg | Antihistamine |
| Phenylephrine hydrochloride 5 mg | Nasal decongestant |

**USES**

- temporarily relieves these symptoms of hay fever or other upper respiratory allergies:
  - headache.
  - sinus congestion and pressure.
  - nasal congestion.
  - runny nose and sneezing.
  - minor aches and pains.
- temporarily relieves these additional symptoms of hay fever:
  - itching of the nose or throat.
  - itchy, watery eyes.
- helps clear nasal passages
- helps decongest sinus openings and passages

**WARNINGS**
**Liver warning**
This product contains acetaminophen. Severe liver damage may occur if you take:

- more than 12 caplets or gelcaps in 24 hours, which is the maximum daily amount
- with other drugs containing acetaminophen
- 3 or more alcoholic drinks every day while using this product

**DO NOT USE**

- with any other drug containing acetaminophen (prescription or nonprescription). If you are not sure whether a drug contains acetaminophen, ask a doctor or pharmacist
- if you are now taking a prescription monoamine oxidase inhibitor (MAOI) (certain drugs for depression, psychiatric or emotional conditions, or Parkinson's disease), or for 2 weeks after stopping the MAOI drug. If you do not know if your prescription drug contains an MAOI, ask a doctor or pharmacist before taking this product

**ASK A DOCTOR BEFORE USE IF YOU HAVE**

- liver disease
- heart disease
- high blood pressure
- thyroid disease
- diabetes
- trouble urinating due to an enlarged prostate gland
- a breathing problem such as emphysema or chronic bronchitis
- glaucoma

**ASK A DOCTOR OR PHARMACIST BEFORE USE IF YOU ARE**

- taking the blood thinning drug warfarin
- taking sedatives or tranquilizers

**WHEN USING THIS PRODUCT**

- do not exceed recommended dosage
- excitability may occur, especially in children

- drowsiness may occur
- alcohol, sedatives, and tranquilizers may increase drowsiness
- avoid alcoholic drinks
- be careful when driving a motor vehicle or operating machinery

### STOP USE AND ASK A DOCTOR IF
- nervousness, dizziness, or sleeplessness occur
- pain or nasal congestion gets worse or lasts more than 7 days
- fever gets worse or lasts more than 3 days
- redness or swelling is present
- new symptoms occur

These could be signs of a serious condition.

**If pregnant or breastfeeding,** ask a health professional before use.

**Keep out of reach of children.**

### OVERDOSE WARNING
Taking more than the recommended dose (overdose) may cause liver damage. In case of overdose, get medical help or contact a Poison Control Center right away. (1-800-222-1222). Quick medical attention is critical for adults as well as for children even if you do not notice any signs or symptoms.

### DIRECTIONS
- do not take more than directed (see overdose warning)

| adults and children 12 years and over | take 2 caplets or gelcaps every 4 hours |
| | swallow whole—do not crush, chew, or dissolve |
| | do not take more than 12 caplets or gelcaps in 24 hours |
| children under 12 years | do not use |
| | this will provide more than the recommended dose (overdose) and may cause liver damage |

### INACTIVE INGREDIENTS (GEL CAPS)
Benzyl alcohol, black iron oxide, butylparaben, carboxymethylcellulose sodium, colloidal silicon dioxide, corn starch, D&C yellow no. 10, D&C yellow no. 10, aluminum lake, edetate, calcium disodium, FD&C red no. 40, FD&C, yellow no. 6, gelatin, hypromellose, methylparaben microcrystalline cellulose, polyethylene glycol, polysorbate 80, powdered cellulose, pregelatinized starch, propylene glycol, propylparaben, red iron oxide, sodium lauryl sulfate, sodium propionate, sodium starch glycolate, stearic acid, titanium dioxide, yellow iron oxide

### INACTIVE INGREDIENTS (CAPLETS)
anhydrous citric acid, carnauba wax, colloidal silicon dioxide*, corn starch, flavors, hypromellose, iron oxide, magnesium stearate, microcrystalline cellulose, polyethylene glycol, polysorbate 80, potassium sorbate, powdered cellulose, pregelatinized starch, propylene glycol, shellac, sodium benzoate, sodium citrate, sodium starch glycolate, stearic acid*, sucralose, titanium dioxide, yellow iron oxide
* may contain one or more of these ingredients

### QUESTIONS OR COMMENTS
Call **1-877-TYLENOL** (English) or **1-888-466-8746** (Spanish)

# TYLENOL ALLERGY MULTI-SYMPTOM NIGHTTIME (acetaminophen, diphenhydramine hydrochloride, and phenylephrine hydrochloride) caplet, film coated

McNeil Consumer Healthcare
Div McNeil-PPC, Inc

## DRUG FACTS

| Active ingredients (in each caplet) | Purpose |
|---|---|
| Acetaminophen 325 mg | Pain reliever |
| Diphenhydramine hydrochloride 25 mg | Antihistamine |
| Phenylephrine hydrochloride 5 mg | Nasal decongestant |

### USES
- temporarily relieves these symptoms of hay fever or other respiratory allergies:
  - headache
  - sinus congestion and pressure
  - nasal congestion
  - runny nose and sneezing
  - minor aches and pains
- temporarily relieves these additional symptoms of hay fever:
  - itching of the nose or throat
  - itchy, watery eyes
- helps clear nasal passages

### WARNINGS
**Alcohol warning**
If you consume 3 or more alcoholic drinks every day, ask your doctor whether you should take acetaminophen or other pain relievers or fever reducers. Acetaminophen may cause liver damage.

### DO NOT USE
- with any other product containing acetaminophen
- with any other product containing diphenhydramine, even one used on skin
- if you are now taking a prescription monoamine oxidase inhibitor (MAOI) (certain drugs for depression, psychiatric or emotional conditions, or Parkinson's disease), or for 2 weeks after stopping the MAOI drug. If you do not know if your prescription drug contains an MAOI, ask a doctor or pharmacist before taking this product

### ASK A DOCTOR BEFORE USE IF YOU HAVE
- liver disease
- heart disease
- high blood pressure
- thyroid disease
- diabetes
- trouble urinating due to an enlarged prostate gland
- a breathing problem such as emphysema or chronic bronchitis
- glaucoma

### ASK A DOCTOR OR PHARMACIST BEFORE USE IF YOU ARE
- taking sedatives or tranquilizers

### WHEN USING THIS PRODUCT
- do not exceed recommended dosage
- excitability may occur, especially in children
- marked drowsiness may occur

- alcohol, sedatives and tranquilizers may increase drowsiness
- avoid alcoholic drinks
- be careful when driving a motor vehicle or operating machinery

## STOP USE AND ASK A DOCTOR IF
- nervousness, dizziness, or sleeplessness occur
- pain or nasal congestion gets worse or lasts more than 7 days
- fever gets worse or lasts more than 3 days
- redness or swelling is present
- new symptoms occur

These could be signs of a serious condition.

**If pregnant or breastfeeding,** ask a health professional before use.

**Keep out of reach of children.**

## OVERDOSE WARNING
Taking more than the recommended dose (overdose) may cause liver damage. In case of overdose, get medical help or contact a Poison Control Center right away (1-800-222-1222). Quick medical attention is critical for adults as well as for children even if you do not notice any signs or symptoms.

## DIRECTIONS
- do not take more than directed (see overdose warning)

| adults and children 12 years and over | take 2 caplets every 4 hours |
| | swallow whole - do not crush, chew or dissolve |
| | do not take more than 12 caplets in 24 hours |
| children under 12 years | do not use |
| | this will provide more than the recommended dose (overdose) and may cause liver damage |

## OTHER INFORMATION
- store between 20-25°C (68-77°F)
- do not use if carton is opened or if blister unit is broken
- see side panel for lot number and expiration date

## INACTIVE INGREDIENTS
anhydrous citric acid, carnauba wax, corn starch, D&C yellow no. 10 aluminum lake, FD&C yellow no. 6, aluminum lake, flavors, hypromellose, iron oxide, magnesium stearate, microcrystalline cellulose, propylene glycol, potassium sorbate, shellac, sodium benzoate, sodium citrate, sodium starch glycolate, sucralose, titanium dioxide, triacetin

## QUESTIONS OR COMMENTS
Call **1-877-895-3665** (English) or **1-888-466-8746** (Spanish)

---

# TYLENOL ARTHRITIS PAIN (acetaminophen)
caplet, film coated, extended release or gelcaps
McNeil Consumer Healthcare, Division of McNeil-PPC, Inc.

## DRUG FACTS

| Active ingredient (in each caplet) | Purpose |
|---|---|
| Acetaminophen 650 mg | Pain reliever/fever reducer |

## USES
- temporarily relieves minor aches and pains due to:
  - arthritis
  - muscular aches
  - backache
  - menstrual cramps
  - the common cold
  - headache
  - toothache
- temporarily reduces fever

## WARNINGS
**Liver warning**
This product contains acetaminophen. Severe liver damage may occur if you take:
- more than 6 caplets or gelcaps in 24 hours, which is the maximum daily amount
- with other drugs containing acetaminophen
- 3 or more alcoholic drinks every day while using this product

## DO NOT USE
- with any other drug containing acetaminophen (prescription or nonprescription). If you are not sure whether a drug contains acetaminophen, ask a doctor or pharmacist

## ASK A DOCTOR BEFORE USE IF YOU HAVE
- liver disease

## ASK A DOCTOR OR PHARMACIST BEFORE USE IF YOU ARE
- taking the blood thinning drug warfarin

## STOP USE AND ASK A DOCTOR IF
- pain gets worse or lasts more than 10 days
- fever gets worse or lasts more than 3 days
- new symptoms occur
- redness or swelling is present

These could be signs of a serious condition.

**If pregnant or breastfeeding,** ask a health professional before use.

**Keep out of the reach of children.**

## OVERDOSE WARNING
Taking more than the recommended dose (overdose) may cause liver damage. In case of overdose, get medical help or contact a Poison Control Center right away (1-800-222-1222). Quick medical attention is critical for adults as well as for children even if you do not notice any signs or symptoms.

## DIRECTIONS
- do not take more than directed (see overdose warning)

| adults | take 2 caplets or gelcaps every 8 hours |
| | swallow whole – do not crush, chew, split or dissolve |
| | do not take more than 6 caplets in 24 hours |
| | do not use for more than 10 days unless directed by a doctor |
| under 18 years of age | ask a doctor |

## OTHER INFORMATION
- store at 20-25°C (68-77°F). Avoid excessive heat 40°C (104°F)
- do not use if carton is opened or neck wrap or foil inner seal imprinted with "Safety Seal" is broken
- see end panel for lot number and expiration date

**INACTIVE INGREDIENTS**
anhydrous citric acid, FD&C blue no. 1, FD&C red no. 40, FD&C
yellow no. 6, flavor, glycerin, propylene glycol, purified water,
sodium benzoate, sorbitol solution, sucralose

**QUESTIONS OR COMMENTS**
Call **1-877-895-3665**

# TYLENOL COLD AND FLU SEVERE
(acetaminophen, dextromethorphan hydrobromide,
guaifenesin, and phenylephrine hydrochloride) liquid
McNeil Consumer Healthcare, Division of McNeil-
PPC, Inc.

## DRUG FACTS

| Active ingredients (in each 15 mL = 1 tablespoon) | Purpose |
| --- | --- |
| Acetaminophen 325 mg | Pain reliever/fever reducer |
| Dextromethorphan hydrobromide 10 mg | Cough suppressant |
| Guaifenesin 200 mg | Expectorant |
| Phenylephrine hydrochloride 5 mg | Nasal decongestant |

## USES
- temporarily relieves the following cold/flu symptoms:
  - minor aches and pains
  - headache
  - sore throat
  - nasal congestion
  - cough
- helps loosen phlegm (mucus) and thin bronchial secretions to make coughs more productive
- temporarily reduces fever

## WARNINGS
**Liver warning**
This product contains acetaminophen. Severe liver damage may occur if you take:
- more than 12 tablespoons in 24 hours, which is the maximum daily amount
- with other drugs containing acetaminophen
- 3 or more alcoholic drinks every day while using this product

**Sore throat warning**
If sore throat is severe, persists for more than 2 days, is accompanied or followed by fever, headache, rash, nausea or vomiting, consult a doctor promptly.

**DO NOT USE**
- with any other drug containing acetaminophen (prescription or nonprescription). If you are not sure whether a drug contains acetaminophen, ask a doctor or pharmacist
- if you are now taking a prescription monoamine oxidase inhibitor (MAOI) (certain drugs for depression, psychiatric or emotional conditions, or Parkinson's disease), or for 2 weeks after stopping the MAOI drug. If you do not know if your prescription drug contains an MAOI, ask a doctor or pharmacist before taking this product
- if you have ever had an allergic reaction to this product or any of its ingredients

**ASK A DOCTOR BEFORE USE IF YOU HAVE**
- liver disease
- heart disease
- high blood pressure
- thyroid disease
- diabetes
- trouble urinating due to an enlarged prostate gland
- persistent or chronic cough such as occurs with smoking, asthma, chronic bronchitis, or emphysema
- cough that occurs with too much phlegm (mucus)

**ASK A DOCTOR OR PHARMACIST BEFORE USE IF YOU ARE**
- taking the blood thinning drug warfarin

**WHEN USING THIS PRODUCT**
- do not exceed recommended dosage

**STOP USE AND ASK A DOCTOR IF**
- nervousness, dizziness, or sleeplessness occur
- pain, nasal congestion or cough gets worse or lasts more than 7 days
- fever gets worse or lasts more than 3 days
- redness or swelling is present
- new symptoms occur
- cough comes back or occurs with rash or headache that lasts

These could be signs of a serious condition.

**If pregnant or breastfeeding,** ask a health professional before use.

**Keep out of reach of children.**

**OVERDOSE WARNING**
Taking more than the recommended dose (overdose) may cause liver damage. In case of overdose, get medical help or contact a Poison Control Center right away. (1-800-222-1222) Quick medical attention is critical for adults as well as for children even if you do not notice any signs or symptoms.

**DIRECTIONS**
- do not take more than directed (see overdose warning)
- use only enclosed dosing cup designed for use with this product. Do not use any other dosing device

| adults and children 12 years and over | take 2 tablespoons (tbsp) or 30 mL in dose cup provided every 4 hours<br><br>do not take more than 12 tbsp or 180 mL in 24 hours |
| --- | --- |
| children under 12 years | do not use<br><br>this will provide more than the recommended dose (overdose) and may cause liver damage |

**OTHER INFORMATION**
- each tablespoon contains: sodium 5 mg
- store between 20-25°C (68-77°F). Do not refrigerate
- do not use if plastic neck wrap or foil inner seal imprinted with "Safety Seal" is broken or missing
- see back label for lot number and expiration date

**INACTIVE INGREDIENTS**
anhydrous citric acid, FD&C blue no. 1, FD&C red no. 40, FD&C yellow no. 6, flavor, glycerin, propylene glycol, purified water, sodium benzoate, sorbitol solution, sucralose

**QUESTIONS OR COMMENTS**
Call **1-877-895-3665**

## TYLENOL COLD SORE THROAT EXTRA STRENGTH (acetaminophen) liquid

McNeil Consumer Healthcare, Division of McNeil-PPC, Inc.

### DRUG FACTS

| Active ingredient (in each 15 mL = 1 tablespoon) | Purpose |
| --- | --- |
| Acetaminophen 500 mg | Pain reliever/fever reducer |

### USES
- temporarily relieves minor aches and pains due to:
  - the common cold
  - headache
  - sore throat
- temporarily reduces fever

### WARNINGS
**Liver warning**
This product contains acetaminophen. Severe liver damage may occur if you take:
- more than 8 tablespoons in 24 hours, which is the maximum daily amount
- with other drugs containing acetaminophen
- 3 or more alcoholic drinks every day while using this product

**Sore throat warning**
If sore throat is severe, persists for more than 2 days, is accompanied or followed by fever, headache, rash, nausea, or vomiting, consult a doctor promptly.

### DO NOT USE
- with any other drug containing acetaminophen (prescription or nonprescription). If you are not sure whether a drug contains acetaminophen, ask a doctor or pharmacist
- if you are allergic to acetaminophen or any of the inactive ingredients in this product

### ASK A DOCTOR BEFORE USE IF YOU HAVE
- liver disease

### ASK A DOCTOR OR PHARMACIST BEFORE USE IF YOU ARE
- taking the blood thinning drug warfarin

### STOP USE AND ASK A DOCTOR IF
- pain gets worse or lasts more than 10 days
- fever gets worse or lasts more than 3 days
- new symptoms occur
- redness or swelling is present

These could be signs of a serious condition.

**If pregnant or breastfeeding,** ask a health professional before use.

**Keep out of reach of children.**

### OVERDOSE WARNING
Taking more than the recommended dose (overdose) may cause liver damage. In case of overdose, get medical help or contact a Poison Control Center right away (1-800-222-1222). Quick medical attention is critical for adults as well as for children even if you do not notice any signs or symptoms.

### DIRECTIONS
- do not take more than directed (see overdose warning)
- use only enclosed dosing cup designed for use with this product. Do not use any other dosing device

| adults and children 12 years and over | take 2 tablespoons (tbsp) or 30 mL in dosing cup provided every 4 to 6 hours |
| --- | --- |
|  | do not take more than 8 tbsp or 120 mL in 24 hours |
|  | do not use for more than 10 days unless directed by a doctor |
| children under 12 years | do not use |
|  | this will provide more than the recommended dose (overdose) and may cause liver damage |

### OTHER INFORMATION
- each tablespoon contains: sodium 11 mg
- store between 20-25°C (68-77°F)
- do not use if neck wrap or foil inner seal imprinted with "Safety Seal" is broken or missing
- see back label for lot number and expiration date

### INACTIVE INGREDIENTS
anhydrous citric acid, carboxymethylcellulose sodium, FD&C blue no. 1, flavors, polyethylene glycol, propylene glycol, purified water, sodium benzoate, sorbitol, sucralose, sucrose

### QUESTIONS OR COMMENTS
Call **1-877-895-3665**

---

## TYLENOL COLD HEAD CONGESTION SEVERE (acetaminophen, dextromethorphan hydrobromide, guaifenesin, and phenylephrine hydrochloride) caplet, film coated

Lil' Drug Store Products, Inc.

### DRUG FACTS

| Active ingredients (in each caplet) | Purpose |
| --- | --- |
| Acetaminophen 325 mg | Pain reliever |
| Dextromethorphan hydrobromide 10 mg | Cough suppressant |
| Guaifenesin 200 mg | Expectorant |
| Phenylephrine hydrochloride 5 mg | Nasal decongestant |

### USES
- for the temporary relief of the following cold symptoms:
  - minor aches and pains
  - headache
  - sore throat
  - nasal congestion
  - cough
  - sinus congestion and pressure
- helps loosen phlegm (mucus) and thin bronchial secretions to make coughs more productive

### WARNINGS
**Liver warning**
This product contains acetaminophen. Severe liver damage may occur if you take:
- more than 12 caplets in 24 hours, which is the maximum daily amount
- with other drugs containing acetaminophen
- 3 or more alcoholic drinks every day while using this product

### Sore throat warning

If sore throat is severe, persists for more than 2 days, is accompanied or followed by fever, headache, rash, nausea or vomiting, consult a doctor promptly.

### DO NOT USE

- with any other product containing acetaminophen (prescription or nonprescription). If you are not sure whether a drug contains acetaminophen, ask a doctor or pharmacist
- if you are now taking a prescription monoamine oxidase inhibitor (MAOI) (certain drugs for depression, psychiatric or emotional conditions, or Parkinson's disease), or for 2 weeks after stopping the MAOI drug. If you do not know if your prescription drug contains an MAOI, ask a doctor or pharmacist before taking this product
- if you have ever had an allergic reaction to this product or any of its ingredients

### ASK A DOCTOR BEFORE USE IF YOU HAVE

- liver disease
- heart disease
- high blood pressure
- thyroid disease
- diabetes
- trouble urinating due to an enlarged prostate gland
- persistent or chronic cough such as occurs with smoking, asthma, chronic bronchitis or emphysema
- cough that occurs with too much phlegm (mucus)

### ASK A DOCTOR OR PHARMACIST BEFORE USE IF YOU ARE

- taking the blood thinning drug warfarin

### WHEN USING THIS PRODUCT

- do not exceed recommended dosage

### STOP USE AND ASK A DOCTOR IF

- nervousness, dizziness, or sleeplessness occur
- pain, nasal congestion or cough gets worse or lasts more than 7 days
- fever gets worse or lasts more than 3 days
- redness or swelling is present
- new symptoms occur
- cough comes back or occurs with rash or headache that lasts

These could be signs of a serious condition.

**If pregnant or breastfeeding,** ask a health professional before use.

**Keep out of reach of children.**

### OVERDOSE WARNING

Taking more than the recommended dose (overdose) may cause liver damage. In case of overdose, get medical help or contact a Poison Control Center right away (1-800-222-1222). Quick medical attention is critical for adults as well as for children even if you do not notice any signs or symptoms.

### DIRECTIONS

- do not take more than directed (see overdose warning)

| adults and children 12 years and over | take 2 caplets every 4 hours |
| | swallow whole - do not crush, chew or dissolve |
| | do not take more than 12 caplets in 24 hours |
| children under 12 years | do not use |
| | this will provide more than the recommended dose (overdose) and may cause liver damage |

### OTHER INFORMATION

- each caplet contains: sodium 3 mg
- store between 20-25°C (68-77°F)
- do not use if carton or pouch is opened or torn
- see bottom panel for lot number and expiration date

### INACTIVE INGREDIENTS

carnauba wax, croscarmellose sodium, FD&C yellow no. 10 aluminum lake, flavor, hydroxypropyl cellulose, hypromellose, iron oxide, magnesium stearate, microcrystalline cellulose, polyethylene glycol, pregelatinized starch, shellac, sucralose, titanium dioxide

### QUESTIONS OR COMMENTS

Call **1-877-895-3665**

---

# TYLENOL COLD MULTI-SYMPTOM
(acetaminophen, dextromethorphan hydrobromide, doxylamine succinate, and phenylephrine hydrochloride) liquid

McNeil Consumer Healthcare, Division of McNeil-PPC, Inc.

## DRUG FACTS

| Active ingredients (in each 15 mL, 1 tablespoon) | Purpose |
| --- | --- |
| Acetaminophen 325 mg | Pain reliever/fever reducer |
| Dextromethorphan hydrobromide 10 mg | Cough suppressant |
| Doxylamine succinate 6.25 mg | Antihistamine |
| Phenylephrine hydrochloride 5 mg | Nasal decongestant |

### USES

- temporarily relieves these common cold/flu symptoms:
  - minor aches and pains
  - headache
  - sore throat
  - nasal congestion
  - runny nose and sneezing
  - cough
  - sinus congestion and pressure
- helps clear nasal passages
- relieves cough to help you sleep
- temporarily reduces fever

### WARNINGS

#### Liver warning

This product contains acetaminophen. Severe liver damage may occur if you take:
- more than 12 tablespoons in 24 hours, which is the maximum daily amount
- with other drugs containing acetaminophen
- 3 or more alcoholic drinks every day while using this product

#### Sore throat warning

If sore throat is severe, persists for more than 2 days, is accompanied or followed by fever, headache, rash, nausea, or vomiting, consult a doctor promptly.

#### DO NOT USE

- with any other drug containing acetaminophen (prescription or nonprescription). If you are not sure whether a drug contains acetaminophen, ask a doctor or pharmacist
- if you are now taking a prescription monoamine oxidase inhibitor (MAOI) (certain drugs for depression, psychiatric

or emotional conditions, or Parkinson's disease), or for 2 weeks after stopping the MAOI drug. If you do not know if your prescription drug contains an MAOI, ask a doctor or pharmacist before taking this product
- if you have ever had an allergic reaction to this product or any of its ingredients

### ASK A DOCTOR BEFORE USE IF YOU HAVE
- liver disease
- heart disease
- high blood pressure
- thyroid disease
- diabetes
- trouble urinating due to an enlarged prostate gland
- a breathing problem such as emphysema or chronic bronchitis
- glaucoma
- persistent or chronic cough such as occurs with smoking, asthma or emphysema
- cough that occurs with too much phlegm (mucus)

### ASK A DOCTOR OR PHARMACIST BEFORE USE IF YOU ARE
- taking the blood thinning drug warfarin
- taking sedatives or tranquilizers

### WHEN USING THIS PRODUCT
- do not exceed recommended dosage
- excitability may occur, especially in children
- marked drowsiness may occur
- alcohol, sedatives and tranquilizers may increase drowsiness
- avoid alcoholic drinks
- be careful when driving a motor vehicle or operating machinery

### STOP USE AND ASK A DOCTOR IF
- nervousness, dizziness, or sleeplessness occur
- pain, nasal congestion or cough gets worse or lasts more than 7 days
- fever gets worse or lasts more than 3 days
- redness or swelling is present
- new symptoms occur
- cough comes back or occurs with rash or headache that lasts

These could be signs of a serious condition.

**If pregnant or breastfeeding,** ask a health professional before use.

**Keep out of reach of children.**

### OVERDOSE WARNING
Taking more than the recommended dose (overdose) may cause liver damage. In case of overdose, get medical help or contact a Poison Control Center right away (1-800-222-1222). Quick medical attention is critical for adults as well as for children even if you do not notice any signs or symptoms.

### DIRECTIONS
- do not take more than directed (see overdose warning)
- use only enclosed dosing cup designed for use with this product. Do not use any other dosing device

| adults and children 12 years and over | take 2 tablespoons (tbsp) or 30 mL in dose cup provided every 4 hours |
| | do not take more than 12 tbsp or 180 mL in 24 hours |
| children under 12 years | do not use |
| | this will provide more than the recommended dose (overdose) and may cause liver damage |

### OTHER INFORMATION
- each tablespoon contains: sodium 5 mg
- store between 20-25°C (68-77°F). Do not refrigerate
- do not use if plastic neck wrap or foil inner seal imprinted with "Safety Seal" is broken or missing
- see back label for lot number and expiration date

### INACTIVE INGREDIENTS
anhydrous citric acid, FD&C blue no. 1, FD&C red no. 40, FD&C yellow no. 6, flavor, glycerin, propylene glycol, purified water, sodium benzoate, sorbitol solution, sucralose

### QUESTIONS OR COMMENTS
Call **1-877-895-3665**

---

# TYLENOL COLD MULTI-SYMPTOM SEVERE
(acetaminophen, dextromethorphan hydrobromide, guaifenesin, and phenylephrine hydrochloride) liquid
McNeil Consumer Healthcare, Division of McNeil-PPC, Inc.

### DRUG FACTS

| Active ingredients (in each 15 mL, 1 tablespoon) | Purpose |
| --- | --- |
| Acetaminophen 325 mg | Pain reliever/fever reducer |
| Dextromethorphan hydrobromide 10 mg | Cough suppressant |
| Guaifenesin 200 mg | Expectorant |
| Phenylephrine hydrochloride 5 mg | Nasal decongestant |

### USES
- for the temporary relief of the following cold/flu symptoms:
  - minor aches and pains
  - headache
  - sore throat
  - nasal congestion
  - cough
- helps loosen phlegm (mucus) and thin bronchial secretions to make coughs more productive
- temporarily reduces fever

### WARNINGS
**Liver warning**
This product contains acetaminophen. Severe liver damage may occur if you take:
- more than 12 tablespoons in 24 hours, which is the maximum daily amount
- with other drugs containing acetaminophen
- 3 or more alcoholic drinks every day while using this product

**Sore throat warning**
If sore throat is severe, persists for more than 2 days, is accompanied or followed by fever, headache, rash, nausea or vomiting, consult a doctor promptly.

### DO NOT USE
- with any other drug containing acetaminophen (prescription or nonprescription). If you are not sure whether a drug contains acetaminophen, ask a doctor or pharmacist
- if you are now taking a prescription monoamine oxidase inhibitor (MAOI) (certain drugs for depression, psychiatric or emotional conditions, or Parkinson's disease), or for 2 weeks after stopping the MAOI drug. If you do not know if your prescription drug contains an MAOI, ask a doctor or pharmacist before taking this product

- if you have ever had an allergic reaction to this product or any of its ingredients

## ASK A DOCTOR BEFORE USE IF YOU HAVE
- liver disease
- heart disease
- high blood pressure
- thyroid disease
- diabetes
- trouble urinating due to an enlarged prostate gland
- persistent or chronic cough such as occurs with smoking, asthma, chronic bronchitis, or emphysema
- cough that occurs with too much phlegm (mucus)

## ASK A DOCTOR OR PHARMACIST BEFORE USE IF YOU ARE
- taking the blood thinning drug warfarin

## WHEN USING THIS PRODUCT
- do not exceed recommended dosage

## STOP USE AND ASK A DOCTOR IF
- nervousness, dizziness, or sleeplessness occur
- pain, nasal congestion or cough gets worse or lasts more than 7 days
- fever gets worse or lasts more than 3 days
- redness or swelling is present
- new symptoms occur
- cough comes back or occurs with rash or headache that lasts

These could be signs of a serious condition.

**If pregnant or breastfeeding,** ask a health professional before use.

**Keep out of reach of children.**

## OVERDOSE WARNING
Taking more than the recommended dose (overdose) may cause liver damage. In case of overdose, get medical help or contact a Poison Control Center right away (1-800-222-1222). Quick medical attention is critical for adults as well as for children even if you do not notice any signs or symptoms.

## DIRECTIONS
- do not take more than directed (see overdose warning)
- use only enclosed dosing cup designed for use with this product. Do not use any other dosing device

| adults and children 12 years and over | take 2 tablespoons (tbsp) or 30 mL in dose cup provided every 4 hours<br><br>do not take more than 12 tbsp or 180 mL in 24 hours |
| --- | --- |
| children under 12 years | ask a doctor |

## OTHER INFORMATION
- each tablespoon contains: sodium 5 mg
- store between 20-25°C (68-77°F). Do not refrigerate
- do not use if plastic neck wrap or foil inner seal imprinted with "safety seal" is broken or missing
- see back label for lot number and expiration date

## INACTIVE INGREDIENTS
alcohol, anhydrous citric acid, FD&C blue no. 1, flavor, glycerin, propylene glycol, purified water, sodium benzoate, sorbitol solution, sucralose

## QUESTIONS OR COMMENTS
Call **1-877-895-3665**

# CHILDREN'S TYLENOL PLUS MULTI-SYMPTOM COLD (acetaminophen, chlorpheniramine maleate, dextromethorphan hydrobromide, and phenylephrine hydrochloride) liquid, suspension
McNeil Consumer Healthcare Division of McNeil-PPC, Inc.

## DRUG FACTS

| Active ingredient (in each teaspoon (5ml) | Purpose |
| --- | --- |
| Acetaminophen 160 mg | Pain reliever/fever reducer |
| Chlorpheniramine maleate 1 mg | Antihistamine |
| Dextromethorphan hydrobromide 5 mg | Cough suppressant |
| Phenylephrine hydrochloride 2.5 mg | Nasal decongestant |

## USES
- temporarily relieves the following cold/flu symptoms:
  - minor aches and pains.
  - headache.
  - sore throat.
  - cough.
  - stuffy nose.
  - sneezing and runny nose.
  - temporarily reduces fever

## WARNINGS
### Liver warning
This product contains acetaminophen. Severe liver damage may occur if your child takes:
- more than 5 doses in 24 hours, which is the maximum daily amount
- with other drugs containing acetaminophen

### Sore throat warning
If sore throat is severe, persists for more than 2 days, is accompanied or followed by fever, headache, rash, nausea, or vomiting, consult a doctor promptly.

## DO NOT USE
- with any other drug containing acetaminophen (prescription or nonprescription). If you are not sure whether a drug contains acetaminophen, ask a doctor or pharmacist
- to make a child sleepy
- in a child who is taking a prescription monoamine oxidase inhibitor (MAOI) (certain drugs for depression, psychiatric, or emotional conditions, or Parkinson's disease), or for 2 weeks after stopping the MAOI drug. If you do not know if your child's prescription drug contains an MAOI, ask a doctor or pharmacist before giving this product

## ASK A DOCTOR BEFORE USE IF THE CHILD HAS
- liver disease
- heart disease
- high blood pressure
- thyroid disease
- diabetes
- persistent or chronic cough such as occurs with asthma
- cough that occurs with too much phlegm (mucus)
- a breathing problem such as chronic bronchitis
- glaucoma

## ASK A DOCTOR OR PHARMACIST BEFORE USE IF YOUR
- child is taking the blood thinning drug warfarin
- taking sedatives or tranquilizers

## WHEN USING THIS PRODUCT
- do not exceed recommended dose (see overdose warning)
- excitability may occur, especially in children
- marked drowsiness may occur
- sedatives and tranquilizers may increase drowsiness

## STOP USE AND ASK A DOCTOR IF
- nervousness, dizziness, or sleeplessness occur
- pain, nasal congestion or cough gets worse or lasts more than 5 days
- fever gets worse or lasts more than 3 days
- redness or swelling is present
- new symptoms occur
- cough comes back or occurs with rash or headache that lasts

These could be signs of a serious condition.

**Keep out of reach of children.**

## OVERDOSE WARNING
Taking more than the recommended dose (overdose) may cause liver damage. In case of overdose, get medical help or contact a Poison Control Center right away. (1-800-222-1222). Quick medical attention is critical for adults as well as for children even if you do not notice any signs or symptoms.

## DIRECTIONS
- this product does not contain directions or complete warnings for adult use
- do not give more than directed (see Overdose Warning)
- shake well before use
- find right dose on chart below. If possible, use weight to dose; otherwise, use age
- use only enclosed dosing cup designed for use with this product. Do not use any other dosing device
- if needed, repeat dose every 4 hours
- do not give more than 5 times in 24 hours

| Weight (lb) | Age (yr) | Dose (tsp or mL) |
|---|---|---|
| under 36 | under 4 years | do not use |
| 36-47 lbs | 4-5 years | do not use unless directed by a doctor |
| 48-95 lbs | 6-11 years | 2 tsp or 10 mL |

## INACTIVE INGREDIENTS (GRAPE FLAVOR)
anhydrous citric acid, D&C red no. 33, FD&C blue no. 1, FD&C red no. 40, flavors, glycerin, microcrystalline cellulose and carboxymethyl cellulose sodium, purified water, sodium benzoate, sorbitol solution, sucrose, xanthan gum

## INACTIVE INGREDIENTS (DYE-FREE GRAPE FLAVOR)
anhydrous citric acid, butylparaben, flavors, glycerin, microcrystalline cellulose and carboxymethyl cellulose sodium, propylene glycol, propylparaben, purified water, sodium citrate, sorbitol solution, sucralose, sucrose, xanthan gum

## OTHER INFORMATION
- store between 20-25°C (68-77°F)
- do not use if bottle wrap, or foil inner seal imprinted with "Safety Seal" is broken or missing
- see package for lot number and expiration date

## QUESTIONS OR COMMENTS
Call **1-877-TYLENOL** (English) or **1-888-466-8746** (Spanish)

# TYLENOL COLD COUGH AND SEVERE CONGESTION (acetaminophen, dextromethorphan hydrobromide, guaifenesin, and phenylephrine hydrochloride) liquid
McNeil Consumer Healthcare, Division of McNeil-PPC, Inc.

## DRUG FACTS

| Active ingredients (in each 15 mL, tablespoon) | Purpose |
|---|---|
| Acetaminophen 325 mg | Pain reliever/fever reducer |
| Dextromethorphan hydrobromide 10 mg | Cough suppressant |
| Guaifenesin 200 mg | Expectorant |
| Phenylephrine hydrochloride 5 mg | Nasal decongestant |

## USES
- temporarily relieves the following cold/flu symptoms:
  - minor aches and pains
  - headache
  - sore throat
  - nasal congestion
  - cough
- helps loosen phlegm (mucus) and thin bronchial secretions to make coughs more productive
- temporarily reduces fever

## WARNINGS
**Alcohol warning**
If you consume 3 or more alcoholic drinks every day, ask your doctor whether you should take acetaminophen or other pain relievers or fever reducers. Acetaminophen may cause liver damage.

**Sore throat warning**
If sore throat is severe, persists for more than 2 days, is accompanied or followed by fever, headache, rash, nausea or vomiting, consult a doctor promptly.

## DO NOT USE
- with any other product containing acetaminophen
- if you are now taking a prescription monoamine oxidase inhibitor (MAOI) (certain drugs for depression, psychiatric or emotional conditions, or Parkinson's disease), or for 2 weeks after stopping the MAOI drug. If you do not know if your prescription drug contains an MAOI, ask a doctor or pharmacist before taking this product

## ASK A DOCTOR BEFORE USE IF YOU HAVE
- heart disease
- high blood pressure
- thyroid disease
- diabetes
- trouble urinating due to an enlarged prostate gland
- persistent or chronic cough such as occurs with smoking, asthma, chronic bronchitis, or emphysema
- cough that occurs with too much phlegm (mucus)

## WHEN USING THIS PRODUCT
- do not exceed recommended dosage

**STOP USE AND ASK A DOCTOR IF**
- nervousness, dizziness, or sleeplessness occur
- pain, nasal congestion or cough gets worse or lasts more than 7 days
- fever gets worse or lasts more than 3 days
- redness or swelling is present
- new symptoms occur
- cough comes back or occurs with rash or headache that lasts

These could be signs of a serious condition.

**If pregnant or breastfeeding,** ask a health professional before use.

**Keep out of reach of children.**

**OVERDOSE WARNING**
Taking more than the recommended dose (overdose) may cause liver damage. In case of overdose, get medical help or contact a Poison Control Center right away. (1-800-222-1222). Quick medical attention is critical for adults as well as for children even if you do not notice any signs or symptoms.

**DIRECTIONS**
- do not take more than directed (see overdose warning)
- use only enclosed dosing cup designed for use with this product. Do not use any other dosing device

| adults and children 12 years and over | take 2 tablespoons (tbsp) or 30 mL in dose cup provided every 4 hours |
| | do not take more than 12 tablespoons (tbsp) or 180 mL in 24 hours |
| children under 12 years | do not use |
| | this will provide more than the recommended dose (overdose) and may cause liver damage |

**OTHER INFORMATION**
- each tablespoon contains: sodium 5 mg
- store between 20-25°C (68-77°F). Do not refrigerate
- do not use if plastic neck wrap or foil inner seal imprinted with "Safety Seal" is broken or missing
- see back label for lot number and expiration date

**INACTIVE INGREDIENTS**
anhydrous citric acid, FD&C blue no. 1, FD&C red no. 40, FD&C yellow no. 6, flavor, glycerin, propylene glycol, purified water, sodium benzoate, sorbitol solution, sucralose

**QUESTIONS OR COMMENTS**
Call **1-877-895-3665** (English) or **1-888-466-8746** (Spanish)

# TYLENOL COUGH AND SORE THROAT
(acetaminophen and dextromethorphan hydrobromide) liquid

McNeil Consumer Healthcare, Division of McNeil-PPC, Inc.

## DRUG FACTS

| Active ingredients (in each 15 mL = 1 tablespoon) | Purpose |
| --- | --- |
| Acetaminophen 500 mg | Pain reliever |
| Dextromethorphan hydrobromide 15 mg | Cough suppressant |

**USES**
- temporarily relieves:
  - minor aches and pains
  - headache
  - sore throat
  - cough due to a cold

**WARNINGS**
**Alcohol warning**
If you consume 3 or more alcoholic drinks every day, ask your doctor whether you should take acetaminophen or other pain relievers or fever reducers. Acetaminophen may cause liver damage.

**Sore throat warning**
If sore throat is severe, persists for more than 2 days, is accompanied or followed by fever, headache, rash, nausea, or vomiting, consult a doctor promptly.

**DO NOT USE**
- with any other product containing acetaminophen
- if you are now taking a prescription monoamine oxidase inhibitor (MAOI) (certain drugs for depression, psychiatric or emotional conditions, or Parkinson's disease), or for 2 weeks after stopping the MAOI drug. If you do not know if your prescription drug contains an MAOI, ask a doctor or pharmacist before taking this product

**ASK A DOCTOR BEFORE USE IF YOU HAVE**
- persistent or chronic cough such as occurs with smoking, asthma or emphysema
- cough that occurs with too much phlegm (mucus)

**STOP USE AND ASK A DOCTOR IF**
- pain or cough gets worse or lasts more than 7 days
- fever gets worse or lasts more than 3 days
- redness or swelling is present
- new symptoms occur
- cough comes back or occurs with rash or headache that lasts

These could be signs of a serious condition.

**If pregnant or breastfeeding,** ask a health professional before use.

**Keep out of reach of children.**

**OVERDOSE WARNING**
Taking more than the recommended dose (overdose) may cause liver damage. In case of overdose, get medical help or contact a Poison Control Center right away (1-800-222-1222). Quick medical attention is critical for adults as well as for children even if you do not notice any signs or symptoms.

**DIRECTIONS**
- do not take more than directed (see overdose warning)
- use only enclosed dosing cup designed for this product. Do not use any other dosing device

| adults and children 12 years and over | take 2 tablespoons in dose cup provided every 6 hours |
| | do not take more than 8 tablespoons in 24 hours |
| children under 12 years | do not use |
| | this will provide more than the recommended dose (overdose) and may cause liver damage |

**OTHER INFORMATION**
- each tablespoon contains: sodium 11 mg
- store between 20-25°C (68-77°F)
- do not use if plastic neck wrap or foil inner seal imprinted "Safety Seal" is broken or missing
- see back label for lot number and expiration date

**INACTIVE INGREDIENTS**
citric acid, FD&C blue no. 1, flavors, polyethylene glycol, propylene glycol, purified water, sodium benzoate, sodium carboxymethylcellulose, sorbitol, sucralose, sucrose

**QUESTIONS OR COMMENTS**
Call **1-877-895-3665** (English) or **1-888-466-8746** (Spanish)

---

# TYLENOL PM EXTRA STRENGTH
(acetaminophen and diphenhydramine hydrochloride) caplet, film coated

McNeil Consumer Healthcare, Division of McNeil-PPC, Inc.

## DRUG FACTS

| Active ingredients (in each caplet) | Purpose |
|---|---|
| Acetaminophen 500 mg | Pain reliever |
| Diphenhydramine hydrochloride 25 mg | Nighttime sleep aid |

**USES**
- temporary relief of occasional headaches and minor aches and pains with accompanying sleeplessness

**WARNINGS**
**Liver warning**
This product contains acetaminophen. Severe liver damage may occur if you take:
- more than 4,000 mg of acetaminophen in 24 hours
- with other drugs containing acetaminophen
- 3 or more alcoholic drinks every day while using this product

**DO NOT USE**
- with any other drug containing acetaminophen (prescription or nonprescription). If you are not sure whether a drug contains acetaminophen, ask a doctor or pharmacist
- with any product containing diphenhydramine, even one used on skin
- in children under 12 years of age
- if you have ever had an allergic reaction to this product or any of its ingredients

**ASK A DOCTOR BEFORE USE IF YOU HAVE**
- liver disease
- a breathing problem such as emphysema or chronic bronchitis
- trouble urinating due to an enlarged prostate gland
- glaucoma

**ASK A DOCTOR OR PHARMACIST BEFORE USE IF YOU ARE**
- taking the blood thinning drug warfarin
- taking sedatives or tranquilizers

**WHEN USING THIS PRODUCT**
- drowsiness will occur
- avoid alcoholic drinks
- do not drive a motor vehicle or operate machinery

**STOP USE AND ASK A DOCTOR IF**
- sleeplessness persists continuously for more than 2 weeks. Insomnia may be a symptom of serious underlying medical illness
- pain gets worse or lasts more than 10 days
- fever gets worse or lasts more than 3 days
- redness or swelling is present
- new symptoms occur

These could be signs of a serious condition.

**If pregnant or breastfeeding,** ask a health professional before use.

**Keep out of reach of children.**

**OVERDOSE WARNING**
Taking more than the recommended dose (overdose) may cause liver damage. In case of overdose, get medical help or contact a Poison Control Center right away (1-800-222-1222). Quick medical attention is critical for adults as well as for children even if you do not notice any signs or symptoms.

**DIRECTIONS**
- do not take more than directed (see overdose warning)

| adults and children 12 years and over | take 2 caplets at bedtime |
| | do not take more than 2 caplets of this product in 24 hours |
| children under 12 years | do not use |
| | this will provide more than the recommended dose (overdose) and may cause liver damage |

**OTHER INFORMATION**
- store between 20°C-25°C (68°F-77°F)
- do not use if carton is opened, or neck wrap or foil inner seal imprinted "Safety Seal" is broken or missing
- see end panel for lot number and expiration date

**INACTIVE INGREDIENTS**
carnauba wax, FD&C blue no. 1 aluminum lake, FD&C blue no. 2 aluminum lake, hypromellose, magnesium stearate, polyethylene glycol, polysorbate 80, powdered cellulose, pregelatinized starch, propylene glycol, shellac, sodium citrate, sodium starch glycolate, titanium dioxide

**QUESTIONS OR COMMENTS**
Call **1-877-895-3665**

---

# TYLENOL SINUS CONGESTION AND PAIN
(acetaminophen and phenylephrine hydrochloride) gelcap, coated

McNeil Consumer Healthcare, Division of McNeil-PPC, Inc.

## DRUG FACTS

| Active ingredients (in each gelcap) | Purpose |
|---|---|
| Acetaminophen 325 mg | Pain reliever |
| Phenylephrine hydrochloride 5 mg | Nasal decongestant |

## USES
- for the temporary relief of:
  - headache
  - sinus congestion and pressure
  - nasal congestion
  - minor aches and pains
- helps decongest sinus openings and passages
- promotes sinus drainage
- helps clear nasal passages

## WARNINGS
**Liver warning**
This product contains acetaminophen. Severe liver damage may occur if you take:
- more than 12 gelcaps in 24 hours, which is the maximum daily amount
- with other drugs containing acetaminophen
- 3 or more alcoholic drinks every day while using this product

## DO NOT USE
- with any other drug containing acetaminophen (prescription or nonprescription). If you are not sure whether a drug contains acetaminophen, ask a doctor or pharmacist
- if you are now taking a prescription monoamine oxidase inhibitor (MAOI) (certain drugs for depression, psychiatric or emotional conditions, or Parkinson's disease), or for 2 weeks after stopping the MAOI drug. If you do not know if your prescription drug contains an MAOI, ask a doctor or pharmacist before taking this product
- if you have ever had an allergic reaction to this product or any of its ingredients

## ASK A DOCTOR BEFORE USE IF YOU HAVE
- liver disease
- heart disease
- high blood pressure
- thyroid disease
- diabetes
- trouble urinating due to an enlarged prostate gland

## ASK A DOCTOR OR PHARMACIST BEFORE USE IF YOU ARE
- taking the blood thinning drug warfarin

## WHEN USING THIS PRODUCT
- do not exceed recommended dosage

## STOP USE AND ASK A DOCTOR IF
- nervousness, dizziness, or sleeplessness occur
- pain or nasal congestion gets worse or lasts more than 7 days
- fever gets worse or lasts more than 3 days
- redness or swelling is present
- new symptoms occur

These could be signs of a serious condition.

**If pregnant or breastfeeding,** ask a health professional before use.

**Keep out of reach of children.**

## OVERDOSE WARNING
Taking more than the recommended dose (overdose) may cause liver damage. In case of overdose, get medical help or contact a Poison Control Center right away (1-800-222-1222). Quick medical attention is critical for adults as well as for children even if you do not notice any signs or symptoms.

## DIRECTIONS
- do not take more than directed (see overdose warning)

| adults and children 12 years and over | take 2 gelcaps every 4 hours |
| | do not take more than 12 gelcaps in 24 hours |
| children under 12 years | do not use |
| | this will provide more than the recommended dose (overdose) and may cause liver damage |

## OTHER INFORMATION
- store between 20°C-25°C (68°F-77°F). Avoid high humidity
- do not use if carton is opened or if blister unit is broken
- see side panel for lot number and expiration date

## INACTIVE INGREDIENTS
benzyl alcohol, black iron oxide, butylparaben, carboxymethylcellulose sodium, colloidal silicon dioxide, corn starch, D&C yellow no. 10, edetate calcium disodium, FD&C blue no. 1, FD&C blue no. 2, FD&C red no. 40, gelatin, hypromellose, methylparaben, microcrystalline cellulose, polyethylene glycol, polysorbate 80, powdered cellulose, pregelatinized starch, propylene glycol, propylparaben, red iron oxide, sodium lauryl sulfate, sodium propionate, sodium starch glycolate, stearic acid, titanium dioxide, yellow iron oxide

## QUESTIONS OR COMMENTS
Call **1-877-895-3665**

---

# TYLENOL SORE THROAT (acetaminophen) liquid
McNeil Consumer Healthcare, Division of McNeil-PPC, Inc.

## DRUG FACTS

| Active ingredient (in each 15 mL = 1 tablespoon) | Purpose |
| --- | --- |
| Acetaminophen 500 mg | Pain reliever/fever reducer |

## USES
- temporarily relieves minor aches and pains due to:
  - the common cold
  - headache
  - sore throat
  - muscular aches
- temporarily reduces fever

## WARNINGS
**Alcohol warning**
If you consume 3 or more alcoholic drinks every day, ask your doctor whether you should take acetaminophen or other pain relievers or fever reducers. Acetaminophen may cause liver damage.

**Sore throat warning**
If sore throat is severe, persists for more than 2 days, is accompanied or followed by fever, headache, rash, nausea or vomiting, consult a doctor promptly.

## DO NOT USE
- with any other drug containing acetaminophen

## STOP USE AND ASK A DOCTOR IF
- pain gets worse or lasts more than 10 days
- fever gets worse or lasts more than 3 days
- new symptoms occur
- redness or swelling is present

These could be signs of a serious condition.

**If pregnant or breastfeeding,** ask a health professional before use.

**Keep out of reach of children.**

### OVERDOSE WARNING
Taking more than the recommended dose (overdose) may cause liver damage. In case of overdose, get medical help or contact a Poison Control Center (1-800-222-1222) right away. Quick medical attention is critical for adults as well as for children even if you do not notice any signs or symptoms.

### DIRECTIONS
- do not take more than directed (see overdose warning)
- do not take for more than 10 days unless directed by a doctor

| adults and children 12 years and over | take 2 tablespoons or 30 mL in dosing cup provided every 4 to 6 hours while symptoms last<br><br>do not take more than 8 tablespoons in 24 hours |
| --- | --- |
| children under 12 years | do not use<br><br>this will provide more than the recommended dose (overdose) and may cause liver damage |

### OTHER INFORMATION
- each tablespoon contains: sodium 11 mg
- do not use if plastic neck wrap or foil inner seal imprinted with "Safety Seal" is broken or missing
- store between 20°C-25°C (68°F-77°F)
- see back label for lot number and expiration date

### INACTIVE INGREDIENTS
citric acid, FD&C blue no. 1, flavors, polyethylene glycol, propylene glycol, purified water, sodium benzoate, sodium carboxymethylcellulose, sorbitol, sucralose, sucrose

### QUESTIONS OR COMMENTS
Call **1-877-895-3665** (English) or **1-888-466-8746** (Spanish)

---

## UNISOM SLEEP GELS (diphenhydramine hydrochloride) softgel, liquid-filled
Chattem, a Sanofi Company

### DRUG FACTS

| Active ingredient (in each softgel) | Purpose |
| --- | --- |
| Diphenhydramine hydrochloride 50 mg | Nighttime sleep-aid |

### USE
- for relief of occasional sleeplessness

### WARNINGS

**DO NOT USE**
- for children under 12 years of age
- with any other product containing diphenhydramine, even one used on skin

**ASK A DOCTOR BEFORE USE IF YOU HAVE**
- a breathing problem such as emphysema or chronic bronchitis
- glaucoma
- trouble urinating due to an enlarged prostate gland

**ASK A DOCTOR OR PHARMACIST BEFORE USE IF YOU ARE**
- taking sedatives or tranquilizers

**WHEN USING THIS PRODUCT**
- avoid alcoholic drinks

**STOP USE AND ASK DOCTOR IF**
- sleeplessness persists continuously for more than 2 weeks. insomnia may be a symptom of serious underlying medical illness

**If pregnant or breastfeeding,** ask a health professional before use.

**Keep out of reach of children.** In case of overdose, get medical help or contact a Poison Control Center right away.

### DIRECTIONS

| adults and children 12 years of age and over | one softgel (50 mg) at bedtime if needed, or as directed by a doctor |
| --- | --- |

### INACTIVE INGREDIENTS
blue 1, gelatin, glycerin, polyethylene glycol, polyvinyl acetate phthalate, propylene glycol, sorbitol, titanium dioxide, and water

---

## URISTAT URINARY PAIN RELIEF TABLETS
(phenazopyridine hydrochloride) tablet
McNeil-PPC, Inc.

### DRUG FACTS

| Active ingredient (in each tablet) | Purpose |
| --- | --- |
| Phenazopyridine hydrochloride 95 mg | Pain relief |

### USES
- relief of pain during urination
- relief of the burning feeling that often accompanies urinary infections
- relief of the urgent need to urinate, even when urine flow is minimal

### WARNINGS

**DO NOT USE**
- if you have liver or kidney trouble
- if you are allergic to phenazopyridine hydrochloride

**WHEN USING THIS PRODUCT**
- you may experience a reddish-orange discoloration of the urine
- may stain your soft contact lenses

**STOP USE AND ASK A DOCTOR IF**
- symptoms do not go away or are severe
- you experience fever, chills, back pain, or bloody urine
- you experience a yellowish tinge of the skin or eyes

**If pregnant or breastfeeding,** ask a health professional before use.

**Keep out of reach of children.** In case of overdose, get medical help or contact a Poison Control Center right away.

## DIRECTIONS

| adults and children 12 years of age and over | swallow 2 tablets with water after meals as needed up to 3 times daily for 2 days maximum |
| | do not use more than 12 tablets in 2 days |
| children under 12 years of age | ask a doctor |

## OTHER INFORMATION

- store at room temperature 15-30°C (59-86°F)
- do not purchase if carton is opened
- do not use if the individual blister unit is open or broken

## INACTIVE INGREDIENT

carnauba wax, colloidal silicon dioxide, corn starch, FD&C blue no. 2, FD&C red no. 40, gelatin, hydrogenated vegetable oil, lactose hydrous, magnesium stearate, povidone, sodium benzoate, sodium starch glycolate, sucrose, titanium dioxide, trichloroethane, white wax

# VAGISIL ANTI-ITCH ORIGINAL (benzocaine and resorcinol) cream
Combe Incorporated

## DRUG FACTS

| Active ingredients | Purpose |
| --- | --- |
| Benzocaine 5% | External analgesic |
| Resorcinol 2% | External analgesic |

## USE

- temporarily relieves itching

## WARNINGS
**For external use only.**

## DO NOT USE

- do not apply over large areas of the body
- avoid contact with eyes

## STOP USE AND ASK A DOCTOR IF

- condition worsens
- if symptoms persist for more than 7 days, or clear up and occur again within a few days

**Keep out of reach of children.** If swallowed, get medical help or contact a Poison Control Center right away.

## DIRECTIONS

| adults and children 2 years and older | apply a fingertip amount (approximately 1-inch strip) to affected area not more than 3 to 4 times daily |
| children under 2 years | consult a doctor |

## INACTIVE INGREDIENTS

water, cetyl alcohol, glyceryl stearate, PEG-100 stearate, mineral oil, isopropyl palmitate, aloe barbadensis leaf juice, tocopheryl acetate, retinyl palmitate, zea mays (corn) oil, cholecalciferol, lanolin alcohol, fragrance, methylparaben, carbomer, isopropyl myristate, isopropyl stearate, sodium sulfite, triethanolamine, trisodium HEDTA

# VAGISIL ANTI-ITCH ORIGINAL MAXIMUM STRENGTH (benzocaine and resorcinol) cream
Combe Incorporated

## DRUG FACTS

| Active ingredients | Purpose |
| --- | --- |
| Benzocaine 20% | External analgesic |
| Resorcinol 3% | External analgesic |

## USE

- temporarily relieves itching

## WARNINGS
**For external use only.**

## DO NOT USE

- do not apply over large areas of the body
- avoid contact with eyes

## STOP USE AND ASK A DOCTOR IF

- condition worsens
- if symptoms persist for more than 7 days, or clear up and occur again within a few days

**Keep out of reach of children.** If swallowed, get medical help or contact a Poison Control Center right away

## DIRECTIONS

| adults and children 12 years and older | apply a fingertip amount (approximately 1-inch strip) to affected area not more than 3 to 4 times daily |
| children under 12 years | consult a doctor |

## INACTIVE INGREDIENTS

water, mineral oil, cetyl alcohol, propylene glycol, glyceryl stearate, PEG-100 stearate, isopropyl palmitate, aloe barbadensis leaf juice, tocopheryl acetate, retinyl palmitate, zea mays (corn) oil, cholecalciferol, lanolin alcohol, fragrance, methylparaben, carbomer, isopropyl myristate, isopropyl stearate, sodium sulfite, triethanolamine, trisodium HEDTA

# VAGISIL MEDICATED WIPES (pramoxine hydrochloride) cloth towelette
Combe Laboratories, Inc.

## DRUG FACTS

| Active ingredients | Purpose |
| --- | --- |
| Pramoxine hydrochloride 1% w/w | External analgesic towelette |

## USE

- temporarily relieves itching

## WARNINGS
**For external use only.**

## DO NOT USE

- avoid contact with eyes

**STOP USE AND ASK A DOCTOR IF**
- condition worsens
- if symptoms persist for more than 7 days or clear up and occur again within a few days

**Keep out of reach of children.** If swallowed, get medical help or contact a Poison Control Center right away.

**DIRECTIONS**

| adults and children 12 years of age and older | unfold towelette and gently pat or wipe external vaginal area from front to back |
| | use each towelette only once and then throw away |
| | apply to affected area not more than 3 to 4 times daily |
| children under 12 years | consult a doctor |

**INACTIVE INGREDIENT**
water, polysorbate 20, glycerin, phenoxyethanol, disodium cocoamphodiacetate, TEA-cocoyl glutamate, methylparaben, fragrance, ethylparaben, disodium EDTA, PEG-7 glyceryl cocoate, aloe barbadensis leaf juice, tocopheryl (Vitamin E) acetate, zea mays (corn) oil, retinyl (Vitamin A) palmitate, cholecalciferol (Vitamin D)

---

# VAGISIL SATIN (hydrocortisone acetate) cream
## Combe Incorporated

**DRUG FACTS**

| Active ingredients | Purpose |
| --- | --- |
| Hydrocortisone acetate 1% | External Analgesic |

**USES**
- temporarily relieves itching associated with minor skin irritation, inflammation and rashes due to:
  - external feminine itching
  - anal itching

**WARNINGS**
**For external use only.**

**DO NOT USE**
- if you have vaginal discharge without consulting a doctor
- for the treatment of diaper rash without consulting a doctor
- avoid contact with eyes

**WHEN USING THIS PRODUCT FOR ANAL ITCHING**
- do not exceed the recommended daily dosage unless directed by a doctor
- in case of bleeding, consult a doctor promptly
- do not put this product in the rectum by using fingers, a mechanical device or applicator

**STOP USE AND ASK A DOCTOR IF**
- condition worsens
- symptoms last more than 7 days or clear up and occur again within a few days

**Keep out of reach of children.** If swallowed, get medical help or contact a Poison Control Center immediately

**DIRECTIONS**
- for external feminine itching

| adults and children 2 years and older | apply to affected area not more than 3 to 4 times daily |
| children under 2 years | do not use; ask a doctor |

- for anal itching

| adults and children 12 years and older | when practical, cleanse the affected area with mild soap and warm water and rinse thoroughly |
| | gently dry by patting or blotting with toilet tissue or soft cloth before application of this product |
| | apply to affected area not more than 3 to 4 times daily |
| children under 12 years | ask a doctor |

**INACTIVE INGREDIENTS**
water, cetyl ethylhexanoate, glycerin, PEG-40 hydrogenated castor oil, glyceryl dilaurate, phenoxyethanol, sodium polyacrylate, dimethicone, ceteareth-20, glyceryl oleate, methylparaben, triethanolamine, acrylates/C10-30 alkyl acrylates crosspolymer, cyclopentasiloxane, fragrance, ethylparaben, trideceth-6, disodium EDTA, PEG/PEG-18/18 dimethicone, tocopheryl (vitamin E) acetate, zea mays (corn) oil, retinyl palmitate (vitamin A) acetate, cholecalciferol (vitamin D3), aloe barbadensis

---

# VAGISTAT (miconazole nitrate) cream, suppository
## Novartis Consumer Health, Inc.

**DRUG FACTS**

| Active ingredients | Purpose |
| --- | --- |
| Miconazole nitrate (200 mg in each suppository) | Vaginal antifungal |
| Miconazole nitrate 2% (external cream) | Vaginal antifungal |

**USES**
- treats vaginal yeast infections
- relieves external itching and irritation due to a vaginal yeast infection

**WARNINGS**
**For vaginal use only.**

**DO NOT USE**
- if you have never had a vaginal yeast infection diagnosed by a doctor

**ASK A DOCTOR BEFORE USE IF YOU HAVE**
- vaginal itching and discomfort for the first time
- lower abdominal, back or shoulder pain, fever, chills, nausea, vomiting, or foul-smelling vaginal discharge. You may have a more serious condition
- vaginal yeast infections often (such as once a month or 3 in 6 months). You could be pregnant or have a serious underlying medical cause for your symptoms, including diabetes or a weakened immune system
- been exposed to the human immunodeficiency virus (HIV) that causes AIDS

**ASK A DOCTOR OR PHARMACIST BEFORE USE IF YOU ARE**
- taking a prescription blood thinning medicine, such as warfarin, because bleeding or bruising may occur

**WHEN USING THIS PRODUCT**
- do not use tampons, douches, spermicides or other vaginal products. Condoms and diaphragms may be damaged and fail to prevent pregnancy or sexually transmitted diseases (STDs)
- do not have vaginal intercourse
- mild increase in vaginal burning, itching or irritation may occur

**STOP USE AND ASK A DOCTOR IF**
- symptoms do not get better in 3 days
- symptoms last more than 7 days
- you get a rash or hives, abdominal pain, fever, chills, nausea, vomiting, or foul-smelling vaginal discharge

**If pregnant or breastfeeding,** ask a health professional before use.

**Keep out of reach of children.** If swallowed, get medical help or contact a Poison Control Center right away.

**DIRECTIONS**

| adults and children 12 years and over | **suppositories:** insert 1 suppository into the vagina at bedtime for 3 nights in a row. Throw applicator away after use |
| | **external cream:** squeeze a small amount of cream onto your fingertip |
| | apply the cream onto the itchy, irritated skin outside the vagina |
| | use 2 times daily for up to 7 days, as needed |
| children under 12 years of age | ask a doctor |

**OTHER INFORMATION**
- do not use if printed suppository wrapper is missing or damaged (each suppository is individually wrapped)
- do not use if seal over tube opening has been punctured or cannot be seen
- do not purchase if carton is open
- store at 20-25°C (68-77°F). Avoid heat over 25°C (77°F)

**INACTIVE INGREDIENTS (SUPPOSITORY)**
**suppository:** hydrogenated vegetable oil

**INACTIVE INGREDIENTS (CREAM)**
**external cream:** benzoic acid, butylated hydroxyanisole, glyceryl stearate, mineral oil, peglicol 5 oleate, pegoxol 7 stearate, purified water

**QUESTIONS OR COMMENTS**
Call **1-888-824-4782**

# VASELINE PETROLEUM JELLY DEEP MOISTURE (petroleum) cream

Conopco Inc. D/B/A Unilever

## DRUG FACTS

| Active ingredient | Purpose |
|---|---|
| White petrolatum, USP (30%) | skin protectant |

**WARNINGS**
**For external use only.**

**DO NOT USE ON**
- deep or puncture wounds
- animal bites
- serious burns

**WHEN USING THIS PRODUCT**
- do not get in eyes

**STOP USE AND ASK A DOCTOR IF**
- condition worsens
- symptoms last more than 7 days or clear up and occur again within a few days

**Keep out of reach of children.** If swallowed get medical help or contact a Poison Control Center right away.

**QUESTIONS OR COMMENTS**
Contact the Consumer Information Center **1-800-457-7084**

# VICKS DAYQUIL COLD & FLU RELIEF LIQUICAPS (acetaminophen, dextromethorphan hydrobromide, and phenylephrine hydrochloride) capsules, liquid filled

Procter & Gamble

## DRUG FACTS

| Active ingredients (in each LiquiCap) | Purpose |
|---|---|
| Acetaminophen 325 mg | Pain reliever/fever reducer |
| Dextromethorphan hydrobromide 10 mg | Cough suppressant |
| Phenylephrine hydrochloride 5 mg | Nasal decongestant |

**USES**
- temporarily relieves common cold and flu symptoms:
  - nasal congestion
  - cough due to minor throat and bronchial irritation
  - sore throat
  - headache
  - minor aches and pains
  - fever

**WARNINGS**
**Liver warning**
This product contains acetaminophen. Severe liver damage may occur if you take:
- more than 4 doses in 24 hours, which is the maximum daily amount for this product
- with other drugs containing acetaminophen
- 3 or more alcoholic drinks daily while using this product

**Sore throat warning:**
If sore throat is severe, lasts for more than 2 days, occurs with or is followed by fever, headache, rash, nausea, or vomiting, see a doctor promptly.

**DO NOT USE**
- with any other drug containing acetaminophen (prescription or nonprescription). If you are not sure whether a drug contains acetaminophen, ask a doctor or pharmacist
- if you are now taking a prescription monoamine oxidase inhibitor (MAOI) (certain drugs for depression, psychiatric or emotional conditions, or Parkinson's disease), or for 2 weeks after stopping the MAOI drug. If you do not know if your prescription drug contains an MAOI, ask a doctor or pharmacist before taking this product

## ASK A DOCTOR BEFORE USE IF YOU HAVE
- liver disease
- heart disease
- thyroid disease
- diabetes
- high blood pressure
- trouble urinating due to enlarged prostate gland
- cough that occurs with too much phlegm (mucus)
- persistent or chronic cough as occurs with smoking, asthma, or emphysema

## ASK A DOCTOR OR PHARMACIST BEFORE USE IF YOU ARE
- taking the blood-thinning drug warfarin

## WHEN USING THIS PRODUCT
- do not use more than directed

## STOP USE AND ASK A DOCTOR IF
- you get nervous, dizzy, or sleepless
- symptoms get worse or last more than 7 days
- fever gets worse or lasts more than 3 days
- redness or swelling is present
- new symptoms occur
- cough comes back, or occurs with rash or headache that lasts

These could be signs of a serious condition.

**If pregnant or breastfeeding,** ask a health professional before use.

**Keep out of reach of children.**

## OVERDOSE WARNING
Taking more than directed can cause serious health problems. In case of overdose, get medical help or contact a Poison Control Center right away. Quick medical attention is critical for adults and for children, even if you do not notice any signs or symptoms.

## DIRECTIONS
- take only as directed—see overdose warning
- do not exceed 4 doses per 24 hours

| adults and children 12 years and over | 2 LiquiCaps with water every 4 hours |
| children 4 to under 12 years | ask a doctor |
| children under 4 years | do not use |

## INACTIVE INGREDIENTS
FD&C red no. 40, FD&C yellow no. 6, gelatin, glycerin, polyethylene glycol, povidone, propylene glycol, purified water, sorbito special, titanium dioxide

## OTHER INFORMATION
- Store at room temperature

## QUESTIONS OR COMMENTS
Call **1-800-251-3374.**

# VICKS DAYQUIL COLD AND FLU
(acetaminophen, dextromethorphan hydrobromide, and phenylephrine hydrochloride) liquid

The Procter & Gamble Manufacturing Company

## DRUG FACTS

| Active ingredients (in each 15 mL tablespoon) | Purpose |
| --- | --- |
| Acetaminophen 325 mg | Pain reliever/fever reducer |
| Dextromethorphan hydrobromide 10 mg | Cough suppressant |
| Phenylephrine hydrochloride 5 mg | Nasal decongestant |

## USES
- temporarily relieves common cold/flu symptoms:
  - nasal congestion
  - cough due to minor throat & bronchial irritation
  - sore throat
  - headache
  - minor aches & pains
  - fever

## WARNINGS
**Liver warning**
This product contains acetaminophen. Severe liver damage may occur if adult/child takes:
- more than 4 doses in 24 hours, which is the maximum daily amount for this product
- with other drugs containing acetaminophen
- adult has 3 or more alcoholic drinks every day while using this product

**Sore throat warning**
If sore throat is severe, lasts for more than 2 days, occurs with or is followed by fever, headache, rash, nausea, or vomiting, see a doctor promptly.

## DO NOT USE
- with any other drug containing acetaminophen (prescription or nonprescription). If you are not sure whether a drug contains acetaminophen, ask a doctor or pharmacist
- if you are now taking a prescription monoamine oxidase inhibitor (MAOI) (certain drugs for depression, psychiatric or emotional conditions, or Parkinson's disease), or for 2 weeks after stopping the MAOI drug. If you do not know if your prescription drug contains an MAOI, ask a doctor or pharmacist before taking this product

## ASK A DOCTOR BEFORE USE IF YOU HAVE
- liver disease
- heart disease
- thyroid disease
- diabetes
- high blood pressure
- trouble urinating due to enlarged prostate gland
- cough that occurs with too much phlegm (mucus)
- persistent or chronic cough as occurs with smoking, asthma, or emphysema
- a sodium-restricted diet

## ASK A DOCTOR OR PHARMACIST BEFORE USE IF YOU ARE
- taking the blood thinning drug warfarin

## WHEN USING THIS PRODUCT
- do not use more than directed

## STOP USE AND ASK A DOCTOR IF
- you get nervous, dizzy or sleepless
- symptoms get worse or last more than 5 days (children) or 7 days (adults)
- fever gets worse or lasts more than 3 days
- redness or swelling is present
- new symptoms occur
- cough comes back, or occurs with rash or headache that lasts. These could be signs of a serious condition

**If pregnant or breastfeeding,** ask a health professional before use.

**Keep out of reach of children.**

## OVERDOSE WARNING
Taking more than directed can cause serious health problems. In case of overdose, get medical help or contact a Poison Control Center right away. Quick medical attention is critical for adults & for children even if you do not notice any signs or symptoms.

## DIRECTIONS
- take only as directed - see Overdose warning
- use dose cup or tablespoon (tbsp)
- do not exceed 4 doses per 24 hrs

| adults and children 12 yrs & over | 30 mL (2 tbsp) every 4 hrs |
|---|---|
| children 6 to under 12 yrs | 15 mL (1 tbsp) every 4 hrs |
| children 4 to under 6 yrs | ask a doctor |
| children under 4 yrs | do not use |

## OTHER INFORMATION
- each tablespoon contains: sodium 50 mg
- store at room temperature

## INACTIVE INGREDIENTS
carboxymethylcellulose sodium, citric acid, disodium EDTA, FD&C Yellow no. 6, flavor, glycerin, propylene glycol, purified water, saccharin sodium, sodium benzoate, sodium chloride, sodium citrate, sorbitol, sucralose

## QUESTIONS OR COMMENTS
Call **1-800-251-3374** or visit www.vicks.com

---

# VICKS DAYQUIL COUGH (dextromethorphan hydrobromide) liquid
The Procter & Gamble Manufacturing Company

## DRUG FACTS

| Active ingredient (in each 15 mL tablespoon) | Purpose |
|---|---|
| Dextromethorphan hydrobromide 15 mg | Cough suppressant |

## USE
- temporarily relieves cough due to minor throat and bronchial irritation

---

## WARNINGS
### DO NOT USE
- if you are now taking a prescription monoamine oxidase inhibitor (MAOI) (certain drugs for depression, psychiatric or emotional conditions, or Parkinson's disease), or for 2 weeks after stopping the MAOI drug. If you do not know if your prescription drug contains an MAOI, ask a doctor or pharmacist before taking this product

## ASK A DOCTOR BEFORE USE IF YOU HAVE
- cough that occurs with too much phlegm (mucus)
- persistent or chronic cough such as occurs with smoking, asthma, or emphysema

## WHEN USING THIS PRODUCT
- do not use more than directed

## STOP USE AND ASK A DOCTOR IF
- cough lasts more than 7 days, comes back, or occurs with fever, rash, or headache that lasts. These could be signs of a serious condition

**If pregnant or breastfeeding,** ask a health professional before use.

**Keep out of reach of children.** In case of overdose, get medical help or contact a Poison Control Center right away.

## DIRECTIONS
- take only as recommended
- use dose cup or tablespoon (tbsp)
- do not exceed 4 doses per 24 hours

| adults and children 12 years and over | 30 mL (2 tbsp) every 6-8 hours |
|---|---|
| children 6 to under 12 years | 15 mL (1 tbsp) every 6-8 hours |
| children 4 to under 6 years | ask a doctor |
| children under 4 years | do not use |

## OTHER INFORMATION
- each tablespoon contains: sodium 15 mg
- store at room temperature

## INACTIVE INGREDIENTS
citric acid, D&C yellow no. 10, FD&C yellow no. 6, flavor, high fructose corn syrup, polyethylene glycol, propylene glycol, purified water, saccharin sodium, sodium citrate

## QUESTIONS OR COMMENTS
Call **1-800-251-3374**

---

# VICKS DAYQUIL MUCUS CONTROL
(guaifenesin) liquid
Procter & Gamble Manufacturing Company

## DRUG FACTS

| Active ingredient (in each 15 ml tablespoon) | Purpose |
|---|---|
| Guaifenesin 200 mg | Expectorant |

## USE
- helps loosen phlegm (mucus) and thin bronchial secretions to rid the bronchial passageways of bothersome mucus

## WARNINGS

### ASK A DOCTOR BEFORE USE IF YOU HAVE
- a sodium-restricted diet
- persistent or chronic cough such as occurs with smoking, asthma, chronic bronchitis, or emphysema
- cough that occurs with too much phlegm (mucus)

### STOP USE AND ASK A DOCTOR IF
- cough lasts more than 7 days, comes back, or occurs with fever, rash, or headache that lasts. These could be signs of a serious condition

**If pregnant or breastfeeding,** ask a health professional before use.

**Keep out of reach of children.** In case of overdose, get medical help or contact a Poison Control Center right away.

### DIRECTIONS
- use dose cup or tablespoon (tbsp)
- do not exceed 6 doses per 24 hours

| adults and children 12 years and over | 30 ml (2 tbsp) every 4 hours |
|---|---|
| children 6 to under 12 years | 15 ml (1 tbsp) every 4 hours |
| children 4 to under 6 years | ask a doctor |
| children under 4 years | do not use |

### OTHER INFORMATION
- each tablespoon contains: sodium 25 mg
- store at room temperature

### INACTIVE INGREDIENTS
carboxymethylcellulose sodium, citric acid, D&C yellow no. 10, FD&C yellow no. 6, flavor, high fructose corn syrup, propylene glycol, purified water, saccharin sodium, sodium benzoate, sodium citrate

### QUESTIONS OR COMMENTS
Call **1-800-251-3374** or visit www.vicks.com

---

# VICKS DAYQUIL MUCUS CONTROL DM
(dextromethorphan hydrobromide and guaifenesin) liquid
Procter & Gamble Manufacturing Company

## DRUG FACTS

| Active ingredients (in each 15 mL tablespoon) | Purpose |
|---|---|
| Dextromethorphan hydrobromide 10 mg | Cough suppressant |
| Guaifenesin 200 mg | Expectorant |

### USES
- temporarily relieves cough associated with the common cold
- helps loosen phlegm and thin bronchial secretions to rid the bronchial passageways of bothersome mucus

### WARNINGS

### DO NOT USE
- if you are now taking a prescription monoamine oxidase inhibitor (MAOI) (certain drugs for depression, psychiatric or emotional conditions, or Parkinson's disease), or for 2 weeks after stopping the MAOI drug. If you do not know if your prescription drug contains an MAOI, ask a doctor or pharmacist before taking this product

### ASK A DOCTOR BEFORE USE IF YOU HAVE
- persistent or chronic cough such as occurs with smoking, asthma, chronic bronchitis, or emphysema
- cough that occurs with too much phlegm (mucus)
- a sodium-restricted diet

### STOP USE AND ASK A DOCTOR IF
- cough lasts more than 7 days, comes back, or occurs with fever, rash, or headache that lasts. These could be signs of a serious condition

**If pregnant or breastfeeding,** ask a health professional before use.

**Keep out of reach of children.** In case of overdose, get medical help or contact a Poison Control Center right away.

### DIRECTIONS
- use dose cup or tablespoon (tbsp)
- do not exceed 6 doses per 24 hours

| adults and children 12 years and over | 30 mL (2 tbsp) every 4 hours |
|---|---|
| children 6 to under 12 years | 15 mL (1 tbsp) every 4 hours |
| children 4 to under 6 years | ask a doctor |
| children under 4 years | do not use |

### OTHER INFORMATION
- each tablespoon contains: sodium 25 mg
- store at room temperature

### INACTIVE INGREDIENTS
carboxymethylcellulose sodium, citric acid, D&C yellow no. 10, FD&C yellow no. 6, flavor, high fructose corn syrup, propylene glycol, purified water, saccharin sodium, sodium benzoate, sodium citrate

### QUESTIONS OR COMMENTS
Call **1-800-251-3374** or visit www.vicks.com

---

# VICKS DAYQUIL SINEX DAYTIME SINUS RELIEF (acetaminophen and phenylephrine hydrochloride) capsule, liquid filled
Procter & Gamble Manufacturing Company

## DRUG FACTS

| Active ingredients (in each LiquiCap) | Purpose |
|---|---|
| Acetaminophen 325 mg | Pain reliever |
| Phenylephrine hydrochloride 5 mg | Nasal decongestant |

### USES
- temporarily relieves sinus symptoms:
  - sinus pain
  - headache
  - nasal & sinus congestion

### WARNINGS
**Liver warning**
This product contains acetaminophen. Severe liver damage may occur if you take:
- more than 4 doses in 24 hrs, which is the maximum daily amount for this product
- with other drugs containing acetaminophen
- 3 or more alcoholic drinks daily while using this product

## DO NOT USE

- with any other drug containing acetaminophen (prescription or nonprescription). If you are not sure whether a drug contains acetaminophen, ask a doctor or pharmacist
- if you are now taking a prescription monoamine oxidase inhibitor (MAOI) (certain drugs for depression, psychiatric or emotional conditions, or Parkinson's disease), or for 2 weeks after stopping the MAOI drug. If you do not know if your prescription drug contains an MAOI, ask a doctor or pharmacist before taking this product

## ASK A DOCTOR BEFORE USE IF YOU HAVE

- liver disease
- heart disease
- thyroid disease
- diabetes
- high blood pressure
- trouble urinating due to enlarged prostate gland

## ASK A DOCTOR OR PHARMACIST BEFORE USE IF YOU ARE

- taking the blood thinning drug warfarin

## WHEN USING THIS PRODUCT

- do not use more than directed

## STOP USE AND ASK A DOCTOR IF

- redness or swelling is present
- you get nervous, dizzy or sleepless
- fever gets worse or lasts more than 3 days
- new symptoms occur
- symptoms do not get better within 7 days or are accompanied by a fever

**If pregnant or breastfeeding,** ask a health professional before use.

**Keep out of reach of children.**

## OVERDOSE WARNING

Taking more than directed can cause serious health problems. In case of overdose, get medical help or contact a Poison Control Center right away. Quick medical attention is critical for adults & for children even if you do not notice any signs or symptoms.

## DIRECTIONS

- take only as directed - see Overdose warning
- do not exceed 4 doses per 24 hrs

| adults & children 12 yrs and over | 2 LiquiCaps with water every 4 hrs |
|---|---|
| children 4 to under 12 yrs | ask a doctor |
| children under 4 yrs | do not use |

## OTHER INFORMATION

- store at room temperature

## INACTIVE INGREDIENTS

FD&C yellow no. 6, gelatin, glycerin, polyethylene glycol, povidone, propylene glycol, purified water, sorbitol special, titanium dioxide

## QUESTIONS OR COMMENTS

Call **1-800-251-3374**

---

# VICKS FORMULA 44 CUSTOM CARE CHESTY COUGH (dextromethorphan hydrobromide, guaifenesin) liquid

Procter & Gamble

## DRUG FACTS

| Active ingredients (in each 15 mL = 1 tablespoon) | Purpose |
|---|---|
| Dextromethorphan hydrobromide 20 mg | Cough suppressant |
| Guaifenesin 200 mg | Expectorant |

## WARNINGS

### DO NOT USE

- if you are now taking a prescription monoamine oxidase inhibitor (MAOI) (certain drugs for depression, psychiatric or emotional conditions, or Parkinson's disease), or for 2 weeks after stopping the MAOI drug. If you do not know if your prescription drug contains an MAOI, ask a doctor or pharmacist before taking this product

### ASK A DOCTOR BEFORE USE IF YOU HAVE:

- a sodium-restricted diet
- persistent or chronic cough such as occurs with smoking, asthma, chronic bronchitis, or emphysema
- cough that occurs with too much phlegm (mucus)

### STOP USE AND ASK A DOCTOR IF

- Cough lasts more than 7 days, comes back, or occurs with fever, rash, or headache that lasts

These could be signs of a serious condition.

**If pregnant or breastfeeding,** ask a health professional before use.

**Keep out of reach of children.** In case of overdose, get medical help or contact a Poison Control Center right away.

## DIRECTIONS

- use dose cup, teaspoon (tsp), or tablespoon (tbsp)
- do not exceed 6 doses per 24 hours

| adults and children 12 years and over | 15 mL (1 tbsp) every 4 hours |
|---|---|
| children 6 to under 12 years | 7½ ml (1½ tsp) every 4 hours |
| children 4 to under 6 years | ask a doctor |
| children under 4 years | do not use |

## INACTIVE INGREDIENTS

carboxymethylcellulose sodium, citric acid, FD&C red no. 40, flavor, high fructose corn syrup, propylene glycol, purified water, saccharin sodium, sodium benzoate, sodium citrate

## OTHER INFORMATION

- each tablespoon contains: sodium 26 mg
- store at room temperature
- do not use if printed shrinkband is missing or broken

## QUESTIONS OR COMMENTS

Call **1-800-342-6844**

# VICKS FORMULA 44 CUSTOM CARE CONGESTION (acetaminophen, chlorpheniramine maleate, dextromethorphan hydrobromide) liquid

Procter & Gamble

## DRUG FACTS

| Active ingredients (in each 15 mL tablespoon) | Purpose |
|---|---|
| Acetaminophen 650 mg | Pain reliever/fever reducer |
| Chlorpheniramine maleate 4 mg | Antihistamine |
| Dextromethorphan hydrobromide 30 mg | Cough suppressant |

## WARNINGS

### Liver warning

This product contains acetaminophen. Severe liver damage may occur if you take:
- more than 4 doses in 24 hours, which is the maximum daily amount for this product
- with other drugs containing acetaminophen
- 3 or more alcoholic drinks every day

### Sore throat warning

If sore throat is severe, lasts for more than 2 days, occurs with or is followed by a fever, headache, rash, nausea, or vomiting, see a doctor promptly.

## DO NOT USE

- with any other drug containing acetaminophen (prescription or nonprescription). If you are not sure whether a drug contains acetaminophen, ask a doctor or pharmacist
- if you are now taking a prescription monoamine oxidase inhibitor (MAOI) (certain drugs for depression, psychiatric or emotional conditions, or Parkinson's disease), or for 2 weeks after stopping the MAOI drug. If you do not know if your prescription drug contains an MAOI, ask a doctor or pharmacist before taking this product
- to make a child sleep

## ASK A DOCTOR BEFORE USE IF YOU HAVE

- liver disease
- glaucoma
- cough that occurs with too much phlegm (mucus)
- a breathing problem or chronic cough that lasts or as occurs with smoking, asthma, chronic bronchitis, or emphysema
- trouble urinating due to enlarged prostate gland

## ASK A DOCTOR OR PHARMACIST BEFORE USE IF YOU ARE

- taking sedatives or tranquilizers
- taking the blood-thinning drug warfarin

## WHEN USING THIS PRODUCT

- do not use more than directed
- excitability may occur, especially in children
- marked drowsiness may occur
- avoid alcoholic drinks
- be careful when driving a motor vehicle or operating machinery
- alcohol, sedatives, and tranquilizers may increase drowsiness

## STOP USE AND ASK A DOCTOR IF

- pain or cough gets worse or lasts more than 7 days
- fever gets worse or lasts more than 3 days
- redness or swelling is present
- new symptoms occur
- cough comes back, or occurs with rash or headache that lasts

These could be signs of a serious condition.

**If pregnant or breastfeeding,** ask a health professional before use.

**Keep out of reach of children.**

## OVERDOSE WARNING

Taking more than directed can cause serious health problems. In case of overdose, get medical help or contact a Poison Control Center right away. Quick medical attention is critical for adults and for children even if you do not notice any signs or symptoms.

## DIRECTIONS

- take only as recommended—see overdose warning
- use dose cup or tablespoon (tbsp)
- do not exceed 4 doses per 24 hours

| adults and children 12 years and over | 15 mL (1 tbsp) every 6 hours |
|---|---|
| children 4 to under 12 years | ask a doctor |
| children under 4 years | do not use |

## INACTIVE INGREDIENTS

acesulfame potassium, carboxymethylcellulose sodium, citric acid. FD&C red no. 40, flavor, high fructose corn syrup, polyethylene glycol, propylene glycol, purified water, saccharin sodium, sodium benzoate, sodium citrate, sucralose

## OTHER INFORMATION

- each tablespoon contains sodium 26 mg
- store at room temperature

## QUESTIONS OR COMMENTS

Call **1-800-342-6844**

# VICKS NYQUIL COLD AND FLU

(acetaminophen, dextromethorphan hydrobromide, and doxylamine succinate) capsule, liquid filled

The Procter & Gamble Manufacturing Company

## DRUG FACTS

| Active ingredients (in each LiquiCap) | Purpose |
|---|---|
| Acetaminophen 325 mg | Pain reliever/fever reducer |
| Dextromethorphan hydrobromide 15 mg | Cough suppressant |
| Doxylamine succinate 6.25 mg | Antihistamine |

## USES

- temporarily relieves common cold/flu symptoms:
  - cough due to minor throat & bronchial irritation
  - sore throat
  - headache
  - minor aches & pains
  - fever
  - runny nose & sneezing

## WARNINGS

**Liver warning**

This product contains acetaminophen. Severe liver damage may occur if you take:

- more than 4 doses in 24 hrs, which is the maximum daily amount for this product
- with other drugs containing acetaminophen
- 3 or more alcoholic drinks daily while using this product

**Sore throat warning**

If sore throat is severe, lasts for more than 2 days, occurs with or is followed by fever, headache, rash, nausea, or vomiting, see a doctor promptly.

## DO NOT USE

- with any other drug containing acetaminophen (prescription or nonprescription). If you are not sure whether a drug contains acetaminophen, ask a doctor or pharmacist
- if you are now taking a prescription monoamine oxidase inhibitor (MAOI) (certain drugs for depression, psychiatric or emotional conditions, or Parkinson's disease), or for 2 weeks after stopping the MAOI drug. If you do not know if your prescription drug contains an MAOI, ask a doctor or pharmacist before taking this product
- to make a child sleep

## ASK A DOCTOR BEFORE USE IF YOU HAVE

- liver disease
- glaucoma
- cough that occurs with too much phlegm (mucus)
- a breathing problem or chronic cough that lasts or as occurs with smoking, asthma, chronic bronchitis or emphysema
- trouble urinating due to enlarged prostate gland

## ASK A DOCTOR OR PHARMACIST BEFORE USE IF YOU ARE

- taking sedatives or tranquilizers
- taking the blood thinning drug warfarin

## WHEN USING THIS PRODUCT

- do not use more than directed
- excitability may occur, especially in children
- marked drowsiness may occur
- avoid alcoholic drinks
- be careful when driving a motor vehicle or operating machinery
- alcohol, sedatives, & tranquilizers may increase drowsiness

## STOP USE AND ASK A DOCTOR IF

- pain or cough gets worse or lasts more than 7 days
- fever gets worse or lasts more than 3 days
- redness or swelling is present
- new symptoms occur
- cough comes back or occurs with rash or headache that lasts. These could be signs of a serious condition

**If pregnant or breastfeeding,** ask a health professional before use.

**Keep out of reach of children.**

## OVERDOSE WARNING

Taking more than directed can cause serious health problems. In case of overdose, get medical help or contact a Poison Control Center right away. Quick medical attention is critical for adults and for children even if you do not notice any signs or symptoms.

## DIRECTIONS

- take only as directed see overdose warning
- do not exceed 4 doses per 24 hrs

| adults & children 12 yrs and over | 2 LiquiCaps with water every 6 hrs |
| children 4 to under 12 yrs | ask a doctor |
| children under 4 yrs | do not use |

## OTHER INFORMATION

- store at room temperature

## INACTIVE INGREDIENTS

D&C yellow no. 10, FD&C blue no. 1, gelatin, glycerin, polyethylene glycol, povidone, propylene glycol, purified water, sorbitol special, titanium dioxide

## QUESTIONS OR COMMENTS

Call **1-800-362-1683**

---

# VICKS NYQUIL COUGH (dextromethorphan hydrobromide and doxylamine succinate) liquid

The Procter & Gamble Manufacturing Company

## DRUG FACTS

| Active ingredients (in each 30 mL dose cup) | Purpose |
| --- | --- |
| Dextromethorphan hydrobromide 30 mg | Cough suppressant |
| Doxylamine succinate 12.5 mg | Antihistamine |

## USES

- temporarily relieves cold symptoms:
  - cough
  - runny nose and sneezing

## WARNINGS

## DO NOT USE

- if you are now taking a prescription monoamine oxidase inhibitor (MAOI) (certain drugs for depression, psychiatric or emotional conditions, or Parkinson's disease), or for 2 weeks after stopping the MAOI drug. If you do not know if your prescription drug contains an MAOI, ask a doctor or pharmacist before taking this product
- to make a child sleep

## ASK A DOCTOR BEFORE USE IF YOU HAVE

- glaucoma
- excessive phlegm (mucus)
- a breathing problem or chronic cough that lasts or as occurs with smoking, asthma, chronic bronchitis or emphysema
- trouble urinating due to enlarged prostate gland
- a sodium-restricted diet

## ASK A DOCTOR OR PHARMACIST BEFORE USE IF YOU ARE

- taking sedatives or tranquilizers

## WHEN USING THIS PRODUCT
- do not use more than directed
- excitability may occur, especially in children
- marked drowsiness may occur
- avoid alcoholic drinks
- be careful when driving a motor vehicle or operating machinery
- alcohol, sedatives, and tranquilizers may increase drowsiness

## STOP USE AND ASK A DOCTOR IF
- cough lasts more than 7 days, comes back, or occurs with fever, rash, or headache that lasts. These could be signs of a serious condition

**If pregnant or breastfeeding,** ask a health professional before use.

**Keep out of reach of children.** In case of overdose, get medical help or contact a Poison Control Center right away.

## DIRECTIONS
- use dose cup or tablespoon (tbsp)
- do not exceed 4 doses per 24 hrs

| adults & children 12 yrs & over | 30 mL (2 tbsp) every 6 hrs |
| --- | --- |
| children 4 to under 12 yrs | ask a doctor |
| children under 4 yrs | do not use |

## OTHER INFORMATION
- each 30 mL dose cup contains: sodium 36 mg
- store at room temperature

## INACTIVE INGREDIENTS
alcohol, citric acid, FD&C blue no. 1, FD&C red no. 40, flavor, high fructose corn syrup, polyethylene glycol, propylene glycol, purified water, saccharin sodium, sodium citrate

## QUESTIONS OR COMMENTS
Call **1-800-362-1683**

---

# VICKS ALCOHOL FREE NYQUIL COLD AND FLU (acetaminophen, chlorpheniramine maleate, and dextromethorphan hydrobromide) liquid
Procter & Gamble Manufacturing Company

## DRUG FACTS

| Active ingredients (in each 30 mL dose cup) | Purpose |
| --- | --- |
| Acetaminophen 650 mg | Pain reliever/fever reducer |
| Chlorpheniramine maleate 4 mg | Antihistamine |
| Dextromethorphan hydrobromide 30 mg | Cough suppressant |

## USES
- temporarily relieves common cold/flu symptoms:
  - cough due to minor throat and bronchial irritation
  - sore throat
  - headache
  - minor aches and pains
  - fever
  - runny nose and sneezing

## WARNINGS
**Liver warning**
This product contains acetaminophen. Severe liver damage may occur if you take:
- more than 4 doses in 24 hours, which is the maximum daily amount for this product
- with other drugs containing acetaminophen
- 3 or more alcoholic drinks daily while using this product

**Sore throat warning**
If sore throat is severe, lasts for more than 2 days, occurs with or is followed by fever, headache, rash, nausea, or vomiting, see a doctor promptly.

## DO NOT USE
- with any other drug containing acetaminophen (prescription or nonprescription). If you are not sure whether a drug contains acetaminophen, ask a doctor or pharmacist
- if you are now taking a prescription monoamine oxidase inhibitor (MAOI) (certain drugs for depression, psychiatric or emotional conditions, or Parkinson's disease), or for 2 weeks after stopping the MAOI drug. If you do not know if your prescription drug contains an MAOI, ask a doctor or pharmacist before taking this product
- to make a child sleep

## ASK A DOCTOR BEFORE USE IF YOU HAVE
- liver disease
- glaucoma
- cough that occurs with too much phlegm (mucus)
- a breathing problem or chronic cough that lasts or as occurs with smoking, asthma, chronic bronchitis or emphysema
- trouble urinating due to enlarged prostate gland
- a sodium-restricted diet

## ASK A DOCTOR OR PHARMACIST BEFORE USE IF YOU ARE
- taking sedatives or tranquilizers
- taking the blood thinning drug warfarin

## WHEN USING THIS PRODUCT
- do not use more than directed
- excitability may occur, especially in children
- marked drowsiness may occur
- avoid alcoholic drinks
- be careful when driving a motor vehicle or operating machinery
- alcohol, sedatives, and tranquilizers may increase drowsiness

## STOP USE AND ASK A DOCTOR IF
- pain or cough gets worse or lasts more than 7 days
- fever gets worse or lasts more than 3 days
- redness or swelling is present
- new symptoms occur
- cough comes back or occurs with rash or headache that lasts. These could be signs of a serious condition

**If pregnant or breastfeeding,** ask a health professional before use.

**Keep out of reach of children.**

## OVERDOSE WARNING
Taking more than directed can cause serious health problems. In case of overdose, get medical help or contact a Poison Control Center right away. Quick medical attention is critical for adults and for children even if you do not notice any signs or symptoms.

## DIRECTIONS
- take only as directed see overdose warning
- use dose cup or tablespoon (tbsp)
- do not exceed 4 doses per 24 hrs

| adults & children 12 yrs and over | 30 mL (2 tbsp) every 6 hrs |
|---|---|
| children 4 to under 12 yrs | ask a doctor |
| children under 4 yrs | do not use |

## OTHER INFORMATION
- each 30 mL dose cup contains: potassium 7 mg, sodium 47 mg
- store at room temperature

## INACTIVE INGREDIENTS
acesulfame potassium, carboxymethylcellulose sodium, citric acid, FD&C red no. 40, flavor, high fructose corn syrup, polyethylene glycol, propylene glycol, purified water, saccharin sodium, sodium benzoate, sodium citrate

## QUESTIONS OR COMMENTS
Call **1-800-362-1683**

---

# VICKS SINEX 12 HOUR DECONGESTANT
## NASAL (oxymetazoline hydrochloride) spray
The Procter & Gamble Manufacturing Company

### DRUG FACTS

| Active ingredient | Purpose |
|---|---|
| Oxymetazoline hydrochloride 0.05% | Nasal decongestant |

### USES
- temporarily relieves nasal congestion due to:
  - colds
  - hay fever
  - upper respiratory allergies

### WARNINGS

**ASK A DOCTOR BEFORE USE IF YOU HAVE**
- heart disease
- thyroid disease
- diabetes
- high blood pressure
- trouble urinating due to enlarged prostate gland

**WHEN USING THIS PRODUCT**
- do not exceed recommended dosage
- use of this container by more than one person may spread infection
- temporary burning, stinging, sneezing, or increased nasal discharge may occur
- frequent or prolonged use may cause nasal congestion to recur or worsen

**STOP USE AND ASK A DOCTOR IF**
- symptoms persist for more than 3 days

**If pregnant or breastfeeding,** ask a health professional before use.

**Keep out of reach of children.** In case of accidental ingestion, get medical help or contact a Poison Control Center right away.

---

## DIRECTIONS

| adults & children 6 yrs and older (with adult supervision) | 2 or 3 sprays in each nostril without tilting your head, not more often than every 10 to 12 hours |
| | do not exceed 2 doses in 24 hours |
| children 2 to under 6 yrs | ask a doctor |
| children under 2 yrs | do not use |

## OTHER INFORMATION
- store at room temperature

## INACTIVE INGREDIENTS
benzalkonium chloride, chlorhexidine gluconate, citric acid, disodium EDTA, fragrance, purified water, sodium citrate, sodium hydroxide, tyloxapol

## QUESTIONS OR COMMENTS
Call **1-800-873-8276** or visit www.vicks.com

---

# VICKS SINEX 12 HOUR DECONGESTANT ULTRA FINE MIST MOISTURIZING
(oxymetazoline hydrochloride) spray
The Procter & Gamble Manufacturing Company

### DRUG FACTS

| Active ingredient | Purpose |
|---|---|
| Oxymetazoline hydrochloride 0.05% | Nasal decongestant |

### USES
- temporarily relieves nasal congestion due to
  - colds
  - hay fever
  - upper respiratory allergies

### WARNINGS

**ASK A DOCTOR BEFORE USE IF YOU HAVE**
- heart disease
- thyroid disease
- diabetes
- high blood pressure
- trouble urinating due to enlarged prostate gland

**WHEN USING THIS PRODUCT**
- do not exceed recommended dosage
- use of this container by more than one person may spread infection
- temporary burning, stinging, sneezing, or increased nasal discharge may occur
- frequent or prolonged use may cause nasal congestion to recur or worsen

**STOP USE AND ASK A DOCTOR IF**
- symptoms persist for more than 3 days

**If pregnant or breastfeeding,** ask a health professional before use.

**Keep out of reach of children.** In case of accidental ingestion, get medical help or contact a Poison Control Center right away.

## DIRECTIONS

- Remove protective cap. Before using for the first time, prime the pump by firmly depressing its rim several times. Hold container with thumb at base and nozzle between first and second fingers. Without tilting your head, insert nozzle into nostril. Fully depress rim with a firm, even stroke and inhale deeply

| adults & children 6 yrs and older (with adult supervision) | 2 or 3 sprays in each nostril, not more often than every 10 to 12 hours |
| --- | --- |
| | do not exceed 2 doses in 24 hours |
| children 2 to under 6 yrs | ask a doctor |
| children under 2 yrs | do not use |

## OTHER INFORMATION

- store at room temperature

## INACTIVE INGREDIENTS

acesulfame potassium, aloe vera, benzalkonium chloride, chlorhexidine gluconate, citric acid, disodium EDTA, fragrance, purified water, sodium citrate, sodium hydroxide, sorbitol, tyloxapol

## QUESTIONS OR COMMENTS

Call **1-800-873-8276** or visit www.vicks.com

---

# VICKS VAPOINHALER (levmetamfetamine)

Procter & Gamble

## DRUG FACTS

| Active ingredient (per inhaler) | Purpose |
| --- | --- |
| Levmetamfetamine 50 mg | Nasal decongestant |

## WARNINGS

### WHEN USING THIS PRODUCT

- do not exceed recommended dosage
- temporary burning, stinging, sneezing, or increased nasal discharge may occur
- use of this container by more than one person may spread infection
- do not use for more than 7 days
- use only as directed
- frequent or prolonged use may cause nasal congestion to recur or worsen

### STOP USE AND ASK A DOCTOR

- if symptoms persist

**If pregnant or breastfeeding,** ask a health professional before use.

**Keep out of reach of children.** If swallowed, get medical help or contact a Poison Control Center right away.

## DIRECTIONS

- the product delivers into each 800 mL of air 0.04 to 0.150 mg of levmetamfetamine
- do not use more often than every 2 hours

| adults and children 12 years and over | 2 inhalations in each nostril |
| --- | --- |
| children 6 to under 12 years (with adult supervision) | 1 inhalation in each nostril |
| children 2 to under 6 years | ask a doctor |
| children under 2 years | do not use |

## OTHER INFORMATION

- store at room temperature
- keep inhaler tightly closed
- this inhaler is effective for a minimum of 3 months after first use

## INACTIVE INGREDIENTS

bornyl acetate, camphor, lavender oil, menthol, methyl salicylate

## QUESTIONS OR COMMENTS

Call **1-800-873-8276**

---

# VICKS VAPOSYRUP (guaifenesin and phenylephrine hydrochloride) liquid

Procter & Gamble

## DRUG FACTS

| Active ingredients (in each 15 ml tablespoon) | Purpose |
| --- | --- |
| Guaifenesin 100 mg | Expectorant |
| Phenylephrine hydrochloride 5 mg | Nasal decongestant |

## USES

- helps loosen phlegm and thin bronchial secretions to rid the bronchial passageways of bothersome mucus
- temporarily relieves nasal congestion due to a cold or hay fever or other upper respiratory allergies

## WARNINGS

### DO NOT USE

- if you are now taking a prescription monoamine oxidase inhibitor (MAOI) (certain drugs for depression, psychiatric or emotional conditions, or Parkinson's disease), or for 2 weeks after stopping the MAOI drug. If you do not know if your prescription drug contains an MAOI, ask a doctor or pharmacist before taking this product

### ASK A DOCTOR BEFORE USE IF YOU HAVE

- heart disease
- thyroid disease
- diabetes
- high blood pressure
- trouble urinating due to enlarged prostate gland
- cough that occurs with too much phlegm (mucus)
- cough that lasts or is chronic such as occurs with smoking, asthma, chronic bronchitis, or emphysema
- a sodium-restricted diet

### WHEN USING THIS PRODUCT

- do not take more than directed

### STOP USE AND ASK A DOCTOR IF

- you get nervous, dizzy or sleepless
- symptoms do not get better within 7 days or are accompanied by fever

- cough lasts more than 7 days, comes back, or occurs with fever, rash, or headache that lasts. These could be signs of a serious condition

**If pregnant or breastfeeding,** ask a health professional before use.

**Keep out of reach of children.** In case of overdose, get medical help or contact a Poison Control Center right away.

## DIRECTIONS
- shake well before use
- use dose cup or tablespoon (tbsp)
- do not exceed 6 doses per 24 hours

| adults and children 12 years and over | 30 ml (2 tbsp) every 4 hours |
|---|---|
| children 4 to under 12 years | ask a doctor |
| children under 4 years | do not use |

## OTHER INFORMATION
- each tablespoon contains: potassium 5 mg, sodium 49 mg
- store at room temperature

## INACTIVE INGREDIENTS
acesulfame potassium, carboxymethylcellulose sodium, citric acid, disodium EDTA, FD&C blue no. 1, flavor, glycerin, propylene glycol, purified water, saccharin sodium, sodium benzoate, sodium chloride, sodium citrate dihydrate, sorbitol

## QUESTIONS OR COMMENTS
1-800-873-8276 or visit www.vicks.com

---

# VISINE A (naphazoline hydrochloride and pheniramine maleate) liquid
Johnson & Johnson Healthcare Products

## DRUG FACTS

| Active ingredients | Purpose |
|---|---|
| Naphazoline hydrochloride 0.025% | Redness reliever |
| Pheniramine maleate 0.3% | Antihistamine |

## USES
- temporarily relieves itchy, red eyes due to:
  - pollen
  - ragweed
  - grass
  - animal hair and dander

## WARNINGS

### DO NOT USE
- if you are sensitive to any ingredient in this product

### ASK A DOCTOR BEFORE USE IF YOU HAVE
- heart disease
- high blood pressure
- narrow angle glaucoma
- trouble urinating due to an enlarged prostate gland

### WHEN USING THIS PRODUCT
- pupils may become enlarged temporarily
- do not touch tip of container to any surface to avoid contamination
- replace cap after each use

---

- remove contact lenses before using
- do not use if this solution changes color or becomes cloudy
- overuse may cause more eye redness

### STOP USE AND ASK A DOCTOR IF
- you feel eye pain
- changes in vision occur
- redness or irritation of the eye lasts
- condition worsens or lasts more than 72 hours

**Keep out of reach of children.** If swallowed, get medical help or contact a Poison Control Center right away. Accidental swallowing by infants and children may lead to coma and marked reduction in body temperature.

## DIRECTIONS

| adults and children 6 years of age and over | put 1 or 2 drops in the affected eye(s) up to four times a day |
|---|---|
| children under 6 years of age | consult a doctor |

## OTHER INFORMATION
- some users may experience a brief tingling sensation
- store between 15° and 25°C (59° and 77°F)

## INACTIVE INGREDIENTS
boric acid and sodium borate buffer system preserved with benzalkonium chloride (0.01%) and edetate disodium (0.1%), sodium hydroxide and/or hydrochloric acid (to adjust pH), purified water

## QUESTIONS OR COMMENTS
Call 1-800-223-0182, weekdays

---

# VISINE L.R. (oxymetazoline hydrochloride) liquid
Johnson & Johnson Healthcare Products Inc.

## DRUG FACTS

| Active ingredient | Purpose |
|---|---|
| Oxymetazoline hydrochloride 0.025% | Redness reliever |

## USE
- for the relief of redness of the eye due to minor eye irritations

## WARNINGS

### ASK A DOCTOR BEFORE USE IF YOU HAVE
- narrow angle glaucoma

### WHEN USING THIS PRODUCT
- overuse may cause more eye redness
- remove contact lenses before using
- do not use if this solution changes color or becomes cloudy
- do not touch tip of container to any surface to avoid contamination
- replace cap after each use

### STOP USE AND ASK A DOCTOR IF
- you feel eye pain
- changes in vision occur
- redness or irritation of the eye lasts
- condition worsens or lasts more than 72 hours

**If pregnant or breastfeeding,** ask a health professional before use.

**Keep out of reach of children.** If swallowed, get medical help or contact a Poison Control Center right away.

## DIRECTIONS

| adults and children 6 years of age and over | put 1 or 2 drops in the affected eye(s) |
| | this may be repeated as needed every 6 hours or as directed by a doctor |
| children under 6 years of age | ask a doctor |

## OTHER INFORMATION
• store at 15°C-25°C (59°F-77°F)

## INACTIVE INGREDIENTS
benzalkonium chloride, boric acid, edetate disodium, purified water, sodium borate, and sodium chloride

## QUESTIONS OR COMMENTS
Call 1-888-734-7648, weekdays

---

## VISINE MAXIMUM REDNESS RELIEF
FORMULA (glycerin, hypromellose, polyethylene glycol 400, and tetrahydrozoline hydrochloride) liquid/drops
Johnson & Johnson Healthcare Products

### DRUG FACTS

| Active ingredients | Purpose |
| --- | --- |
| Glycerin 0.2% | Lubricant |
| Hypromellose 0.36% | Lubricant |
| Polyethylene glycol 400 1% | Lubricant |
| Tetrahydrozoline hydrochloride 0.05% | Redness reliever |

## USES
• for the relief of redness of the eye due to minor eye irritations
• for the temporary relief of burning and discomfort due to dryness of the eye or exposure to wind or sun
• for protection against further irritation

## WARNINGS

### ASK A DOCTOR BEFORE USE IF YOU HAVE
• narrow angle glaucoma

### WHEN USING THIS PRODUCT
• pupils may become enlarged temporarily
• overuse may cause more eye redness
• remove contact lenses before using
• do not use if this solution changes color or becomes cloudy
• do not touch tip of container to any surface to avoid contamination
• replace cap after each use

### STOP USE AND ASK A DOCTOR IF
• you feel eye pain
• changes in vision occur
• redness or irritation of the eye lasts
• condition worsens or lasts more than 72 hours

If pregnant or breastfeeding, ask a health professional before use.

Keep out of reach of children. If swallowed, get medical help or contact a Poison Control Center right away.

## DIRECTIONS
• put 1 to 2 drops in the affected eye(s) up to 4 times daily
• children under 6 years of age: ask a doctor

## OTHER INFORMATION
• store at 15°C-25°C (59°F-77°F)

## INACTIVE INGREDIENTS
benzalkonium chloride, boric acid, edetate disodium, purified water, sodium chloride, sodium citrate

## QUESTIONS OR COMMENTS
Call 1-888-734-7468, weekdays

---

## VISINE SUMMER SPECTRUM RELIEF
(tetrahydrozoline hydrochloride, polyethylene glycol 400, povidone, and dextran 70) liquid
Johnson & Johnson Healthcare Products Inc.

### DRUG FACTS

| Active ingredients | Purpose |
| --- | --- |
| Dextran 70 0.1% | Lubricant |
| Polyethylene glycol 400 1% | Lubricant |
| Povidone 1% | Lubricant |
| Tetrahydrozoline hydrochloride 0.05% | Redness reliever |

## USES
• for the relief of redness of the eye due to minor eye irritations
• for use as a protectant against further irritation or to relieve dryness of the eye

## WARNINGS

### ASK A DOCTOR BEFORE USE IF YOU HAVE
• narrow angle glaucoma

### WHEN USING THIS PRODUCT
• pupils may become enlarged temporarily
• overuse may cause more eye redness
• remove contact lenses before using
• do not use if this solution changes color or becomes cloudy
• do not touch tip of container to any surface to avoid contamination
• replace cap after each use

### STOP USE AND ASK A DOCTOR IF
• you feel eye pain
• changes in vision occur
• redness or irritation of the eye lasts
• condition worsens or lasts more than 72 hours

If pregnant or breastfeeding, ask a health professional before use.

Keep out of reach of children. If swallowed, get medical help or contact a Poison Control Center right away.

## DIRECTIONS
• put 1 to 2 drops in the affected eye(s) up to 4 times daily
• children under 6 years of age: ask a doctor

## OTHER INFORMATION
• store at 15°C-25°C (59°F-77°F)

## INACTIVE INGREDIENTS
benzalkonium chloride, boric acid, edetate disodium, purified water, sodium borate, sodium chloride

## QUESTIONS OR COMMENTS
Call 1-800-223-0182, weekdays, 9 AM-5 PM EST

## VISINE TEARS DRY EYE RELIEF (glycerin, hypromellose, and polyethylene glycol)

Johnson & Johnson Healthcare Products, Division of McNeil-PPC, Inc.

### DRUG FACTS

| Active ingredients | Purpose |
|---|---|
| Glycerin 0.2% | Lubricant |
| Hypromellose 0.2% | Lubricant |
| Polyethylene glycol 400 1% | Lubricant |

### USES
- for the temporary relief of burning and irritation due to dryness of the eye
- for protection against further irritation

### WHEN USING THIS PRODUCT
- remove contact lenses before using
- do not use if this solution changes color or becomes cloudy
- do not touch tip of container to any surface to avoid contamination
- replace cap after each use

### STOP USE AND ASK A DOCTOR IF
- you feel eye pain
- changes in vision occur
- redness or irritation of the eye lasts
- condition worsens or lasts more than 72 hours

**If pregnant or breastfeeding ask,** a health professional before use.

**Keep out of reach of children.** If swallowed, get medical help or contact a Poison Control Center right away.

### OTHER INFORMATION
- store at 15°C-25°C (59°F-77°F)

### INACTIVE INGREDIENTS
ascorbic acid, benzalkonium chloride, boric acid, dextrose, disodium phosphate, glycine, magnesium chloride, potassium chloride, purified water, sodium borate, sodium chloride, sodium citrate, and sodium lactate

### DIRECTIONS
- put 1 or 2 drops in the affected eye(s) as needed
- children under 5 years of age ask a doctor

### QUESTIONS OR COMMENTS
Call **1-888-734-7648**, weekdays or TTY users can call 880-722-1322 (Monday to Friday, 8 AM to 8 PM EST).

## VISINE TIRED EYE RELIEF LUBRICANT
(glycerin, hypromellose, and polyethylene glycol 400) liquid/drops

Johnson & Johnson Healthcare Products, Division of McNeil-PPC, Inc.

### DRUG FACTS

| Active ingredients | Purpose |
|---|---|
| Glycerin 0.2% | Lubricant |
| Hypromellose 0.36% | Lubricant |
| Polyethylene glycol 400 1% | Lubricant |

### USES
- for the temporary relief of burning, irritation, and discomfort due to dryness of the eye or exposure to wind or sun
- for protection against further irritation

### WARNINGS
### WHEN USING THIS PRODUCT
- remove contact lenses before using
- do not use if this solution changes color or becomes cloudy
- do not touch tip of container to any surface to avoid contamination
- replace cap after each use

### STOP USE AND ASK A DOCTOR IF
- you feel eye pain
- changes in vision occur
- redness or irritation of the eye lasts
- condition worsens or lasts more than 72 hours

**If pregnant or breastfeeding,** ask a health professional before use.

**Keep out of reach of children.** If swallowed, get medical help or contact a Poison Control Center right away.

### DIRECTIONS
- put 1 or 2 drops in the affected eye(s) as needed
- children under 6 years of age: ask a doctor

### OTHER INFORMATION
- store at 15°C-25°C (59°F-77°F)

### INACTIVE INGREDIENTS
ascorbic acid, benzalkonium chloride, boric acid, dextrose, glycine, magnesium chloride, potassium chloride, purified water, sodium borate, sodium chloride, sodium citrate, sodium lactate, and sodium phosphate dibasic

### QUESTIONS OR COMMENTS
Call **1-800-734-3648**, weekdays

## VIVARIN (caffeine) tablet/caplet
GlaxoSmithKline Consumer Healthcare LP

### DRUG FACTS

| Active ingredient (in each tablet) | Purpose |
|---|---|
| Caffeine 200 mg | Alertness aid |

### USE
- helps restore mental alertness or wakefulness when experiencing fatigue or drowsiness

### WARNINGS
**For occasional use only**

### DO NOT USE
- in children under 12 years
- as a substitute for sleep

### WHEN USING THIS PRODUCT
- limit the use of caffeine containing medications, foods, or beverages because too much caffeine may cause nervousness, irritability, sleeplessness, and occasionally, rapid heartbeat
- The recommended dose of this product contains about as much caffeine as a cup of coffee

### STOP USE AND ASK A DOCTOR
- if fatigue or drowsiness persists or continues to recur

**If pregnant or breastfeeding,** ask a health professional before use.

**Keep out of reach of children.** In case of overdose, get medical help or contact a Poison Control Center right away.

## DIRECTIONS (tablets)
- adults and children 12 years and over
- take 1 tablet not more often than every 3 to 4 hours

## DIRECTIONS (caplets)
- adults and children 12 years and over
- take 1 caplet not more often than every 3 to 4 hours

## OTHER INFORMATION
- store at room temperature
- avoid excessive heat (greater than 100°F) or humidity

## INACTIVE INGREDIENTS
carnauba wax, colloidal silicon dioxide, D&C yellow no. 10 aluminum lake, dextrose, FD&C yellow no. 6 aluminum lake, hypromellose, magnesium stearate, microcrystalline cellulose, polyethylene glycol, polysorbate 80, starch, titanium dioxide

## QUESTIONS OR COMMENTS
Call toll-free **1-800-245-1040** weekdays or visit www.vivarin.com

---

# ZADITOR ANTIHISTAMINE EYE DROPS
(ketotifen fumarate) solution
Novartis Pharmaceuticals Corporation

## DRUG FACTS

| Active ingredient | Purpose |
|---|---|
| Ketotifen (0.025%) (equivalent to ketotifen fumarate 0.035%) | Antihistamine |

## USE
- temporarily relieves itchy eyes due to pollen, ragweed, grass, animal hair and dander

## WARNINGS

## DO NOT USE
- if solution changes color or becomes cloudy
- if you are sensitive to any ingredient in this product
- to treat contact lens related irritation

## WHEN USING THIS PRODUCT
- do not touch tip of container to any surface to avoid contamination
- remove contact lenses before use
- wait at least 10 minutes before reinserting contact lenses after use
- replace cap after each use

## STOP USE AND ASK A DOCTOR
- if you experience any of the following:
  - eye pain
  - changes in vision
  - redness of the eye
  - itching worsens or lasts for more than 72 hours

## DIRECTIONS

| adults and children 3 years of age and older | put 1 drop in the affected eye(s) twice daily, every 8-12 hours, no more than twice per day |
|---|---|
| children under 3 years of age | consult a doctor |

## OTHER INFORMATION
- only for use in the eye
- store between 4°C-25°C (39°F-77°F)

## INACTIVE INGREDIENTS
benzalkonium chloride 0.01%, glycerol, sodium hydroxide and/or hydrochloric acid, purified water

## QUESTIONS OR COMMENTS
Call toll-free **1-866-393-6336,** weekdays, 8:30 AM-5:00 PM EST. Serious side effects associated with use of this product may be reported to this number.

---

# ZANTAC 75 TABLETS (ranitidine) tablet, coated
Boehringer Ingelheim Pharmaceuticals, Inc.

## DRUG FACTS

| Active ingredient (in each tablet) | Purpose |
|---|---|
| Ranitidine 75 mg (as ranitidine hydrochloride 84 mg) | Acid reducer |

## USES
- relieves heartburn associated with acid indigestion and sour stomach
- prevents heartburn associated with acid indigestion and sour stomach brought on by certain foods and beverages

## WARNINGS
**Allergy alert**
Do not use if you are allergic to ranitidine or other acid reducers

## DO NOT USE
- if you have trouble or pain swallowing food, vomiting with blood, or bloody or black stools. These may be signs of a serious condition. See your doctor
- with other acid reducers

## ASK A DOCTOR BEFORE USE IF YOU HAVE
- frequent chest pain
- frequent wheezing, particularly with heartburn
- unexplained weight loss
- nausea or vomiting
- stomach pain
- had heartburn over 3 months. This may be a sign of a more serious condition
- heartburn with lightheadedness, sweating or dizziness
- chest pain or shoulder pain with shortness of breath; sweating; pain spreading to arms, neck or shoulders; or lightheadedness

## STOP USE AND ASK A DOCTOR IF
- your heartburn continues or worsens
- you need to take this product for more than 14 days

**If pregnant or breastfeeding,** ask a health professional before use.

**Keep out of reach of children.** In case of overdose, get medical help or contact a Poison Control Center right away.

## DIRECTIONS

| adults and children 12 years and over | to relieve symptoms, swallow 1 tablet with a glass of water |
| | to prevent symptoms, swallow 1 tablet with a glass of water 30 to 60 minutes before eating food or drinking beverages that cause heartburn |
| | can be used up to twice daily (do not take more than 2 tablets in 24 hours) |
| children under 12 years | ask a doctor |

## OTHER INFORMATION
- blister: do not use if individual blister unit is open or torn
- bottle: do not use of printed foil under bottle cap is open or torn
- store at 20-25°C (68-77°F)
- avoid excessive heat or humidity
- this product is sodium and sugar free

## INACTIVE INGREDIENTS
hypromellose, magnesium stearate, microcrystalline cellulose, synthetic red iron oxide, titanium dioxide, triacetin

## QUESTIONS OR COMMENTS
Call **1-888-285-9159** or visit www.zantacotc.com

# ZANTAC 150 COOL MINT TABLETS (ranitidine)
tablet, coated

Boehringer Ingelheim Pharmaceuticals, Inc.

## DRUG FACTS

| Active ingredient (in each tablet) | Purpose |
|---|---|
| Ranitidine 150 mg (as ranitidine hydrochloride 168 mg) | Acid reducer |

## USES
- relieves heartburn associated with acid indigestion and sour stomach
- prevents heartburn associated with acid indigestion and sour stomach brought on by certain foods and beverages

## WARNINGS
**Allergy alert**
Do not use if you are allergic to ranitidine or other acid reducers.

## DO NOT USE
- with other acid reducers
- if you have kidney disease, except under the advice and supervision of a doctor
- if you have trouble or pain swallowing food, vomiting with blood, or bloody or black stools

These may be signs of a serious condition. See your doctor.

## ASK A DOCTOR BEFORE USE IF YOU HAVE
- nausea or vomiting
- stomach pain
- unexplained weight loss
- frequent chest pain
- frequent wheezing, particularly with heartburn
- had heartburn over 3 months. This may be a sign of a more serious condition
- heartburn with lightheadedness, sweating or dizziness

- chest pain or shoulder pain with shortness of breath; sweating; pain spreading to arms, neck or shoulders; or lightheadedness

## STOP USE AND ASK A DOCTOR IF
- your heartburn continues or worsens
- you need to take this product for more than 14 days

**If pregnant or breastfeeding,** ask a health professional before use.

**Keep out of reach of children.** In case of overdose, get medical help or contact a Poison Control Center right away.

## DIRECTIONS

| adults and children 12 years and over | to relieve symptoms, swallow 1 tablet with a glass of water |
| | to prevent symptoms, swallow 1 tablet with a glass of water 30 to 60 minutes before eating food or drinking beverages that cause heartburn |
| | can be used up to twice daily (do not take more than 2 tablets in 24 hours) |
| | do not chew tablet |
| children under 12 years | ask a doctor |

## OTHER INFORMATION
- blister: do not use if individual blister unit is open or torn
- bottle: do not use of printed foil under bottle cap is open or torn
- store at 20-25°C (68-77°F)
- avoid excessive heat or humidity
- this product is sodium and sugar free
- keep carton. It contains important information

## INACTIVE INGREDIENTS
carrageenan, FD&C blue no.1, flavors, hypromellose, magnesium stearate, microcrystalline cellulose, polyethylene glycol, polysorbate, sucralose, titanium dioxide

## QUESTIONS OR COMMENTS
Call **1-888-285-9159** or visit www.zantacotc.com

# ZEASORB (miconazole nitrate) powder
Stiefel Laboratories Inc.

## DRUG FACTS

| Active ingredient | Purpose |
|---|---|
| Miconazole nitrate 2% | Antifungal |

## USES
- for the cure of most athlete's foot
- for the cure of most jock itch

## WARNINGS
**For external use only.**

## DO NOT USE
- on children under 2 years of age unless directed by a doctor
- avoid contact with the eyes

## STOP USE AND ASK A DOCTOR IF (Athlete's foot)
- irritation occurs or there is no improvement within 4 weeks

## STOP USE AND ASK A DOCTOR IF (Jock itch)
• irritation occurs or there is no improvement within 2 weeks

**Keep out of reach of children.** If swallowed, get medical help or contact a Poison Control Center right away.

## DIRECTIONS (Athlete's foot)
• clean the affected area and dry thoroughly
• apply a thin layer of the product over affected area twice daily (morning and night) or as directed by a doctor
• supervise children in the use of this product
• pay special attention to spaces between the toes; wear well-fitting, ventilated shoes, and change shoes and socks at least once daily
• use daily for 4 weeks
• if condition persists longer, consult a doctor
• this product is not effective on the scalp or nails

## DIRECTIONS (Jock itch)
• clean the affected area and dry thoroughly
• apply a thin layer of the product over affected area twice daily (morning and night) or as directed by a doctor
• supervise children in the use of this product
• use daily for 2 weeks
• if condition persists longer, consult a doctor
• this product is not effective on the scalp or nails

## OTHER INFORMATION
• product settles during shipment. Package contains full net weight

## INACTIVE INGREDIENTS
acrylamide/sodium acrylate copolymer, aldioxa, chloroxylenol, fragrance, imidurea, microporous cellulose, talc; contains no starch

## QUESTIONS OR COMMENTS
Call **1-888-438-7426**. Side effects should be reported to this number. www.zeasorb.com

## ZICAM ULTRA RAPID MELTS COLD
**REMEDY** (zinc acetate anhydrous and zinc gluconate) tablet, multilayer

Matrixx Initiatives, Inc.

Capricorn Pharma Inc.

### DRUG FACTS

| Active ingredients (in each tablet) | Purpose |
|---|---|
| Zincum aceticum 2x Zincum gluconicum 1x | Reduces duration and severity of the common cold |

## USES
• reduces duration of the common cold
• reduces severity of cold symptoms:
  • sore throat
  • stuffy nose
  • sneezing
  • coughing
  • congestion

## WARNINGS

### STOP USE AND ASK A DOCTOR
• if symptoms persist or are accompanied by fever

## ASK A DOCTOR OR PHARMACIST BEFORE USE IF YOU ARE
• allergic or sensitive to zinc

**If pregnant or breastfeeding,** ask a health professional before use.

**Keep out of reach of children.**

## DIRECTIONS
• For best results, use at the first sign of a cold and continue to use until symptoms completely subside

| adults and children 12 years of age and older | take 1 tablet at the onset of symptoms |
|---|---|
| | dissolve entire tablet in mouth. Do not chew. Do not swallow whole |
| | repeat every 4-6 hours, not to exceed 4 tablets in 24 hours |
| | to avoid minor stomach upset, do not take on an empty stomach |
| | do not eat or drink for 15 minutes after use |
| | do not eat or drink citrus fruits or juices for 30 minutes before or after use; otherwise, drink plenty of fluids |
| children under 12 years of age | consult a doctor before use |

## OTHER INFORMATION
• store at room temperature 15-29°C (59-84°F)

## INACTIVE INGREDIENTS
acesulfame K, crospovidone, FD&C red no. 40 aluminum lake, hypromellose, magnesium stearate, maltodextrin, mannitol, microcrystalline cellulose, modified food starch, natural & artificial flavors, polyethylene glycol, polysorbate 80, povidone, silicon dioxide, sodium lauryl sulphate, sodium starch glycolate, sorbitan monostearate, stearic acid, sucralose, talc

## QUESTIONS OR COMMENTS
Call **877-942-2626** toll-free or visit www.zicam.com

## ZILACTIN-B (benzocaine) gel
Balirex Laboratories

### DRUG FACTS

| Active ingredient | Purpose |
|---|---|
| Benzocaine 10% | Oral reliever |

## USES
• temporarily relieves pain caused by:
  • canker sores
  • minor mouth sores and gum irritations
  • denture and brace pain

## WARNINGS
• flammable: keep away from fire or flame
• apply only to affected areas
• do not exceed recommended dosage
• avoid contact with the eyes
• do not use for more than 7 days unless directed by a physician or dentist

**STOP USE AND ASK A PHYSICIAN IF:**
- sore mouth symptoms do not improve in 7 days
- swelling, rash or fever develops
- irritation, pain or redness persists or worsens

**Keep out of reach of children.** If swallowed, get medical help or contact a Poison Control Center immediately.

### DIRECTIONS

| adults and children 2 years and older | dry affected area. Apply a thin coat of gel with cotton swab or clean finger up to 4 times daily allow to dry 30-60 seconds |
|---|---|
| children under 12 | adult supervision should be given in the use of this product |
| children under 2 years | do not use consult a physician or dentist |

### OTHER INFORMATION
- do not peel off protective film. Attempting to peel off film may result in skin irritation or tenderness. To remove film, first apply another coat of Zilactin-B to film and immediately wipe the area with a moist gauze pad or tissue
- contains alcohol 70% by volume
- store at 15-20°C (59-86°F)

### INACTIVE INGREDIENTS:
boric acid, hydroxypropylcellulose, propylene glycol, purified water, salicylic acid, SD alcohol 38-B, tannic acid

# ZOSTRIX ORIGINAL STRENGTH (capsaicin)
cream

Health Care Products

### DRUG FACTS

| Active ingredient | Purpose |
|---|---|
| Capsaicin 0.025% | Topical analgesic |

### USES
- for the temporary relief of minor aches and pains of muscles and joints associated with arthritis, simple backache, strains and sprains
- for use in treating neuralgias, consult a physician

### WARNINGS
**For external use only.**

**Do not apply to wounds or to damaged or irritated skin.**

### WHEN USING THIS PRODUCT
- you may experience a burning sensation which is normal and related to the way the product works. With regular use, this sensation generally disappears within several days
- do not get it on mucous membranes, into eyes, or on contact lenses. If this occurs, rinse the affected area thoroughly with water
- do not apply immediately before or after activities such as bathing, swimming, sun bathing, or strenuous exercise
- do not apply heat to the treated areas immediately before or after use
- do not tightly wrap or bandage the treated area
- avoid inhaling airborne material from dried residue. This can result in coughing, sneezing, tearing, throat or respiratory irritation

**STOP USE AND ASK A DOCTOR IF**
- condition worsens or does not improve after regular use
- blistering occurs
- difficulty breathing or swallowing occurs
- severe burning persists

**Keep out of reach of children.** If swallowed, get medical help or contact a Poison Control Center immediately.

### DIRECTIONS
- for persons under 18 years of age, ask a doctor before using
- apply a thin film of cream to the affected area and gently rub in until fully absorbed
- for optimum relief, apply 3 to 4 times daily
- best results typically occur after 2 to 4 weeks of continuous use
- unless treating hands, wash hands thoroughly with soap and water immediately after use
- see package insert for more information

### OTHER INFORMATION
- store at 15-30°C (59-86°F)

### INACTIVE INGREDIENTS
benzyl alcohol, cetyl alcohol, glyceryl stearate, isopropyl myristate, PEG-100 stearate, purified water, sorbitol solution, white petrolatum

### QUESTIONS OR COMMENTS
Call: **1-800-899-3116**, Mon-Thurs 9:00 AM-5:00 PM EST, Fri 9:00 AM-2:30 PM EST. Serious side effects associated with use of this product may be reported to this number.

# ZOSTRIX FOOT PAIN RELIEF (capsaicin) cream

Health Care Products

### DRUG FACTS

| Active ingredient | Purpose |
|---|---|
| Capsaicin 0.075% | Topical analgesic |

### USES
- for the temporary relief of minor aches and pains of the muscle joints associated with:
  - strains
  - sprains
  - bruises
  - arthritis

### WARNINGS
**For external use only.**

**Do not apply to wounds or to damaged or irritated skin.**

### WHEN USING THIS PRODUCT
- you may experience a burning sensation which is normal and related to the way the product works. With regular use, this sensation generally disappears within several days
- avoid contact with eyes. Do not get it on mucous membranes, into eyes, or on contact lenses. If this occurs, rinse the affected area thoroughly with water
- do not apply immediately before or after activities such as bathing, swimming, sun bathing, or strenuous exercise
- do not apply heat to the treated areas immediately before or after use
- do not tightly wrap or bandage the treated area
- avoid inhaling airborne material from dried residue. This can result in coughing, sneezing, tearing, throat or respiratory irritation

## STOP USE AND ASK A DOCTOR IF
- condition worsens, or if symptoms persist for more than 7 days or clear up and occur again within a few days
- blistering occurs
- difficulty breathing or swallowing occurs
- severe burning persists

**Keep out of reach of children.** If swallowed, get medical help or contact a Poison Control Center immediately.

## DIRECTIONS
- for persons under 18 years of age, ask a doctor before using
- to avoid getting cream on hands use applicator pad to apply a thin film of cream to the affected area and gently rub in until fully absorbed. Discard applicator pad after use
- for optimum relief, apply 3 to 4 times daily
- best results typically occur after 2 to 4 weeks of continuous use
- unless treating hands, wash hands thoroughly with soap and water immediately after use
- see package insert for more information

## OTHER INFORMATION
- store at 15-30°C (59-86°F)

## INACTIVE INGREDIENTS
benzyl alcohol, cetyl alcohol, glyceryl stearate, isopropyl myristate, PEG-100 stearate, purified water, sorbitol solution, white petrolatum

## QUESTIONS OR COMMENTS
Call: **1-800-899-3116**, Mon-Thurs 9:00 AM-5:00 PM EST, Fri. 9:00 AM-2:30 PM EST. Serious side effects associated with the use of this product may be reported to this number.

---

## ZYRTEC (cetirizine hydrochloride) capsule, film coated
McNeil Consumer Healthcare, Division of McNeil-PPC, Inc.

### DRUG FACTS

| Active ingredient (in each tablet) | Purpose |
|---|---|
| Cetirizine hydrochloride 10 mg | Antihistamine |

## USES
- temporarily relieves these symptoms due to hay fever or other upper respiratory allergies:
  - runny nose
  - sneezing
  - itchy, watery eyes
  - itching of the nose or throat

## WARNINGS

### DO NOT USE
- if you have ever had an allergic reaction to this product or any of its ingredients or to an antihistamine containing hydroxyzine

### ASK A DOCTOR BEFORE USE IF YOU HAVE
- liver or kidney disease. Your doctor should determine if you need a different dose

### ASK A DOCTOR OR PHARMACIST BEFORE USE IF YOU ARE
- taking tranquilizers or sedatives

### WHEN USING THIS PRODUCT
- drowsiness may occur
- avoid alcoholic drinks
- alcohol, sedatives, and tranquilizers may increase drowsiness

- be careful when driving a motor vehicle or operating machinery

## STOP USE AND ASK A DOCTOR IF
- an allergic reaction to this product occurs. Seek medical help right away

**If pregnant or breastfeeding:** ask a health professional before use.

**Keep out of reach of children.** In case of overdose, get medical help or contact a Poison Control Center right away. (1-800-222-1222)

## DIRECTIONS

| adults and children 6 years and over | one 10 mg tablet once daily; do not take more than one 10 mg tablet in 24 hours. A 5 mg product may be appropriate for less severe symptoms |
|---|---|
| adults 65 years and over | ask a doctor |
| children under 6 years of age | ask a doctor |
| consumers with liver or kidney disease | ask a doctor |

## OTHER INFORMATION
- store between 20°C-25°C (68°F-77°F)
- avoid high humidity and excessive heat above 40°C (104°F)
- do not use if imprinted foil inner seal on bottle is broken or missing

## INACTIVE INGREDIENTS
gelatin, glycerin, mannitol, pharmaceutical ink, polyethylene glycol 400, purified water, sodium hydroxide, sorbitan, sorbitol

## QUESTIONS OR COMMENTS
Call **1-800-343-7805**

---

## CHILDREN'S ZYRTEC (cetirizine hydrochloride) tablet, chewable
McNeil Consumer Healthcare, Division of McNeil-PPC, Inc.

### DRUG FACTS

| Active ingredient (in each chewable tablet) | Purpose |
|---|---|
| Cetirizine hydrochloride 5 mg | Antihistamine |

## USES
- temporarily relieves these symptoms due to hay fever or other upper respiratory allergies:
  - runny nose
  - sneezing
  - itchy, watery eyes
  - itching of the nose or throat

## WARNINGS

### DO NOT USE
- if you have ever had an allergic reaction to this product or any of its ingredients or to an antihistamine containing hydroxyzine

### ASK A DOCTOR BEFORE USE IF YOU HAVE
- liver or kidney disease. Your doctor should determine if you need a different dose

**ASK A DOCTOR OR PHARMACIST BEFORE USE IF YOU ARE**
- taking tranquilizers or sedatives

**WHEN USING THIS PRODUCT**
- drowsiness may occur
- avoid alcoholic drinks
- alcohol, sedatives, and tranquilizers may increase drowsiness
- be careful when driving a motor vehicle or operating machinery

**STOP USE AND ASK A DOCTOR IF**
- an allergic reaction to this product occurs. Seek medical help right away

**If pregnant or breastfeeding:** not recommended; ask a health professional before use.

**Keep out of reach of children.** In case of overdose, get medical help or contact a Poison Control Center right away. (1-800-222-1222)

**DIRECTIONS**
- may be taken with or without water

| adults and children 6 years and over | 1 to 2 tablets once daily depending upon severity of symptoms; do not take more than 2 tablets in 24 hours |
|---|---|
| adults 65 years and over | 1 tablet once a day; do not take more than 1 tablet in 24 hours |
| children under 6 years of age | ask a doctor |
| consumers with liver or kidney disease | ask a doctor |

**OTHER INFORMATION**
- store between 20°C-25°C (68°F-77°F)
- do not use if blister unit is open or torn
- see bottom panel for lot number and expiration date

**INACTIVE INGREDIENTS**
acesulfame potassium, betacyclodextrin, calcium silicate, carmine, colloidial silicon dioxide, disodium inosinate/guanylate, ethyl acetate, FD&C blue no. 2 aluminum lake, flavors, lactose monohydrate, magnesium stearate, maltodextrin, mannitol, microcrystalline cellulose, modified cornstarch, sorbitol

**QUESTIONS OR COMMENTS**
Call **1-800-343-7805**

---

## CHILDREN'S ZYRTEC (cetirizine hydrochloride)
syrup

McNeil Consumer Healthcare, Division of McNeil-PPC, Inc.

### DRUG FACTS

| Active ingredient (in each 5 mL teaspoonful) | Purpose |
|---|---|
| Cetirizine hydrochloride 5 mg | Antihistamine |

**USES**
- temporarily relieves these symptoms due to hay fever or other upper respiratory allergies:
  - runny nose
  - sneezing
  - itchy, watery eyes
  - itching of the nose or throat

**WARNINGS**

**DO NOT USE**
- if you have ever had an allergic reaction to this product or any of its ingredients or to an antihistamine containing hydroxyzine

**ASK A DOCTOR BEFORE USE**
- if you have liver or kidney disease. Your doctor should determine if you need a different dose

**ASK A DOCTOR OR PHARMACIST BEFORE USE**
- if you are taking tranquilizers or sedatives

**WHEN USING THIS PRODUCT**
- drowsiness may occur
- avoid alcoholic drinks
- alcohol, sedatives, and tranquilizers may increase drowsiness
- be careful when driving a motor vehicle or operating machinery

**STOP USE AND ASK A DOCTOR IF**
- an allergic reaction to this product occurs. Seek medical help right away

**If pregnant or breastfeeding:** not recommended; ask a health professional before use.

**Keep out of reach of children.** In case of overdose, get medical help or contact a Poison Control Center right away. (1-800-222-1222)

**DIRECTIONS**
- use only with enclosed dosing cup

| adults and children 6 years and over | 1 teaspoonful (5 mL) or 2 teaspoonfuls (10 mL) once daily depending upon severity of symptoms; do not take more than 2 teaspoonfuls (10 mL) in 24 hours |
|---|---|
| adults 65 years and over | 1 teaspoonful (5 mL) once daily; do not take more than 1 teaspoonful (5 mL) in 24 hours |
| children 2 to under 6 years of age | ½ teaspoonful (2.5 mL) once daily. If needed, dose can be increased to a maximum of 1 teaspoonful (5 mL) once daily or ½ teaspoonful (2.5 mL) every 12 hours. Do not give more than 1 teaspoonful (5 mL) in 24 hours |
| children under 2 years of age | ask a doctor |
| consumers with liver or kidney disease | ask a doctor |

**OTHER INFORMATION**
- store between 20°C-25°C (68°F-77°F)
- do not use if carton is opened; or if bottle wrap or foil inner seal printed with "Safety Seal" is broken or missing
- see bottom panel for lot number and expiration date

**INACTIVE INGREDIENTS**
anhydrous citric acid, flavors, propylene glycol, purified water, sodium benzoate, sorbitol solution, sucralose

**QUESTIONS OR COMMENTS**
Call **1-800-343-7805**

# ZYRTEC-D ALLERGY AND CONGESTION

(cetirizine hydrochloride and pseudoephedrine hydrochloride) tablet, extended release

McNeil Consumer Healthcare, Division of McNeil-PPC, Inc.

## DRUG FACTS

| Active ingredients (in each extended release tablet) | Purpose |
|---|---|
| Cetirizine hydrochloride 5 mg | Antihistamine |
| Pseudoephedrine hydrochloride 120 mg | Nasal decongestant |

## USES

- temporarily relieves these symptoms due to hay fever or other upper respiratory allergies:
  - runny nose
  - sneezing
  - itchy, watery eyes
  - itching of the nose or throat
  - nasal congestion
- reduces swelling of nasal passages
- temporarily relieves sinus congestion and pressure
- temporarily restores freer breathing through the nose

## WARNINGS

### DO NOT USE

- if you have ever had an allergic reaction to this product or any of its ingredients or to an antihistamine containing hydroxyzine
- if you are now taking a prescription monoamine oxidase inhibitor (MAOI) (certain drugs for depression, psychiatric, or emotional conditions, or Parkinson's disease), or for 2 weeks after stopping the MAOI drug. If you do not know if your prescription drug contains an MAOI, ask a doctor or pharmacist before taking this product

### ASK A DOCTOR BEFORE USE IF YOU HAVE

- heart disease
- thyroid disease
- diabetes
- glaucoma
- high blood pressure
- trouble urinating due to an enlarged prostate gland
- liver or kidney disease. Your doctor should determine if you need a different dose

### ASK A DOCTOR OR PHARMACIST BEFORE USE IF YOU ARE

- taking tranquilizers or sedatives

### WHEN USING THIS PRODUCT

- do not use more than directed
- drowsiness may occur
- avoid alcoholic drinks
- alcohol, sedatives, and tranquilizers may increase drowsiness
- be careful when driving a motor vehicle or operating machinery

### STOP USE AND ASK A DOCTOR IF

- an allergic reaction to this product occurs. Seek medical help right away
- you get nervous, dizzy, or sleepless
- symptoms do not improve within 7 days or are accompanied by fever

**If pregnant or breastfeeding:** not recommended; ask a health professional before use.

**Keep out of reach of children.** In case of overdose, get medical help or contact a Poison Control Center right away. (1-800-222-1222)

## DIRECTIONS

- do not break or chew tablet; swallow tablet whole

| adults and children 12 years and over | take 1 tablet every 12 hours; do not take more than 2 tablets in 24 hours |
|---|---|
| adults 65 years and over | ask a doctor |
| children under 12 years of age | ask a doctor |
| consumers with liver or kidney disease | ask a doctor |

## OTHER INFORMATION

- store between 20°C-25°C (68°F-77°F)
- do not use if individual blister unit is open or torn
- see back panel for lot number and expiration date

## INACTIVE INGREDIENTS

colloidal silicon dioxide, croscarmellose sodium, hypromellose, lactose monohydrate, magnesium stearate, microcrystalline cellulose, polyethylene glycol, titanium dioxide

## QUESTIONS OR COMMENTS

Call **1-800-343-7805**

# ZYRTEC ITCHY EYE (ketotifen fumarate) solution/drops

McNeil Consumer Healthcare Division of McNeil-PPC, Inc.

## DRUG FACTS

| Active ingredient | Purpose |
|---|---|
| Ketotifen (0.025%) (equivalent to ketotifen fumarate 0.035%) | Antihistamine |

## USE

- temporarily relieves itchy eyes due to pollen, ragweed, grass, animal hair and dander

## WARNINGS

### DO NOT USE

- if solution changes color or becomes cloudy
- if you are sensitive to any ingredient in this product
- to treat contact lens related irritation

### WHEN USING THIS PRODUCT

- do not touch tip of container to any surface to avoid contamination
- remove contact lenses before use
- wait at least 10 minutes before reinserting contact lenses after use
- replace cap after each use

### STOP USE AND ASK A DOCTOR IF

- you experience any of the following:
  - eye pain
  - changes in vision
  - redness of the eye
  - itching worsens or lasts for more than 72 hours

**Keep out of reach of children.** If swallowed, get medical help or contact a Poison Control Center right away. (1-800-222-1222)

## DIRECTIONS

| adults and children 3 years of age and older | put 1 drop in the affected eye(s) twice daily, every 8-12 hours, no more than twice per day |
|---|---|
| children under 3 years of age | consult a doctor |

## OTHER INFORMATION
- only for use in the eye
- do not use if outer package is torn or opened
- store at 20-25°C (68-77°F)

## INACTIVE INGREDIENTS
benzalkonium chloride 0.01%, glycerol, sodium hydroxide, hydrochloric acid, water for injection

## QUESTIONS OR COMMENTS
Call **1-800-343-7805**

# CHILDREN'S ZYRTEC HIVES RELIEF (cetirizine hydrochloride) syrup
McNeil Consumer Healthcare

## DRUG FACTS

| Active ingredient (in each 5 mL teaspoonful) | Purpose |
|---|---|
| Cetirizine hydrochloride 5 mg | Antihistamine |

## USES
- relieves itching due to hives (urticaria)
- this product will not prevent hives or an allergic skin reaction from occurring

## WARNINGS
**Severe allergy warning**
Get emergency help **immediately** if you have hives along with any of the following symptoms:

- trouble swallowing
- dizziness or loss of consciousness
- swelling of tongue
- swelling in or around mouth
- trouble speaking
- drooling
- wheezing or problems breathing

These symptoms may be signs of anaphylactic shock.

This condition can be life threatening if not treated by a health professional **immediately.** Symptoms of anaphylactic shock may occur when hives first appear or up to a few hours later.

**Not a substitute for epinephrine.**
If your doctor has prescribed an epinephrine injector for "anaphylaxis" or severe allergy symptoms that could occur with your hives, never use this product as a substitute for the epinephrine injector. If you have been prescribed an epinephrine injector, you should carry it with you at all times.

## DO NOT USE
- to prevent hives from any known cause such as:
  - foods
  - insect stings
  - medicines
  - latex or rubber gloves

because this product will not stop hives from occurring. Avoiding the cause of your hives is the only way to prevent them. Hives can sometimes be serious. If you do not know the cause of your hives, see your doctor for a medical exam. Your doctor may be able to help you find a cause.

- if you have ever had an allergic reaction to this product or any of its ingredients or to an antihistamine containing hydroxyzine

## ASK A DOCTOR BEFORE USE IF YOU HAVE
- liver or kidney disease. Your doctor should determine if you need a different dose
- hives that are an unusual color, look bruised or blistered
- hives that do not itch

## ASK A DOCTOR OR PHARMACIST BEFORE USE IF YOU ARE
- taking tranquilizers or sedatives

## WHEN USING THIS PRODUCT
- drowsiness may occur
- avoid alcoholic drinks
- alcohol, sedatives, and tranquilizers may increase drowsiness
- be careful when driving a motor vehicle or operating machinery

## STOP USE AND ASK A DOCTOR IF
- an allergic reaction to this product occurs. Seek medical help right away
- symptoms do not improve after 3 days of treatment
- the hives have lasted more than 6 weeks

**If pregnant or breastfeeding:** not recommended; ask a health professional before use.

**Keep out of reach of children.** In case of overdose, get medical help or contact a Poison Control Center right away. (1-800-222-1222)

## DIRECTIONS
- use only with enclosed dosing cup

| adults and children 6 years and over | 1 teaspoonful (5 mL) or 2 teaspoonfuls (10 mL) once daily depending upon severity of symptoms; do not take more than 2 teaspoonfuls (10 mL) in 24 hours |
|---|---|
| adults 65 years and over | 1 teaspoonful (5 mL) once daily; do not take more than 1 teaspoonful (5 mL) in 24 hours |
| children under 6 years of age | ask a doctor |
| consumers with liver or kidney disease | ask a doctor |

## OTHER INFORMATION
- store between 20°C-25°C (68°F-77°F)
- do not use if carton is opened, or if bottle wrap printed with "Safety Seal" is broken or missing
- see bottom panel for lot number and expiration date

## INACTIVE INGREDIENTS
anhydrous citric acid, flavors, propylene glycol, purified water, sodium benzoate, sorbitol solution, sucralose

## QUESTIONS OR COMMENTS
Call **1-800-343-7805**

# POISON CONTROL CENTERS

The American Association of Poison Control Centers (AAPCC) uses a single, nationwide **emergency** number to automatically link callers with their regional poison center. This toll-free number, **800-222-1222**, also works for **teletype lines (TTY)** for the hearing-impaired and **telecommunication devices (TTD)** for individuals who are deaf. However, a few local poison centers and the ASPCA/Animal Poison Control Center are not part of this nationwide system and continue to use separate numbers.

Most of the centers listed below are accredited by the AAPCC. **Certified centers are marked by an asterisk after the name.** Each has to meet certain criteria. It must, for example, serve a large geographic area; it must be open 24 hours a day and provide direct-dial or toll-free access; it must be supervised by a medical director; and it must have registered pharmacists or nurses available to answer questions from the public.

Within each state, centers are listed alphabetically by city. Some state poison centers also list their original emergency numbers (including TTY/TDD) that only work within that state. For these listings, callers may use either the state number or the nationwide 800 number.

## ALABAMA

### BIRMINGHAM

**Regional Poison Control Center (\*)**
**The Children's Hospital of Alabama**

1600 7th Ave. South
Birmingham, AL 35233-1711
Business:     205-939-9201
**Emergency:** 800-222-1222
www.chsys.org

### TUSCALOOSA

**Alabama Poison Center (\*)**

2503 Phoenix Dr.
Tuscaloosa, AL 35405
Business:     205-345-0600
**Emergency:** 800-222-1222
              800-462-0800 (AL)
www.alapoisoncenter.org

## ALASKA

### JUNEAU

**Alaska Poison Control System**
**Section of Community Health and EMS**

410 Willoughby Ave., Room 109
Box 110616
Juneau, AK 99811-0616
Business:     907-465-3027
**Emergency:** 800-222-1222
www.chems.alaska.gov

### (PORTLAND, OR)

**Oregon Poison Center (\*)**
**Oregon Health and Science University**

3181 SW Sam Jackson Park Rd.
CB550
Portland, OR 97239
Business:     503-494-8600
**Emergency:** 800-222-1222
www.ohsu.edu/poison

## ARIZONA

### PHOENIX

**Banner Poison Control Center (\*)**
**Banner Good Samaritan Medical Center**

901 E. Willetta St.
Phoenix, AZ 85006
Business:     602-495-6360
**Emergency:** 800-222-1222

              800-362-0101 (AZ)
              800-253-3334 (AZ)
www.bannerpoisoncontrol.com

### TUCSON

**Arizona Poison and Drug Information Center (\*)**
**Arizona Health Science Center**

1501 N. Campbell Ave.
Room 1156
Tucson, AZ 85724
Business:     520-626-7899
**Emergency:** 800-222-1222
www.pharmacy.arizona.edu/
outreach/poison

## ARKANSAS

### LITTLE ROCK

**Arkansas Poison and Drug Information Center (\*)**
**College of Pharmacy - UAMS**

4301 West Markham St.
Mail Slot 522-2
Little Rock, AR 72205-7122
Business:     501-686-5540
**Emergency:** 800-222-1222
              800-376-4766 (AR)
TDD/TTY:     800-641-3805
www.uams.edu/cop/

## ASPCA/
## ANIMAL POISON CONTROL
## CENTER

1717 South Philo Rd.
Suite 36
Urbana, IL 61802
Business:     217-337-5030
**Emergency:** 888-426-4435
              800-548-2423
http://www.aspcapro.org/animal-poison-control.
php

## CALIFORNIA

### FRESNO/MADERA

**California Poison Control System-Fresno/Madera Div. (\*)**
**Children's Hospital Central California**

9300 Valley Children's Place, MB 15
Madera, CA 93638-8762
Business:     559-622-2300
**Emergency:** 800-222-1222
              800-876-4766 (CA)
TDD/TTY:     800-972-3323
www.calpoison.org

### SACRAMENTO

**California Poison Control System-Sacramento Div. (\*)**
**UC Davis Medical Center**

Room HSF1024

2315 Stockton Blvd.
Sacramento, CA 95817
Business:     916-227-1400
**Emergency:** 800-222-1222
              800-876-4766 (CA)
TDD/TTY:     800-972-3323
www.calpoison.org

### SAN DIEGO

**California Poison Control System-San Diego Div. (\*)**
**UC San Diego Medical Center**

200 West Arbor Dr.
San Diego, CA 92103-8925
Business:     858-715-6300
**Emergency:** 800-222-1222
              800-876-4766 (CA)
TDD/TTY:     800-972-3323
www.calpoison.org

## SAN FRANCISCO

**California Poison Control System-San Francisco Div. (*)**
**San Francisco Hospital University of California San Francisco**

Box 1369
San Francisco, CA 94143-1369
Business:       415-502-6000
**Emergency:**   800-222-1222
                 800-876-4766 (CA)
TDD/TTY:        800-972-3323
www.calpoison.org

# COLORADO

## DENVER

**Rocky Mountain Poison and Drug Center (*)**

777 Bannock St., Mail Code 0180
Denver, CO  80204-4507
Business:       303-389-1100
**Emergency:**   800-222-1222
TDD/TTY:        303-739-1127 (CO)
www.RMPDC.org

# CONNECTICUT

## FARMINGTON

**Connecticut Regional Poison Control Center (*)**
**University of Connecticut Health Center**

263 Farmington Ave.
Farmington, CT  06030-5365
Business:       860-679-4540
**Emergency:**   800-222-1222
TDD/TTY:        866-218-5372
http://poisoncontrol.uchc.edu

# DELAWARE

## (PHILADELPHIA, PA)

**The Poison Control Center (*)**
**Children's Hospital of Philadelphia**

34th St. & Civic Center Blvd.
Philadelphia, PA 19104-4399
Business:       215-590-2003
**Emergency:**   800-222-1222
                 800-722-7112 (DE)
TDD/TTY:        215-590-8789
www.chop.edu

# DISTRICT OF COLUMBIA

## WASHINGTON, DC

**National Capital Poison Center (*)**

3201 New Mexico Ave., NW
Suite 310
Washington, DC  20016
Business:       202-362-3867
**Emergency:**   800-222-1222
www.poison.org

# FLORIDA

## JACKSONVILLE

**Florida Poison Information Center-Jacksonville (*)**
**SHANDS Hospital**

655 West 8th St.
Jacksonville, FL 32209
Business:       904-244-4465
**Emergency:**  800-222-1222
http://fpicjax.org

## MIAMI

**Florida Poison Information Center (*)-Miami**
**University of Miami, Department of Pediatrics**

P.O. Box 016960 (R-131)
Miami, FL 33101
Business:       305-585-5250
**Emergency:**   800-222-1222
www.med.miami.edu/poisoncontrol

## TAMPA

**Florida Poison Information Center (*)-Tampa**
**Tampa General Hospital**

P.O. Box 1289
Tampa, FL  33601-1289
Business:       813-844-7044
**Emergency:**   800-222-1222
www.poisoncentertampa.org

# GEORGIA

## ATLANTA

**Georgia Poison Center (*)**
**Hughes Spalding Children's Hospital, Grady Health System**

80 Jesse Hill Jr. Dr., SE
P.O. Box 26066
Atlanta, GA  30303-3050
Business:       404-616-9237
**Emergency:**   800-222-1222
                 404-616-9000 (Atlanta)
TDD:            404-616-9287
www.georgiapoisoncenter.org

# HAWAII

## (DENVER, CO)

**Rocky Mountain Poison and Drug Center (*)**

777 Bannock St., Mail Code 0180
Denver, CO  80204-4507
Business:       303-389-1100
**Emergency:**   800-222-1222
TDD/TTY:        303-739-1127 (CO)
www.RMPDC.org

# IDAHO

## (DENVER, CO)

**Rocky Mountain Poison and Drug Center (*)**

777 Bannock St., Mail Code 0180
Denver, CO  80204-4507
Business:       303-389-1100
**Emergency:**   800-222-1222
TDD/TTY:        303-739-1127 (CO)
www.RMPDC.org

# ILLINOIS

## CHICAGO

**Illinois Poison Center (*)**

222 South Riverside Plaza
Suite 1900
Chicago, IL  60606
Business:       312-906-6136
**Emergency:**   800-222-1222
TDD/TTY:        312-906-6185
http://illinoispoisoncenter.org/

# INDIANA

## INDIANAPOLIS

**Indiana Poison Control Center (*)**
**Clarian Health Partners Methodist Hospital**

I-65 at 21st St.
Indianapolis, IN  46206-1367
Business:       317-962-2335
**Emergency:**   800-222-1222
                 800-382-9097
                 317-962-2323
                 (Indianapolis)
www.clarian.org/poisoncontrol

# IOWA

## SIOUX CITY

**Iowa Statewide Poison Control Center (*)**
**Iowa Health System and the University of Iowa Hospitals and Clinics**

2910 Hamilton Blvd., Suite 101
Sioux City, IA  51104
Business:       712-279-3710
**Emergency:**   800-222-1222
                 712-277-2222 (IA)
www.iowapoison.org

# KANSAS

## KANSAS CITY

**Mid-America Poison Control**
**University of Kansas Medical Center**

3901 Rainbow Blvd.
Room B-400
Kansas City, KS  66160-7231
Business:       913-588-6638
**Emergency:**   800-222-1222
                 800-332-6633 (KS)

TDD:            913-588-6639
www.kumed.com/poison

## KENTUCKY

### LOUISVILLE

**Kentucky Regional Poison Center (*)**

PO Box 35070
Louisville, KY 40232-5070
Business:     502-629-7246
**Emergency:** 800-222-1222
              502-589-8222
              (Louisville)
www.krpc.com

## LOUISIANA

### MONROE

**Louisiana Drug and Poison Information Center (*)**
**University of Louisiana at Monroe**

700 University Ave.
Monroe, LA 71209-6430
Business:     318-342-3648
**Emergency:** 800-222-1222
www.lapcc.org

## MAINE

### PORTLAND

**Northern New England Poison Center (*)**
**Maine Medical Center**

22 Bramhall St.
Portland, ME 04102
Business:     207-662-7220
**Emergency:** 800-222-1222
TDD/TTY:      877-299-4447 (ME)
www.nnepc.org

## MARYLAND

### BALTIMORE

**Maryland Poison Center (*)**
**University of Maryland at Baltimore School of Pharmacy**

20 North Pine St., PH 772
Baltimore, MD 21201
Business:     410-706-7604
**Emergency:** 800-222-1222
              207-871-2879 (ME)
TDD:          410-706-1858
www.mdpoison.com

### (WASHINGTON, DC)

**National Capital Poison Center (*)**

3201 New Mexico Ave., NW
Suite 310
Washington, DC 20016
Business:     202-362-3867
**Emergency:** 800-222-1222
TDD/TTY:      202-362-8563 (MD)
www.poison.org

## MASSACHUSETTS

### BOSTON

**Regional Center for Poison Control and Prevention (*)**
**(Serving Massachusetts and Rhode Island)**

300 Longwood Ave.
Boston, MA 02115
Business:     617-355-6609
**Emergency:** 800-222-1222
TDD/TTY:      888-244-5313
www.maripoisoncenter.com

## MICHIGAN

### DETROIT

**Regional Poison Control Center (*)**
**Children's Hospital of Michigan**

4160 John R. Harper Professional Office Bldg.
Suite 616
Detroit, MI 48201
Business:     313-745-5335
**Emergency:** 800-222-1222
TDD/TTY:      800-356-3232
www.mitoxic.org/pcc

## MINNESOTA

### MINNEAPOLIS

**Minnesota Poison Control System**
**Hennepin County Medical Center**

701 Park Ave.
Mail Code RL
Minneapolis, MN 55415
Business:     612-873-3141
**Emergency:** 800-222-1222
www.mnpoison.org

## MISSISSIPPI

### JACKSON

**Mississippi Regional Poison Control Center**
**University of Mississippi Medical Center**

2500 North State St.
Jackson, MS 39216
Business:     601-984-1675
**Emergency:** 800-222-1222
http://poisoncontrol.umc.edu

## MISSOURI

### ST. LOUIS

**Missouri Regional Poison Center (*)**
**Cardinal Glennon Children's Medical Center**

1465 S. Grand Blvd.
St. Louis, MO 63104-1095
Business:     314-577-5610
**Emergency:** 800-222-1222
              314-577-5610
www.cardinalglennon.com

## MONTANA

### (DENVER, CO)

**Rocky Mountain Poison and Drug Center (*)**

777 Bannock St., Mail Code 0180
Denver, CO 80204-4507
Business:     303-389-1100
**Emergency:** 800-222-1222
TDD/TTY:      303-739-1127 (CO)
www.RMPDC.org

## NEBRASKA

### OMAHA

**The Poison Center (*)**
**Children's Hospital**

8200 Dodge St.
Omaha, NE 68114
Business:     402-955-5555
**Emergency:** 800-222-1222
www.nebraskapoison.com

## NEVADA

### (DENVER, CO)

**Rocky Mountain Poison and Drug Center (*)**

777 Bannock St., Mail Code 0180
Denver, CO 80204-4507
Business:     303-389-1100
**Emergency:** 800-222-1222
TDD/TTY:      303-739-1127 (CO)
www.RMPDC.org

### PORTLAND (OR)

**Oregon Poison Center (*)**
**Oregon Health Sciences University**

3181 SW Sam Jackson Park Rd.
Portland, OR 97201
Business:     503-494-8600
**Emergency:** 800-222-1222
www.ohsu.edu/poison

## NEW HAMPSHIRE

### (PORTLAND, ME)

**Northern New England Poison Center (*)**

Maine Medical Center
22 Bramhall St.
Portland, ME 04102
Business:     207-662-7220
**Emergency:** 800-222-1222
TDD/TTY:      877-299-4447 (ME)
www.nnepc.org

## NEW JERSEY

### NEWARK

**New Jersey Poison Information and Education System (*)**
**UMDNJ**

65 Bergen St.
Newark, NJ 07101

Business:      973-972-9280
**Emergency:**  800-222-1222
TDD/TTY:      973-926-8008
www.njpies.org

## NEW MEXICO

### ALBUQUERQUE

**New Mexico Poison and Drug Information Center (*)**

MSC09/5080
1 University of New Mexico
Albuquerque, NM 87131-0001
Business:      505-272-4261
**Emergency:**  800-222-1222
http://hsc.unm.edu/pharmacy/poison

## NEW YORK

### MINEOLA

**Long Island Regional Poison and Drug Information Center (*)**
**Winthrop University Hospital**

259 First St.
Mineola, NY 11501
Business:      516-663-2650
**Emergency:**  800-222-1222
TDD:          516-747-3323
              (Nassau)
              516-924-8811
              (Suffolk)
www.winthrop.org

### NEW YORK CITY

**New York City Poison Control Center (*)**
**NYC Department Public Health**

455 First Ave., Room 123
New York, NY 10016
Business:      212-447-8152
**Emergency:**  800-222-1222
(English)      212-340-4494
              212-POISONS
              (212-764-7667)
**Emergency:**  212-venenos
(Spanish)      (212-836-3667)
TDD:          212-689-9014
www.nyc.gov/html/doh/html/poison/poison.shtml

### ROCHESTER

**Fingerlakes Regional Poison and Drug Information Center (*)**
**University of Rochester Medical Center**

601 Elmwood Ave.
Box 321
Rochester, NY 14642
Business:      585-273-4155
**Emergency:**  800-222-1222
TTY:          585-273-3854
www.fingerlakespoison.org

### SYRACUSE

**Upstate New York Poison Center (*)**
**SUNY-Upstate Medical University**

750 East Adams St.
Syracuse, NY 13210
Business:      315-464-7078
**Emergency:**  800-222-1222
TTY:          315-464-5424
www.upstate.edu/poison/contactus/

## NORTH CAROLINA

### CHARLOTTE

**Carolinas Poison Center (*)**
**Carolina Medical Center**

PO Box 32861
Charlotte, NC 28232
Business:      704-395-3795
**Emergency:**  800-222-1222
TDD:          800-735-8262
TYY:          800-735-2962
www.ncpoisoncenter.org

## NORTH DAKOTA

### (MINNEAPOLIS, MN)

**Minnesota Poison Control System**
**Hennepin County Medical Center**

701 Park Ave.
Mail Code RL
Minneapolis, MN 55415
Business:      612-873-3141
**Emergency:**  800-222-1222
www.mnpoison.org

## OHIO

### CINCINNATI

**Cincinnati Drug and Poison Information Center (*)**
**Regional Poison Control System**

3333 Burnet Ave.
Vermon Place, 3rd Floor
Cincinnati, OH 45229
Business:      513-636-5111
**Emergency:**  800-222-1222
TTY:          800-253-7955
www.cincinnatichildrens.org/dpic

### CLEVELAND

**Greater Cleveland**
**Poison Control Center**
**University Hospitals**

11100 Euclid Ave.
B261 MP 6007
Cleveland, OH 44106-6007
Business:      216-844-1573
**Emergency:**  800-222-1222
              216-231-4455 (OH)
www.uhhospitals.org/
rainbowchildren/tabid/195/
Default.aspx

## COLUMBUS

**Central Ohio Poison Center (*)**
**Nationwide Children's Hospital**

700 Children's Dr.
Room L032
Columbus, OH 43205-2696
Business:      614-722-2635
**Emergency:**  800-222-1222
              614-228-1323
              937-222-2227
              (Dayton region)
TTY:          614-228-2272
www.bepoisonsmart.com

## OKLAHOMA

### OKLAHOMA CITY

**Oklahoma Poison Control**
**Center (*)**
**Children's Hospital at OU Health Sciences Center**

940 NE 13th St.
Room 3510
Oklahoma City, OK 73104
Business:      405-271-5062
**Emergency:**  800-222-1222
www.oklahomapoison.org

## OREGON

### PORTLAND

**Oregon Poison Center (*)**
**Oregon Health Sciences University**

3181 SW Sam Jackson Park Rd.
CB550
Portland, OR 97239
Business:      503-494-8600
**Emergency:**  800-222-1222
www.ohsu.edu/poison

## PENNSYLVANIA

### PHILADELPHIA

**The Poison Control Center (*)**
**Children's Hospital of Philadelphia**

34th St. & Civic Center Blvd.
Philadelphia, PA 19104-4399
Business:      215-590-2003
**Emergency:**  800-222-1222
              800-722-7112 (DE)
TDD/TTY:      215-590-8789
www.chop.edu

### PITTSBURGH

**Pittsburgh Poison Center (*)**
**University of Pittsburgh Medical Center**

200 Lothrop Street
Pittsburgh, PA 15213
Business:      412-390-3300
**Emergency:**  800-222-1222
              412-681-6669
www.upmc.com/services/
poisoncenter

## PUERTO RICO

**Puerto Rico Poison Control Center, Inc.**
**Administracion de Servicios Medicos de P.R.**
**(ASEM),**

Centro Medico de Puerto Rico
Barrio Monacillo Carr. #22,
Paseo Dr. Jose Celso Barbosa
Rio Piedras Pu 935
**Emergency:** 800-222-1222

## RHODE ISLAND

### (BOSTON, MA)

**Regional Center for Poison Control and Prevention (*)**

300 Longwood Ave.
Boston, MA 02115
**Business:** 617-355-6609
**Emergency:** 800-222-1222
**TDD/TTY:** 888-244-5313
www.maripoisoncenter.com

## SOUTH CAROLINA

### COLUMBIA

**Palmetto Poison Center (*)**
**University of South Carolina-College of Pharmacy**

USC Columbia, SC 29208
**Business:** 803-777-7909
**Emergency:** 800-222-1222
http://poison.sc.edu

## SOUTH DAKOTA

### (MINNEAPOLIS, MN)

**Minnesota Poison Control System**
**Hennepin County Medical Center**

701 Park Ave.
Mail Code RL
Minneapolis, MN 55415
**Business:** 612-873-3141
**Emergency:** 800-222-1222
www.mnpoison.org

### SIOUX FALLS

**Sanford Poison Center**

Sanford Health USD Medical Center
1305 W 18th Street - PO Box 5039
Sioux Falls, SD 57117-5039
**Business:** 605-333-6638
**Emergency:** 800-222-1222
www.sdpoison.org

## TENNESSEE

### NASHVILLE

**Tennessee Poison Center (*)**

1161 21st Ave. South
501 Oxford House
Nashville, TN 37232-4632
**Business:** 615-936-0760
**Emergency:** 800-222-1222
www.tnpoisoncenter.org

## TEXAS

### AMARILLO

**Texas Panhandle Poison Center (*)**

1501 S. Coulter Dr.
Amarillo, TX 79106
**Business:** 806-354-1630
**Emergency:** 800-222-1222
www.poisoncontrol.org

### DALLAS

**North Texas Poison Center (*)**
**Texas Poison Center Network**
**Parkland Health & Hospital System**

5201 Harry Hines Blvd.
Dallas, TX 75235
**Business:** 214-590-9011
**Emergency:** 800-222-1222
www.poisoncontrol.org

### EL PASO

**West Texas Regional Poison Center (*)**
**Thomason Hospital**

4815 Alameda Ave.
El Paso, TX 79905
**Business:** 915-534-3800
**Emergency:** 800-222-1222
www.poisoncontrol.org

### GALVESTON

**Southeast Texas Poison Center (*)**
**The University of Texas Medical Branch**

301 University Blvd.
3.112 Trauma Bldg.
Galveston, TX 77555-1175
**Business:** 409-766-4403
**Emergency:** 800-222-1222
www.utmb.edu/setpc

### SAN ANTONIO

**South Texas Poison Center (*)**
**The University of Texas Health Science Center–San Antonio**

7703 Floyd Curl Dr., MSC 7849
Trauma Bldg.
San Antonio, TX 78229-3900
**Business:** 210-567-5762
**Emergency:** 800-222-1222
**TTY:** 800-222-1222
www.texaspoison.com

## TEMPLE

**Central Texas Poison Center (*)**
**Scott & White Healthcare**

2401 South 31st St.
Temple, TX 76508
**Business:** 254-724-2111
**Emergency:** 800-222-1222
http://www.sw.org/web/
patientsAndVisitors/iwcontent/
public/poison/en_us/html/poison.jsp

## UTAH

### SALT LAKE CITY

**Utah Poison Control Center (*)**
**University of Utah**

585 Komas Dr. Suite #200
Salt Lake City, UT 84108-1234
**Business:** 801-581-7504
**Emergency:** 800-222-1222
http://uuhsc.utah.edu/poison

## VERMONT

### (PORTLAND, ME)

**Northern New England Poison Center (*)**
**Maine Medical Center**

22 Bramhall St.
Portland, ME 04102
**Business:** 207-662-7220
**Emergency:** 800-222-1222
**TDD/TTY:** 877-299-4447 (ME)
www.nnepc.org

## VIRGINIA

### CHARLOTTESVILLE

**Blue Ridge Poison Center (*)**
**University of Virginia-School of Medicine**

PO Box 800774
Charlottesville, VA 22908
**Business:** 434-924-5118
**Emergency:** 800-222-1222
800-451-1418 (VA)
www.healthsystem.virginia.edu/brpc

### RICHMOND

**Virginia Poison Center (*)**
**Virginia Commonwealth University-Medical Center**

P.O. Box 980522
Richmond, VA 23298-0522
**Business:** 804-828-4780
**Emergency:** 800-222-1222
804-828-9123
**TDD/TYY:** 804-828-9123
www.poison.vcu.edu

## WASHINGTON

### SEATTLE

**Washington Poison Center (*)**

155 NE 100th St., Suite 400
Seattle, WA  98125-8007
Business:        206-517-2351
**Emergency:**   800-222-1222
                 206-526-2121 (WA)
TDD:             800-572-0638 (WA)
                 206-517-2394
                 (Seattle)
www.wapc.org

## WEST VIRGINIA

### CHARLESTON

**West Virginia Poison Center (*)**
**WVU Robert C. Byrd Health Sciences Center**

3110 MacCorkle Ave. SE
Charleston, WV  25304
Business:        304-347-1212
**Emergency:**   800-222-1222
www.wvpoisoncenter.org

## WISCONSIN

### MILWAUKEE

**Wisconsin Poison Center (*)**
**Children's Hospital of Wisconsin**

9000 W. Wisconsin Ave.
P.O. Box 1997, Mail Station 677A
Milwaukee, WI  53201
Business:        414-266-2000
**Emergency:**   800-222-1222
TDD/TYY:         414-964-3497
www.wisconsinpoison.org

## WYOMING

### (OMAHA, NE)

**The Poison Center (*)**
**Children's Hospital**

8200 Dodge St.
Omaha, NE  68114
Business:        402-955-5555
**Emergency:**   800-222-1222
www.nebraskapoison.com

# PRODUCT COMPARISON TABLES

This section offers a graphic overview of the most-used OTC drugs for select categories or conditions, as well as information that may be helpful in selecting or recommending appropriate products.

- Antipyretic Products
- Insomnia Products
- Smoking Cessation Products
- Weight Management Products
- Antifungal Products
- Contact Dermatitis Products
- Diaper Rash Products
- Psoriasis Products
- Wound Care Products

- Antacid and Heartburn Products
- Antidiarrheal Products
- Laxative Products
- Allergic Rhinitis Products
- Is It a Cold, the Flu, or an Allergy?
- Cough-Cold-Flu Products
- Analgesic Products
- Dietary Calcium Intake

## Table 1. ANTIPYRETIC PRODUCTS

| BRAND NAME | INGREDIENT/STRENGTH | DOSE |
|---|---|---|
| **ACETAMINOPHEN** | | |
| Anacin Extra Strength Aspirin Free Tablets | Acetaminophen 500mg | **Adults & Peds ≥12 yrs:** 2 tabs q6h. **Max:** 8 tabs q24h. |
| FeverAll Childrens' Suppositories | Acetaminophen 120mg | **Peds 3-6 yrs:** 1 supp q4-6h. **Max:** 6 supp q24h. |
| FeverAll Infants' Suppositories | Acetaminophen 80mg | **Peds 6-11 months:** 1 supp q6h. **12-36 months:** 1 supp q4h. **Max:** 6 supp q24h. |
| FeverAll Jr. Strength Suppositories | Acetaminophen 325mg | **Peds 6-12 yrs:** 1 supp q4-6h. **Max:** 6 supp q24h. |
| Tylenol 8 Hour Caplets | Acetaminophen 650mg | **Adults & Peds ≥12 yrs:** 2 tabs q8h prn. **Max:** 6 tabs q24h. |
| Tylenol Arthritis Caplets | Acetaminophen 650mg | **Adults:** 2 tabs q8h prn. **Max:** 6 tabs q24h. |
| Tylenol Arthritis Gelcaps | Acetaminophen 650mg | **Adults:** 2 caps q8h prn. **Max:** 6 caps q24h. |
| Tylenol Arthritis Geltabs | Acetaminophen 650mg | **Adults:** 2 tabs q8h prn. **Max:** 6 tabs q24h. |
| Tylenol Children's Meltaways Tablets* | Acetaminophen 80mg | **Peds 2-3 yrs (24-35 lbs):** 2 tabs. **4-5 yrs (36-47 lbs):** 3 tabs. **6-8 yrs (48-59 lbs):** 4 tabs. **9-10 yrs (60-71 lbs):** 5 tabs. **11 yrs (72-95 lbs):** 6 tabs. May repeat q4h. **Max:** 5 doses q24h. |
| Tylenol Children's Suspension* | Acetaminophen 160mg/5mL | **Peds 2-3 yrs (24-35 lbs):** 1 tsp (5mL). **4-5 yrs (36-47 lbs):** 1.5 tsp (7.5mL). **6-8 yrs (48-59 lbs):** 2 tsp (10mL). **9-10 yrs (60-71 lbs):** 2.5 tsp (12.5mL). **11 yrs (72-95 lbs):** 3 tsp (15mL). May repeat q4h. **Max:** 5 doses q24h. |
| Tylenol Extra Strength Caplets | Acetaminophen 500mg | **Adults & Peds ≥12 yrs:** 2 tabs q4-6h prn. **Max:** 8 tabs q24h. |
| Tylenol Extra Strength Cool Caplets | Acetaminophen 500mg | **Adults & Peds ≥12 yrs:** 2 tabs q4-6h prn. **Max:** 8 tabs q24h. |

*(Continued)*

## Table 1. ANTIPYRETIC PRODUCTS (cont.)

| BRAND NAME | INGREDIENT/STRENGTH | DOSE |
|---|---|---|
| Tylenol Extra Strength EZ Tablets | Acetaminophen 500mg | **Adults & Peds ≥12 yrs:** 2 tabs q4-6h prn. **Max:** 8 tabs q24h. |
| Tylenol Extra Strength Rapid Blast Liquid | Acetaminophen 500mg/15mL | **Adults & Peds ≥12 yrs:** 2 tbl (30mL) q4-6h prn. **Max:** 8 tbl (120mL) q24h. |
| Tylenol Extra Strength Rapid Release Gelcaps | Acetaminophen 500mg | **Adults & Peds ≥12 yrs:** 2 caps q4-6h prn. **Max:** 8 caps q24h. |
| Tylenol Infants' Drops* | Acetaminophen 160mg/1.6mL | **Peds 2-3 yrs (24-35 lbs):** 1.6 mL q4h prn. **Max:** 5 doses (8mL) q24h. |
| Tylenol Junior Meltaways Tablets* | Acetaminophen 160mg | **Peds 6-8 yrs (48-59 lbs):** 2 tabs. **9-10 yrs (60-71 lbs):** 2.5 tabs. **11 yrs (72-95 lbs):** 3 tabs. **12 yrs (≥96 lbs):** 4 tabs. May repeat q4h. **Max:** 5 doses q24h. |
| Tylenol Regular Strength Tablets | Acetaminophen 325mg | **Adults & Peds ≥12 yrs:** 2 tabs q4-6h prn. **Max:** 12 tabs q24h. **Peds 6-11 yrs:** 1 tab q4-6h. **Max:** 5 tabs q24h. |
| **NONSTEROIDAL ANTI-INFLAMMATORY DRUGS (NSAIDS)** | | |
| Advil Caplets | Ibuprofen 200mg | **Adults & Peds ≥12 yrs:** 1-2 tabs q4-6h. **Max:** 6 tabs q24h. |
| Advil Children's Suspension | Ibuprofen 100mg/5mL | **Peds 2-3 yrs (24-35 lbs):** 1 tsp (5mL). **4-5 yrs (36-47 lbs):** 1.5 tsp (7.5mL). **6-8 yrs (48-59 lbs):** 2 tsp (10mL). **9-10 yrs (60-71 lbs):** 2.5 tsp (12.5mL). **11 yrs (72-95 lbs):** 3 tsp (15mL). May repeat q6-8h. **Max:** 4 doses q24h. |
| Advil Gel Caplets | Ibuprofen 200mg | **Adults & Peds ≥12 yrs:** 1-2 tabs q4-6h. **Max:** 6 tabs q24h. |
| Advil Infants' Concentrated Drops* | Ibuprofen 50mg/1.25mL | **Peds 6-11 months (12-17 lbs):** 1.25mL. **12-23 months (18-23 lbs):** 1.875mL. May repeat q6-8h. **Max:** 4 doses q24h. |
| Advil Liqui-Gels | Ibuprofen 200mg | **Adults & Peds ≥12 yrs:** 1-2 caps q4-6h. **Max:** 6 caps q24h. |

## Table 1. ANTIPYRETIC PRODUCTS (cont.)

| BRAND NAME | INGREDIENT/STRENGTH | DOSE |
| --- | --- | --- |
| Advil Tablets | Ibuprofen 200mg | **Adults & Peds ≥12 yrs:** 1-2 tabs q4-6h. **Max:** 6 tabs q24h. |
| Aleve Caplets | Naproxen Sodium 220mg | **Adults & Peds ≥12 yrs:** 1 tab q8-12h. May take 1 additional tab within 1 hour of first dose. **Max:** 2 tabs q8-12h or 3 tabs q24h. |
| Aleve Liquid Gels | Naproxen Sodium 220mg | **Adults & Peds ≥12 yrs:** 1 cap q8-12h. May take 1 additional cap within 1 hour of first dose. **Max:** 2 caps q8-12h or 3 caps q24h. |
| Aleve Tablets | Naproxen Sodium 220mg | **Adults & Peds ≥12 yrs:** 1 tab q8-12h. May take 1 additional tab within 1 hour of first dose. **Max:** 2 tabs q8-12h or 3 tabs q24h. |
| Motrin Children's Suspension*† | Ibuprofen 100mg/5mL | **Peds 2-3 yrs (24-35 lbs):** 1 tsp (5mL). **4-5 yrs (36-47 lbs):** 1.5 tsp (7.5mL). **6-8 yrs (48-59 lbs):** 2 tsp (10mL). **9-10 yrs (60-71 lbs):** 2.5 tsp (12.5mL). **11 yrs (72-95 lbs):** 3 tsp (15mL). May repeat q6-8h. **Max:** 4 doses q24h. |
| Motrin IB Caplets | Ibuprofen 200mg | **Adults & Peds ≥12 yrs:** 1-2 tabs q4-6h. **Max:** 6 tabs q24h. |
| Motrin IB Tablets | Ibuprofen 200mg | **Adults & Peds ≥12 yrs:** 1-2 tabs q4-6h. **Max:** 6 tabs q24h. |
| Motrin Infants' Drops*† | Ibuprofen 50mg/1.25mL | **Peds 6-11 months (12-17 lbs):** 1.25mL. **12-23 months (18-23 lbs):** 1.875mL. May repeat q6-8h. **Max:** 4 doses q24h. |
| Motrin Junior Strength Caplets*† | Ibuprofen 100mg | **Peds 6-8 yrs (48-59 lbs):** 2 tabs. **9-10 yrs (60-71 lbs):** 2.5 tabs. **11 yrs (72-95 lbs):** 3 tabs. May repeat q6-8h. **Max:** 4 doses q24h. |

*(Continued)*

## Table 1. ANTIPYRETIC PRODUCTS (cont.)

| BRAND NAME | INGREDIENT/STRENGTH | DOSE |
|---|---|---|
| Motrin Junior Strength Chewable Tablets*† | Ibuprofen 100mg | **Peds 2-3 yrs (24-35 lbs):** 1 tab. **4-5 yrs (36-47 lbs):** 1.5 tabs. **6-8 yrs (48-59 lbs):** 2 tabs. **9-10 yrs (60-71 lbs):** 2.5 tabs. **11 yrs (72-95 lbs):** 3 tabs. May repeat q6-8h. **Max:** 4 doses q24h. |
| **SALICYLATES** | | |
| Bayer Aspirin Extra Strength Caplets | Aspirin 500mg | **Adults & Peds ≥12 yrs:** 1-2 tabs q4-6h. **Max:** 8 tabs q24h. |
| Bayer Aspirin Safety Coated Caplets | Aspirin 325mg | **Adults & Peds ≥12 yrs:** 1-2 tabs q4h. **Max:** 12 tabs q24h. |
| Bayer Genuine Aspirin Tablets | Aspirin 325mg | **Adults & Peds ≥12 yrs:** 1-2 tabs q4h or 3 tabs q6h. **Max:** 12 tabs q24h. |
| Bayer Low-Dose Aspirin Chewable Tablets* | Aspirin 81mg | **Adults & Peds ≥12 yrs:** 4-8 tabs q4h. **Max:** 48 tabs q24h. |
| Bayer Low-Dose Aspirin Safety Coated Tablets | Aspirin 81mg | **Adults & Peds ≥12 yrs:** 4-8 tabs q4h. **Max:** 48 tabs q24h. |
| Ecotrin Low Strength Tablets | Aspirin 81mg | **Adults:** 4-8 tabs q4h. **Max:** 48 tabs q24h. |
| Ecotrin Regular Strength Tablets | Aspirin 325mg | **Adults & Peds ≥12 yrs:** 1-2 tabs q4h. **Max:** 12 tabs q24h. |
| Halfprin 162mg Tablets | Aspirin 162mg | **Adults & Peds ≥12 yrs:** 2-4 tabs q4h. **Max:** 24 tabs q24h. |
| Halfprin 81mg Tablets | Aspirin 81mg | **Adults & Peds ≥12 yrs:** 4-8 tabs q4h. **Max:** 48 tabs q24h. |
| St. Joseph Aspirin Chewable Tablets | Aspirin 81mg | **Adults & Peds ≥12 yrs:** 4-8 tabs q4h. **Max:** 48 tabs q24h. |
| St. Joseph Enteric Safety-Coated Tablets | Aspirin 81mg | **Adults & Peds ≥12 yrs:** 4-8 tabs q4h. **Max:** 48 tabs q24h. |
| **SALICYLATES, BUFFERED** | | |
| Bayer Extra Strength Plus Caplets | Aspirin 500mg Buffered with Calcium Carbonate | **Adults & Peds ≥12 yrs:** 1-2 tabs q4-6h. **Max:** 8 tabs q24h. |
| Bayer Women's Low Dose Aspirin Caplets | Aspirin 81mg Buffered with Calcium Carbonate 777mg | **Adults & Peds ≥12 yrs:** 4-8 tabs q4h. **Max:** 10 tabs q24h. |

## Table 1. ANTIPYRETIC PRODUCTS (cont.)

| BRAND NAME | INGREDIENT/STRENGTH | DOSE |
|---|---|---|
| Bufferin Extra Strength Tablets | Aspirin 500mg Buffered with Calcium Carbonate/Magnesium Oxide/ Magnesium Carbonate | **Adults & Peds ≥12 yrs:** 2 tabs q6h. **Max:** 8 tabs q24h. |
| Bufferin Tablets | Aspirin 325mg Buffered with Benzoic Acid/Citric Acid | **Adults & Peds ≥12 yrs:** 2 tabs q4h. **Max:** 12 tabs q24h. |
| Bufferin Low Dose Tablets | Aspirin 81mg Buffered with Calcium Carbonate/Magnesium Oxide/ Magnesium Carbonate | **Adults & Peds ≥12 yrs:** 4-8 tabs q4h. **Max:** 48 tabs q24h. |

*Multiple flavors available.
†Product currently on recall, available in generic form.

## Table 2. INSOMNIA PRODUCTS

| BRAND NAME | INGREDIENT/STRENGTH | DOSE |
| --- | --- | --- |
| **DIPHENHYDRAMINE** | | |
| Nytol Quick Caps Caplets | Diphenhydramine 25mg | **Adults & Peds ≥12 yrs:** 2 tabs qhs. |
| Simply Sleep Nighttime Sleep Aid Caplets | Diphenhydramine 25mg | **Adults & Peds ≥12 yrs:** 2 tabs qhs. |
| Sominex Original Formula | Diphenhydramine 25mg | **Adults & Peds ≥12 yrs:** 2 tabs qhs. |
| Sominex Maximum Strength Formula | Diphenhydramine 50mg | **Adults & Peds ≥12 yrs:** 1 tab qhs. |
| Unisom Nighttime Sleep-Aid Sleep Gels | Diphenhydramine 50mg | **Adults & Peds ≥12 yrs:** 1 cap qhs. |
| Unisom Sleep Melts | Diphenhydramine 25mg | **Adults & Peds ≥12 yrs:** 2 tabs qhs. |
| **DIPHENHYDRAMINE COMBINATION** | | |
| Advil PM Caplets | Ibuprofen/Diphenhydramine Citrate 200mg-38mg | **Adults & Peds ≥12 yrs:** 2 tabs qhs. |
| Advil PM Liqui-Gels | Ibuprofen/Diphenhydramine HCl 200mg-25mg | **Adults & Peds ≥12 yrs:** 2 caps qhs. |
| Bayer PM Relief Caplets | Aspirin/Diphenhydramine Citrate 500mg-38.3mg | **Adults & Peds ≥12 yrs:** 2 tabs qhs. |
| Doan's Extra Strength PM Caplets | Magnesium Salicylate Tetrahydrate/ Diphenhydramine 580mg-25mg | **Adults & Peds ≥12 yrs:** 2 tabs qhs. |
| Excedrin PM Caplets | Acetaminophen/Diphenhydramine Citrate 500mg-38mg | **Adults & Peds ≥12 yrs:** 2 tabs qhs. |
| Excedrin PM Express Gels | Acetaminophen/Diphenhydramine Citrate 500mg-38mg | **Adults & Peds ≥12 yrs:** 2 caps qhs. |
| Goody's PM Powder | Acetaminophen/Diphenhydramine Citrate 1000mg-76mg/dose | **Adults & Peds ≥12 yrs:** 1 packet (2 powders) qhs. |
| Motrin PM Caplets | Ibuprofen/Diphenhydramine Citrate 200-38mg | **Adults & Peds ≥12 yrs:** 2 tabs qhs. |
| Tylenol PM Caplets | Acetaminophen/Diphenhydramine HCl 500mg-25mg | **Adults & Peds ≥12 yrs:** 2 tabs qhs. |
| Tylenol PM Rapid Release Gelcaps | Acetaminophen/Diphenhydramine HCl 500mg-25mg | **Adults & Peds ≥12 yrs:** 2 caps qhs. |

*(Continued)*

## Table 2. INSOMNIA PRODUCTS (cont.)

| BRAND NAME | INGREDIENT/STRENGTH | DOSE |
|---|---|---|
| Tylenol PM Geltabs | Acetaminophen/Diphenhydramine HCl 500mg-25mg | **Adults & Peds ≥12 yrs:** 2 tabs qhs. |
| Tylenol PM Liquid | Acetaminophen/Diphenhydramine HCl 1000mg-50mg/30mL | **Adults & Peds ≥12 yrs:** 2 tbl (30mL) qhs. |
| Unisom PM Pain SleepCaps | Acetaminophen/Diphenhydramine HCl 325mg-50mg | **Adults & Peds ≥12 yrs:** 1 cap qhs. |
| **DOXYLAMINE** | | |
| Unisom Nighttime Sleep-Aid Sleep Tabs | Doxylamine Succinate 25mg | **Adults & Peds ≥12 yrs:** 1 tab 30 min before hs. |

## Table 3. SMOKING CESSATION PRODUCTS

| BRAND NAME | INGREDIENT/STRENGTH | DOSE |
| --- | --- | --- |
| NicoDerm CQ Step 1 Clear Patch | Nicotine 21mg | **Adults:** If smoking >10 cigarettes/day. **Weeks 1 to 6:** Apply one 21mg patch/day. **Weeks 7 to 8:** Apply one 14mg patch/day. **Weeks 9 to 10:** Apply one 7mg patch/day. |
| NicoDerm CQ Step 2 Clear Patch | Nicotine 14mg | **Adults:** If smoking >10 cigarettes/day. **Weeks 1 to 6:** Apply one 21mg patch/day. **Weeks 7 to 8:** Apply one 14mg patch/day. **Weeks 9 to 10:** Apply one 7mg patch/day. If smoking ≤10 cigarettes/day. **Weeks 1 to 6:** Apply one 14mg patch/day. **Weeks 7 to 8:** Apply one 7mg patch/day. |
| NicoDerm CQ Step 3 Clear Patch | Nicotine 7mg | **Adults:** Apply 1 patch qd Weeks 9 to 10 if smoking >10 cigarettes/day or Weeks 7 to 8 if smoking <10 cigarettes/day. |
| Nicorette 2mg | Nicotine Polacrilex 2mg | **Adults:** If smoking <25 cigarettes/day use 2mg gum. **Weeks 1 to 6:** 1 piece q1-2h. **Weeks 7 to 9:** 1 piece q2-4h. **Weeks 10 to 12:** 1 piece q4-8h. **Max:** 24 pieces/day. |
| Nicorette 4mg | Nicotine Polacrilex 4mg | **Adults:** If smoking ≥25 cigarettes/day use 4mg gum. **Weeks 1 to 6:** 1 piece q1-2h. **Weeks 7 to 9:** 1 piece q2-4h. **Weeks 10 to 12:** 1 piece q4-8h. **Max:** 24 pieces/day. |
| Nicorette Stop Smoking 2mg Lozenges | Nicotine Polacrilex 2mg | **Adults:** If smoking first cigarette >30 minutes after waking up use 2mg lozenge. **Weeks 1 to 6:** 1 lozenge q1-2h. **Weeks 7 to 9:** 1 lozenge q2-4h. **Weeks 10 to 12:** 1 lozenge q4-8h. **Max:** 5 lozenges/6 hours; 20 lozenges/day. Stop using at the end of 12 weeks. |

*(Continued)*

## Table 3. SMOKING CESSATION PRODUCTS (cont.)

| BRAND NAME | INGREDIENT/STRENGTH | DOSE |
|---|---|---|
| Nicorette Stop Smoking 4mg Lozenges | Nicotine Polacrilex 4mg | **Adults:** If smoking first cigarette within 30 minutes after waking up use 4mg lozenge. **Weeks 1 to 6:** 1 lozenge q1-2h. **Weeks 7 to 9:** 1 lozenge q2-4h. **Weeks 10 to 12:** 1 lozenge q4-8h. **Max:** 5 lozenges/6 hours; 20 lozenges/ day. Stop using at the end of 12 weeks. |
| Habitrol Nicotine Transdermal System Patch Step 1 | Nicotine 21mg/24hr | **Adults:** If smoking >10 cigarettes/day. **Weeks 1 to 4:** Apply one 21mg patch/day. **Weeks 5 to 6:** Apply one 14mg patch/day. **Weeks 7 to 8:** Apply one 7mg patch/day. |
| Habitrol Nicotine Transdermal System Patch Step 2 | Nicotine 14mg/24hr | **Adults:** If smoking >10 cigarettes/day. **Weeks 1 to 4:** Apply one 21mg patch/day. **Weeks 5 to 6:** Apply one 14mg patch/day. **Weeks 7 to 8:** Apply one 7mg patch/day. If smoking ≤10 cigarettes/day. **Weeks 1 to 6:** Apply one 14 mg patch/day. **Weeks 7 to 8:** Apply one 7mg patch/day. |
| Habitrol Nicotine Transdermal System Patch Step 3 | Nicotine 7mg/24hr | **Adults:** If smoking >10 cigarettes/day. **Weeks 1 to 4:** Apply one 21mg patch/day. **Weeks 5 to 6:** Apply one 14mg patch/day. **Weeks 7 to 8:** Apply one 7mg patch/day. If smoking ≤10 cigarettes/day. **Weeks 1 to 6:** Apply one 14mg patch/day. **Weeks 7 to 8:** Apply one 7mg patch/day. |

## Table 4. WEIGHT MANAGEMENT PRODUCTS

| BRAND NAME | DOSE |
|---|---|
| Alli Weight-Loss Aid | **Adults:** 1 cap with each fat-containing meal. **Max:** 3 caps per day. |
| Applied Nutrition Carb Blocker | **Adults:** Take 2 caps with meals bid. |
| Applied Nutrition Green Tea Fat Burner | **Adults:** Take 2 caps with meals bid. |
| Applied Nutrition Green Tea Triple Fat Burner | **Adults:** Take 2 caps with meals bid. |
| Applied Nutrition Natural Fat Burner Capsules | **Adults:** Take 2 caps with meals bid. |
| Applied Nutrition Resveratol Rapid Calorie Burn | **Adults:** Take 2 tabs qam and 2 tabs qpm. |
| Aqua-Ban Maximum Strength Diuretic Tablets | **Adults:** Take 1 tab qid. **Max:** 4 tabs q24h. |
| BioMD Nutraceuticals Metabolism T3 Capsules | **Adults:** Take 2 caps with meals bid-tid. **Max:** 6 caps q24h. |
| Biotest Hot-Rox Capsules | **Adults:** Take 1-2 caps bid. **Max:** 6 caps q24h. |
| Carb Cutter Original Formula Tablets | **Adults:** Take 1-2 tabs with a glass of water 15 mins prior to carbohydrate foods. |
| Carb Cutter Phase 2 Starch Neutralizer Tablets | **Adults:** Take 1-2 tabs with meals bid. |
| Dexatrim Max | **Adults:** Take 1-2 caps with water, one in AM and one in afternoon. **Max:** 2 caps q24h. |
| Dexatrim Max Daytime Appetite Control | **Adults:** Take 1-2 caps daily. **Max:** 2 caps q24h. |
| Dexatrim Max Slim Packs | **Adults:** Dissolve 1 packet in 16.9 ounces of water. **Max:** 6 packs q24h. |
| Dexatrim Natural Extra Energy Formula Caplets | **Adults:** Take 1 tab with meals tid. **Max:** 3 tabs q24h. |
| Dexatrim Natural Green Tea Formula Caplets | **Adults:** Take 1 tab with meals tid. **Max:** 3 tabs q24h. |
| Dexatrim Max Complex 7 | **Adults:** Take 2 caps qam. Second serving mid-afternoon. **Max:** 4 caps q24h. |
| EAS CLA Capsules | **Adults:** Take 2 caps with meals tid. |
| Estrin-D Capsules | **Adults:** Take 2 caps 30 min before meals. **Max:** 6 caps q24h. |
| Isatori MX-LS7 Maximum Strength Lean System 7 | **Adults: Men/Women <200 lbs:** Day 1 to 6: 2 caps bid. Day 7 & on: 3 caps bid. **Men >200 lbs:** Day 1 to 6: 2 caps bid. Day 7 to 14: 3 caps bid. Day 14 & on: 4 caps bid. **Max:** 4 caps q4h. |
| Metabolife Break Through | **Adults:** Take 2 tabs 1 hr before meals tid, at least 3-4 hrs apart. **Max:** 6 tabs q24h. |

*(Continued)*

## Table 4. WEIGHT MANAGEMENT PRODUCTS (cont.)

| Brand Name | Dose |
| --- | --- |
| Metabolife Extreme Energy | **Adults:** Take 1-2 tabs tid at least 3-4 hrs apart. **Max:** 4 tabs q8h. |
| Metabolife Ultra Caplets | **Adults:** Take 2 tabs tid 30-60 min before meals, at least 3-4 hrs apart. **Max:** 6 tabs q24h. |
| Metabolife Caffeine Free Caplets | **Adults:** Take 2 tabs tid 30-60 min before meals, at least 3-4 hrs apart. **Max:** 6 tabs q24h. |
| Metabolife Green Tea | **Adults:** Take 2 tabs tid 30-60 min before meals, at least 3-4 hrs apart. **Max:** 6 tabs q24h. |
| MHP TakeOff, Hi-Energy Fat Burner Capsules | **Adults:** Take 2 caps qd or bid. |
| Natrol Carb Intercept with Phase 2 Starch Neutralizer Capsules | **Adults:** Take 2 caps before carbohydrate-containing meals. |
| Natrol Green Tea 500mg Capsules | **Adults:** Take 1 cap with meals qd. |
| Natural Balance Fat Magnet Capsules | **Adults:** Take 2 caps with meals bid. |
| Nature Made Chromium Picolinate, Extra Strength | **Adults:** Take 1 tab qd. |
| Nunaturals LevelRight for Blood Sugar Management Capsules | **Adults:** Take 1 cap with meals tid. |
| Prolab Enhanced CLA | **Adults:** Take 3 caps with meals qd. |
| Stacker 2 Ephedra Free Capsules | **Adults:** Take 1 cap after meals. **Max:** 3 caps q24h. |
| Stacker 3 Ephedra Free Formula with Chitosan Capsules | **Adults:** Take 1 cap after meals. **Max:** 3 caps q24h. |
| Stacker 3 XPLC Extreme Performance Formula Ephedra Free | **Adults:** Take 1 cap after meals. **Max:** 3 caps q24h. |
| Tetrazene ES-50 Ultra High-Energy Weight Loss Catalyst Capsules | **Adults:** Take 2 caps with meals tid. **Max:** 6 caps q24h. |
| Tetrazene KGM-90 Rapid Weight Loss Catalyst Capsules | **Adults:** Take 2 caps with meals tid. **Max:** 6 caps q24h. |
| Twinlab CLA Fuel | **Adults:** Take 1 cap tid. |
| Twinlab GTF Chromium | **Adults:** Take 1 tab qd. |
| Twinlab Mega L-Carnitine | **Adults:** Take 1 tab daily on an empty stomach |
| Twinlab Metabolift, Ephedra Free Formula Capsules | **Adults:** Take 2 caps before each meal. **Max:** 6 caps q24h. |
| Twinlab Ripped Fuel 5X | **Adults:** Take 1 tab before meals bid. |

## Table 4. WEIGHT MANAGEMENT PRODUCTS (cont.)

| Brand Name | Dose |
|---|---|
| Twinlab Ripped Fuel Ephedra Free | **Adults:** Take 2 caps before each meal. **Max:** 6 caps q24h. |
| Twinlab Ripped Fuel Extreme | **Adults:** Take 2 caps bid. |
| Twinlab Ripped Fuel Xtendr | **Adults:** Take 2 tabs 30 min before meals. **Max:** 6 tabs q24h. |
| Twinlab 7-Keto Fuel | **Adults:** Take 2-4 caps daily. |
| Ultra Diet Pep Tablets | **Adults:** Take 1 tab with meals bid. |
| XtremeLean Advanced Formula, Ephedra Free Capsules | **Adults:** Take 2 caps before meals bid. |
| Zantrex 3, Ephedrine Free | **Adults:** Take 2 caps with meals qd. **Max:** 6 caps q24h. |
| Zantrex 3 High Energy Fat Burner | **Adults:** Take 2 caps qam and 2 caps with main meal. **Max:** 4 caps q24h. |
| Zantrex 3 Power Crystals | **Adults:** Add 1 packet to 16 oz of water. **Max:** 3 packets q24h. |

## Table 5. ANTIFUNGAL PRODUCTS

| BRAND NAME | INGREDIENT/STRENGTH | DOSE |
| --- | --- | --- |
| **BUTENAFINE** | | |
| Lotrimin Ultra Athlete's Foot Cream | Butenafine HCl 1% | **Adults & Peds ≥12 yrs:** Athlete's Foot: Apply bid for 1 week or qd for 4 weeks. Jock Itch/Ringworm: Apply qd for 2 weeks. |
| Lotrimin Ultra Jock Itch Cream | Butenafine HCl 1% | **Adults & Peds ≥12 yrs:** Apply qd for 2 weeks. |
| **CLOTRIMAZOLE** | | |
| Desenex Antifungal Cream | Clotrimazole 1% | **Adults & Peds ≥2 yrs:** Athlete's Foot/Ringworm: Apply bid for 4 weeks. Jock Itch: Apply bid for 2 weeks. |
| FungiCure Anti-Fungal Liquid Pump Spray | Clotrimazole 1% | **Adults & Peds ≥2 yrs:** Athlete's Foot/Ringworm: Apply bid for 4 weeks. Jock Itch: Apply bid for 2 weeks. |
| FungiCure Intensive Anti-Fungal Treatment | Clotrimazole 1% | **Adults & Peds ≥2 yrs:** Athlete's Foot/Ringworm: Apply bid for 4 weeks. Jock Itch: Apply bid for 2 weeks. |
| Lotrimin AF Athlete's Foot Cream | Clotrimazole 1% | **Adults & Peds ≥2 yrs:** Athlete's Foot/Ringworm: Apply bid for 4 weeks. Jock Itch: Apply bid for 2 weeks. |
| Lotrimin AF For Her Athlete's Foot Cream | Clotrimazole 1% | **Adults & Peds ≥2 yrs:** Apply bid for 4 weeks. |
| Lotrimin AF Jock Itch Cream | Clotrimazole 1% | **Adults & Peds ≥2 yrs:** Apply bid for 2 weeks. |
| Lotrimin AF Ringworm Cream | Clotrimazole 1% | **Adults & Peds ≥2 yrs:** Apply bid for 4 weeks. |
| **MICONAZOLE** | | |
| Clearly Confident Antifungal Cream | Miconazole Nitrate 2% | **Adults & Peds ≥2 yrs:** Apply bid for 4 weeks. |
| Desenex Antifungal Liquid Spray | Miconazole Nitrate 2% | **Adults & Peds ≥2 yrs:** Apply bid for 4 weeks. |

*(Continued)*

## Table 5. ANTIFUNGAL PRODUCTS (cont.)

| BRAND NAME | INGREDIENT/STRENGTH | DOSE |
|---|---|---|
| Desenex Antifungal Powder | Miconazole Nitrate 2% | **Adults & Peds ≥2 yrs:** Athlete's Foot/Ringworm: Apply bid for 4 weeks. Jock Itch: Apply bid for 2 weeks. |
| Desenex Antifungal Spray Powder | Miconazole Nitrate 2% | **Adults & Peds ≥2 yrs:** Apply bid for 4 weeks. |
| Lotrimin AF Athlete's Foot Deodorant Powder Spray | Miconazole Nitrate 2% | **Adults & Peds ≥2 yrs:** Athlete's Foot/Ringworm: Apply bid for 4 weeks. Jock Itch: Apply bid for 2 weeks. |
| Lotrimin AF Athlete's Foot Liquid Spray | Miconazole Nitrate 2% | **Adults & Peds ≥2 yrs:** Athlete's Foot/Ringworm: Apply bid for 4 weeks. Jock Itch: Apply bid for 2 weeks. |
| Lotrimin AF Athlete's Foot Powder | Miconazole Nitrate 2% | **Adults & Peds ≥2 yrs:** Athlete's Foot/Ringworm: Apply bid for 4 weeks. Jock Itch: Apply bid for 2 weeks. |
| Lotrimin AF Athlete's Foot Powder Spray | Miconazole Nitrate 2% | **Adults & Peds ≥2 yrs:** Athlete's Foot/Ringworm: Apply bid for 4 weeks. Jock Itch: Apply bid for 2 weeks. |
| Lotrimin AF Jock Itch Powder Spray | Miconazole Nitrate 2% | **Adults & Peds ≥2 yrs:** Apply bid for 2 weeks. |
| Micatin Cream | Miconazole Nitrate 2% | **Adults & Peds ≥2 yrs:** Athlete's Foot/Ringworm: Apply bid for 4 weeks. Jock Itch: Apply bid for 2 weeks. |
| Miranel AF Antifungal Treatment | Miconazole Nitrate 2% | **Adults & Peds ≥12 yrs:** Athlete's Foot: Apply bid for 4 weeks. |
| Ting Spray Powder | Miconazole Nitrate 2% | **Adults & Peds ≥2 yrs:** Athlete's Foot/Ringworm: Apply bid for 4 weeks. Jock Itch: Apply bid for 2 weeks. |
| Zeasorb-AF Antifungal Drying Gel | Miconazole Nitrate 2% | **Adults & Peds ≥2 yrs:** Athlete's Foot/Ringworm: Apply bid for 4 weeks. Jock Itch: Apply bid for 2 weeks. |

## Table 5. ANTIFUNGAL PRODUCTS (cont.)

| BRAND NAME | INGREDIENT/STRENGTH | DOSE |
|---|---|---|
| Zeasorb-AF Super Absorbent Antifungal Powder | Miconazole Nitrate 2% | **Adults & Peds ≥2 yrs:** Athlete's Foot/Ringworm: Apply bid for 4 weeks. Jock Itch: Apply bid for 2 weeks. |
| **TERBINAFINE** | | |
| Lamisil AT Antifungal Continuous Spray, Athlete's Foot | Terbinafine HCl 1% | **Adults & Peds ≥12 yrs:** Athlete's Foot (between toes): Apply bid for 1 week. Jock Itch/Ringworm: Apply qd for 1 week. |
| Lamisil AT Antifungal Continuous Spray, Jock Itch | Terbinafine HCl 1% | **Adults & Peds >12 yrs:** Apply qd for 1 week. |
| Lamisil AT Athlete's Foot Treatment Cream | Terbinafine HCl 1% | **Adults & Peds ≥12 yrs:** Athlete's Foot (between toes): Apply bid for 1 week. Athlete's Foot (on side or bottom of foot): Apply bid for 2 weeks. Jock Itch/Ringworm: Apply qd for 1 week. |
| Lamisil AT Athlete's Foot Treatment Gel | Terbinafine HCl 1% | **Adults & Peds ≥12 yrs:** Athlete's Foot (between toes): Apply qhs for 1 week. Jock Itch/Ringworm: Apply qd for 1 week. |
| **TOLNAFTATE** | | |
| Flexitol Medicated Foot Cream | Tolnaftate 1% | **Adults & Peds ≥2 yrs:** Apply bid for 4 weeks. |
| Tinactin Athlete's Foot Cream | Tolnaftate 1% | **Adults & Peds ≥2 yrs:** Apply bid for 4 weeks. |
| Tinactin Deodorant Powder Spray | Tolnaftate 1% | **Adults & Peds ≥2 yrs:** Athlete's Foot: Apply bid for 4 weeks. Prevention: Apply qd-bid. |
| Tinactin Jock Itch Cream | Tolnaftate 1% | **Adults & Peds ≥2 yrs:** Apply bid for 2 weeks. |
| Tinactin Jock Itch Powder Spray | Tolnaftate 1% | **Adults & Peds ≥2 yrs:** Apply bid for 2 weeks. |
| Tinactin Liquid Spray | Tolnaftate 1% | **Adults & Peds ≥2 yrs:** Athlete's Foot: Apply bid for 4 weeks. Prevention: Apply qd-bid. |

*(Continued)*

## Table 5. ANTIFUNGAL PRODUCTS (cont.)

| BRAND NAME | INGREDIENT/STRENGTH | DOSE |
| --- | --- | --- |
| Tinactin Powder Spray | Tolnaftate 1% | **Adults & Peds ≥2 yrs:** Athlete's Foot: Apply bid for 4 weeks. Prevention: Apply qd-bid. |
| Tinactin Pump Spray | Tolnaftate 1% | **Adults & Peds ≥2 yrs:** Athlete's Foot: Apply bid for 4 weeks. Prevention: Apply qd-bid. |
| Tinactin Super Absorbent Powder | Tolnaftate 1% | **Adults & Peds ≥2 yrs:** Athlete's Foot: Apply bid for 4 weeks. Prevention: Apply qd-bid. |
| Ting Antifungal Cream | Tolnaftate 1% | **Adults & Peds ≥2 yrs:** Athlete's Foot/Ringworm: Apply bid for 4 weeks. Jock Itch: Apply bid for 2 weeks. |
| Ting Spray Liquid | Tolnaftate 1% | **Adults & Peds ≥2 yrs:** Apply bid for 4 weeks. |
| **UNDECYLENIC ACID** | | |
| DiabetiDerm Toenail & Foot Fungus Antifungal Cream | Undecylenic Acid 10% | **Adults & Peds ≥2 yrs:** Athlete's Foot/Ringworm: Apply bid for 4 weeks. Jock Itch: Apply bid for 2 weeks. |
| Flexitol Anti-Fungal Liquid | Undecylenic Acid 25% | **Adults & Peds ≥2 yrs:** Athlete's Foot/Ringworm: Apply bid. |
| Fungi Nail Anti-Fungal Solution | Undecylenic Acid 25% | **Adults & Peds ≥2 yrs:** Athlete's Foot/Ringworm: Apply bid. |
| Fungi Nail Anti-Fungal Pen | Undecylenic Acid 25% | **Adults & Peds ≥2 yrs:** Athlete's Foot/Ringworm: Apply bid. |
| FungiCure Extra Strength Anti-Fungal Liquid | Undecylenic Acid 10% | **Adults & Peds ≥2 yrs:** Athlete's Foot/Ringworm: Apply bid for 4 weeks. |
| FungiCure Professional Formula Anti-Fungal Liquid | Undecylenic Acid 15% | **Adults & Peds ≥2 yrs:** Athlete's Foot/Ringworm: Apply bid for 4 weeks. |
| Tineacide Antifungal Cream | Undecylenic Acid 13% | **Adults & Peds ≥12 yrs:** Athlete's Foot (between toes): Apply bid for 4 weeks. Jock Itch/ Ringworm: Apply bid for 2 weeks. |

## Table 6. CONTACT DERMATITIS PRODUCTS

| Brand Name | Ingredient/Strength | Dose |
|---|---|---|
| **ANTIHISTAMINE** | | |
| Benadryl Itch Stopping Extra Strength Gel | Diphenhydramine HCl 2% | **Adults & Peds ≥2 yrs:** Apply to affected area tid-qid. |
| **ANTIHISTAMINE COMBINATION** | | |
| Benadryl Extra Strength Itch Stopping Cream | Diphenhydramine HCl/Zinc Acetate 2%-0.1% | **Adults & Peds ≥2 yrs:** Apply to affected area tid-qid. |
| Benadryl Extra Strength Spray | Diphenhydramine HCl/Zinc Acetate 2%-0.1% | **Adults & Peds ≥2 yrs:** Apply to affected area tid-qid. |
| Benadryl Extra Strength Itch Relief Stick | Diphenhydramine HCl/Zinc Acetate 2%-0.1% | **Adults & Peds ≥2 yrs:** Apply to affected area tid-qid. |
| Benadryl Original Strength Itch Stopping Cream | Diphenhydramine HCl/Zinc Acetate 1%-0.1% | **Adults & Peds ≥2 yrs:** Apply to affected area tid-qid. |
| Benadryl Readymist Itch Stopping Spray | Diphenhydramine/Zinc Acetate 2%-0.1% | **Adults & Peds ≥2 yrs:** Apply to affected area tid-qid. |
| CalaGel Anti-Itch Gel | Diphenhydramine HCl/Zinc Acetate/ Benzenthonium Chloride 2%-0.215%-0.15% | **Adults & Peds ≥2 yrs:** Apply to affected area no more than tid |
| Ivarest Double Relief Formula | Diphenhydramine HCl/Benzyl Alcohol/ Calamine 2%-10.5%-14% | **Adults & Peds ≥2 yrs:** Apply to affected area tid-qid. |
| **ASTRINGENT** | | |
| Domeboro Astringent Solution Powder Packets | Aluminum Acetate (combination of Calcium Acetate 952mg and Aluminum Sulfate 1347mg) | **Adults & Peds:** Dissolve 1-3 pkts and apply to affected area for 15-30 min tid. |
| Ivy-Dry Cream | Zinc Acetate/Benzyl Alcohol 2%-10% | **Adults & Peds ≥6 yrs:** Apply to affected area tid. |
| **ASTRINGENT COMBINATION** | | |
| Aveeno Calamine and Pramoxine HCl Anti-Itch Cream | Calamine/Camphor/Pramoxine HCl 3%-0.5%-1% | **Adults & Peds ≥2 yrs:** Apply to affected area tid-qid. |
| Aveeno Anti-Itch Concentrated Lotion | Calamine/Camphor/Pramoxine HCl 3%-0.47%-1% | **Adults & Peds ≥2 yrs:** Apply to affected area qid. |
| Caladryl Clear Anti-Itch Lotion | Zinc Acetate/Pramoxine HCl 0.1%-1% | **Adults & Peds ≥2 yrs:** Apply to affected area tid-qid. |
| Caladryl Anti-Itch Lotion | Calamine/Pramoxine HCl 8%-1% | **Adults & Peds ≥2 yrs:** Apply to affected area tid-qid. |

*(Continued)*

## Table 6. CONTACT DERMATITIS PRODUCTS (cont.)

| BRAND NAME | INGREDIENT/STRENGTH | DOSE |
|---|---|---|
| Calamine Lotion (generic) | Calamine/Zinc Oxide 8%-8% | **Adults & Peds:** Apply to affected area prn. |
| Cortaid Poison Ivy Care Treatment Kit | (Scrub) Water, polyethylene, laureth-4, sodium lauryl sarcosinate, glycol distearate, acrylates/C10-30, alkyl acrylate crosspolymer, cocoglucoside, sodium hydroxide, microcrystalline wax, tetrasodium EDTA, glyceryl oleate, glyceryl stearate, quaternium-15, chromium hydroxide green, tocopherol (Spray) Zinc Acetate/Pramoxine 0.12%-1% | **Adults & Peds:** (Scrub) Apply quarter-sized amount into hand and rub onto affected area for 30 seconds. Rinse area thoroughly and pat dry. (Spray) Apply to affected area tid-qid. |

### CLEANSER

| | | |
|---|---|---|
| Cortaid Poison Ivy Care Toxin Removal Cloths | Water, laureth-4, sodium lauryl sarcosinate, glycerin, DMDM, hydantoin, methylparaben, tetrasodium EDTA, *Aloe barbadensis* leaf extract, citric acid | **Adults & Peds:** Wipe affected area at least 15 seconds. Rinse or wipe dry. |
| Ivarest Poison Ivy Cleansing Foam | Menthol 1% | **Adults & Peds ≥2 yrs:** Gently rub into affected area and rinse under running water. |

### CORTICOSTEROID

| | | |
|---|---|---|
| Aveeno 1% Hydrocortisone Anti-Itch Cream | Hydrocortisone 1% | **Adults & Peds ≥2 yrs:** Apply to affected area tid-qid. |
| Cortaid Advanced 12-Hour Anti-Itch Cream | Hydrocortisone 1% | **Adults & Peds ≥2 yrs:** Apply to affected area tid-qid. |
| Cortaid Intensive Therapy Cooling Spray | Hydrocortisone 1% | **Adults & Peds ≥2 yrs:** Apply to affected area tid-qid. |
| Cortaid Intensive Therapy Moisturizing Cream | Hydrocortisone 1% | **Adults & Peds ≥2 yrs:** Apply to affected area tid-qid. |
| Cortaid Maximum Strength Cream | Hydrocortisone 1% | **Adults & Peds ≥2 yrs:** Apply to affected area tid-qid. |
| Cortaid Maximum Strength Ointment | Hydrocortisone 1% | **Adults & Peds ≥2 yrs:** Apply to affected area tid-qid. |
| Cortizone-10 Easy Relief Applicator | Hydrocortisone 1% | **Adults & Peds ≥2 yrs:** Apply to affected area tid-qid. |
| Cortizone-10 Cooling Relief Gel | Hydrocortisone 1% | **Adults & Peds ≥2 yrs:** Apply to affected area tid-qid. |

## Table 6. CONTACT DERMATITIS PRODUCTS (cont.)

| BRAND NAME | INGREDIENT/STRENGTH | DOSE |
|---|---|---|
| Cortizone-10 Creme | Hydrocortisone 1% | **Adults & Peds ≥2 yrs:** Apply to affected area tid-qid. |
| Cortizone-10 Ointment | Hydrocortisone 1% | **Adults & Peds ≥2 yrs:** Apply to affected area tid-qid. |
| Cortizone-10 Creme Plus | Hydrocortisone 1% | **Adults & Peds ≥2 yrs:** Apply to affected area tid-qid. |
| Cortizone-10 Intensive Healing Formula | Hydrocortisone 1% | **Adults & Peds ≥2 yrs:** Apply to affected area tid-qid. |
| Cortizone-10 Intensive Healing Eczema Lotion | Hydrocortisone 1% | **Adults & Peds ≥2 yrs:** Apply to affected area tid-qid. |
| Cortizone-10 Hydraintensive Anti-Itch Soothing Lotion | Hydrocortisone 1% | **Adults & Peds ≥2 yrs:** Apply to affected area tid-qid. |
| Cortizone-10 Hydraintensive Anti-Itch Healing Lotion | Hydrocortisone 1% | **Adults & Peds ≥2 yrs:** Apply to affected area tid-qid. |
| Corticool 1% Hydrocortisone Anti-Itch Gel | Hydrocortisone 1% | **Adults & Peds ≥2 yrs:** Apply to affected area tid-qid. |
| **COUNTERIRRITANT** | | |
| Gold Bond Medicated Maximum Strength Anti-Itch Cream | Menthol/Pramoxine HCl 1%-1% | **Adults & Peds ≥2 yrs:** Apply to affected area tid-qid. |
| Ivy Block Lotion | Bentoquatam 5% | **Adults & Peds ≥6 yrs:** Apply 15 minutes before exposure risk and q4h for continued protection. |
| **LOCAL ANESTHETIC** | | |
| Solarcaine Aloe Extra Burn Relief Gel | Lidocaine HCl 0.5% | **Adults & Peds ≥2 yrs:** Apply to affected area tid-qid. |
| Solarcaine Aloe Extra Burn Relief Spray | Lidocaine HCl 0.5% | **Adults & Peds ≥2 yrs:** Apply to affected area tid-qid. |
| Solarcaine First Aid Medicated Spray | Benzocaine/Triclosan 20%-0.13% | **Adults & Peds ≥2 yrs:** Apply to affected area qd-tid. |
| **LOCAL ANESTHETIC COMBINATION** | | |
| Bactine Pain Relieving Cleansing Spray | Lidocaine HCl/Benzalkonium Chloride 2.5%-0.13% | **Adults & Peds ≥2 yrs:** Apply to affected area qd-tid. |
| Bactine Original First Aid Liquid | Lidocaine HCl/Benzalkonium Chloride 2.5%-0.13% | **Adults & Peds ≥2 yrs:** Apply to affected area qd-tid. |

*(Continued)*

## Table 6. CONTACT DERMATITIS PRODUCTS (cont.)

| BRAND NAME | INGREDIENT/STRENGTH | DOSE |
|---|---|---|
| Lanacane Maximum Strength Cream | Benzocaine/Benzethonium Chloride 20%-0.2% | **Adults & Peds ≥2 yrs:** Apply to affected area qd-tid. |
| Lanacane Antibacterial First Aid Spray | Benzocaine/Benzethonium Chloride 20%-0.2% | **Adults & Peds ≥2 yrs:** Apply to affected area qd-tid. |
| **SKIN PROTECTANT** | | |
| Aveeno Skin Relief Moisturizing Cream | Dimethicone 2.5% | **Adults & Peds ≥2 yrs:** Apply to affected area prn. |
| Aveeno Skin Relief Moisturizing Lotion | Dimethicone 1.3% | **Adults & Peds:** Apply to affected area prn. |
| Vaseline Intensive Rescue Clinical Therapy Lotion | Dimethicone 1% | **Adults & Peds:** Apply to affected area prn. |
| **SKIN PROTECTANT COMBINATION** | | |
| Gold Bond Extra Strength Medicated Body Lotion | Dimethicone/Menthol 5%-0.5% | **Adults & Peds:** Apply to affected area tid-qid. |
| Gold Bond Medicated Body Lotion | Dimethicone/Menthol 5%-0.15% | **Adults & Peds:** Apply to affected area prn. |
| Gold Bond Medicated Powder | Zinc Oxide/Menthol 1%-0.15% | **Adults & Peds ≥2 yrs:** Apply to affected area tid-qid. |
| Gold Bond Extra Strength Medicated Powder | Zinc Oxide/Menthol 5%-0.8% | **Adults & Peds ≥2 yrs:** Apply to affected area tid-qid. |
| Gold Bond Medicated Baby Powder | Cornstarch/Kaolin/Zinc Oxide 79%-4%-15% | **Adults & Peds ≥2 yrs:** Apply to affected area tid-qid. |

## Table 7. DIAPER RASH PRODUCTS

| BRAND NAME | INGREDIENT/STRENGTH | DOSE |
|---|---|---|
| **WHITE PETROLATUM** | | |
| Balmex Multi-Purpose Healing Ointment | White Petrolatum 51.1% | **Peds:** Apply prn. |
| Desitin Multi-Purpose Skin Protectant and Diaper Rash Ointment | White Petrolatum 60.4% | **Peds:** Apply prn. |
| Vaseline Petroleum Jelly | White Petrolatum 100% | **Peds:** Apply prn. |
| **ZINC OXIDE** | | |
| Aveeno Baby Soothing Relief Diaper Rash Cream | Zinc Oxide 13% | **Peds:** Apply prn. |
| Balmex Prevention Baby Powder with ActivGuard | Zinc Oxide 11.3% | **Adults & Peds ≥2 yrs:** Apply tid-qid. **Peds <2 yrs:** Apply prn. |
| Boudreaux's Butt Paste, Diaper Rash Ointment | Zinc Oxide 16% | **Peds:** Apply prn. |
| California Baby Calming Diaper Rash Cream | Zinc Oxide 12% | **Peds:** Apply prn. |
| Canus Li'l Goat's Milk Ointment | Zinc Oxide 40% | **Peds:** Apply prn. |
| Desitin Rapid Relief Cream | Zinc Oxide 13% | **Peds:** Apply prn. |
| Desitin Maximum Strength Original Paste | Zinc Oxide 40% | **Peds:** Apply prn. |
| Johnson's Baby Powder Medicated with Aloe & Vitamin E Medicated | Zinc Oxide 10% | **Peds:** Apply prn. |
| Mustela Bebe Vitamin Barrier Cream | Zinc Oxide 10% | **Peds:** Apply prn. |
| Triple Paste Medicated Ointment | Zinc Oxide 12.8% | **Peds:** Apply prn. |
| **COMBINATION PRODUCTS** | | |
| A+D Original Ointment | Petrolatum/Lanolin 53.4%-15.5% | **Peds:** Apply prn. |
| A+D Zinc Oxide Cream | Dimethicone/Zinc Oxide 1%-10% | **Peds:** Apply prn. |
| Balmex Diaper Rash Cream with ActivGuard | Cornstarch/Zinc Oxide 83.6%-11.3% | **Peds:** Apply prn. |
| Lansinoh Diaper Rash Ointment | Dimethicone/USP Modified Lanolin/ Zinc Oxide 5.0%-15.5%-5.5% | **Peds:** Apply prn. |

## Table 8. PSORIASIS PRODUCTS

| BRAND NAME | INGREDIENT/STRENGTH | DOSE |
|---|---|---|
| **COAL TAR** | | |
| DHS Tar Gel Shampoo | Coal Tar 0.5% | Use at least biw. |
| DHS Tar Shampoo | Coal Tar 0.5% | Use at least biw. |
| Ionil Plus Shampoo | Coal Tar 2% | Use at least biw. |
| Ionil-T Plus Shampoo | Coal Tar 2% | Use at least biw. |
| Ionil-T Shampoo | Coal Tar 2% | Use at least biw. |
| MG217 Medicated Tar Lotion | Coal Tar 1% | Apply to affected area qd-qid. |
| MG217 Medicated Tar Ointment | Coal Tar 2% | Apply to affected area qd-qid. |
| MG217 Medicated Tar Shampoo | Coal Tar 3% | Use at least biw. |
| Neutrogena T/Gel Shampoo Extra Strength | Coal Tar 1% | Use at least biw. |
| Neutrogena T/Gel Shampoo Original Formula | Coal Tar 0.5% | Use at least biw. |
| Neutrogena T/Gel Shampoo Stubborn Itch Control | Coal Tar 0.5% | Use at least biw. |
| Psoriasin Gel | Coal Tar 1.25% | **Adults:** Apply to affected area qd-qid. |
| Psoriasin Liquid For Skin & Scalp | Coal Tar 0.66% | **Adults:** Apply to affected area qd-qid. |
| Psoriasin Ointment | Coal Tar 2% | **Adults:** Apply to affected area qd-qid. |
| **CORTICOSTEROID** | | |
| Aveeno 1% Hydrocortisone Anti-Itch Cream | Hydrocortisone 1% | **Adults & Peds ≥2 yrs:** Apply to affected area tid-qid. |
| Cortaid Advanced 12-Hour Anti-Itch Cream | Hydrocortisone 1% | **Adults & Peds ≥2 yrs:** Apply to affected area tid-qid. |
| Cortaid Intensive Therapy Cooling Spray | Hydrocortisone 1% | **Adults & Peds ≥2 yrs:** Apply to affected area tid-qid. |
| Cortaid Intensive Therapy Moisturizing Cream | Hydrocortisone 1% | **Adults & Peds ≥2 yrs:** Apply to affected area tid-qid. |
| Cortaid Maximum Strength Cream | Hydrocortisone 1% | **Adults & Peds ≥2 yrs:** Apply to affected area tid-qid. |

*(Continued)*

## Table 8. PSORIASIS PRODUCTS (cont.)

| BRAND NAME | INGREDIENT/STRENGTH | DOSE |
|---|---|---|
| Cortaid Maximum Strength Ointment | Hydrocortisone 1% | **Adults & Peds ≥2 yrs:** Apply to affected area tid-qid. |
| Corticool 1% Hydrocortisone Anti-Itch Gel | Hydrocortisone 1% | **Adults & Peds ≥2 yrs:** Apply to affected area tid-qid. |
| Cortizone-10 Cooling Relief Gel | Hydrocortisone 1% | **Adults & Peds ≥2 yrs:** Apply to affected area tid-qid. |
| Cortizone-10 Creme | Hydrocortisone 1% | **Adults & Peds ≥2 yrs:** Apply to affected area tid-qid. |
| Cortizone-10 Creme Plus | Hydrocortisone 1% | **Adults & Peds ≥2 yrs:** Apply to affected area tid-qid. |
| Cortizone-10 Ointment | Hydrocortisone 1% | **Adults & Peds ≥2 yrs:** Apply to affected area tid-qid. |
| Cortizone-10 Easy Relief Applicator | Hydrocortisone 1% | **Adults & Peds ≥2 yrs:** Apply to affected area tid-qid. |
| Cortizone-10 Intensive Healing Formula | Hydrocortisone 1% | **Adults & Peds ≥2 yrs:** Apply to affected area tid-qid. |
| **SALICYLIC ACID** | | |
| Dermarest Psoriasis Medicated Moisturizer | Salicylic Acid 2% | **Adults & Peds:** Apply to affected area qd-qid. |
| Dermarest Psoriasis Medicated Scalp Treatment | Salicylic Acid 3% | **Adults & Peds:** Apply to affected area qd-qid. |
| Dermarest Psoriasis Medicated Shampoo Plus Conditioner | Salicylic Acid 3% | **Adults & Peds:** Use at least biw. |
| Dermarest Psoriasis Medicated Skin Treatment | Salicylic Acid 3% | **Adults & Peds:** Apply to affected area qd-qid. |
| DHS Sal Shampoo | Salicylic Acid 3% | **Adults & Peds:** Use at least biw. |
| MG217 Sal-Acid Ointment | Salicylic Acid 3% | **Adults & Peds:** Apply to affected area qd-qid. |
| Neutrogena T/Gel Therapeutic Conditioner | Salicylic Acid 2% | **Adults & Peds:** Use at least biw. |
| Neutrogena T/Sal Therapeutic Shampoo | Salicylic Acid 3% | **Adults & Peds:** Use at least tiw. |
| Psoriasin Therapeutic Shampoo and Body Wash | Salicylic Acid 3% | **Adults & Peds:** Use at least biw. |

## Table 9. WOUND CARE PRODUCTS

| BRAND NAME | INGREDIENT/STRENGTH | DOSE |
|---|---|---|
| **NEOMYCIN/POLYMYXIN B/BACITRACIN COMBINATIONS** | | |
| Bacitracin Ointment | Bacitracin 500 U | **Adults & Peds:** Apply to affected area qd-tid. |
| Neosporin First Aid Antibiotic Ointment | Neomycin/polymyxin B/bacitracin 3.5mg-5,000 U-400 U | **Adults & Peds:** Apply to affected area qd-tid. |
| Neosporin Neo To Go! Single Use Packets | Neomycin/polymyxin B/bacitracin 3.5mg-5,000 U-400 U | **Adults & Peds:** Apply to affected area qd-tid. |
| Neosporin Plus Pain Relief Cream | Neomycin/polymyxin B/pramoxine HCl 3.5mg-10,000 U-10mg | **Adults & Peds ≥2 yrs:** Apply to affected area qd-tid. |
| Neosporin Plus Pain Relief Ointment | Neomycin/polymyxin B/bacitracin/ pramoxine HCl 3.5mg-10,000 U-400 U-10mg | **Adults & Peds ≥2 yrs:** Apply to affected area qd-tid. |
| Polysporin First Aid Antibiotic Ointment | Polymyxin B/bacitracin 10,000 U-500 U | **Adults & Peds:** Apply to affected area qd-tid. |
| Polysporin First Aid Antibiotic Powder | Polymyxin B/bacitracin 10,000 U-500 U | **Adults & Peds:** Apply to affected area qd-tid. |
| **BENZALKONIUM CHLORIDE COMBINATIONS** | | |
| Bactine Original First Aid Liquid | Benzalkonium chloride/lidocaine HCl 0.13%-2.5% | **Adults & Peds ≥2 yrs:** Use to clean affected area qd-tid. |
| Bactine Pain Relieving Cleansing Spray | Benzalkonium chloride/lidocaine HCl 0.13%-2.5% | **Adults & Peds ≥2 yrs:** Use to clean affected area qd-tid. |
| Band-Aid Hurt Free Antiseptic Wash | Benzalkonium chloride/lidocaine HCl 0.13%-2% | **Adults & Peds ≥2 yrs:** Use to clean affected area qd-tid. |
| Neosporin Neo To Go! First Aid Antiseptic/Pain Relieving Spray | Benzalkonium chloride/pramoxine HCl 0.13%-1% | **Adults & Peds ≥2 yrs:** Use to clean affected area qd-tid. |
| **BENZETHONIUM CHLORIDE COMBINATIONS** | | |
| Gold Bond Quick Spray | Benzethonium chloride/menthol 0.13%-1% | **Adults & Peds ≥2 yrs:** Apply to affected area qd-tid. |
| Lanacane Anti-Bacterial First Aid Spray | Benzethonium chloride/benzocaine 0.2%-20% | **Adults & Peds ≥2 yrs:** Apply to affected area qd-tid. |
| Lanacane Maximum Strength Pain & Intense Itch Anti-Itch Cream | Benzethonium chloride/benzocaine 0.2%-20% | **Adults & Peds ≥2 yrs:** Apply to affected area qd-tid. |
| Lanacane Original Strength Itch & Irritation Anti-Itch Cream | Benzethonium chloride/benzocaine 0.2%-6% | **Adults & Peds ≥2 yrs:** Apply to affected area qd-tid. |

*(Continued)*

## Table 9. WOUND CARE PRODUCTS (cont.)

| Brand Name | Ingredient/Strength | Dose |
|---|---|---|
| **CHLORHEXIDINE GLUCONATE** | | |
| Hibiclens | Chlorhexidine gluconate 4% | **Adults:** Apply sparingly to affected area and wash. |
| Hibistat | Chlorhexidine gluconate/isopropyl alcohol 0.5%-70% | **Adults:** Rub vigorously with the towelette for about 15 seconds. |
| **IODINE** | | |
| Betadine Skin Cleanser | Povidone-iodine 7.5% | **Adults & Peds:** Apply to affected area, wash vigorously for 15 seconds, rinse and dry. |
| Betadine Solution | Povidone-iodine 10% | **Adults & Peds:** Apply to affected area qd-tid. |
| **MISCELLANEOUS** | | |
| Aquaphor Healing Ointment | Petrolatum (41%), mineral oil, ceresin, lanolin alcohol, panthenol, glycerin, bisabolol | **Adults & Peds:** Apply to affected area prn. |
| Wound Wash Saline | Sterile 0.9% sodium chloride solution | **Adults & Peds:** Use to clean affected area prn. |

## Table 10. ANTACID AND HEARTBURN PRODUCTS

| BRAND NAME | INGREDIENT/STRENGTH | DOSE |
|---|---|---|
| **ANTACID** | | |
| Alka-Seltzer Gold Tablets | Citric Acid/Potassium Bicarbonate/ Sodium Bicarbonate 1000mg-344mg-1050mg | **Adults ≥60 yrs:** 2 tabs q4h prn. **Max:** 6 tabs q24h. **Adults & Peds ≥12 yrs:** 2 tabs q4h prn. **Max:** 8 tabs q24h. **Peds ≤12 yrs:** 1 tab q4h prn. **Max:** 4 tabs q24h. |
| Alka-Seltzer Heartburn Relief Tablets | Citric Acid/Sodium Bicarbonate 1000mg-1940mg | **Adults ≥60 yrs:** 2 tabs q4h prn. **Max:** 4 tabs q24h. **Adults & Peds ≥12 yrs:** 2 tabs q4h prn. **Max:** 8 tabs q24h. |
| Alka-Seltzer Lemon Lime Tablets | Aspirin/Citric Acid/Sodium Bicarbonate 325mg-1000mg-1700mg | **Adults ≥60 yrs:** 2 tabs q4h prn. **Max:** 4 tabs q24h. **Adults & Peds >12 yrs:** 2 tabs q4h prn. **Max:** 8 tabs q24h. |
| Alka-Seltzer Tablets, Extra-Strength | Aspirin/Citric Acid/Sodium Bicarbonate 500mg-1000mg-1985mg | **Adults ≥60 yrs:** 2 tabs q6h prn. **Max:** 3 tabs q24h. **Adults & Peds ≥12 yrs:** 2 tabs q6h prn. **Max:** 7 tabs q24h. |
| Alka Seltzer Tablets, Original | Aspirin/Citric Acid/Sodium Bicarbonate 325mg-1000mg-1916mg | **Adults ≥60 yrs:** 2 tabs q4h prn. **Max:** 4 tabs q24h. **Adults & Peds ≥12 yrs:** 2 tabs q4h prn. **Max:** 8 tabs q24h. |
| Brioschi Powder | Sodium Bicarbonate/Tartaric Acid 2.69g-2.43g/dose | **Adults & Peds ≥12 yrs:** 1 capful (6g) dissolved in 4-6 oz water q1h. **Max:** 6 doses q24h. **Adults ≥60 yrs:** 1 capful (6g) dissolved in 4-6 oz water q1h. **Max:** 3 doses q24h. |
| Gaviscon Extra Strength Liquid | Aluminum Hydroxide/Magnesium Carbonate 254mg-237.5mg/5mL | **Adults:** 2-4 tsp (10-20mL) qid. |
| Gaviscon Extra Strength Tablets | Aluminum Hydroxide/Magnesium Carbonate 160mg-105mg | **Adults:** 2-4 tabs qid. **Max:** 16 doses q24h. |
| Gaviscon Regular Strength Liquid | Aluminum Hydroxide/Magnesium Carbonate 95mg-358mg/15mL | **Adults:** 1-2 tbl (15-30mL) qid. **Max:** 8 tbl q24h. |
| Gaviscon Regular Strength Tablets | Aluminum Hydroxide/Magnesium Trisilicate 80mg-14.2mg | **Adults:** 2-4 tabs qid. **Max:** 16 tabs q24h. |

*(Continued)*

## Table 10. ANTACID AND HEARTBURN PRODUCTS (cont.)

| BRAND NAME | INGREDIENT/STRENGTH | DOSE |
|---|---|---|
| Maalox Children's Relief Chewables | Calcium Carbonate 400mg | **Peds 6-11 yrs (48-95 lbs):** 2 tabs prn. **Max:** 6 tabs q24h. **Peds 2-5 yrs (24-47 lbs):** 1 tab prn. **Max:** 3 tabs q24h. |
| Maalox Regular Strength Chewable Tablets | Calcium Carbonate 600mg | **Adults:** 1-2 tabs prn. **Max:** 12 tabs q24h. |
| Mylanta, Children's | Calcium Carbonate 400mg | **Peds 6-11 yrs (48-95 lbs):** Take 2 tabs prn. **Max:** 6 tabs q24h. **Peds 2-5 yrs (24-47 lbs):** Take 1 tab prn. **Max:** 3 tabs q24h. |
| Mylanta Supreme Antacid Liquid | Calcium Carbonate/Magnesium Hydroxide 400mg-135mg/5mL | **Adults:** 2-4 tsp (10-20mL) qid (between meals & hs). **Max:** 18 tsp (90mL) q24h. |
| Mylanta Ultimate Strength Chewable Tablets | Calcium Carbonate/Magnesium Hydroxide 700mg-300mg | **Adults:** 2-4 tabs qid (between meals & hs). **Max:** 10 tabs q24h for ≤2 weeks. |
| Mylanta Ultimate Strength Liquid | Aluminum Hydroxide/Magnesium Hydroxide 500mg-500mg/5mL | **Adults & Peds ≥12 yrs:** 2-4 tsp (10-20mL) qid (between meals & hs). **Max:** 9 tsp (45mL) q24h for ≤2 weeks. |
| Pepto Bismol Children's Pepto Chewable Tablets | Calcium Carbonate 400mg | **Peds 6-11 yrs (48-95 lbs):** Take 2 tabs prn. **Max:** 6 tabs q24h. **Peds 2-5 yrs (24-47 lbs):** Take 1 tab prn. **Max:** 3 tabs q24h. |
| Rolaids Extra Strength Softchews | Calcium Carbonate 1177mg | **Adults:** 2-3 chews q1h prn. **Max:** 6 chews q24h. |
| Rolaids Extra Strength Tablets | Calcium Carbonate/Magnesium Hydroxide 675mg-135mg | **Adults:** 2-4 tabs q1h prn. **Max:** 10 tabs q24h. |
| Rolaids Regular Strength Tablets | Calcium Carbonate/Magnesium Hydroxide 550mg-110mg | **Adults:** 2-4 tabs q1h prn. **Max:** 12 tabs q24h. |
| Titralac Instant Relief Tablets | Calcium Carbonate 420mg | **Adults:** 2 tabs q2-3h prn. **Max:** 19 tabs q24h. |
| Tums Regular Strength Tablets | Calcium Carbonate 500mg | **Adults:** 2-4 tabs prn. **Max:** 15 tabs q24h. |
| Tums E-X 750 Chewable Tablets | Calcium Carbonate 750mg | **Adults:** 2-4 tabs prn. **Max:** 10 tabs q24h. |
| Tums E-X 750 Sugar Free Chewable Tablets | Calcium Carbonate 750mg | **Adults:** 2-4 tabs prn. **Max:** 9 tabs q24h. |

## Table 10. ANTACID AND HEARTBURN PRODUCTS (cont.)

| Brand Name | Ingredient/Strength | Dose |
|---|---|---|
| Tums Kids Chewable Tablets | Calcium Carbonate 750mg | **Peds 5-11 yrs:** 1 tab prn. **Max:** 4 tabs q24h. **Peds 2-4 yrs:** ½ tab prn. **Max:** 2 tabs q24h. |
| Tums Smoothies Tablets | Calcium Carbonate 750mg | **Adults:** 2-4 tabs prn. **Max:** 10 tabs q24h. |
| Tums Ultra 1000 Chewable Tablets | Calcium Carbonate 1000mg | **Adults:** 2-3 tabs prn. **Max:** 7 tabs q24h for ≤2 weeks. |

### ANTACID/ANTIFLATULENT

| Brand Name | Ingredient/Strength | Dose |
|---|---|---|
| Gelusil Chewable Tablets | Aluminum Hydroxide/Magnesium Hydroxide/Simethicone 200mg-200mg-25mg | **Adults:** 2-4 tabs q1h prn. **Max:** 12 tabs q24h. |
| Maalox Advanced Maximum Strength Chewable Tablets | Calcium Carbonate/Simethicone 1000mg-60mg | **Adults & Peds ≥12 yrs:** 1-2 tabs prn. **Max:** 8 tabs q24h. |
| Maalox Advanced Maximum Strength Liquid | Aluminum Hydroxide/Magnesium Hydroxide/Simethicone 400mg-400mg-40mg/5mL | **Adults & Peds ≥12 yrs:** 2-4 tsp (10-20mL) bid. **Max:** 8 tsp (40mL) q24h. |
| Maalox Advanced Regular Strength Liquid | Aluminum Hydroxide/Magnesium Hydroxide/Simethicone 200mg-200mg-20mg/5mL | **Adults & Peds ≥12 yrs:** 2-4 tsp (10-20mL) qid. **Max:** 16 tsp (80mL) q24h. |
| Maalox Junior Relief Chewables | Calcium Carbonate/Simethicone 400mg-24mg | **Peds 6–11 yrs:** 2 tabs prn. **Max:** 6 tabs q24h. |
| Mylanta Maximum Strength Liquid | Aluminum Hydroxide/Magnesium Hydroxide/Simethicone 400mg-400mg-40mg/5mL | **Adults & Peds ≥12 yrs:** 2-4 tsp (between meals and hs) (10-20mL) qid. **Max:** 12 tsp (60mL) q24h. |
| Mylanta Regular Strength Liquid | Aluminum Hydroxide/Magnesium Hydroxide/Simethicone 200mg-200mg-20mg/5mL | **Adults & Peds ≥12 yrs:** 2-4 tsp (between meals and hs) (10-20mL) qid. **Max:** 24 tsp (120mL) q24h. |
| Rolaids Extra Strength Plus Gas Soft Chews | Calcium Carbonate/Simethicone 1177mg-80mg | **Adults:** 2-3 chews q1h prn. **Max:** 6 chews q24h. |
| Rolaids Multi-Symptom Chewable Tablets | Calcium Carbonate/Magnesium Hydroxide/Simethicone 675mg-135mg-60mg | **Adults:** 2-4 tabs q1h prn. **Max:** 8 tabs q24h. |
| Titralac Plus Chewable Tablets | Calcium Carbonate/Simethicone 420mg-21mg | **Adults:** 2 tabs q2-3h prn. **Max:** 19 tabs q24h. |

*(Continued)*

## Table 10. ANTACID AND HEARTBURN PRODUCTS (cont.)

| Brand Name | Ingredient/Strength | Dose |
| --- | --- | --- |
| **BISMUTH SUBSALICYLATE** | | |
| Maalox Total Relief Maximum Strength Liquid | Bismuth Subsalicylate 525mg/15mL | **Adults & Peds ≥12 yrs:** 2 tbl (30mL) q1h prn. **Max:** 8 tbl (120mL) q24h. |
| Pepto Bismol Caplets | Bismuth Subsalicylate 262mg | **Adults & Peds ≥12 yrs:** 2 tabs q½-1h prn. **Max:** 8 doses q24h. |
| Pepto Bismol Chewable Tablets | Bismuth Subsalicylate 262mg | **Adults & Peds ≥12 yrs:** 2 tabs q½-1h prn. **Max:** 8 doses q24h. |
| Pepto Bismol Liquid | Bismuth Subsalicylate 262mg/15mL | **Adults & Peds ≥12 yrs:** 2 tbl (30mL) q½-1h prn. **Max:** 8 doses (240mL) q24h. |
| Pepto Bismol Liquid Max | Bismuth Subsalicylate 525mg/15mL | **Adults & Peds ≥12 yrs:** 2 tbl (30mL) q1h prn. **Max:** 4 doses (120mL) q24h. |
| **H$_2$-RECEPTOR ANTAGONIST** | | |
| Axid AR | Nizatidine 75mg | **Adults & Peds ≥12 yrs:** 1 tab qd. **Max:** 2 tabs q24h. |
| Pepcid AC Maximum Strength EZ Chews | Famotidine 20mg | **Adults & Peds ≥12 yrs:** 1 tab qd. **Max:** 2 tabs q24h. |
| Pepcid AC Maximum Strength Tablets | Famotidine 20mg | **Adults & Peds ≥12 yrs:** 1 tab qd. **Max:** 2 tabs q24h. |
| Pepcid AC Tablets | Famotidine 10mg | **Adults & Peds ≥12 yrs:** 1 tab qd. **Max:** 2 tabs q24h. |
| Tagamet HB Tablets | Cimetidine 200mg | **Adults & Peds ≥12 yrs:** 1 tab qd. **Max:** 2 tabs q24h. |
| Zantac 75 Tablets | Ranitidine 75mg | **Adults & Peds ≥12 yrs:** 1 tab qd. **Max:** 2 tabs q24h. |
| Zantac 150 Tablets | Ranitidine 150mg | **Adults & Peds ≥12 yrs:** 1 tab qd. **Max:** 2 tabs q24h. |
| **H$_2$-RECEPTOR ANTAGONIST/ANTACID** | | |
| Pepcid Complete Chewable Tablets | Famotidine/Calcium Carbonate/ Magnesium Hydroxide 10mg-800mg-165mg | **Adults & Peds ≥12 yrs:** 1 tab qd. **Max:** 2 tabs q24h. |
| Tums Dual Action | Famotidine/Calcium Carbonate/ Magnesium Hydroxide 10mg-800mg-165mg | **Adults & Peds ≥12 yrs:** 1 tab qd. **Max:** 2 tabs q24h. |

## Table 10. ANTACID AND HEARTBURN PRODUCTS (cont.)

| BRAND NAME | INGREDIENT/STRENGTH | DOSE |
|---|---|---|
| **PROTON PUMP INHIBITOR** | | |
| Prevacid 24HR | Lansoprazole 15mg | **Adults:** 1 cap qd x 14 days. May repeat 14-day course q4 months. |
| Prilosec OTC Tablets | Omeprazole 20mg | **Adults:** 1 tab qd x 14 days. May repeat 14-day course q4 months. |
| Zegerid OTC | Omeprazole/Sodium bicarbonate 20mg-1100mg | **Adults:** 1 cap qd x 14 days. May repeat 14-day course q4 months. |

## Table 11. ANTIDIARRHEAL PRODUCTS

| BRAND NAME | INGREDIENT/STRENGTH | DOSE |
|---|---|---|
| **ABSORBENT AGENTS** | | |
| Equalactin Chewable Tablets | Calcium Polycarbophil 625mg | **Adults & Peds ≥12 yrs:** 2 tabs/dose. **Max:** 8 tabs q24h. **Peds 6-12 yrs:** 1 tab/dose. **Max:** 4 tabs q24h. **Peds 2 to ≤6 yrs:** 1 tab/dose. **Max:** 2 tabs q24h. |
| Fibercon Caplets | Calcium Polycarbophil 625mg | **Adults & Peds ≥12 yrs:** 2 tabs qd. **Max:** 8 tabs q24h. |
| Konsyl Fiber Caplets | Calcium Polycarbophil 625mg | **Adults & Peds ≥12 yrs:** 2 tabs qd-qid. **Peds 6-12 yrs:** 1 tab qd-tid. **Max:** 8 tabs q24h. |
| **ANTIPERISTALTIC AGENTS** | | |
| Imodium A-D Caplets | Loperamide HCl 2mg | **Adults & Peds ≥12 yrs:** 2 tabs after first loose stool; 1 tab after each subsequent loose stool. **Max:** 4 tabs q24h. **Peds 9-11 yrs (60-95 lbs):** 1 tab after first loose stool; ½ tab after each subsequent loose stool. **Max:** 3 tabs q24h. **Peds 6-8 yrs (48-59 lbs):** 1 tab after first loose stool; ½ tab after each subsequent loose stool. **Max:** 2 tabs q24h. |
| Imodium A-D E-Z Chews | Loperamide HCl 2mg | **Adults & Peds ≥12 yrs:** 2 tabs after first loose stool; 1 tab after each subsequent loose stool. **Max:** 4 tabs q24h. **Peds 9-11 yrs (60-95 lbs):** 1 tab after first loose stool; ½ tab after each subsequent loose stool. **Max:** 3 tabs q24h. **Peds 6-8 yrs (48-59 lbs):** 1 tab after first loose stool; ½ tab after each subsequent loose stool. **Max:** 2 tabs q24h. |

*(Continued)*

## Table 11. ANTIDIARRHEAL PRODUCTS (cont.)

| BRAND NAME | INGREDIENT/STRENGTH | DOSE |
|---|---|---|
| Imodium A-D Liquid | Loperamide HCl 1mg/7.5mL | **Adults & Peds ≥12 yrs:** 4 tsp (20mL) after first loose stool; 2 tsp (10mL) after each subsequent loose stool. **Max:** 8 tsp (40mL) q24h. **Peds 9-11 yrs (60-95 lbs):** 2 tsp (10mL) after the first loose stool; 1 tsp (5mL) after each subsequent loose stool. **Max:** 6 tsp (30mL) q24h. **Peds 6-8 yrs (48-59 lbs):** 2 tsp (10mL) after the first loose stool; 1 tsp (5mL) after each subsequent loose stool. **Max:** 4 tsp (20mL) q24h. |
| Imodium A-D Liquid For Use In Children (Mint Flavor) | Loperamide HCl 1mg/7.5mL | **Adults & Peds ≥12 yrs:** 6 tsp (30mL) after first loose stool; 3 tsp (15mL) after each subsequent loose stool. **Max:** 12 tsp (60mL) q24h. **Peds 9-11 yrs (60-95 lbs):** 3 tsp (15mL) after the first loose stool; 1½ tsp (7.5mL) after each subsequent loose stool. **Max:** 9 tsp (45mL) q24h. **Peds 6-8 yrs (48-59 lbs):** 3 tsp (15mL) after first loose stool; 1½ tsp (7.5mL) after each subsequent loose stool. **Max:** 6 tsp (30mL) q24h. |
| **ANTIPERISTALTIC/ANTIFLATULENT AGENTS** | | |
| Imodium Multi-Symptom Relief Caplets | Loperamide HCl/Simethicone 2mg-125mg | **Adults & Peds ≥12 yrs:** 2 tabs after first loose stool; 1 tab after each subsequent loose stool. **Max:** 4 tabs q24h. **Peds 9-11 yrs (60-95 lbs):** 1 tab after first loose stool; ½ tab after each subsequent loose stool. **Max:** 3 tabs q24h. **6-8 yrs (48-59 lbs):** 1 tab after first loose stool; ½ tab after each subsequent loose stool. **Max:** 2 tabs q24h. |

## Table 11. ANTIDIARRHEAL PRODUCTS (cont.)

| BRAND NAME | INGREDIENT/STRENGTH | DOSE |
|---|---|---|
| Imodium Multi-Symptom Relief Chewable Tablets | Loperamide HCl/Simethicone 2mg-125mg | **Adults & Peds ≥12 yrs:** 2 tabs with 4-8 oz water after first loose stool; 1 tab with 4-8 oz water after each subsequent loose stool. **Max:** 4 tabs q24h. **Peds 9-11 yrs (60-95 lbs):** 1 tab with 4-8 oz water after first loose stool; ½ tab after each subsequent loose stool. **Max:** 3 tabs q24h. **Peds 6-8 yrs (48-59 lbs):** 1 tab with 4-8 oz water after first loose stool; ½ tab with 4-8 oz water after each subsequent loose stool. **Max:** 2 tabs q24h. |
| **BISMUTH SUBSALICYLATE** | | |
| Kaopectate Extra Strength Liquid | Bismuth Subsalicylate 525mg/15mL | **Adults & Peds ≥12 yrs:** 2 tbl (30mL) q1h prn. **Max:** 4 doses (8 tbl) q24h. |
| Kaopectate Liquid | Bismuth Subsalicylate 262mg/15mL | **Adults & Peds ≥12 yrs:** 2 tbl (30mL) q½-1h prn. **Max:** 8 doses (16 tbl) q24h. |
| Maalox Total Relief Liquid | Bismuth Subsalicylate 525mg/15mL | **Adults & Peds ≥12 yrs:** 2 tbl (30mL) q1h prn. **Max:** 4 doses (8 tbl) q24h. |
| Pepto Bismol Caplets | Bismuth Subsalicylate 262mg | **Adults & Peds ≥12 yrs:** 2 tabs q½-1h. **Max:** 8 doses (16 tabs) q24h. |
| Pepto Bismol Chewable Tablets | Bismuth Subsalicylate 262mg | **Adults & Peds ≥12 yrs:** 2 tabs q½-1h. **Max:** 8 doses (16 tabs) q24h. |
| Pepto Bismol Liquid | Bismuth Subsalicylate 262mg/15mL | **Adults & Peds ≥12 yrs:** 2 tbl (30mL) q½-1h prn. **Max:** 8 doses (16 tbl) q24h. |
| Pepto Bismol Liquid Max | Bismuth Subsalicylate 525mg/15mL | **Adults & Peds ≥12 yrs:** 2 tbl (30mL) q1h prn. **Max:** 4 doses (8 tbl) q24h. |

## Table 12. LAXATIVE PRODUCTS

| BRAND NAME | INGREDIENT/STRENGTH | DOSE |
|---|---|---|
| **BULK-FORMING** | | |
| Citrucel Caplets | Methylcellulose 500mg | **Adults & Peds ≥12 yrs:** 2 tabs qd prn. **Max:** 12 tabs q24h. **Peds 6-11 yrs:** 1 tab qd prn. **Max:** 6 tabs q24h. |
| Citrucel Sugar Free Powder | Methylcellulose 2g/tbl | **Adults & Peds ≥12 yrs:** 1 tbl (11.5g) qd-tid. **Peds 6-11 yrs:** ½ tbl (5.75g) qd. |
| Equalactin Chewable Tablets | Calcium Polycarbophil 625mg | **Adults & Peds ≥12 yrs:** 2 tabs qd. **Max:** 8 tabs q24h. **Peds 6-11 yrs:** 1 tab qd. **Max:** 4 tabs q24h. **Peds 2-5 yrs:** 1 tab qd. **Max:** 2 tabs q24h. |
| Fibercon Caplets | Calcium Polycarbophil 625mg | **Adults & Peds ≥12 yrs:** 2 tabs qd. **Max:** 8 tabs qd. |
| Konsyl Easy Mix Powder | Psyllium 4.3g/tsp | **Adults & Peds ≥12 yrs:** 1 tsp qd-tid. **Peds 6-11 yrs:** ½ tsp qd-tid. |
| Konsyl Fiber Caplets | Calcium Polycarbophil 625mg | **Adults:** 2 tabs qd-qid. **Max:** 8 tabs q24h. **Peds 6-12 yrs:** 1 tab qd-tid. **Max:** 3 tabs q24h. |
| Konsyl Orange Powder | Psyllium 3.4g/tbl | **Adults & Peds ≥12 yrs:** 1 tbl qd-tid. **Peds 6-11 yrs:** ½ tbl qd-tid. |
| Konsyl Original Powder | Psyllium 6g/tsp | **Adults & Peds ≥12 yrs:** 1 tsp qd-tid. **Peds 6-11 yrs:** ½ tsp qd-tid. |
| Konsyl-D Powder | Psyllium 3.4g/tsp | **Adults & Peds ≥12 yrs:** 1 tsp qd-tid. **Peds 6-11 yrs:** ½ tsp qd-tid. |
| Metamucil Capsules | Psyllium 0.52g | **Adults & Peds ≥12 yrs:** 5 caps qd-tid. |
| Metamucil Original Texture Powder (multi-flavor) | Psyllium 3.4g/tbl | **Adults & Peds ≥12 yrs:** 1 tbl up to tid. **Peds 6-11 yrs:** ½ tbl up to tid. |
| Metamucil Smooth Texture Powder (multi-flavor) | Psyllium 3.4g/tbl | **Adults & Peds ≥12 yrs:** 1 tbl up to tid. **Peds 6-11 yrs:** ½ tbl up to tid. |

*(Continued)*

## Table 12. LAXATIVE PRODUCTS (cont.)

| BRAND NAME | INGREDIENT/STRENGTH | DOSE |
|---|---|---|
| Metamucil Wafers | Psyllium 3.4g/dose | **Adults & Peds ≥12 yrs:** 2 wafers qd-tid. **Peds 6-11 yrs:** 1 wafer qd-tid. |
| **HYPEROSMOTICS** | | |
| Colace Glycerin Suppositories for Adults and Children | Glycerin 2.1g | **Adults & Peds ≥6 yrs:** 1 supp **Max:** 1 supp q24h. |
| Colace Glycerin Suppositories for Infants and Children | Glycerin 1.2g | **Peds 2-5 yrs:** 1 supp **Max:** 1 supp q24h. |
| Dulcolax Balance | Polyethylene Glycol 3350, 17g | **Adults & Peds ≥17 yrs:** 1 capful (17g) qd. **Max:** 7 days. |
| Fleet Glycerin Suppositories | Glycerin 2g | **Adults & Peds ≥6 yrs:** 1 supp ud. |
| Fleet Liquid Glycerin Suppositories | Glycerin 5.6g | **Adults & Peds ≥6 yrs:** 1 supp ud. |
| Fleet Mineral Oil Enema | Mineral Oil 118mL | **Adults & Peds ≥12 yrs:** 1 bottle (118mL). **Peds 2-11 yrs:** ½ bottle (59mL). |
| Fleet Pedia-Lax Glycerin Suppositories | Glycerin 1g | **Peds 2-6 yrs:** 1 supp ud. |
| Fleet Pedia-Lax Liquid Glycerin Suppositories | Glycerin 2.8g | **Peds 2-6 yrs:** 1 supp ud. |
| **SALINES** | | |
| Fleet Enema | Monobasic Sodium Phosphate/Dibasic Sodium Phosphate 19g-7g/118mL | **Adults & Peds ≥12 yrs:** 1 bottle (118mL). |
| Fleet Enema Extra | Monobasic Sodium Phosphate/Dibasic Sodium Phosphate 19g-7g/197mL | **Adults & Peds ≥12 yrs:** 1 bottle (197mL). |
| Fleet Pedia-Lax Chewable Tablets | Magnesium Hydroxide 400mg | **Peds 6-<12 yrs:** 3-6 tabs qd. **Max:** 6 tabs q24h. **Peds 2-<6 yrs:** 1-3 tabs qd. **Max:** 3 tabs q24h. |
| Fleet Pedia-Lax Enema | Monobasic Sodium Phosphate/Dibasic Sodium Phosphate 9.5g-3.5g/59mL | **Peds 5-11 yrs:** 1 bottle (59mL). **Peds 2-<5 yrs:** ½ bottle (29.5mL). |
| Magnesium Citrate Solution | Magnesium Citrate 1.75g/30mL | **Adults & Peds ≥12 yrs:** 300mL. **Peds 6-<12 yrs:** 90-210mL. **Peds 2-<6 yrs:** 60mL. |

## Table 12. LAXATIVE PRODUCTS (cont.)

| BRAND NAME | INGREDIENT/STRENGTH | DOSE |
|---|---|---|
| Little Phillips' Milk of Magnesia Safe and Gentle | Magnesium Hydroxide 800mg/5mL | **Adults & Peds ≥12 yrs:** 3-6 tsp qd. **Peds 6-11 yrs:** 1.5-3 tsp qd. **Peds 2-5 yrs:** 1/2-1.5 tsp qd. |
| Phillips' Antacid/Laxative Chewable Tablets | Magnesium Hydroxide 311mg | **Adults & Peds ≥12 yrs:** 8 tabs qd. **Peds 6-11 yrs:** 4 tabs qd. **Peds 3-5 yrs:** 2 tabs qd. |
| Phillips' Laxative Caplets | Magnesium 500mg | **Adults & Peds ≥12 yrs:** Take 2-4 tabs qd. **Max:** 4 tabs q24h. |
| Phillips' M-O | Magnesium Hydroxide 300mg/5mL | **Adults & Peds ≥12 yrs:** 3-4 tbl qd. **Peds 6-11 yrs:** 4-6 tsp qd. |
| Phillips' Concentrated Milk of Magnesia Liquid | Magnesium Hydroxide 800mg/5mL | **Adults & Peds ≥12 yrs:** 1-2 tbl qd. **Peds 6-11 yrs:** ½-1 tbl qd. |
| Phillips' Milk of Magnesia Liquid | Magnesium Hydroxide 400mg/5mL | **Adults & Peds ≥12 yrs:** 2-4 tbl qd. **Peds 6-11 yrs:** 1-2 tbl qd. |
| **SALINE COMBINATION** | | |
| Phillips' M-O Liquid | Magnesium Hydroxide/Mineral Oil 300mg-1.25mL/5ml | **Adults & Peds ≥12 yrs:** 3-4 tbl qd. **Peds 6-11 yrs:** 4-6 tsp qd. |
| **STIMULANTS** | | |
| Alophen Enteric Coated Stimulant Laxative Pills | Bisacodyl 5mg | **Adults & Peds ≥12 yrs:** Take 1-3 tabs qd. **Peds 6-11 yrs:** Take 1 tab qd. |
| Carter's Laxative, Sodium Free Pills | Bisacodyl 5mg | **Adults & Peds ≥12 yrs:** Take 1-3 tabs (usually 2 tabs) qd. **Peds 6-<12 yrs:** Take 1 tab qd. |
| Castor Oil | Castor Oil | **Adults & Peds ≥12 yrs:** 15-60mL. **Peds 2-<12 yrs:** 5-15mL. **Peds <2 yrs:** 1-5 mL. |
| Dulcolax Suppository | Bisacodyl 10mg | **Adults & Peds ≥12 yrs:** 1 supp qd. **Peds 6-<12 yrs:** ½ supp qd. |
| Dulcolax Tablets | Bisacodyl 5mg | **Adults & Peds ≥12 yrs:** 1-3 tabs qd. **Peds 6-<12 yrs:** 1 tab qd. |
| Ex-Lax Maximum Strength Tablets | Sennosides 25mg | **Adults & Peds ≥12 yrs:** 2 tabs qd-bid. **Peds 6-<12 yrs:** 1 tab qd-bid. |

*(Continued)*

## Table 12. LAXATIVE PRODUCTS (cont.)

| BRAND NAME | INGREDIENT/STRENGTH | DOSE |
|---|---|---|
| Ex-Lax Tablets | Sennosides 15mg | **Adults & Peds ≥12 yrs:** 2 tabs qd-bid. **Peds 6-<12 yrs:** 1 tab qd-bid. |
| Ex-Lax Ultra Stimulant Laxative Tablets | Bisacodyl 5mg | **Adults & Peds ≥12 yrs:** 1-3 tabs qd. **Peds 6-<12 yrs:** 1 tab qd-bid. |
| Fleet Bisacodyl Enema | Bisacodyl 10mg/30mL | **Adults & Peds ≥12 yrs:** 1 bottle (30mL). |
| Fleet Bisacodyl Suppositories | Bisacodyl 10mg | **Adults & Peds ≥12 yrs:** 1 supp qd. **Peds 6-<12 yrs:** ½ supp qd. |
| Fleet Pedia-Lax Quick Dissolve Strips · | Sennosides 8.6mg | **Peds 6-<12 yrs:** 2 strips. **Max:** 4 strips q24h. **Peds 2-<6 yrs:** 1 strip. **Max:** 2 strips q24h. |
| Fleet Stimulant Laxative Tablets | Bisacodyl 5mg | **Adults & Peds ≥12 yrs:** 1-3 tabs qd. **Peds 6-<12 yrs:** 1 tab qd. |
| Perdiem Overnight Relief Tablets | Sennosides 15mg | **Adults & Peds ≥12 yrs:** 2 tabs qd-bid. **Peds 6-<12 yrs:** 1 tab qd-bid. |
| Senokot Tablets | Sennosides 8.6mg | **Adults & Peds ≥12 yrs:** 2 tabs qd. **Max:** 4 tabs bid. **Peds 6-<12 yrs:** 1 tab qd. **Max:** 2 tabs bid. **Peds 2-<6 yrs:** ½ tab qd. **Max:** 1 tab bid. |
| SenokotXTRA Tablets | Sennosides 17.2mg | **Adults & Peds ≥6 yrs:** Starting dose 1 tab qd. **Max:** 2 tabs bid. **Peds 2-<6 yrs:** ½ tab qd. **Max:** 1 tab bid. |
| **STIMULANT COMBINATIONS** | | |
| Peri-Colace Tablets | Sennosides/Docusate 8.6mg-50mg | **Adults & Peds ≥12 yrs:** 2-4 tabs qd. **Peds 6-<12 yrs:** 1-2 tabs qd. **Peds 2-5 yrs:** 1 tab qd. |
| Senna Prompt | Psyllium/Sennosides 500mg-9mg | **Adults & Peds ≥12 yrs:** 1-5 caps qd-bid. |

## Table 12. LAXATIVE PRODUCTS (cont.)

| BRAND NAME | INGREDIENT/STRENGTH | DOSE |
|---|---|---|
| Senokot S Tablets | Sennosides/Docusate 8.6mg-50mg | **Adults ≥12 yrs:** 2 tabs qd. **Max:** 4 tabs bid. **Peds 6-<12 yrs:** 1 tab qd. **Max:** 2 tabs bid. **Peds 2-<6 yrs:** ½ tab qd. **Max:** 1 tab bid. |
| **SURFACTANTS (STOOL SOFTENERS)** | | |
| Colace Capsules | Docusate Sodium 100mg | **Adults & Peds ≥12 yrs:** 1-3 caps qd. **Peds 2-<12 yrs:** 1 cap qd. |
| Colace Capsules | Docusate Sodium 50mg | **Adults & Peds ≥12 yrs:** 1-6 caps qd. **Peds 2-<12 yrs:** 1-3 caps qd. |
| Colace Liquid | Docusate Sodium 10mg/mL | **Adults & Peds ≥12 yrs:** 5-15mL qd-bid. **Peds 2-<12 yrs:** 5-15mL qd. |
| Colace Syrup | Docusate Sodium 60mg/15mL | **Adults & Peds ≥12 yrs:** 1-6 tbl qd. **Peds 2-<12 yrs:** 1-2½ tbl qd. |
| Docusol Constipation Relief, Mini Enemas | Docusate Sodium 283mg | **Adults & Peds ≥12 yrs:** Take 1-3 units qd. **Peds 6-12 yrs:** Take 1 unit qd. |
| Dulcolax Stool Softener Capsules | Docusate Sodium 100mg | **Adults & Peds ≥12 yrs:** 1-3 caps qd. **Peds 2-<12 yrs:** 1 cap qd. |
| Fleet Pedia-Lax Liquid Stool Softener | Docusate 50mg/15mL | **Peds 2-12 yrs:** 1-3 tbl qd. **Max:** 3 tbl q24h. |
| Fleet Sof-Lax | Docusate 100mg | **Adults & Peds ≥12 yrs:** 1-3 caps qd. **Peds 2-<12 yrs:** 1 cap qd. |
| Kaopectate Liqui-Gels | Docusate Calcium 240mg | **Adults & Peds ≥12 yrs:** 1 cap qd until normal bowel movement. |
| Phillips' Stool Softener Capsules | Docusate Sodium 100mg | **Adults & Peds ≥12 yrs:** 1-3 caps qd. **Peds 6-<12 yrs:** 1 cap qd. |

## Table 13. ALLERGIC RHINITIS PRODUCTS

| BRAND NAME | INGREDIENT/STRENGTH | DOSE |
|---|---|---|
| **ANTIHISTAMINE** | | |
| Alavert Quick Dissolving Tablets | Loratadine 10mg | **Adults & Peds ≥6 yrs:** 1 tab qd. **Max:** 1 tab q24h. |
| Alavert For Kids 6+ | Loratadine 10mg | **Adults & Peds ≥6 yrs:** 1 tab qd. **Max:** 1 tab q24h. |
| Benadryl Allergy Quick Dissolve Strips | Diphenhydramine HCl 25mg | **Adults & Peds ≥12 yrs:** Dissolve 1-2 strips on tongue q4-6h. **Peds 6-<12 yrs:** Dissolve 1 strip on tongue q4-6h. **Max:** 6 doses q24h. |
| Benadryl Allergy Kapgels | Diphenhydramine HCl 25mg | **Adults & Peds ≥12 yrs:** 1-2 caps q4-6h. **Peds 6-<12 yrs:** 1 cap q4-6h. **Max:** 6 doses q24h. |
| Benadryl Allergy Ultratab Tablets | Diphenhydramine HCl 25mg | **Adults & Peds ≥12 yrs:** 1-2 tabs q4-6h. **Peds 6-<12 yrs:** 1 tab q4-6h. **Max:** 6 doses q24h. |
| Benadryl Dye-Free Allergy Liqui-Gels | Diphenhydramine HCl 25mg | **Adults & Peds ≥12 yrs:** 1-2 caps q4-6h. **Peds 6-<12 yrs:** 1 cap q4-6h. **Max:** 6 doses q24h. |
| Children's Benadryl Allergy Fastmelt Tablets | Diphenhydramine HCl 12.5mg | **Adults & Peds ≥12 yrs:** 2-4 tabs q4-6h. **Peds 6-<12 yrs:** 1-2 tabs q4-6h. **Max:** 6 doses q24h. |
| Children's Benadryl Perfect Measure Pre-Filled Single Use Spoons | Diphenhydramine HCl 12.5mg/5mL | **Adults & Peds ≥12 yrs:** 2-4 pre-filled spoons (10-20mL) q4-6h. **Peds 6-<12 yrs:** 1-2 pre-filled spoons (5-10mL) q4-6h. **Max:** 6 doses q24h. |
| Children's Benadryl Allergy Liquid | Diphenhydramine HCl 12.5mg/5mL | **Peds 6-<12 yrs:** 1-2 tsp (5-10mL) q4-6h. **Max:** 6 doses q24h. |
| Children's Benadryl Dye-Free Allergy Liquid | Diphenhydramine HCl 12.5mg/5mL | **Peds 6-<12 yrs:** 1-2 tsp (5-10mL) q4-6h. **Max:** 6 doses q24h. |
| Claritin Tablets | Loratadine 10mg | **Adults & Peds ≥6 yrs:** 1 tab qd. **Max:** 1 tab q24h. |
| Claritin Liqui-Gels | Loratadine 10mg | **Adults & Peds ≥6 yrs:** 1 cap qd. **Max:** 1 cap q24h. |

*(Continued)*

## Table 13. ALLERGIC RHINITIS PRODUCTS (cont.)

| BRAND NAME | INGREDIENT/STRENGTH | DOSE |
|---|---|---|
| Claritin RediTabs 24-Hour | Loratadine 10mg | **Adults & Peds ≥6 yrs:** 1 tab qd. **Max:** 1 tab q24h. |
| Claritin 12-Hour RediTabs | Loratadine 5mg | **Adults & Peds ≥6 yrs:** 1 tab q12h. **Max:** 2 tabs q24h. |
| Claritin 24-Hour RediTabs For Kids | Loratadine 10mg | **Adults & Peds ≥6 yrs:** 1 tab qd. **Max:** 1 tab q24h. |
| Claritin 12-Hour RediTabs For Kids | Loratadine 5mg | **Adults & Peds ≥6 yrs:** 1 tab q12h. **Max:** 2 tabs q24h. |
| Children's Claritin Chewables | Loratadine 5mg | **Adults & Peds ≥6 yrs:** 2 tabs qd. **Max:** 2 tabs q24h. **Peds 2-<6 yrs:** 1 tab qd. **Max:** 1 tab q24h. |
| Children's Claritin Syrup | Loratadine 5mg/5mL | **Adults & Peds ≥6 yrs:** 2 tsp (10mL) qd. **Max:** 2 tsp q24h. **Peds 2-<6 yrs:** 1 tsp (5mL) qd. **Max:** 1 tsp q24h. |
| Zyrtec Tablets | Cetirizine HCl 10mg | **Adults & Peds 6-<65 yrs:** 1 tab qd. **Max:** 1 tab q24h. |
| Children's Zyrtec Chewable 10mg | Cetirizine HCl 10mg | **Adults & Peds 6-<65 yrs:** 1 tab qd. **Max:** 1 tab q24h. |
| Children's Zyrtec Perfect Measure | Cetirizine HCl 5mg/5mL | **Adults & Peds 6-<65 yrs:** 1-2 prefilled spoons (5-10mL) qd. **Max:** 2 prefilled spoons q24h. **Adults ≥65 yrs:** 1 pre-filled spoon (5mL) qd. **Max:** 1 pre-filled spoon q24h. |
| Children's Zyrtec Allergy Syrup | Cetirizine HCl 5mg/5mL | **Adults & Peds 6-<65 yrs:** 1-2 tsp (5-10mL) qd. **Max:** 2 tsp q24h. **Adults ≥65 yrs:** 1 tsp qd. **Max:** 1 tsp q24h. **Peds 2-<6 yrs:** ½-1 tsp (2.5-5mL) qd or ½ tsp q12h. **Max:** 1 tsp q24h. |
| **ANTIHISTAMINE COMBINATIONS** | | |
| Advil Allergy Sinus Caplets | Chlorpheniramine Maleate/ Ibuprofen/Pseudoephedrine HCl 2mg-200mg-30mg | **Adults & Peds ≥12 yrs:** 1 tab q4-6h. **Max:** 6 tabs q24h. |
| Alavert Allergy & Sinus D-12 | Loratadine/Pseudoephedrine Sulfate 5mg-120mg | **Adults & Peds ≥12 yrs:** 1 tab q12h. **Max:** 2 tabs q24h. |

## Table 13. ALLERGIC RHINITIS PRODUCTS (cont.)

| BRAND NAME | INGREDIENT/STRENGTH | DOSE |
|---|---|---|
| Allerest PE | Chlorpheniramine Maleate/ Phenylephrine HCl 4mg-10mg | **Adults & Peds ≥12 yrs:** 1 tab q4h. **Peds 6-<12 yrs:** ½ tab q4h **Max:** 6 doses q24h. |
| Benadryl-D Allergy Plus Sinus | Diphenhydramine HCl/ Phenylephrine HCl 25mg-10mg | **Adults & Peds ≥12 yrs:** 1 tab q4h. **Max:** 6 tabs q24h. |
| Benadryl Severe Allergy Plus Sinus Headache Caplets | Diphenhydramine HCl/ Acetaminophen/Phenylephrine HCl 25mg-325mg-5mg | **Adults & Peds ≥12 yrs:** 2 tabs q4h. **Max:** 12 tabs q24h. |
| Benadryl Severe Allergy Plus Sinus Headache Kapgels | Diphenhydramine HCl/ Acetaminophen/Phenylephrine HCl 12.5mg-325mg-5mg | **Adults & Peds ≥12 yrs:** 2 caps q4h. **Max:** 12 caps q24h. |
| Benadryl Severe Allergy Plus Cold Kapgels | Diphenhydramine HCl/ Acetaminophen/Phenylephrine HCl 12.5mg-325mg-5mg | **Adults & Peds ≥12 yrs:** 2 caps q4h. **Max:** 12 caps q24h. |
| Children's Benadryl-D Allergy & Sinus Liquid | Diphenhydramine HCl/ Phenylephrine HCl 12.5mg-5mg/5mL | **Adults & Peds ≥12 yrs:** 2 tsp (10mL) q4h. **Peds 6-<12 yrs:** 1 tsp (5mL) q4h. **Max:** 6 doses q24h. |
| Claritin-D 12 Hour | Loratadine/Pseudoephedrine Sulfate 5mg-120mg | **Adults & Peds ≥12 yrs:** 1 tab q12h. **Max:** 2 tabs q24h. |
| Claritin-D 24 Hour | Loratadine/Pseudoephedrine Sulfate 10mg-240mg | **Adults & Peds ≥12 yrs:** 1 tab qd. **Max:** 1 tab q24h. |
| Children's Dimetapp Cold & Allergy Chewable Tablets | Brompheniramine Maleate/ Phenylephrine HCl 1mg-2.5mg | **Peds 6-<12 yrs:** 2 tabs q4h. **Max:** 6 doses q24h. |
| Children's Dimetapp Cold & Allergy Syrup | Brompheniramine Maleate/ Phenylephrine HCl 1mg-2.5mg/5mL | **Adults & Peds ≥12 yrs:** 4 tsp (20mL) q4h. **Peds 6-<12 yrs:** 2 tsp (10mL) q4h. **Max:** 6 doses q24h. |
| Zyrtec-D Tablets | Cetirizine HCl/ Pseudoephedrine HCl 5mg-120mg | **Adults & Peds 12-<65 yrs:** 1 tab q12h. **Max:** 2 tabs q24h. |
| **TOPICAL NASAL DECONGESTANTS** | | |
| 4-Way Fast Acting Nasal Decongestant Spray | Phenylephrine HCl 1% | **Adults & Peds ≥12 yrs:** Instill 2-3 sprays per nostril q4h. |
| 4-Way Mentholated Nasal Decongestant Spray | Phenylephrine HCl 1% | **Adults & Peds ≥12 yrs:** Instill 2-3 sprays per nostril q4h. |

*(Continued)*

## Table 13. ALLERGIC RHINITIS PRODUCTS (cont.)

| BRAND NAME | INGREDIENT/STRENGTH | DOSE |
|---|---|---|
| Afrin Original 12 Hour Pump Mist | Oxymetazoline HCl 0.05% | **Adults & Peds ≥6 yrs:** Instill 2-3 sprays per nostril q10-12h. **Max:** 2 doses q24h. |
| Afrin Extra Moisturizing 12 Hour Pump Mist | Oxymetazoline HCl 0.05% | **Adults & Peds ≥6 yrs:** Instill 2-3 sprays per nostril q10-12h. **Max:** 2 doses q24h. |
| Afrin All Night 12 Hour Pump Mist | Oxymetazoline HCl 0.05% | **Adults & Peds ≥6 yrs:** Instill 2-3 sprays per nostril q10-12h. **Max:** 2 doses q24h. |
| Afrin Sinus 12 Hour Pump Mist | Oxymetazoline HCl 0.05% | **Adults & Peds ≥6 yrs:** Instill 2-3 sprays per nostril q10-12h. **Max:** 2 doses q24h. |
| Afrin Severe Congestion 12 Hour Pump Mist | Oxymetazoline HCl 0.05% | **Adults & Peds ≥6 yrs:** Instill 2-3 sprays per nostril q10-12h. **Max:** 2 doses q24h. |
| Benzedrex Inhaler | Propylhexedrine 250mg | **Adults & Peds ≥6 yrs:** Inhale 2 sprays per nostril q2h. **Max:** Do not use >3 days. |
| Dristan 12-hr Nasal Spray | Oxymetazoline HCl 0.05% | **Adults & Peds ≥12 yrs:** Instill 2-3 sprays per nostril q10-12h. **Max:** 2 doses q24h. |
| Little Noses Decongestant Nose Drops | Phenylephrine HCl 0.125% | **Peds 2-<6 yrs:** Instill 2-3 sprays per nostril q4h. **Max:** 2 doses q24h. |
| Mucinex Moisture Smart Nasal Spray | Oxymetazoline HCl 0.05% | **Adults & Peds ≥6 yrs:** Instill 2-3 sprays per nostril q10-12h. **Max:** 2 doses q24h. |
| Mucinex Full Force Nasal Spray | Oxymetazoline HCl 0.05% | **Adults & Peds ≥6 yrs:** Instill 2-3 sprays per nostril q10-12h. **Max:** 2 doses q24h. |
| Neo-Synephrine Regular Strength Nasal Spray | Phenylephrine HCl 0.5% | **Adults & Peds ≥12 yrs:** Instill 2-3 sprays per nostril q4h. |
| Neo-Synephrine Extra Strength Nasal Spray | Phenylephrine HCl 1% | **Adults & Peds ≥12 yrs:** Instill 2-3 sprays per nostril q4h. |
| Neo-Synephrine Nighttime Nasal Spray | Oxymetazoline HCl 0.05% | **Adults & Peds ≥6 yrs:** Instill 2-3 sprays per nostril q10-12h. **Max:** 2 doses q24h. |

## Table 13. ALLERGIC RHINITIS PRODUCTS (cont.)

| Brand Name | Ingredient/Strength | Dose |
|---|---|---|
| Nostrilla Fast Relief | Oxymetazoline HCl 0.05% | **Adults & Peds ≥6 yrs:** Instill 2-3 sprays per nostril q10-12h. **Max:** 2 doses q24h. |
| Nostrilla Complete Congestion Relief | Oxymetazoline HCl 0.05% | **Adults & Peds ≥6 yrs:** Instill 2-3 sprays per nostril q10-12h. **Max:** 2 doses q24h. |
| Privine Nasal Drops | Naphazoline HCl 0.05% | **Adults & Peds ≥12 yrs:** Instill 1-2 sprays per nostril q6h. |
| Privine Nasal Spray | Naphazoline HCl 0.05% | **Adults & Peds ≥12 yrs:** Instill 1-2 sprays per nostril q6h. |
| Sudafed OM Sinus Congestion Spray | Oxymetazoline HCl 0.05% | **Adults & Peds ≥6 yrs:** Instill 2-3 sprays per nostril q10-12h. **Max:** 2 doses q24h. |
| Vicks Sinex 12-Hour Decongestant UltraFine Mist | Oxymetazoline HCl 0.05% | **Adults & Peds ≥6 yrs:** Instill 2-3 sprays per nostril q10-12h. **Max:** 2 doses q24h. |
| Vicks Sinex VapoSpray 12-Hour Decongestant Nasal Spray | Oxymetazoline HCl 0.05% | **Adults & Peds >6 yrs:** Instill 2-3 sprays per nostril q10-12h. **Max:** 2 doses q24h. |
| Vicks VapoInhaler | Levmetamfetamine 50mg | **Adults & Peds ≥12 yrs:** Inhale 2 sprays per nostril q2h. **Peds 6-<12 yrs:** Inhale 1 spray per nostril q2h. |
| Zicam Extreme Congestion Relief Nasal Gel | Oxymetazoline HCl 0.05% | **Adults & Peds ≥6 yrs:** Instill 2-3 sprays per nostril q10-12h. **Max:** 2 doses q24h. |
| Zicam Intense Sinus Relief Nasal Gel | Oxymetazoline HCl 0.05% | **Adults & Peds ≥6 yrs:** Instill 2-3 sprays per nostril q10-12h. **Max:** 2 doses q24h. |
| **TOPICAL NASAL MOISTURIZERS** | | |
| 4-Way Saline Moisturizing Mist | Water, Boric Acid, Glycerin, Sodium Chloride, Sodium Borate, Eucalyptol, Menthol, Polysorbate 80, Benzalkonium Chloride | **Adults & Peds ≥2 yrs:** Instill 2-3 sprays per nostril prn. |

*(Continued)*

## Table 13. ALLERGIC RHINITIS PRODUCTS (cont.)

| Brand Name | Ingredient/Strength | Dose |
|---|---|---|
| Afrin PureSea Medium Stream | Sea Water | **Adults & Peds ≥2 yrs:** Use to rinse nostrils qid. |
| Afrin PureSea Gentle Mist | Sea Water | **Adults & Peds ≥2 yrs:** Use to rinse nostrils qid. |
| Afrin PureSea Ultra-Gentle Mist | Sea Water | **Peds ≥6 mos:** Use to rinse nostrils qid. |
| Ayr Saline Nasal Mist | Sodium Chloride 0.65% | **Adults & Peds:** Instill 1 spray per nostril prn. |
| Ayr Saline Nasal Drops | Sodium Chloride 0.65% | **Adults & Peds:** Instill 2-6 drops per nostril prn |
| Ayr Allergy & Sinus Hypertonic Saline Nasal Mist | Sodium Chloride 2.65% | **Adults & Peds:** Instill 2 sprays per nostril bid-tid |
| Baby Ayr Saline Nose Spray/Drops | Sodium Chloride 0.65% | **Peds:** Instill 2-6 drops per nostril. |
| Ayr Saline Nasal Gel No-Drip Sinus Spray | Water, Sodium Carbomethyl Starch, Propylene Glycol, Glycerin, *Aloe Barbadensis* Leaf Juice (Aloe Vera), Sodium Chloride, Cetylpyridinium Chloride, Citric Acid, Disodium EDTA, *Glycine Soja* (Soybean) Oil, Tocopheryl Acetate, Benzyl Alcohol, Benzalkonium Chloride, *Geranium Maculatum* Oil | **Adults & Peds:** Instill 1 spray per nostril. |
| Ayr Saline Nasal Gel | Water, Methyl Gluceth-10, Propylene Glycol, Glycerin, Glyceryl Polymethacrylate, Triethanolamine, *Aloe Barbadensis* Leaf Juice (Aloe Vera Gel), PEG/PPG-18/18 Dimethicone, Carbomer, Poloxamer 184, Sodium Chloride, Xanthan Gum, Diazolidinyl Urea, Methylparaben, Propylparaben, *Glycine Soja* (Soybean) Oil, *Geranium Maculatum* Oil, Tocopheryl Acetate, Blue 1 | **Adults & Peds:** Apply around nostrils and under nose prn. |

## Table 13. ALLERGIC RHINITIS PRODUCTS (cont.)

| BRAND NAME | INGREDIENT/STRENGTH | DOSE |
|---|---|---|
| Ayr Saline Nasal Gel Swabs | Water, Methyl Gluceth-10, Propylene Glycol, Glycerin, Glyceryl Polymethacrylate, Triethanolamine, *Aloe Barbadensis* Leaf Juice (Aloe Vera Gel), PEG/PPG-18/18 Dimethicone, Carbomer, Poloxamer 184, Sodium Chloride, Xanthan Gum, Diazolidinyl Urea, Methylparaben, Propylparaben, *Glycine Soja* (Soybean) Oil, *Geranium Maculatum* Oil, Tocopheryl Acetate, Blue 1 | **Adults & Peds:** Apply around nostrils and under nose prn. |
| Little Noses Saline Spray/Drops | Sodium Chloride 0.65% | **Adults & Peds:** Instill 2-6 drops/sprays per nostril prn. |
| Little Noses Sterile Saline Nasal Mist | Sodium Chloride 0.9% | **Adults & Peds:** Instill 1-3 short sprays per nostril prn. |
| Nostrilla Conditioning Double-Moisture | Benzalkonium Chloride Solution, Carboxymethylcellulose Sodium, Eucalyptol, Glycine, Hyaluronic Acid Sodium, Polyethylene Glycol, Povidone, Propylene Glycol, Sodium Chloride (as 1.9% saline solution), Spearmint Oil, Wintergreen Oil, Water | **Adults & Peds:** Instill 1-2 sprays per nostril bid. |
| Ocean Gel Ultra Moisturizing Gel | Purified water, Glycerin, Carbomer 940, Trolamine, Hyaluranon, Methlyparaben, Propylparaben | **Adults & Peds:** Apply around nostrils and under nose prn. |
| Ocean Complete Sinus Irrigation | Purified Water, Glycerin, Sodium Chloride, Monobasic Sodium Phosphate, Dibasic Sodium Phosphate, Potassium Chloride, Calcium Chloride, Magnesium Chloride | **Adults & Peds:** Attach white actuator and spray into each nostril prn. |
| Ocean Ultra Sterile Saline Mist | Purified Water, Glycerin, Sodium Chloride, Monobasic Sodium Phosphate, Sodium Hyaluronan, Dibasic Sodium Phosphate, Potassium Chloride, Calcium Chloride, Magnesium Chloride | **Adults & Peds:** Spray into each nostril prn. |
| Ocean for Kids Premium Saline Nasal Spray | Sodium Chloride 0.65%, Purified Water, Glycerin, Sodium Phosphate Monobasic, Sodium Hydroxide, Benzalkonium Chloride | **Peds:** Instill 2 sprays per nostril prn. |

*(Continued)*

## Table 13. ALLERGIC RHINITIS PRODUCTS (cont.)

| Brand Name | Ingredient/Strength | Dose |
|---|---|---|
| Ocean Premium Saline Nasal Spray | Sodium Chloride 0.65% | **Adults & Peds:** Instill 2 sprays per nostril prn. |
| Simply Saline Nasal Mist | Sodium Chloride 0.9% | **Adults & Peds:** Spray into each nostril prn. |
| Baby Simply Saline Sterile Saline Mist | Sodium Chloride 0.9% | **Peds:** Spray into each nostril prn. |
| Simply Saline Nasal Moist Gel | Propylene Glycol, Hydroxyethyl-cellulose, Aloe Vera, Sodium Chloride, Allantoin, Methylparaben, Propylparaben, Purified Water | **Adults & Peds:** Apply around nostrils and under nose prn. |
| **MISCELLANEOUS** | | |
| NasalCrom Nasal Spray | Cromolyn Sodium 5.2 mg | **Adults & Peds ≥2 yrs:** Instill 1 spray per nostril q4-6h. **Max:** 6 doses q24h. |
| Similasan Relief Nasal Spray | *Cardiospermum* 6X, *Galphimia glauca* 6X, *Luffa operculata* 6X, *Sabadilla* 6X | **Adults & Peds:** Instill 1-3 sprays per nostril prn. |
| SinoFresh Nasal & Sinus Care | *Eucalyptus Globulus* 20x, *Kalium Bichromicum* 30x | **Adults:** Instill 1-2 sprays per nostril every morning and evening. Gently sniff to distribute solution. Blow nose to clear it of loosened debris and mucus. Re-apply 1 spray to each nostril. |
| Zicam Allergy Relief Nasal Gel | *Luffa Operculata* (4x, 12x, 30x), *Galphimia Glauca* (12x, 30x), *Histaminum Hydrochloricum* (12x, 30x, 200x), *Sulphur* (12x, 30x, 200x) | **Adults & Peds ≥12 yrs:** Instill 1 spray per nostril q4h. |
| Zicam Allergy Relief Gel Swabs | *Galphimia Glauca* (12x, 30x), *Histaminum Hydrochloricum* (12x, 30x, 200x), *Luffa Operculata* (4x, 12x, 30x), *Sulphur* (12x, 30x, 200x) | **Adults & Peds ≥6 yrs:** Apply medication just inside first nostril. Remove swab and press lightly on the outside of first nostril for 5 sec. Re-dip swab in tube and repeat with 2nd nostril. |

## Table 14. IS IT A COLD, THE FLU, OR AN ALLERGY?

| | COLD | FLU | AIRBORNE ALLERGY |
|---|---|---|---|
| **SYMPTOMS** | | | |
| Chest discomfort | Mild to moderate | Common; can become severe | Sometimes |
| Cough | Common (hacking cough) | Sometimes | Sometimes |
| Diarrhea | Never | Sometimes (more common in children) | Never |
| Duration | 3-14 days | Days to weeks | Weeks (eg, 6 weeks for ragweed or grass pollen seasons) |
| Extreme exhaustion | Never | Early and prominent | Never |
| Fatigue, weakness | Sometimes | Can last up to 2-3 weeks | Sometimes |
| Fever | Rare | Characteristic, high (100-102°F); lasts 3-4 days | Never |
| General aches, pains | Slight | Usual; often severe | Never |
| Headache | Rare | Common | Sometimes |
| Itchy eyes | Rare or never | Rare or never | Common |
| Runny nose | Common | Common | Common |
| Sneezing | Usual | Sometimes | Usual |
| Sore throat | Common | Sometimes | Sometimes |
| Stuffy nose | Common | Sometimes | Common |
| Vomiting | Never | Sometimes (more common in children) | Never |
| **TREATMENT** | | | |
| | Antihistamines* | Amantadine | Antihistamines* |
| | Decongestants* | Rimantadine | Nasal steroids* |
| | Nonsteroidal anti-inflammatories* | Oseltamivir | Decongestants* |
| | | Zanamivir | |

*(Continued)*

## Table 14. IS IT A COLD, THE FLU, OR AN ALLERGY? (cont.)

|  | COLD | FLU | AIRBORNE ALLERGY |
|---|---|---|---|
| **PREVENTION** | | | |
|  | Wash your hands often; avoid close contact with anyone with a cold | Annual vaccination<br>Amantadine<br>Rimantadine<br>Oseltamivir | Avoid allergens such as pollen, house flies, dust mites, mold, pet dander, cockroaches |
| **COMPLICATIONS** | | | |
|  | Sinus infection | Bronchitis | Sinus infections |
|  | Middle ear infection | Pneumonia | Asthma |
|  | Asthma | Can be life-threatening | |

Adapted from the National Institute of Allergy and Infectious Diseases, November 2008 and CDC.gov.

*Used only for temporary relief of cold symptoms.

## Table 15. COUGH-COLD-FLU

| Brand Name | Analgesic | Antihistamine | Decongestant | Cough Suppressant | Expectorant | Dose |
|---|---|---|---|---|---|---|
| **ANTIHISTAMINE + DECONGESTANT** | | | | | | |
| Actifed Cold & Allergy Tablets | | Chlorpheniramine Maleate 4mg | Phenylephrine HCl 10mg | | | **Adults & Peds ≥12 yrs:** 1 tab q4h. **Max:** 6 tabs q24h. |
| Benadryl-D Allergy Plus Sinus | | Diphenhydramine HCl 25mg | Phenylephrine HCl 10mg | | | **Adults & Peds ≥12 yrs:** 1 tab q4h. **Max:** 6 tabs q24h. |
| Children's Benadryl-D Allergy & Sinus Liquid | | Diphenhydramine HCl 12.5mg/5mL | Phenylephrine HCl 5mg/5mL | | | **Adults ≥12 yrs:** 2 tsp (10mL) q4h. **Peds 6-<12 yrs:** 1 tsp (5mL) q4h. **Max:** 6 doses q24h. |
| Children's Dimetapp Cold & Allergy Chewable Tablets | | Brompheniramine Maleate 1mg | Phenylephrine HCl 2.5mg | | | **Peds ≥12 yrs:** 4 tabs q4h. **6-<12 yrs:** 2 tabs q4h. **Max:** 6 doses q24h. |
| Children's Dimetapp Cold & Allergy Syrup | | Brompheniramine Maleate 1mg/5mL | Phenylephrine HCl 2.5mg/5mL | | | **Adults & Peds ≥12 yrs:** 4 tsp (20mL) q4h. **Peds 6-<12 yrs:** 2 tsp (10mL) q4h. **Max:** 6 doses q24h. |
| Children's Dimetapp Nighttime Cold & Congestion Liquid | | Diphenhydramine HCl 6.25mg/5mL | Phenylephrine HCl 2.5mg/5mL | | | **Adults & Peds ≥12 yrs:** 4 tsp (20mL) q4h. **Peds 6-<12 yrs:** 2 tsp (10mL) q4h. **Max:** 6 doses q24h. |
| Pediacare Children's Allergy & Cold | | Diphenhydramine HCl 12.5mg/5mL | Phenylephrine HCl 5mg/5mL | | | **Peds 6-11 yrs:** 1 tsp (5mL) q4h. **Max:** 6 doses q24h. |
| Robitussin Night Time Cough & Cold | | Diphenhydramine HCl 6.25mg/5mL | Phenylephrine HCl 2.5mg/5mL | | | **Adults & Peds ≥12 yrs:** 4 tsp (20mL) q4h. **Max:** 6 doses q24h. |
| Sudafed PE Maximum Strength Sinus & Allergy Tablets | | Chlorpheniramine Maleate 4mg | Phenylephrine HCl 10mg | | | **Adults & Peds ≥12 yrs:** 1 tab q4h. **Max:** 6 tabs q24h. |
| Night Time Triaminic Thin Strips Cold & Cough | | Diphenhydramine HCl 12.5mg/strip | Phenylephrine HCl 5mg/strip | | | **Peds 6-12 yrs:** 1 strip q4h. **Max:** 6 strips q24h. |
| Triaminic Night Time Cold & Cough | | Diphenhydramine HCl 6.25mg/5mL | Phenylephrine HCl 2.5mg/5mL | | | **Peds 6-<12 yrs:** 2 tsp (10mL) q4h. **Max:** 6 doses q24h. |
| Triaminic Syrup Cold & Allergy | | Chlorpheniramine Maleate 1mg/5mL | Phenylephrine HCl 2.5mg/5mL | | | **Peds 6-<12 yrs:** 2 tsp (10mL) q4h. **Max:** 6 doses q24h. |
| **ANTIHISTAMINE + DECONGESTANT + ANALGESIC** | | | | | | |
| Advil Allergy Sinus Caplets | Ibuprofen 200mg | Chlorpheniramine Maleate 2mg | Pseudoephedrine HCl 30mg | | | **Adults & Peds ≥12 yrs:** 1 tab q4-6h. **Max:** 6 tabs q24h. |
| Alka-Seltzer Plus Cold Formula Effervescent Tablets | Aspirin 325mg | Chlorpheniramine Maleate 2mg | Phenylephrine Bitartrate 7.8mg | | | **Adults & Peds ≥12 yrs:** 2 tabs q4h. **Max:** 8 tabs q24h. |

*(Continued)*

# Table 15. COUGH-COLD-FLU (cont.)

| Brand Name | Analgesic | Antihistamine | Decongestant | Cough Suppressant | Expectorant | Dose |
|---|---|---|---|---|---|---|
| Alka-Seltzer Plus Fast Crystal Packs | Acetaminophen 650mg/packet | Chlorpheniramine Maleate 4mg/packet | Phenylephrine HCl 10mg/packet | | | **Adults & Peds ≥12 yrs:** 1 pkt q4h. **Max:** 6 pkts q24h. |
| Benadryl Severe Allergy Plus Cold Kapgels | Acetaminophen 325mg | Diphenhydramine HCl 12.5mg | Phenylephrine HCl 5mg | | | **Adults & Peds ≥12 yrs:** 2 caps q4h. **Max:** 12 caps q24h. |
| Benadryl Severe Allergy Plus Sinus Headache Caplets | Acetaminophen 325mg | Diphenhydramine HCl 25mg | Phenylephrine HCl 5mg | | | **Adults & Peds ≥12 yrs:** 2 tabs q4h. **Max:** 12 tabs q24h. |
| Benadryl Severe Allergy Plus Sinus Headache Kapgels | Acetaminophen 325mg | Diphenhydramine HCl 12.5mg | Phenylephrine HCl 5mg | | | **Adults & Peds ≥12 yrs:** 2 caps q4h. **Max:** 12 caps q24h. |
| Comtrex Severe Cold & Sinus Caplets | Acetaminophen 325mg | Chlorpheniramine Maleate 2mg | Phenylephrine HCl 5mg | | | **Adults & Peds ≥12 yrs:** 2 tabs q4h. **Max:** 12 tabs q24h. |
| Contac Cold Plus Flu | Acetaminophen 500mg | Chlorpheniramine Maleate 2mg | Phenylephrine HCl 5mg | | | **Adults & Peds ≥12 yrs:** 2 tabs q4-6h. **Max:** 8 tabs q24h. |
| Dristan Cold Multi-Symptom Formula Tablets | Acetaminophen 325mg | Chlorpheniramine Maleate 2mg | Phenylephrine HCl 5mg | | | **Adults & Peds ≥12 yrs:** 2 tabs q4h. **Max:** 12 tabs q24h. |
| Sudafed PE Severe Cold Formula Caplets | Acetaminophen 325mg | Diphenhydramine HCl 12.5mg | Phenylephrine HCl 5mg | | | **Adults & Peds ≥12 yrs:** 2 tabs q4h. **Peds 6-<12 yrs:** 1 tab q4h. **Max:** 5 tabs q24h. |
| Theraflu Cold & Sore Throat Hot Liquid | Acetaminophen 325mg/packet | Pheniramine Maleate 20mg/packet | Phenylephrine HCl 10mg/packet | | | **Adults & Peds ≥12 yrs:** 1 pkt q4h. **Max:** 6 pkts q24h. |
| Theraflu Nighttime Severe Cold & Cough Hot Liquid | Acetaminophen 650mg/packet | Diphenhydramine HCl 25mg/packet | Phenylephrine HCl 10mg/packet | | | **Adults & Peds ≥12 yrs:** 1 pkt q4h. **Max:** 6 pkts q24h. |
| Theraflu Sugar Free Nighttime Severe Cold & Cough Hot Liquid | Acetaminophen 650mg/packet | Diphenhydramine HCl 25mg/packet | Phenylephrine HCl 10mg/packet | | | **Adults & Peds ≥12 yrs:** 1 pkt q4h. **Max:** 6 pkts q24h. |
| Theraflu Flu & Sore Throat Hot Liquid | Acetaminophen 650mg/packet | Pheniramine Maleate 20mg/packet | Phenylephrine HCl 10mg/packet | | | **Adults & Peds ≥12 yrs:** 1 pkt q4h. **Max:** 6 pkts q24h. |
| Theraflu Warming Relief Nighttime Severe Cough & Cold | Acetaminophen 325mg/15mL | Diphenhydramine HCl 12.5mg/15mL | Phenylephrine HCl 5mg/15mL | | | **Adults & Peds ≥12 yrs:** 2 tbl (30mL) q4h. **Max:** 6 doses (12 tbl or 180mL) q24h. |
| Theraflu Warming Relief Flu & Sore Throat | Acetaminophen 325mg/15mL | Diphenhydramine HCl 12.5mg/15mL | Phenylephrine HCl 5mg/15mL | | | **Adults & Peds ≥12 yrs:** 2 tbl (30mL) q4h. **Max:** 6 doses (12 tbl or 180mL) q24h. |
| Children's Tylenol Plus Cold | Acetaminophen 160mg/5mL | Chlorpheniramine Maleate 1mg/5mL | Phenylephrine HCl 2.5mg/5mL | | | **Peds 6-11 yrs (48-95 lbs):** 2 tsp (10mL) q4h. **Max:** 5 doses q24h. |

## Table 15. COUGH-COLD-FLU (cont.)

| Brand Name | Analgesic | Antihistamine | Decongestant | Cough Suppressant | Expectorant | Dose |
|---|---|---|---|---|---|---|
| Children's Tylenol Plus Cold and Allergy | Acetaminophen 160mg/5mL | Diphenhydramine HCl 12.5mg/5mL | Phenylephrine HCl 2.5mg/5mL | | | **Peds 6-11 yrs (48-95 lbs):** 2 tsp (10mL) q4h. **Max:** 5 doses q24h. |
| Tylenol Allergy Multi-Symptom* | Acetaminophen 325mg | Chlorpheniramine Maleate 2mg | Phenylephrine HCl 5mg | | | **Adults & Peds ≥12 yrs:** 2 tabs q4h. **Max:** 12 tabs q24h. |
| Tylenol Allergy Multi-Symptom Nighttime* | Acetaminophen 325mg | Diphenhydramine HCl 25mg | Phenylephrine HCl 5mg | | | **Adults & Peds ≥12 yrs:** 2 tabs q4h. **Max:** 12 tabs q24h. |
| Tylenol Sinus Congestion & Pain Nighttime* | Acetaminophen 325mg | Chlorpheniramine Maleate 2mg | Phenylephrine HCl 5mg | | | **Adults & Peds ≥12 yrs:** 2 tabs q4h. **Max:** 12 tabs q24h. |
| Vicks NyQuil Sinex LiquiCaps | Acetaminophen 325mg | Doxylamine Succinate 6.25mg | Phenylephrine HCl 5mg | | | **Adults & Peds ≥12 yrs:** 2 caps q4h. **Max:** 4 doses q24h. |
| **COUGH SUPPRESSANT** | | | | | | |
| Children's Delsym Cough Medicine | | | | Dextromethorphan HBr 30mg/5mL | | **Adults & Peds ≥12 yrs:** 2 tsp (10mL) q12h. **Max:** 4 tsp (20mL) q24h. **Peds 6-<12 yrs:** 1 tsp (5mL) q12h. **Max:** 2 tsp (10mL) q24h. **Peds 4-<6 yrs:** ½ tsp (2.5mL) q12h. **Max:** 1 tsp (5mL) q24h. |
| Delsym Cough Medicine | | | | Dextromethorphan HBr 30mg/5mL | | **Adults & Peds ≥12 yrs:** 2 tsp (10mL) q12h. **Max:** 4 tsp (20mL) q24h. **Peds 6-<12 yrs:** 1 tsp (5mL) q12h. **Max:** 2 tsp (10mL) q24h. **Peds 4-<6 yrs:** ½ tsp (2.5mL) q12h. **Max:** 1 tsp (5mL) q24h. |
| Children's Robitussin Cough Long-Acting | | | | Dextromethorphan HBr 7.5mg/5mL | | **Adults & Peds ≥12 yrs:** 4 tsp (20mL) q6-8h. **Peds 6-<12 yrs:** 2 tsp (10mL) q6-8h. **Peds 4-<6 yrs:** 1 tsp (5mL) q6-8h. **Max:** 4 doses q24h. |
| Robitussin Cough Long-Acting | | | | Dextromethorphan HBr 15mg/5mL | | **Adults & Peds ≥12 yrs:** 2 tsp (10mL) q6-8h. **Max:** 4 doses q24h. |
| Robitussin CoughGels | | | | Dextromethorphan HBr 15mg | | **Adults & Peds ≥12 yrs:** 2 caps q6-8h. **Max:** 8 caps q24h. |
| Triaminic Long-Acting Cough | | | | Dextromethorphan HBr 7.5mg/5mL | | **Peds 6-<12 yrs:** 2 tsp (10mL) q6-8h. **Peds 4-<6 yrs:** 1 tsp (5mL) q6-8h. **Max:** 4 doses q24h. |
| Triaminic Thin Strips Long-Acting Cough | | | | Dextromethorphan HBr 7.5mg/strip | | **Peds 6-<12 yrs:** 2 strips q6-8h. **Peds 4-<6 yrs:** 1 strip q6-8h. **Max:** 4 doses q24h. |

*(Continued)*

## Table 15. COUGH-COLD-FLU (cont.)

| Brand Name | Analgesic | Antihistamine | Decongestant | Cough Suppressant | Expectorant | Dose |
|---|---|---|---|---|---|---|
| Vicks DayQuil Cough | | | | Dextromethorphan HBr 15mg/15mL | | **Adults & Peds ≥12 yrs:** 2 tbl (30mL) q6-8h. **Peds 6-12 yrs:** 1 tbl (15mL) q6-8h. **Max:** 4 doses q24h. |
| Vicks Formula 44 Custom Care Dry Cough Suppressant | | | | Dextromethorphan HBr 30mg/15mL | | **Adults & Peds ≥12 yrs:** 1 tbl (15mL) q6-8h. **Peds 6-<12 yrs:** 1½ tsp (7.5mL) q6-8h. **Max:** 4 doses q24h. |
| Vicks BabyRub | | | | Petrolatum, fragrance, aloe extract, eucalyptus oil, lavender oil, rosemary oil | | **Peds:** Gently massage on the chest, neck, and back to help soothe and comfort. |
| Vicks VapoRub Topical Cream | | | | Camphor 5.2%, Menthol 2.8%, Eucalyptus 1.2% | | **Adults & Peds ≥2 yrs:** Apply to chest and throat. **Max:** tid per 24h. |
| Vicks VapoRub Topical Ointment | | | | Camphor 4.8%, Menthol 2.6%, Eucalyptus 1.2% | | **Adults & Peds ≥2 yrs:** Apply to chest and throat. **Max:** tid per 24h. |
| Vicks VapoSteam | | | | Camphor 6.2% | | **Adults & Peds ≥2 yrs:** 1 tbl/quart q8h or 1½ tsp/pint q8h (for use in a hot steam vaporizer). **Max:** tid per 24h. |
| Vicks Vapodrops | | | | Menthol 1.7mg (cherry), Menthol 3.3mg (menthol) | | **Peds ≥5 years:** 3 drops (cherry). **Peds >5 years:** 2 drops (menthol). |
| **COUGH SUPPRESSANT + ANTIHISTAMINE** | | | | | | |
| Coricidin HBP Cough & Cold | | Chlorpheniramine Maleate 4mg | | Dextromethorphan HBr 30mg | | **Adults & Peds ≥12 yrs:** 1 tab q6h. **Max:** 4 tabs q24h. |
| Children's Dimetapp Long-Acting Cough Plus Cold | | Chlorpheniramine Maleate 1mg/5mL | | Dextromethorphan HBr 7.5mg/5mL | | **Adults & Peds ≥12 yrs:** 4 tsp (20mL) q6h. **6-<12 yrs:** 2 tsp (10mL) q6h. **Max:** 4 doses q24h. |
| Children's Robitussin Cough & Cold Long-Acting | | Chlorpheniramine Maleate 1mg/5mL | | Dextromethorphan HBr 7.5mg/5mL | | **Adults & Peds ≥12 yrs:** 4 tsp (20mL) q6h. **Peds 6-<12 yrs:** 2 tsp (10mL) q6h. **Max:** 4 doses q24h. |
| Robitussin Cough & Cold Long-Acting | | Chlorpheniramine Maleate 2mg/5mL | | Dextromethorphan HBr 15mg/5mL | | **Adults & Peds ≥12 yrs:** 2 tsp (10mL) q6h. **Max:** 4 doses q24h. |
| Triaminic Softchews Cough and Runny Nose | | Chlorpheniramine Maleate 1mg | | Dextromethorphan HBr 5mg | | **Peds 6-<12 yrs:** 2 tabs q4-6h. **Max:** 5 doses q24h. |
| Vicks Children's NyQuil | | Chlorpheniramine Maleate 2mg/15mL | | Dextromethorphan HBr 15mg/15mL | | **Adults & Peds ≥12 yrs:** 2 tbl (30mL) q6h. **Peds 6-11 yrs:** 1 tbl (15mL) q6h. **Max:** 4 doses q24h. |

## Table 15. COUGH-COLD-FLU (cont.)

| Brand Name | Analgesic | Antihistamine | Decongestant | Cough Suppressant | Expectorant | Dose |
|---|---|---|---|---|---|---|
| Vicks NyQuil Cough | | Doxylamine Succinate 6.25mg/15mL | | Dextromethorphan HBr 15mg/15mL | | **Adults & Peds ≥12 yrs:** 2 tbl (30mL) q6h. **Max:** 4 doses q24h. |
| **COUGH SUPPRESSANT + ANALGESIC** | | | | | | |
| Pediacare Children's Fever Reducer Plus Cough and Sore Throat with APAP | Acetaminophen 160mg/5mL | | | Dextromethorphan 5mg/5mL | | **6-11 yrs (48-95 lbs):** 2 tsp (10ml) q4h. **Max:** 5 times in 24 hrs. |
| Triaminic Cough & Sore Throat | Acetaminophen 160mg/5mL | | | Dextromethorphan HBr 5mg/5mL | | **Peds 6-<12 yrs:** 2 tsp (10mL) q4h. **Peds 4-<6 yrs:** 1 tsp (5mL) q4h. **Max:** 5 doses q24h. |
| Children's Tylenol Plus Cough and Sore Throat | Acetaminophen 160mg/5mL | | | Dextromethorphan HBr 5mg/5mL | | **Peds 6-11 yrs (48-95 lbs):** 2 tsp (10mL) q4h. **Peds 4-5 yrs (36-47 lbs):** 1 tsp (5mL) q4h. **Max:** 5 doses q24h. |
| Tylenol Cough & Sore Throat Daytime* | Acetaminophen 1000mg/30mL | | | Dextromethorphan HBr 30mg/30mL | | **Adults & Peds ≥12 yrs:** 2 tbl (30mL) q6h. **Max:** 8 tbl q24h. |
| **COUGH SUPPRESSANT + ANTIHISTAMINE + ANALGESIC** | | | | | | |
| Alka-Seltzer Plus Flu Formula Effervescent Tablets | Aspirin 500mg | Chlorpheniramine Maleate 2mg | | Dextromethorphan HBr 15mg | | **Adults & Peds ≥12 yrs:** 2 tabs q6h. **Max:** 8 tabs q24h. |
| Coricidin HBP Day & Night Multi-Symptom Cold | Acetaminophen 500mg (nighttime dose only) | Chlorpheniramine Maleate 2mg (nighttime dose only) | | Dextromethorphan HBr 10mg (daytime dose), 15mg (nighttime dose) | Guaifenesin 200 mg (daytime dose only) | **Adults & Peds ≥12 yrs:** 2 tabs hs and q6h prn. **Max:** 4 tabs q12h. |
| Coricidin HBP Maximum Strength Flu | Acetaminophen 500mg | Chlorpheniramine Maleate 2mg | | Dextromethorphan HBr 15mg | | **Adults & Peds ≥12 yrs:** 2 tabs q6h. **Max:** 8 tabs q24h. |
| Coricidin HBP Nighttime Multi-Symptom Cold Relief Liquid | Acetaminophen 500mg/15mL | Doxylamine 6.25mg/15mL | | Dextromethorphan HBr 15mg/15mL | | **Adults & Peds ≥12 yrs:** 2 tbl (30mL) q6h. **Max:** 4 doses q24h. |
| Pediacare Children's Fever Reducer Plus Cough and Runny Nose with Acetaminophen | Acetaminophen 160mg/5mL | Chlorpheniramine Maleate 1mg/5mL | | Dextromethorphan HBr 5mg/5mL | | **6-11 yrs (48-95 lbs):** 2 tsp (10ml) q4h. **Max:** 5 times in 24 hrs. |
| Triaminic Multisymptom Fever | Acetaminophen 160mg/5mL | Chlorpheniramine Maleate 1mg/5mL | | Dextromethorphan HBr 7.5mg/5mL | | **Peds 6-<12 yrs:** 2 tsp (10mL) q6h. **Max:** 4 doses q24h. |
| Children's Tylenol Plus Cough & Runny Nose | Acetaminophen 160mg/5mL | Chlorpheniramine Maleate 1mg/5mL | | Dextromethorphan HBr 5mg/5mL | | **Peds 6-11 yrs (48-95 lbs):** 2 tsp (10mL) q4h. **Max:** 5 doses q24h. |
| Tylenol Cold and Cough Nighttime Liquid Burst | Acetaminophen 500mg/15mL | Doxylamine 6.25mg/15mL | | Dextromethorphan HBr 15mg/15mL | | **Adults & Peds ≥12 yrs:** 2 tbl (30mL) q6h. **Max:** 8 tbl q24h. |

(Continued)

## Table 15. COUGH-COLD-FLU (cont.)

| Brand Name | Analgesic | Antihistamine | Decongestant | Cough Suppressant | Expectorant | Dose |
|---|---|---|---|---|---|---|
| Vicks Formula 44 Custom Care Cough & Cold PM | Acetaminophen 650mg/15mL | Chlorpheniramine Maleate 4mg/15mL | | Dextromethorphan HBr 30mg/15mL | | **Adults & Peds** ≥**12 yrs:** 1 tbl q6h. **Max:** 4 doses q24h. |
| Vicks NyQuil Cold & Flu Relief Liquid | Acetaminophen 500mg/15mL | Doxylamine Succinate 6.25mg/15mL | | Dextromethorphan HBr 15mg/15mL | | **Adults & Peds** ≥**12 yrs:** 2 tbl (30mL) q6h. **Max:** 4 doses q24h. |
| Vicks NyQuil Cold & Flu Relief LiquiCaps | Acetaminophen 325mg | Doxylamine Succinate 6.25mg | | Dextromethorphan HBr 15mg | | **Adults & Peds** ≥**12 yrs:** 2 caps q6h. **Max:** 4 doses q24h. |
| Vicks NyQuil Cold & Flu Symptom Relief Plus Vitamin C | Acetaminophen 325mg | Doxylamine Succinate 6.25mg | | Dextromethorphan HBr 15mg | | **Adults & Peds** ≥**12 yrs:** 2 caps q6h. **Max:** 4 doses q24h. |
| Alcohol Free NyQuil, Cold and Flu Relief Liquid | Acetaminophen 325mg/15mL | Chlorpheniramine Maleate 2mg/15mL | | Dextromethorphan 15mg/15mL | | **Adults & Peds** ≥**12 yrs:** 2 tbl (30mL) q6h. **Max:** 4 doses q24h. |
| **COUGH SUPPRESSANT + ANTIHISTAMINE + ANALGESIC + DECONGESTANT** | | | | | | |
| Alka-Seltzer Plus Cold & Cough Formula Effervescent Tablets | Aspirin 325mg | Chlorpheniramine Maleate 2mg | Phenylephrine Bitartrate 7.8mg | Dextromethorphan HBr 10mg | | **Adults & Peds** ≥**12 yrs:** 2 tabs q4h. **Max:** 8 tabs q24h. |
| Alka-Seltzer Plus Cold & Cough Formula Liquid Gels | Acetaminophen 325mg | Chlorpheniramine Maleate 2mg | Phenylephrine HCl 5mg | Dextromethorphan HBr 10mg | | **Adults & Peds** ≥**12 yrs:** 2 caps q4h. **Max:** 12 caps q24h. |
| Alka-Seltzer Plus Night Cold Formula Effervescent Tablets | Aspirin 500mg | Doxylamine Succinate 6.25mg | Phenylephrine Bitartrate 7.8mg | Dextromethorphan HBr 10mg | | **Adults & Peds** ≥**12 yrs:** 2 tabs q4-6h. **Max:** 8 tabs q24h. |
| Alka-Seltzer Plus Night Cold Formula Liquid Gels | Acetaminophen 325mg | Doxylamine Succinate 6.25mg | Phenylephrine HCl 5mg | Dextromethorphan HBr 10mg | | **Adults & Peds** ≥**12 yrs:** 2 caps q4h. **Max:** 12 caps q24h. |
| Comtrex Nighttime Cough & Cold Caplets | Acetaminophen 325mg | Chlorpheniramine Maleate 2mg | Phenylephrine HCl 5mg | Dextromethorphan HBr 10mg | | **Adults & Peds** ≥**12 yrs:** 2 tabs q4h. **Max:** 12 tabs q24h. |
| Robitussin Night Time Cough, Cold & Flu | Acetaminophen 160mg/5mL | Chlorpheniramine Maleate 1mg/5mL | Phenylephrine HCl 2.5mg/5mL | Dextromethorphan HBr 5mg/5mL | | **Adults & Peds** ≥**12 yrs:** 4 tsp (20mL) q4h. **Max:** 6 doses q24h. |
| Theraflu Nighttime Severe Cold & Cough Caplets | Acetaminophen 325mg | Chlorpheniramine Maleate 2mg | Phenylephrine HCl 5mg | Dextromethorphan HBr 10mg | | **Adults & Peds** ≥**12 yrs:** 2 tabs q4h. **Max:** 12 tabs q24h. |
| Children's Tylenol Plus Multi-Symptom Cold | Acetaminophen 160mg/5mL | Chlorpheniramine Maleate 1mg/5mL | Phenylephrine HCl 2.5mg/5mL | Dextromethorphan HBr 5mg/5mL | | **Peds 6-11 yrs (48-95 lbs):** 2 tsp (10mL) q4h. **Max:** 5 doses q24h. |
| Tylenol Cold Head Congestion Nighttime | Acetaminophen 325mg | Chlorpheniramine Maleate 2mg | Phenylephrine HCl 5mg | Dextromethorphan HBr 10mg | | **Adults & Peds** ≥**12 yrs:** 2 tabs q4h. **Max:** 12 tabs q24h. |
| Tylenol Cold Multi-Symptom Nighttime Gelcaps | Acetaminophen 325mg | Chlorpheniramine Maleate 2mg | Phenylephrine HCl 5mg | Dextromethorphan HBr 10mg | | **Adults & Peds** ≥**12 yrs:** 2 tabs q4h. **Max:** 12 tabs q24h. |
| Tylenol Cold Multi-Symptom Nighttime Liquid | Acetaminophen 325mg/15mL | Doxylamine Succinate 6.25mg/30mL | Phenylephrine HCl 5mg/15mL | Dextromethorphan HBr 10mg/15mL | | **Adults & Peds** ≥**12 yrs:** 2 tbl (30mL) q4h. **Max:** 12 tbl (180mL) q24h. |

## Table 15. COUGH-COLD-FLU (cont.)

| Brand Name | Analgesic | Antihistamine | Decongestant | Cough Suppressant | Expectorant | Dose |
|---|---|---|---|---|---|---|
| Vicks NyQuil D | Acetaminophen 500mg/15mL | Doxylamine Succinate 6.25mg/15mL | Pseudoephedrine HCl 30mg/15mL | Dextromethorphan HBr 15mg/15mL | | **Adults & Peds ≥12 yrs:** 2 tbl (30mL) q6h. **Max:** 4 doses q24h. |
| **COUGH SUPPRESSANT + ANTIHISTAMINE + DECONGESTANT** | | | | | | |
| Children's Dimetapp Cold & Cough | | Brompheniramine Maleate 1mg/5mL | Phenylephrine HCl 2.5mg/5mL | Dextromethorphan HBr 5mg/5mL | | **Adults & Peds ≥12 yrs:** 4 tsp (20mL) q4h. **Peds 6–<12 yrs:** 2 tsp (10mL) q4h. **Max:** 6 doses q24h. |
| Theraflu Cold & Cough Hot Liquid | | Pheniramine Maleate 20mg/packet | Phenylephrine HCl 10mg/packet | Dextromethorphan HBr 20mg/packet | | **Adults & Peds ≥12 yrs:** 1 pkt q4h. **Max:** 6 pkts q24h. |
| Triaminic-D Multi-Symptom Cold | | Chlorpheniramine Maleate 1mg/5mL | Pseudoephedrine HCl 15mg/5mL | Dextromethorphan HBr 7.5mg/5mL | | **Peds 6–<12 yrs:** 2 tsp q6h. **Max:** 4 doses q24h. |
| **COUGH SUPPRESSANT + DECONGESTANT** | | | | | | |
| PediaCare Children's Multi-Symptom Cold | | | Phenylephrine HCl 2.5mg/5mL | Dextromethorphan HBr 5mg/5mL | | **Peds 6-11 yrs:** 2 tsp (10mL) q4h. **Peds 4-5 yrs:** 1 tsp (5mL) q4h. **Max:** 6 doses q24h. |
| Children's Sudafed PE Cold & Cough Liquid | | | Phenylephrine HCl 2.5mg/5mL | Dextromethorphan HBr 5mg/5mL | | **Peds 6-11 yrs:** 2 tsp (10mL) q4h. **Peds 4-5 yrs:** 1 tsp (5mL) q4h. **Max:** 6 doses q24h. |
| Day Time Triaminic Thin Strips Cold & Cough | | | Phenylephrine HCl 2.5mg/strip | Dextromethorphan HBr 5mg/strip | | **Peds 6–<12 yrs:** 2 strips q4h. **Peds 4–<6 yrs:** 1 strip q4h. **Max:** 6 doses q24h. |
| Triaminic Day Time Cold & Cough | | | Phenylephrine HCl 2.5mg/5mL | Dextromethorphan HBr 5mg/5mL | | **Peds 6–<12 yrs:** 2 tsp (10mL) q4h. **Peds 4–<6 yrs:** 1 tsp (5mL) q4h. **Max:** 6 doses q24h. |
| Vicks Formula 44 Custom Care Congestion | | | Phenylephrine HCl 10mg/15mL | Dextromethorphan HBr 20mg/15mL | | **Adults & Peds ≥12 yrs:** 1 tbl (15mL) q4h. **Peds 6–<12 yrs:** 1½ tsp (7.5mL) q4h. **Max:** 6 doses q24h. |
| **COUGH SUPPRESSANT + DECONGESTANT + ANALGESIC** | | | | | | |
| Alka-Seltzer Plus Day Non-Drowsy Cold Formula Liquid Gels | Acetaminophen 325mg | | Phenylephrine HCl 5mg | Dextromethorphan HBr 10mg | | **Adults & Peds ≥12 yrs:** 2 caps q4h. **Max:** 12 caps q24h. |
| Alka-Seltzer Plus Day & Night Cold Formula Liquid Gels | Acetaminophen 325mg | Doxylamine 6.25mg (nighttime dose only) | Phenylephrine HCl 5mg | Dextromethorphan HBr 10mg | | **Adults & Peds ≥12 yrs:** 2 caps q4h. **Max:** 12 caps q24h. |
| Alka-Seltzer Plus Day & Night Cold Formula Effervescent Tablets | Aspirin 325mg | Doxylamine 6.25mg (nighttime dose only) | Phenylephrine Bitartrate 7.8mg | Dextromethorphan HBr 10mg | | **Adults & Peds ≥12 yrs:** 2 tabs q4h. **Max:** 8 tabs q24h. |

*(Continued)*

## Table 15. COUGH-COLD-FLU (cont.)

| Brand Name | Analgesic | Antihistamine | Decongestant | Cough Suppressant | Expectorant | Dose |
|---|---|---|---|---|---|---|
| Theraflu Daytime Severe Cold & Cough Caplets | Acetaminophen 325mg | | Phenylephrine HCl 5mg | Dextromethorphan HBr 10mg | | **Adults & Peds ≥12 yrs:** 2 tabs q4h. **Max:** 12 tabs q24h. |
| Theraflu Daytime Severe Cold & Cough Hot Liquid | Acetaminophen 650mg/packet | | Phenylephrine HCl 10mg/packet | Dextromethorphan HBr 20mg/packet | | **Adults & Peds ≥12 yrs:** 1 pkt q4h. **Max:** 6 pkts q24h. |
| Theraflu Warming Relief Daytime Severe Cough & Cold | Acetaminophen 325mg/15mL | | Phenylephrine HCl 5mg/15mL | Dextromethorphan HBr 10mg/15mL | | **Adults & Peds ≥12 yrs:** 2 tbl (30mL) q4h. **Max:** 6 doses q24h. |
| Children's Tylenol Plus Cold & Cough | Acetaminophen 160mg/5mL | | Phenylephrine HCl 2.5mg/5mL | Dextromethorphan HBr 5mg/5mL | | **Peds 6-11 yrs (48-95 lbs):** 2 tsp (10mL) q4h. **Peds 4-5 yrs (36-47 lbs):** 1 tsp (5mL) q4h. **Max:** 5 doses q24h. |
| Tylenol Cold Head Congestion Daytime | Acetaminophen 325mg | | Phenylephrine HCl 5mg | Dextromethorphan HBr 10mg | | **Adults & Peds ≥12 yrs:** 2 caps q4h. **Max:** 12 caps q24h. |
| Tylenol Cold Multi-Symptom Daytime Gelcaps/Caplets | Acetaminophen 325mg | | Phenylephrine HCl 5mg | Dextromethorphan HBr 10mg | | **Adults & Peds ≥12 yrs:** 2 caps q4h. **Max:** 12 caps q24h. |
| Tylenol Cold Multi-Symptom Daytime Liquid | Acetaminophen 325mg/15mL | | Phenylephrine HCl 5mg/15mL | Dextromethorphan HBr 10mg/15mL | | **Adults & Peds ≥12 yrs:** 2 tbl (30mL) q4h. **Max:** 12 tbl (180mL) q24h. |
| Vicks DayQuil Cold & Flu Relief LiquiCaps | Acetaminophen 325mg | | Phenylephrine HCl 5mg | Dextromethorphan HBr 10mg | | **Adults & Peds ≥12 yrs:** 2 doses q4h. **Max:** 6 doses q24h. |
| Vicks DayQuil Cold & Flu Relief Liquid | Acetaminophen 325mg/15mL | | Phenylephrine HCl 5mg/15mL | Dextromethorphan HBr 10mg/15mL | | **Adults & Peds ≥12 yrs:** 2 tbl (30 mL) q4h. **Max:** 6 doses q24h. **Peds 6-<12 yrs:** 1 tbl (15mL) q4h. **Max:** 5 doses q24h. |
| Vicks DayQuil Cold & Flu Symptom Relief Plus Vitamin C | Acetaminophen 325mg | | Phenylephrine HCl 5mg | Dextromethorphan HBr 15mg | | **Adults & Peds ≥12 yrs:** 2 caps q4h. **Max:** 6 doses q24h. |
| **COUGH SUPPRESSANT + DECONGESTANT + EXPECTORANT** | | | | | | |
| Children's Robitussin Cough & Cold CF | | | Phenylephrine HCl 2.5mg/5mL | Dextromethorphan HBr 5mg/5mL | Guaifenesin 50mg/5mL | **Adults & Peds ≥12 yrs:** 4 tsp (20mL) q4h. **Peds 6-<12 yrs:** 2 tsp (10mL) q4h. **Peds 4-<6 yrs:** 1 tsp (5mL) q4h. **Max:** 6 doses q24h. |
| Robitussin Cough & Cold CF | | | Phenylephrine HCl 5mg/5mL | Dextromethorphan HBr 10mg/5mL | Guaifenesin 100mg/5mL | **Adults & Peds ≥12 yrs:** 2 tsp (10mL) q4h. **Max:** 6 doses q24h. |
| Children's Mucinex, Multi-Symptom Cold Liquid (Very Berry Flavor) | | | Phenylephrine 2.5mg | Dextromethorphan 5mg | Guaifenesin 100mg | **Peds 6-<12 yrs:** 10mL q4h. **Peds 4-6 yrs:** 5mL q4h. |

## Table 15. COUGH-COLD-FLU (cont.)

| Brand Name | Analgesic | Antihistamine | Decongestant | Cough Suppressant | Expectorant | Dose |
|---|---|---|---|---|---|---|
| Robitussin To Go Cough & Cold CF | | | Phenylephrine HCl 10mg/10mL | Dextromethorphan HBr 20mg/10mL | Guaifenesin 200mg/10mL | **Adults & Peds ≥12 yrs:** 1 pre-filled spoon (10 mL) q4h. **Max:** 6 doses q24h. |
| **COUGH SUPPRESSANT + DECONGESTANT + EXPECTORANT + ANALGESIC** | | | | | | |
| Sudafed PE Cold & Cough Caplets | Acetaminophen 325mg | | Phenylephrine HCl 5mg | Dextromethorphan HBr 10mg | Guaifenesin 100mg | **Adults & Peds ≥12 yrs:** 2 tabs q4h. **Max:** 12 tabs q24h. |
| Tylenol Cold Multi-Symptom Severe Liquid | Acetaminophen 325mg/15mL | | Phenylephrine HCl 5mg/15mL | Dextromethorphan HBr 10mg/15mL | Guaifenesin 200mg/15mL | **Adults & Peds ≥12 yrs:** 2 tb (30mL) q4h. **Max:** 12 tbl (180mL) q24h. |
| Tylenol Cold Severe Head Congestion | Acetaminophen 325mg | | Phenylephrine HCl 5mg | Dextromethorphan HBr 10mg | Guaifenesin 200mg | **Adults & Peds ≥12 yrs:** 2 tabs q4h. **Max:** 12 tabs q24h. |
| **COUGH SUPPRESSANT + EXPECTORANT** | | | | | | |
| Alka-Seltzer Plus Mucus & Congestion Liquid Gels | | | | Dextromethorphan HBr 10mg | Guaifenesin 200mg | **Adults & Peds ≥12 yrs:** 2 caps q4h. **Max:** 12 caps q24h. |
| Coricidin HBP Chest Congestion & Cough | | | | Dextromethorphan HBr 10mg | Guaifenesin 200mg | **Adults & Peds ≥12 yrs:** 1-2 caps q4h. **Max:** 12 caps q24h. |
| Maximum Strength Mucinex DM | | | | Dextromethorphan HBr 60mg | Guaifenesin 1200mg | **Adults & Peds ≥12 yrs:** 1 tab q12h. **Max:** 2 tabs q24h. |
| Mucinex Cough Liquid (Cherry Flavor) | | | | Dextromethorphan HBr 5mg/5mL | Guaifenesin 100mg/5mL | **Peds 6-<12 yrs:** 1-2 tsp (5-10mL) q4h. **Peds 4-<6yrs:** ½-1 tsp (2.5-5mL) q4h. **Max:** 6 doses q24h. |
| Mucinex Cough Mini-Melts (Orange Crème Flavor) | | | | Dextromethorphan HBr 5mg | Guaifenesin 100mg | **Adults & Peds ≥12 yrs:** 2-4 pkts q4h. **Peds 6-<12 yrs:** 1-2 pkts q4h. **Peds 4-<6yrs:** 1 pkt q4h. **Max:** 6 doses q24h. |
| Mucinex DM | | | | Dextromethorphan HBr 30mg | Guaifenesin 600mg | **Adults & Peds ≥12 yrs:** 1-2 tabs q12h. **Max:** 4 tabs q24h. |
| Robitussin Cough & Chest Congestion DM Max | | | | Dextromethorphan HBr 10mg/5mL | Guaifenesin 200mg/5mL | **Adults & Peds ≥12 yrs:** 2 tsp (10mL) q4h. **Max:** 6 doses q24h. |
| Robitussin Cough & Chest Congestion DM | | | | Dextromethorphan HBr 10mg/5mL | Guaifenesin 100mg/5mL | **Adults & Peds ≥12 yrs:** 2 tsp (10mL) q4h. **Max:** 6 doses q24h. |
| Robitussin Cough & Chest Congestion Sugar-Free DM | | | | Dextromethorphan HBr 10mg/5mL | Guaifenesin 100mg/5mL | **Adults & Peds ≥12 yrs:** 2 tsp (10mL) q4h. **Max:** 6 doses q24h. |
| Robitussin To Go Cough & Chest Congestion DM | | | | Dextromethorphan HBr 20mg/10mL | Guaifenesin 200mg/10mL | **Adults & Peds ≥12 yrs:** 1 pre-filled spoon (10mL) q4h. **Max:** 6 doses q24h. |

*(Continued)*

## Table 15. COUGH-COLD-FLU (cont.)

| Brand Name | Analgesic | Antihistamine | Decongestant | Cough Suppressant | Expectorant | Dose |
|---|---|---|---|---|---|---|
| Vicks DayQuil Mucus Control DM | | | | Dextromethorphan HBr 10mg/15mL | Guaifenesin 200mg/15mL | **Adults & Peds ≥12 yrs:** 2 tbl (30mL) q4h. **Peds 6-12 yrs:** 1 tbl (15mL) q4h. **Max:** 6 doses q24h. |
| Vicks Formula 44 Custom Care Chesty Cough | | | | Dextromethorphan HBr 20mg/15mL | Guaifenesin 200mg/15mL | **Adults & Peds ≥12 yrs:** 1 tbl (15mL) q4h. **Peds 6-<12 yrs:** 1½ tsp (7.5mL) q4h. **Max:** 6 doses q24h. |
| **DECONGESTANT** | | | | | | |
| Contac-D Cold Decongestant Tablets | | | Phenylephrine HCl 10mg | | | **Adults & Peds ≥12 yrs:** 1 tab q4h. **Max:** 6 tabs q24h. |
| Mucinex Moisture Smart Nasal Spray | | | Oxymetazoline HCl 0.05% | | | **Adults & Peds ≥12 yrs:** 2-3 sprays in each nostril q10-12h. **Max:** 2 doses q24h. |
| Mucinex Full Force Nasal Spray | | | Oxymetazoline HCl 0.05% | | | **Adults & Peds ≥12 yrs:** 2-3 sprays in each nostril q10-12h. **Max:** 2 doses q24h. |
| PediaCare Children's Decongestant | | | Phenylephrine HCl 2.5mg/5mL | | | **Peds 6-11 yrs:** 2 tsp (10mL) q4h. **Peds 4-5 yrs:** 1 tsp (5mL) q4h. **Max:** 6 doses q24h. |
| Children's Sudafed Nasal Decongestant Liquid | | | Pseudoephedrine HCl 15mg/5mL | | | **Peds 6-11 yrs:** 2 tsp (10mL) q4-6h. **Peds 4-5 yrs:** 1 tsp (5mL) q4-6h. **Max:** 4 doses q24h. |
| Children's Sudafed PE Nasal Decongestant Liquid | | | Phenylephrine HCl 2.5mg/5mL | | | **Peds 6-11 yrs:** 2 tsp (10mL) q4h. **Peds 4-5 yrs:** 1 tsp (5mL) q4h. **Max:** 6 doses q24h. |
| Sudafed 12-Hour Tablets | | | Pseudoephedrine HCl 120mg | | | **Adults & Peds ≥12 yrs:** 1 tab q12h. **Max:** 2 tabs q24h. |
| Sudafed 24-Hour Tablets | | | Pseudoephedrine HCl 240mg | | | **Adults & Peds ≥12 yrs:** 1 tab q24h. **Max:** 1 tab q24h. |
| Sudafed Nasal Decongestant Tablets | | | Pseudoephedrine HCl 30mg | | | **Adults ≥12 yrs:** 2 tabs q4-6h. **Max:** 8 tabs q24h. **Peds 6-12 yrs:** 1 tab q4-6h. **Max:** 4 tabs q24h. |
| Sudafed OM Sinus Congestion Spray | | | Oxymetazoline HCl 0.05% | | | **Adults & Peds ≥6 yrs:** 2-3 sprays in each nostril q10-12h. **Max:** 2 doses q24h. |
| Sudafed PE Nasal Decongestant Tablets | | | Phenylephrine HCl 10mg | | | **Adults & Peds ≥12 yrs:** 1 tab q4h. **Max:** 6 tabs q24h. |

## Table 15. COUGH-COLD-FLU (cont.)

| Brand Name | Antihistamine | Analgesic | Decongestant | Cough Suppressant | Expectorant | Dose |
|---|---|---|---|---|---|---|
| Triaminic Thin Strips Cold with Stuffy Nose | | | Phenylephrine HCl 2.5mg/strip | | | **Peds 6-<12 yrs:** 2 strips q4h. **Peds 4-<6 yrs:** 1 strip q4h. **Max:** 6 doses q24h. |
| Vicks Sinex VapoSpray 4-Hour* | | | Phenylephrine HCl 0.5% | | | **Adults & Peds ≥12 yrs:** Instill 2-3 sprays per nostril q4h. |
| Vicks Sinex VapoSpray 12-Hour Decongestant Nasal Spray | | | Oxymetazoline HCl 0.05% | | | **Adults & Peds ≥6 yrs:** Instill 2-3 sprays per nostril q10-12h. **Max:** 2 doses q24h. |
| Vicks Sinex VapoSpray 12-Hour Decongestant UltraFine Mist | | | Oxymetazoline HCl 0.05% | | | **Adults & Peds ≥6 yrs:** Instill 2-3 sprays per nostril q10-12h. **Max:** 2 doses q24h. |
| Vicks VapoInhaler | | | Levmetamfetamine 50mg | | | **Adults & Peds ≥12 yrs:** 2 inhalations q2h. **Max:** 24 inhalations q24h. **Peds 6-<12 yrs:** 1 inhalation q2h. |
| **DECONGESTANT + ANALGESIC** | | | | | | |
| Children's Advil Cold Suspension | | Ibuprofen 100mg/5mL | Pseudoephedrine HCl 15mg/5mL | | | **Peds 6-11 yrs (48-95 lbs):** 2 tsp (10mL) q6h. **2-5 yrs (24-47 lbs):** 1 tsp (5mL) q6h. **Max:** 4 doses q24h. |
| Advil Cold & Sinus Caplets/Liqui-Gels | | Ibuprofen 200mg | Pseudoephedrine HCl 30mg | | | **Adults & Peds ≥12 yrs:** 1-2 caps q4-6h. **Max:** 6 caps q24h. |
| Alka-Seltzer Plus Sinus Formula Effervescent Tablets | | Aspirin 325mg | Phenylephrine Bitartrate 7.8mg | | | **Adults & Peds ≥12 yrs:** 2 tabs q4h. **Max:** 8 tabs q24h. |
| Contac Cold Plus Flu | | Acetaminophen 500mg | Phenylephrine HCl 5mg | | | **Adults & Peds ≥12 yrs:** 2 tabs q4-6h. **Max:** 8 tabs q24h. |
| Children's Motrin Cold* | | Ibuprofen 100mg/5mL | Pseudoephedrine HCl 15mg/5m_ | | | **Peds 6-11 yrs (48-95 lbs):** 2 tsp (10mL) q6h. **2-5 yrs (24-47 lbs):** 1 tsp (5mL) q6h. **Max:** 4 doses q24h. |
| Sinutab Sinus Caplets | | Acetaminophen 325mg | Phenylephrine HCl 5mg | | | **Adults & Peds ≥12 yrs:** 2 tabs q4h. **Max:** 12 tabs q24h. |
| Sudafed PE Sinus Headache Caplets | | Acetaminophen 325mg | Phenylephrine HCl 5mg | | | **Adults & Peds ≥12 yrs:** 2 tabs q4h. **Max:** 12 tabs q24h. |
| Sudafed Sinus Pain 12 Hour Caplets | | Naproxen Sodium 220mg | Pseudoephedrine HCl 120mg | | | **Adults & Peds ≥12 yrs:** 1 tab q12h. **Max:** 2 tabs q24h. |

*(Continued)*

## Table 15. COUGH-COLD-FLU (cont.)

| Brand Name | Analgesic | Antihistamine | Decongestant | Cough Suppressant | Expectorant | Dose |
|---|---|---|---|---|---|---|
| Children's Tylenol Plus Cold & Stuffy Nose | Acetaminophen 160mg/5mL | | Phenylephrine HCl 2.5mg/5mL | | | **Peds 6-11 yrs (48-95 lbs):** 2 tsp (10mL) q4h. **Peds 4-5 yrs (36-47 lbs):** 1 tsp (5mL) q4h. **Max:** 5 doses q24h. |
| Tylenol Sinus Congestion & Pain Daytime | Acetaminophen 325mg | | Phenylephrine HCl 5mg | | | **Adults & Peds ≥12 yrs:** 2 caps q4h. **Max:** 12 caps q24h. |
| **DECONGESTANT + EXPECTORANT** | | | | | | |
| Maximum Strength Mucinex D | | | Pseudoephedrine HCl 120mg | | Guaifenesin 1200mg | **Adults & Peds ≥12 yrs:** 1 tab q12h. **Max:** 2 tabs q24h. |
| Mucinex Cold Liquid (Mixed Berry Flavor) | | | Phenylephrine HCl 2.5mg/5mL | | Guaifenesin 100mg/5mL | **Peds 6-<12 yrs:** 2 tsp (10mL) q4h. **Peds 4-<6 yrs:** 1 tsp (5mL) q4h. **Max:** 6 doses q24h. |
| Mucinex D | | | Pseudoephedrine HCl 60mg | | Guaifenesin 600mg | **Adults & Peds ≥12 yrs:** 2 tabs q12h. **Max:** 4 tabs q24h. |
| Sudafed PE Non-Drying Sinus Caplets | | | Phenylephrine HCl 5mg | | Guaifenesin 200mg | **Adults & Peds ≥12 yrs:** 2 tabs q4h. **Max:** 12 tabs q24h. |
| Triaminic Chest & Nasal Congestion | | | Phenylephrine HCl 2.5mg/5mL | | Guaifenesin 50mg/5mL | **Peds 6-<12 yrs:** 2 tsp (10mL) q4h. **Peds 4-<6 yrs:** 1 tsp (5mL) q4h. **Max:** 6 doses q24h. |
| **DECONGESTANT + EXPECTORANT + ANALGESIC** | | | | | | |
| Sudafed PE Triple Action Caplets | Acetaminophen 325mg | | Phenylephrine HCl 5mg | | Guaifenesin 200mg | **Adults & Peds ≥12 yrs:** 2 tabs q4h. **Max:** 12 tabs q24h. |
| Sudafed Triple Action Caplets | Acetaminophen 325mg | | Pseudoephedrine HCl 30mg | | Guaifenesin 200mg | **Adults & Peds ≥12 yrs:** 2 tabs q4-6h. **Max:** 8 tabs q24h. |
| Theraflu Warming Relief Cold & Chest Congestion | Acetaminophen 325mg/15mL | | Phenylephrine HCl 5mg/15mL | | Guaifenesin 200mg/15mL | **Adults & Peds ≥12 yrs:** 2 tbl (30mL) q4h. **Max:** 6 doses q24h. |
| Tylenol Sinus Severe Congestion & Pain* | Acetaminophen 325mg | | Phenylephrine HCl 5mg | | Guaifenesin 200mg | **Adults & Peds ≥12 yrs:** 2 tabs q4h. **Max:** 12 tabs q24h. |
| Tylenol Sinus Severe Congestion Daytime* | Acetaminophen 325mg | | Pseudoephedrine HCl 30mg | | Guaifenesin 200mg | **Adults & Peds ≥12 yrs:** 2 tabs q4-6h. **Max:** 8 tabs q24h. |
| **EXPECTORANT** | | | | | | |
| Maximum Strength Mucinex | | | | | Guaifenesin 1200mg | **Adults & Peds ≥12 yrs:** 1 tab q12h. **Max:** 2 tabs q24h. |
| Mucinex | | | | | Guaifenesin 600mg | **Adults & Peds ≥12 yrs:** 1-2 tabs q12h. **Max:** 4 tabs q24h. |

## Table 15. COUGH-COLD-FLU (cont.)

| Brand Name | Analgesic | Antihistamine | Decongestant | Cough Suppressant | Expectorant | Dose |
|---|---|---|---|---|---|---|
| Mucinex Liquid (Grape Flavor) | | | | | Guaifenesin 100mg/5mL | **Peds 6-<12 yrs:** 1-2 tsp (5-10mL) q4h. **Peds 4-<6 yrs:** ½-1 tsp (2.5-5mL) q4h. **Max:** 6 doses q24h. |
| Mucinex Mini-Melts (Bubble Gum Flavor) | | | | | Guaifenesin 100mg/pkt | **Adults & Peds ≥12 yrs:** 2-4 pkts q4h. **Peds 6-<12 yrs:** 1-2 pkts q4h. **Peds 4-<6 yrs:** 1 pkt q4h. **Max:** 6 doses q24h. |
| Mucinex Mini-Melts (Grape Flavor) | | | | | Guaifenesin 50mg/pkt | **Peds 6-<12 yrs:** 2-4 pkts q4h. **Peds 4-<6 yrs:** 1-2 pkts q4h. **Max:** 6 doses q24h. |
| Robitussin Chest Congestion | | | | | Guaifenesin 100mg/5mL | **Adults & Peds ≥12 yrs:** 2-4 tsp (10-20mL) q4h. **Max:** 6 doses q24h. |
| Vicks DayQuil Mucus Control Liquid | | | | | Guaifenesin 200mg/15mL | **Adults & Peds ≥12 yrs:** 2 tbl (30mL) q4h. **Peds 6-<12 yrs:** 1 tbl (15mL) q4h. **Max:** 6 doses q24h. |

### EXPECTORANT + ANALGESIC

| Brand Name | Analgesic | Antihistamine | Decongestant | Cough Suppressant | Expectorant | Dose |
|---|---|---|---|---|---|---|
| Comtrex Deep Chest Cold Caplets | Acetaminophen 325mg | | | | Guaifenesin 200mg | **Adults & Peds ≥12 yrs:** 2 tabs q4h. **Max:** 12 tabs q24h. |
| Theraflu & Chest Congestion Hot Liquid | Acetaminophen 1000mg/packet | | | | Guaifenesin 400mg/packet | **Adults & Peds ≥12 yrs:** 1 pkt q6h. **Max:** 4 pkts q24h. |

### ANTIHISTAMINE + ANALGESIC

| Brand Name | Analgesic | Antihistamine | Decongestant | Cough Suppressant | Expectorant | Dose |
|---|---|---|---|---|---|---|
| Advil PM Caplets/Liqui-Gels | Ibuprofen 200mg | Diphenhydramine Citrate 38mg | | | | **Adults & Peds ≥12 yrs:** 2 caps hs. **Max:** 2 caps q24h. |
| Coricidin HBP Cold & Flu | Acetaminophen 325mg | Chlorpheniramine Maleate 2mg | | | | **Adults & Peds ≥12 yrs:** 2 tabs q4-6h. **Max:** 12 tabs q24h. **Peds 6-<12 yrs:** 1 tab q4-6h. **Max:** 5 tabs q24h. |
| Motrin PM | Ibuprofen 200mg | Diphenhydramine Citrate 38mg | | | | **Adults & Peds ≥12 yrs:** 2 tabs hs. **Max:** 2 tabs q24h. |
| Tylenol Severe Allergy* | Acetaminophen 500mg | Diphenhydramine HCl 12.5mg | | | | **Adults & Peds ≥12 yrs:** 2 tabs q4-6h. **Max:** 8 tabs q24h. |

*Product currently on recall but generic forms may be available.

## Table 16. ANALGESIC PRODUCTS

| BRAND NAME | INGREDIENT/STRENGTH | DOSE |
|---|---|---|
| **ACETAMINOPHEN** | | |
| Anacin Extra Strength Aspirin Free Tablets | Acetaminophen 500mg | **Adults & Peds ≥12 yrs:** 2 tabs q6h. **Max:** 8 tabs q24h. |
| FeverAll Children's Suppositories | Acetaminophen 120mg | **Peds 3-6 yrs:** 1 supp q4-6h. **Max:** 6 supp q24h. |
| FeverAll Infants' Suppositories | Acetaminophen 80mg | **Peds 6-11 months:** 1 supp q6h. **12-36 months:** 1 supp q4h. **Max:** 6 supp q24h. |
| FeverAll Jr. Strength Suppositories | Acetaminophen 325mg | **Peds 6-12 yrs:** 1 supp q4-6h. **Max:** 6 supp q24h. |
| Tylenol 8 Hour Caplets | Acetaminophen 650mg | **Adults & Peds ≥12 yrs:** 2 tabs q8h prn. **Max:** 6 tabs q24h. |
| Tylenol Arthritis Caplets | Acetaminophen 650mg | **Adults:** 2 tabs q8h prn. **Max:** 6 tabs q24h. |
| Tylenol Arthritis Gelcaps | Acetaminophen 650mg | **Adults:** 2 caps q8h prn. **Max:** 6 caps q24h. |
| Tylenol Arthritis Geltabs | Acetaminophen 650mg | **Adults:** 2 tabs q8h prn. **Max:** 6 tabs q24h. |
| Tylenol Children's Meltaways Tablets* | Acetaminophen 80mg | **Peds 2-3 yrs (24-35 lbs):** 2 tabs. **4-5 yrs (36-47 lbs):** 3 tabs. **6-8 yrs (48-59 lbs):** 4 tabs. **9-10 yrs (60-71 lbs):** 5 tabs. **11 yrs (72-95 lbs):** 6 tabs. May repeat q4h. **Max:** 5 doses q24h. |
| Tylenol Children's Suspension* | Acetaminophen 160mg/5mL | **Peds 2-3 yrs (24-35 lbs):** 1 tsp (5mL). **4-5 yrs (36-47 lbs):** 1.5 tsp (7.5mL). **6-8 yrs (48-59 lbs):** 2 tsp (10mL). **9-10 yrs (60-71 lbs):** 2.5 tsp (12.5mL). **11 yrs (72-95 lbs):** 3 tsp (15mL). May repeat q4h. **Max:** 5 doses q24h. |
| Tylenol Extra Strength Caplets | Acetaminophen 500mg | **Adults & Peds ≥12 yrs:** 2 tabs q4-6h prn. **Max:** 8 tabs q24h. |
| Tylenol Extra Strength Cool Caplets | Acetaminophen 500mg | **Adults & Peds ≥12 yrs:** 2 tabs q4-6h prn. **Max:** 8 tabs q24h. |
| Tylenol Extra Strength Rapid Release Gelcaps | Acetaminophen 500mg | **Adults & Peds ≥12 yrs:** 2 caps q4-6h prn. **Max:** 8 caps q24h. |

*(Continued)*

## Table 16. ANALGESIC PRODUCTS (cont.)

| Brand Name | Ingredient/Strength | Dose |
|---|---|---|
| Tylenol Extra Strength Rapid Blast Liquid | Acetaminophen 500mg/15mL | **Adults & Peds ≥12 yrs:** 2 tbl (30mL) q4-6h prn. **Max:** 8 tbl (120mL) q24h. |
| Tylenol Extra Strength EZ Tablets | Acetaminophen 500mg | **Adults & Peds ≥12 yrs:** 2 tabs q4-6h prn. **Max:** 8 tabs q24h. |
| Tylenol Infants' Drops* | Acetaminophen 160mg/1.6mL | **Peds 2-3 yrs (24-35 lbs):** 1.6 mL q4h prn. **Max:** 5 doses (8mL) q24h. |
| Tylenol Junior Meltaways Tablets* | Acetaminophen 160mg | **Peds 6-8 yrs (48-59 lbs):** 2 tabs. **9-10 yrs (60-71 lbs):** 2.5 tabs. **11 yrs (72-95 lbs):** 3 tabs. **12 yrs (≥96 lbs):** 4 tabs. May repeat q4h. **Max:** 5 doses q24h. |
| Tylenol Regular Strength Tablets | Acetaminophen 325mg | **Adults & Peds ≥12 yrs:** 2 tabs q4-6h prn. **Max:** 12 tabs q24h. **Peds 6-11 yrs:** 1 tab q4-6h. **Max:** 5 tabs q24h. |
| **ACETAMINOPHEN COMBINATIONS** | | |
| Excedrin Back & Body Caplets | Acetaminophen/Aspirin Buffered 250mg-250mg | **Adults & Peds ≥12 yrs:** 2 tabs q6h. **Max:** 8 tabs q24h. |
| Excedrin Extra Strength Caplets | Acetaminophen/Aspirin/Caffeine 250mg-250mg-65mg | **Adults & Peds ≥12 yrs:** 2 tabs q6h. **Max:** 8 tabs q24h. |
| Excedrin Extra Strength Geltabs | Acetaminophen/Aspirin/Caffeine 250mg-250mg-65mg | **Adults & Peds ≥12 yrs:** 2 tabs q6h. **Max:** 8 tabs q24h. |
| Excedrin Extra Strength Express Gels | Acetaminophen/Aspirin/Caffeine 250mg-250mg-65mg | **Adults & Peds ≥12 yrs:** 2 tabs q6h. **Max:** 8 tabs q24h. |
| Excedrin Extra Strength Tablets | Acetaminophen/Aspirin/Caffeine 250mg-250mg-65mg | **Adults & Peds ≥12 yrs:** 2 tabs q6h. **Max:** 8 tabs q24h. |
| Excedrin Menstrual Complete Express Gels | Acetaminophen/Aspirin/Caffeine 250mg-250mg-65mg | **Adults & Peds ≥12 yrs:** 2 tabs q4-6h. **Max:** 8 tabs q24h. |
| Excedrin Migraine Caplets | Acetaminophen/Aspirin/Caffeine 250mg-250mg-65mg | **Adults:** 2 tabs prn. **Max:** 2 tabs q24h. |
| Excedrin Migraine Geltabs | Acetaminophen/Aspirin/Caffeine 250mg-250mg-65mg | **Adults:** 2 tabs prn. **Max:** 2 tabs q24h. |
| Excedrin Migraine Tablets | Acetaminophen/Aspirin/Caffeine 250mg-250mg-65mg | **Adults:** 2 tabs prn. **Max:** 2 tabs q24h. |

## Table 16. ANALGESIC PRODUCTS (cont.)

| Brand Name | Ingredient/Strength | Dose |
|---|---|---|
| Excedrin Sinus Headache Caplets | Acetaminophen/Phenylephrine HCl 325mg-5mg | **Adults & Peds ≥12 yrs:** 2 tabs q4h. **Max:** 12 tabs q24h. |
| Excedrin Tension Headache Caplets | Acetaminophen/Caffeine 500mg-65mg | **Adults & Peds ≥12 yrs:** 2 tabs q6h. **Max:** 8 tabs q24h. |
| Excedrin Tension Headache Express Gels | Acetaminophen/Caffeine 500mg-65mg | **Adults & Peds ≥12 yrs:** 2 caps q6h. **Max:** 8 caps q24h. |
| Excedrin Tension Headache Geltabs | Acetaminophen/Caffeine 500mg-65mg | **Adults & Peds ≥12 yrs:** 2 tabs q6h. **Max:** 8 tabs q24h. |
| Goody's Body Pain Powder | Acetaminophen/Aspirin 325mg-500mg | **Adults & Peds ≥12 yrs:** 1 powder q4-6h. **Max:** 4 powders q24h. |
| Goody's Cool Orange | Acetaminophen/Aspirin/Caffeine 325mg-500mg-65mg | **Adults & Peds ≥12 yrs:** 1 powder q6h. **Max:** 4 powders q24h. |
| Goody's Extra Strength Headache Powder | Acetaminophen/Aspirin/Caffeine 260mg-520mg-32.5mg | **Adults & Peds ≥12 yrs:** 1 powder q4-6h. **Max:** 4 powders q24h. |
| Midol Menstrual Complete Caplets | Acetaminophen/Caffeine/ Pyrilamine Maleate 500mg-60mg-15mg | **Adults & Peds ≥12 yrs:** 2 tabs q6h. **Max:** 8 tabs q24h. |
| Midol Menstrual Complete Gelcaps | Acetaminophen/Caffeine/ Pyrilamine Maleate 500mg-60mg-15mg | **Adults & Peds ≥12 yrs:** 2 caps q6h. **Max:** 8 caps q24h. |
| Midol Teen Formula Caplets | Acetaminophen/Pamabrom 500mg-25mg | **Adults & Peds ≥12 yrs:** 2 tabs q6h. **Max:** 8 tabs q24h. |
| Pamprin Cramp Caplets | Acetaminophen/Magnesium Salicylate/ Pamabrom 250mg-250mg-25mg | **Adults & Peds ≥12 yrs:** 2 tabs q4-6h. **Max:** 8 tabs q24h. |
| Pamprin Max Caplets | Acetaminophen/Aspirin/Caffeine 250mg-250mg-65mg | **Adults & Peds ≥12 yrs:** 2 tabs q4-6h. **Max:** 8 tabs q24h. |
| Pamprin Multi-Symptom Caplets | Acetaminophen/Pamabrom/Pyrilamine 500mg-25mg-15mg | **Adults & Peds ≥12 yrs:** 2 tabs q4-6h. **Max:** 8 tabs q24h. |
| Premsyn PMS Caplets | Acetaminophen/Pamabrom/Pyrilamine 500mg-25mg-15mg | **Adults & Peds ≥12 yrs:** 2 tabs q4-6h. **Max:** 8 tabs q24h. |
| Vanquish Caplets | Acetaminophen/Aspirin/Caffeine 194mg-227mg-33mg | **Adults & Peds ≥12 yrs:** 2 tabs q6h. **Max:** 8 tabs q24h. |

*(Continued)*

## Table 16. ANALGESIC PRODUCTS (cont.)

| Brand Name | Ingredient/Strength | Dose |
|---|---|---|
| **ACETAMINOPHEN/SLEEP AIDS** | | |
| Excedrin PM Caplets | Acetaminophen/Diphenhydramine Citrate 500mg-38mg | **Adults & Peds ≥12 yrs:** 2 tabs qhs. **Max:** 2 tabs q24h. |
| Excedrin PM Express Gels | Acetaminophen/Diphenhydramine Citrate 500mg-38mg | **Adults & Peds ≥12 yrs:** 2 tabs qhs. **Max:** 2 tabs q24h. |
| Goody's PM Powder | Acetaminophen/Diphenhydramine 1000mg-76mg/dose | **Adults & Peds ≥12 yrs:** 1 packet (2 powders) qhs. |
| Tylenol PM Caplets | Acetaminophen/Diphenhydramine 500mg-25mg | **Adults & Peds ≥12 yrs:** 2 tabs qhs. **Max:** 2 tabs q24h. |
| Tylenol PM Rapid Release Gels | Acetaminophen/Diphenhydramine 500mg-25mg | **Adults & Peds ≥12 yrs:** 2 caps qhs. **Max:** 2 caps q24h. |
| Tylenol PM Geltabs | Acetaminophen/Diphenhydramine 500mg-25mg | **Adults & Peds ≥12 yrs:** 2 tabs qhs. **Max:** 2 tabs q24h. |
| **NSAIDs** | | |
| Advil Caplets | Ibuprofen 200mg | **Adults & Peds ≥12 yrs:** 1-2 tabs q4-6h. **Max:** 6 tabs q24h. |
| Advil Children's Suspension | Ibuprofen 100mg/5mL | **Peds 2-3 yrs (24-35 lbs):** 1 tsp (5mL). **4-5 yrs (36-47 lbs):** 1.5 tsp (7.5mL). **6-8 yrs (48-59 lbs):** 2 tsp (10mL). **9-10 yrs (60-71 lbs):** 2.5 tsp (12.5mL). **11 yrs (72-95 lbs):** 3 tsp (15mL). May repeat q6-8h. **Max:** 4 doses q24h. |
| Advil Gel Caplets | Ibuprofen 200mg | **Adults & Peds ≥12 yrs:** 1-2 tabs q4-6h. **Max:** 6 tabs q24h. |
| Advil Infants' Concentrated Drops | Ibuprofen 50mg/1.25mL | **Peds 6-11 months (12-17 lbs):** 1.25mL. **12-23 months (18-23 lbs):** 1.875mL. May repeat q6-8h. **Max:** 4 doses q24h. |
| Advil Liqui-Gels | Ibuprofen 200mg | **Adults & Peds ≥12 yrs:** 1-2 caps q4-6h. **Max:** 6 caps q24h. |
| Advil Migraine Capsules | Ibuprofen 200mg | **Adults:** 2 caps prn. **Max:** 2 caps q24h. |
| Advil Tablets | Ibuprofen 200mg | **Adults & Peds ≥12 yrs:** 1-2 tabs q4-6h. **Max:** 6 tabs q24h. |

## Table 16. ANALGESIC PRODUCTS (cont.)

| BRAND NAME | INGREDIENT/STRENGTH | DOSE |
| --- | --- | --- |
| Aleve Caplets | Naproxen Sodium 220mg | **Adults & Peds ≥12 yrs:** 1 tab q8-12h. May take 1 additional tab within 1h of first dose. **Max:** 2 tabs q8-12h or 3 tabs q24h. |
| Aleve Liquid Gels | Naproxen Sodium 220mg | **Adults & Peds ≥12 yrs:** 1 cap q8-12h. May take 1 additional cap within 1h of first dose. **Max:** 2 caps q8-12h or 3 caps q24h. |
| Aleve Tablets | Naproxen Sodium 220mg | **Adults & Peds ≥12 yrs:** 1 tab q8-12h. May take 1 additional tab within 1h of first dose. **Max:** 2 tabs q8-12h or 3 tabs q24h. |
| Midol Liquid Gels | Ibuprofen 200mg | **Adults & Peds ≥12 yrs:** 1-2 caps q4-6h. **Max:** 6 caps q24h. |
| Midol Extended Relief Caplets | Naproxen Sodium 220mg | **Adults & Peds ≥12 yrs:** 1-2 tabs q8-12h. **Max:** 2 tabs q8-12h or 3 tabs q24h. |
| Motrin Children's Suspension** | Ibuprofen 100mg/5mL | **Peds 2-3 yrs (24-35 lbs):** 1 tsp (5mL). **4-5 yrs (36-47 lbs):** 1.5 tsp (7.5mL). **6-8 yrs (48-59 lbs):** 2 tsp (10mL). **9-10 yrs (60-71 lbs):** 2.5 tsp (12.5mL). **11 yrs (72-95 lbs):** 3 tsp (15mL). May repeat q6-8h. **Max:** 4 doses q24h. |
| Motrin IB Caplets | Ibuprofen 200mg | **Adults & Peds ≥12 yrs:** 1-2 tabs q4-6h. **Max:** 6 tabs q24h. |
| Motrin IB Tablets | Ibuprofen 200mg | **Adults & Peds ≥12 yrs:** 1-2 tabs q4-6h. **Max:** 6 tabs q24h. |
| Motrin Infants' Drops** | Ibuprofen 50mg/1.25mL | **Peds 6-11 months (12-17 lbs):** 1.25mL. **12-23 months (18-23 lbs):** 1.875mL. May repeat q6-8h. **Max:** 4 doses q24h. |
| Motrin Junior Strength Caplets** | Ibuprofen 100mg | **Peds 6-8 yrs (48-59 lbs):** 2 tabs. **9-10 yrs (60-71 lbs):** 2.5 tabs. **11 yrs (72-95 lbs):** 3 tabs. May repeat q6-8h. **Max:** 4 doses q24h. |

*(Continued)*

## Table 16. ANALGESIC PRODUCTS (cont.)

| Brand Name | Ingredient/Strength | Dose |
|---|---|---|
| Motrin Junior Strength Chewable Tablets** | Ibuprofen 100mg | **Peds 2-3 yrs (24-35 lbs):** 1 tab. **4-5 yrs (36-47 lbs):** 1.5 tabs. **6-8 yrs (48-59 lbs):** 2 tabs. **9-10 yrs (60-71 lbs):** 2.5 tabs. **11 yrs (72-95 lbs):** 3 tabs. May repeat q6-8h. **Max:** 4 doses q24h. |
| Pamprin All Day Caplets | Naproxen Sodium 220mg | **Adults & Peds ≥12 yrs:** 1-2 tabs q8-12h. **Max:** 2 tabs q8-12h or 3 tabs q24h. |
| **NSAID SLEEP AIDS** | | |
| Advil PM Caplets | Ibuprofen/Diphenhydramine Citrate 200mg-38mg | **Adults & Peds ≥12 yrs:** 2 tabs qhs. **Max:** 2 tabs q24h. |
| Advil PM Liqui-Gels | Ibuprofen/Diphenhydramine 200mg-25mg | **Adults & Peds ≥12 yrs:** 2 caps qhs. **Max:** 2 caps q24h. |
| Motrin PM Caplets | Ibuprofen/Diphenhydramine Citrate 200mg-38mg | **Adults & Peds ≥12 yrs:** 2 tabs qhs. **Max:** 2 tabs q24h. |
| **SALICYLATES** | | |
| Bayer Aspirin Extra Strength Caplets | Aspirin 500mg | **Adults & Peds ≥12 yrs:** 1-2 tabs q4-6h. **Max:** 8 tabs q24h. |
| Bayer Aspirin Safety Coated Caplets | Aspirin 325mg | **Adults & Peds ≥12 yrs:** 1-2 tabs q4h. **Max:** 12 tabs q24h. |
| Bayer Low Dose Aspirin Chewable Tablets* | Aspirin 81mg | **Adults & Peds ≥12 yrs:** 4-8 tabs q4h. **Max:** 48 tabs q24h. |
| Bayer Low Dose Aspirin Safety Coated Tablets | Aspirin 81mg | **Adults & Peds ≥12 yrs:** 4-8 tabs q4h. **Max:** 48 tabs q24h. |
| Bayer Genuine Aspirin Tablets | Aspirin 325mg | **Adults & Peds ≥12 yrs:** 1-2 tabs q4h or 3 tabs q6h. **Max:** 12 tabs q24h. |
| Doan's Extra Strength Caplets | Magnesium Salicylate Tetrahydrate 580mg | **Adults & Peds ≥12 yrs:** 2 tabs q6h. **Max:** 8 tabs q24h. |
| Ecotrin Low Strength Tablets | Aspirin 81mg | **Adults:** 4-8 tabs q4h. **Max:** 48 tabs q24h. |
| Ecotrin Regular Strength Tablets | Aspirin 325mg | **Adults & Peds ≥12 yrs:** 1-2 tabs q4h. **Max:** 12 tabs q24h. |
| Halfprin 162mg Tablets | Aspirin 162mg | **Adults & Peds ≥12 yrs:** 2-4 tabs q4h. **Max:** 24 tabs q24h. |

## Table 16. ANALGESIC PRODUCTS (cont.)

| BRAND NAME | INGREDIENT/STRENGTH | DOSE |
|---|---|---|
| Halfprin 81mg Tablets | Aspirin 81mg | **Adults & Peds ≥12 yrs:** 4-8 tabs q4h. **Max:** 48 tabs q24h. |
| St. Joseph Chewable Aspirin Tablets | Aspirin 81mg | **Adults & Peds ≥12 yrs:** 4-8 tabs q4h. **Max:** 48 tabs q24h. |
| St. Joseph Enteric Safety-Coated Tablets | Aspirin 81mg | **Adults & Peds ≥12 yrs:** 4-8 tabs q4h. **Max:** 48 tabs q24h. |
| **SALICYLATES, BUFFERED** | | |
| Alka-Seltzer Lemon-Lime Tablets | Aspirin/Citric Acid/Sodium Bicarbonate 325mg-1000mg-1700mg | **Adults & Peds ≥12 yrs:** 2 tabs q4h. **Max:** 8 tabs q24h. **≥60 yrs: Max:** 4 tabs q24h. |
| Alka-Seltzer Original Effervescent Tablets | Aspirin/Citric Acid/Sodium Bicarbonate 325mg-1000mg-1916mg | **Adults & Peds ≥12 yrs:** 2 tabs q4h. **Max:** 8 tabs q24h. **≥60 yrs: Max:** 4 tabs q24h. |
| Alka-Seltzer Extra Strength Effervescent Tablets | Aspirin/Citric Acid/Sodium Bicarbonate 500mg-1000mg-1985mg | **Adults & Peds ≥12 yrs:** 2 tabs q6h. **Max:** 7 tabs q24h. **≥60 yrs: Max:** 3 tabs q24h. |
| Ascriptin Maximum Strength Tablets | Aspirin 500mg Buffered with Aluminum Hydroxide/Calcium Carbonate/ Magnesium Hydroxide | **Adults:** 2 tabs q6h. **Max:** 8 tabs q24h. |
| Ascriptin Regular Strength Tablets | Aspirin 325mg Buffered with Aluminum Hydroxide/Calcium Carbonate/ Magnesium Hydroxide | **Adults:** 2 tabs q4h. **Max:** 12 tabs q24h. |
| Bayer Extra Strength Plus Caplets | Aspirin 500mg Buffered with Calcium Carbonate | **Adults & Peds ≥12 yrs:** 1-2 tabs q4-6h. **Max:** 8 tabs q24h. |
| Bayer Women's Low Dose Aspirin Caplets | Aspirin 81mg Buffered with Calcium Carbonate 777mg | **Adults & Peds ≥12 yrs:** 4-8 tabs q4h. **Max:** 10 tabs q24h. |
| Bufferin Extra Strength Tablets | Aspirin 500mg Buffered with Calcium Carbonate/Magnesium Oxide/ Magnesium Carbonate | **Adults & Peds ≥12 yrs:** 2 tabs q6h. **Max:** 8 tabs q24h. |
| Bufferin Tablets | Aspirin 325mg Buffered with Benzoic Acid/Citric Acid | **Adults & Peds ≥12 yrs:** 2 tabs q4h. **Max:** 12 tabs q24h. |
| **SALICYLATE COMBINATIONS** | | |
| Anacin Max Strength Tablets | Aspirin/Caffeine 500mg-32mg | **Adults & Peds ≥12 yrs:** 2 tabs q6h. **Max:** 8 tabs q24h. |
| Anacin Regular Strength Caplets | Aspirin/Caffeine 400mg-32mg | **Adults & Peds ≥12 yrs:** 2 tabs q6h. **Max:** 8 tabs q24h. |

*(Continued)*

## Table 16. ANALGESIC PRODUCTS (cont.)

| Brand Name | Ingredient/Strength | Dose |
|---|---|---|
| Anacin Tablets | Aspirin/Caffeine 400mg-32mg | **Adults & Peds ≥12 yrs:** 2 tabs q6h. **Max:** 8 tabs q24h. |
| Bayer Back & Body Pain Caplets | Aspirin/Caffeine 500mg-32.5mg | **Adults & Peds ≥12 yrs:** 2 tabs q6h. **Max:** 8 tabs q24h. |
| Bayer AM Extra Strength Tablets | Aspirin/Caffeine 500mg-65mg | **Adults & Peds ≥12 yrs:** 2 tabs q6h. **Max:** 8 tabs q24h. |
| BC Arthritis Strength Powders | Aspirin/Caffeine 1000mg-65mg | **Adults & Peds ≥12 yrs:** 1 powder q6h. **Max:** 4 powders q24h. |
| BC Original Formula Powders | Aspirin/Caffeine 845mg-65mg | **Adults & Peds ≥12 yrs:** 1 powder q6h. **Max:** 4 powders q24h. |
| **SALICYLATE/SLEEP AID** | | |
| Bayer PM Caplets | Aspirin/Diphenhydramine Citrate 500mg-38.3mg | **Adults & Peds ≥12 yrs:** 2 tabs qhs. |
| Doan's Extra Strength PM Caplets | Magnesium Salicylate Tetrahydrate/Diphenhydramine 580mg-25mg | **Adults & Peds ≥12 yrs:** 2 tabs qhs. |

*Multiple flavors available
**Currently on recall, generics available

## Table 17. DIETARY CALCIUM INTAKE

### RECOMMENDED CALCIUM INTAKES*

| AGE | DAILY INTAKE (MG) |
|---|---|
| Birth-6 months | 210 |
| 6 months-1 year | 270 |
| 1-3 years | 500 |
| 4-8 years | 800 |
| 9-18 years | 1,300 |
| 19-50 years | 1,000 |
| Over 50 years | 1,200 |
| **PREGNANT OR LACTATING** | |
| 14-18 years | 1,300 |
| 19-50 years | 1,000 |

*Source: National Institute of Arthritis and Musculoskeletal and Skin Diseases (NIAMS); National Institutes of Health

### Estimating Daily Dietary Calcium Intake

**Step 1:** Estimate calcium intake from calcium-rich foods.*

| Product | Servings/Day | Calcium/Serving (mg) | | Calcium (mg) |
|---|---|---|---|---|
| Milk (8 oz) | _____ | × 300 | = | _____ |
| Yogurt (8 oz) | _____ | × 300 | = | _____ |
| Cheese (1 oz, or 1 cubic inch) | _____ | × 200 | = | _____ |
| Fortified foods or juices | _____ | × 80-1,000** | = | _____ |

**Step 2:** Total from above + 250 mg for nondairy sources = total dietary calcium.

* About 75-80% of the calcium consumed in American diets is from dairy products.

** Calcium content of fortified foods varies.

### Factors related to vitamin D that may affect calcium absorption:

- National Osteoporosis Foundation recommends an intake of 800 to 1,000 International Units (IU) of vitamin $D_3$ per day for adults over age 50 and 400 to 800 IU of Vitamin $D_3$ for <50 years of age
- Desired level for the average adult's serum 25(OH)D concentration is 30 ng/mL (75 nmol/L) or higher
- Safe upper limit for vitamin D intake for normal adult population was set at 4,000 IU per day
- Patients with malabsorption (eg, celiac disease) or chronic renal insufficiency, or those who are housebound, chronically ill, or have limited sun exposure, may need vitamin D supplements

**Source:** National Institute of Arthritis and Musculoskeletal and Skin Diseases (NIAMS), National Institutes of Health, National Osteoporosis Foundation.

# PRODUCT NAME INDEX

This section identifies the page number for each product in the book, by brand name.

# PRODUCT NAME INDEX

## C

## J

## K

## L

## T